MR AND CT IMAGING OF THE HEAD, NECK, AND SPINE

SECOND EDITION

MR and CT Imaging of the Head, Neck, and Spine

EDITED BY

RICHARD E. LATCHAW, M.D.
Neuroradiologist
Radiology Imaging Associates, P.C., and Colorado
  Neurological Institute
Englewood, Colorado
Clinical Professor of Radiology
University of Colorado
Denver Colorado

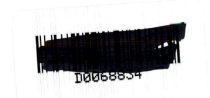
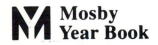

Mosby
Year Book

St. Louis   Baltimore   Boston   Chicago   London   Philadelphia   Sydney   Toronto

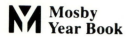
Mosby
Year Book
Dedicated to Publishing Excellence

Sponsoring Editors: James D. Ryan/Anne S. Patterson
Associate Managing Editor, Manuscript Services: Deborah
  Thorp
Production Project Coordinator: Carol A. Reynolds
Proofroom Manager: Barbara Kelly

Mosby–Year Book, Inc.
11830 Westline Industrial Drive
St. Louis. MO 63146

1 2 3 4 5 6 7 8 9 0 CL PC 95 94 93 92 91

Library of Congress Cataloging-in-Publication Data
MR and CT imaging of the head, neck, and spine / [edited by Richard E.
  Latchaw.—2nd ed.
       p.   cm.
    Rev. ed. of: Computed tomography of the head, neck, and spine.
  c1985.
    Includes bibliographical references.
    Includes index.
    ISBN 0-8151-5330-9
    1. Central nervous system—Magnetic resonance imaging. 2. Central
nervous system—Tomography. 3. Head—Imaging. 4. Neck—Imaging.
5. Spine—Imaging.
    [DNLM: 1. Head—anatomy & histology. 2. Head—radiography.
3. Magnetic Resonance Imaging. 4. Neck—anatomy & histology.
5. Neck—radiography. 6. Spine—anatomy & histology. 7. Spine—
radiography. 8. Tomography. X-Ray Computed. WE 141 M9385]
RC386.6.M34M75   1991   90-6587
616.8′047572—dc20   CIP
DNLM/DLC
for Library of Congress

This book is dedicated to Dr. Lou Wener: unparalleled in MRI, a caring individual. . . he was my friend.

STEPHEN A. BERMAN, M.D., PH.D.
Fellow in EMG
Spinal Cord Injury Service
West Roxbury Veterans Administration Medical Center
Boston, Massachusetts

JAMES A. BRUNBERG, M.D.
Assistant Professor of Radiology, Neurology, and
  Neurosurgery
University of Michigan
Director, Division of MR Imaging
Co-director, Division of Neuroradiology
Department of Radiology
University of Michigan Hospitals
Ann Arbor, Michigan

R. NICK BRYAN, M.D., PH.D.
Profesor of Radiology and Neurosurgery
Johns Hopkins University
Director, Division of Neuroradiology
Department of Radiology
Johns Hopkins Hospital
Baltimore, Maryland

GLEN E. BURMEISTER, M.D.
Radiologist, Radiology Imaging Associates, P.C.,
  Musculoskeletal Radiologist and Swedish Medical
  Center
Englewood, Colorado

GEORGE F. CARR, D.M.D.
Prosthodontist
Allentown, Pennsylvania
Faculty Member
Michigan Implant Institute
Dearborn, Michigan

SYLVESTER H. S. CHUANG, M.D.C.M., D.A.B.R.,
C.S.P.Q., F.R.C.P.C.
Associate Professor of Radiology
University of Toronto
Neuroradiologist, Department of Radiology
Hospital for Sick Children
Toronto, Ontario, Canada

HUGH D. CURTIN, M.D.
Professor of Radiology and Otolaryngology
Chief, Department of Radiology
Eye and Ear Hospital
Medical and Health Care Division
University of Pittsburgh
Pittsburgh, Pennsylvania

RICHARD H. DAFFNER, M.D.
Professor of Radiologic Sciences
Medical College of Pennsylvania (Western Campus)
Clinical Professor of Radiology
University of Pittsburgh
Senior Staff Radiologist
Department of Radiology
Allegheny General Hospital
Pittsburgh, Pennsylvania

MONY J. DE LEON, B.A, M.A., M.ED., ED.D.
Associate Professor of Psychiatry
New York University
Director of the Neuroimaging Research Laboratory
New York University Medical Center
New York, New York

BURTON P. DRAYER, M.D.
Director, Magnetic Resonance Imaging and Research
Chairman, Division of Neuroimaging Research-
  Education
Barrow Neurological Institute
Phoenix, Arizona

ELIZABETH A. EELKEMA, M.D.
Radiologist, Department of Radiology
St. Clair Hospital
Pittsburgh, Pennsylvania

CHARLES R. FITZ, M.D.
Professor of Radiology and Pediatrics
George Washington University
Neuroradiologist, Department of Radiology
Children's National Medical Center
Washington, D.C.

AJAX E. GEORGE, M.D.
Professor of Radiology
New York University
Senior Attending Neuroradiologist
New York University Medical Center
New York, New York

ROBERT I. GROSSMAN, M.D.
Professor of Radiology and Neurosurgery
University of Pennsylvania
Chief of Neuroradiology
Department of Radiology
Hospital of the University of Pennsylvania
Philadelphia, Pennsylvania

DAVID GUR, SC.D.
Professor of Radiology and Radiation Health
Director, Division of Radiological Imaging
Department of Radiology
Medical and Health Care Division
University of Pittsburgh
Pittsburgh, Pennsylvania

L. ANNE HAYMAN, M.D.
Research Professor of Radiology
Baylor College of Medicine
Director of Neuroradiology
Department of Radiology
Ben Taub General Hospital
Houston, Texas

STEPHEN T. HECHT, M.D.
Assistant Professor of Radiology and Neurosurgery
University of California—Davis
Neuroradiologist, Department of Radiology
University of California Medical Center—Davis
Sacramento, California

ROBERT J. HERFKENS, M.D.
Associate Professor of Radiology
Stanford University School of Medicine
Chief of Body MRI
Stanford University Hospital
Stanford, California

VINCENT C. HINCK, M.D.
Emeritus, Professor of Radiology
Baylor College of Medicine
Houston, Texas

WILLIAM L. HIRSCH, JR., M.D.
Assistant Professor of Radiology
Neuroradiologist, Department of Radiology
Medical and Health Care Division
University of Pittsburgh
Pittsburgh, Pennsylvania

JEFFERY P. HOGG, M.D.
Assistant Professor of Radiology
Neuroradiologist, Department of Radiology
Medical and Health Care Division
University of Pittsburgh
Pittsburgh, Pennsylvania

BARRY HOROWITZ, M.D.
Director of Neuroradiology
The Methodist Hospital
Clinical Associate Professor of Radiology
Baylor College of Medicine
Houston, Texas

JOSEPH A. HORTON, M.D.
Professor of Radiology and Neurological Surgery
Chief, Division of Neuroradiology
Department of Radiology
Medical and Health Care Division
University of Pittsburgh
Pittsburgh, Pennsylvania

DAVID JENKINS, M.D.
Staff Radiologist
Department of Radiology
Lafayette General Hospital
Lafayette, Louisiana

DAVID W. JOHNSON, M.D.
Assistant Professor of Radiology
Neuroradiologist, Department of Radiology
Medical and Health Care Division
University of Pittsburgh
Pittsburgh, Pennsylvania

CHARLES A. JUNGREIS, M.D.
Assistant Professor of Radiology and Neurological
  Surgery
Neuroradiologist, Department of Radiology
Medical and Health Care Division
University of Pittsburgh
Pittsburgh, Pennsylvania

EMANUEL KANAL, M.D.
Assistant Professor of Radiology
Chief, Division of Magnetic Resonance Imaging
Department of Radiology
Director, The Pittsburgh NMR Institute
Medical and Health Care Division
University of Pittsburgh
Pittsburgh, Pennsylvania

SUSAN S. KEMP, M.D.
Assistant Professor of Radiology
Neuroradiologist, Department of Radiology
Medical and Health Care Division
University of Pittsburgh
Pittsburgh, Pennsylvania

JOEL B. KIRKPATRICK, M.D.
Professor of Neuropathology
Department of Pathology
Baylor College of Medicine
Houston, Texas

RICHARD E. LATCHAW, M.D.
Neuroradiologist
Radiology Imaging Associates, P.C., and Colorado
  Neurological Institute
Englewood, Colorado
Clinical Professor of Radiology
University of Colorado
Denver, Colorado
Formerly:
Professor of Radiology and
  Neurological Surgery
Interim Chairman and Chief
  of Neuroradiology
Department of Radiology
Medical and Health Care Division
University of Pittsburgh
Pittsburgh, Pennsylvania

L. DADE LUNSFORD, M.D.
Professor of Neurological Surgery, Radiology, and
  Radiation Oncology
Neurosurgeon, Department of Neurological Surgery
Medical and Health Care Division
University of Pittsburgh
Pittsburgh, Pennsylvania

CHARLES W. McCLUGGAGE, M.D.
*Neuroradiologist, Texas Children's and St. Luke's
 Episcopal Hospitals
Clinical Assistant Professor of Radiology
Baylor College of Medicine
Houston, Texas*

THOMAS J. MASARYK, M.D.
*Head, Section of Neuroradiology
Division of Radiology
Cleveland Clinic Foundation
Cleveland, Ohio*

JOHN J. PAGANI, M.D.
*Staff Radiologist
Department of Radiology
Park Plaza Hospital
Houston, Texas*

MICHAEL J. PAINTER, M.D.
*Associate Professor of Pediatrics and Neurology
Chief, Department of Neurology
Children's Hospital of Neurology
Medical and Health Care Division
University of Pittsburgh
Pittsburgh, Pennsylvania*

STANLEY M. PERL, M.D.
*Radiologist and Medical Director
Magnetic Resonance Imaging Associates
Clinton, Maryland*

MARK J. PFLEGER, M.D.
*Resident, Radiology
Department of Radiology
Baylor College of Medicine
Houston, Texas*

ROBERT M. QUENCER, M.D.
*Professor of Radiology, Neurological Surgery, and
 Ophthalmology
Medical Director
Division of Magnetic Resonance Imaging
Department of Radiology
University of Miami School of Medicine
Miami, Florida*

JEFFREY M. ROGG, M.D.
*Clinical Instructor
Radiation Medicine
Brown University
Director of Magnetic Resonance Imaging
Rhode Island Hospital
Providence, Rhode Island*

HELEN M. N. ROPPOLO, M.D.
*Clinical Associate Professor of Radiology
Neuroradiologist, Department of Radiology
Medical and Health Care Division
University of Pittsburgh
Pittsburgh, Pennsylvania*

WILLIAM E. ROTHFUS, M.D.
*Associate Professor of Radiologic Science
Medical College of Pennsylvania (Western Campus)
Senior Staff Radiologist
Department of Radiology
Allegheny General Hospital
Pittsburgh, Pennsylvania*

JOACHIM F. SEEGER, M.D.
*Professor of Radiology
University of Arizona
Head, Section of Neuroradiology
Department of Radiology
University of Arizona Health Sciences Center
Tucson, Arizona*

CHARLES E. SEIBERT, M.D.
*Neuroradiologist
Radiology Imaging Associates, P.C., Swedish Medical
 Center and Colorado Neurological Institute
Englewood, Colorado
Clinical Associate Professor of Radiology
University of Colorado
Denver, Colorado*

KATHERINE SHAFFER, M.D.
*Associate Professor of Radiology and Otolarygology
Medical College of Wisconsin
Radiologist, Department of Radiology
Milwaukee County Medical Complex
Milwaukee, Wisconsin*

ELLEN K. TABOR, M.D.
*Assistant Professor of Radiology
Head and Neck Radiologist, Department of Radiology
Medical and Health Care Division
University of Pittsburgh
Pittsburgh, Pennsylvania*

ROBERT W. TARR, M.D.
*Assistant Professor of Radiology
Case-Western Reserve University
Neuroradiologist, Department of Radiology
University Hospitals
Cleveland, Ohio*

FELIX W. WEHRLI, PH.D.
*Professor of Radiologic Science
University of Pennsylvania
Director of MR Education
Hospital of the University of Pennsylvania
Philadelphia, Pennsylvania*

MEREDITH A. WEINSTEIN, M.D.
*Staff Radiologist
Hill and Thomas
Cleveland, Ohio*

LOUIS WENER, M.D. (DECEASED)
*Formerly:
Radiologist and Medical Director
Magnetic Resonance Imaging Associates
Clinton, Maryland*

GERALD L. WOLF, PH.D., M.D.
*Professor of Radiology
Harvard Medical School
Director, Center for Imaging and Pharmaceutical
 Research
Massachusetts General Hospital
Boston, Massachusetts*

HOWARD YONAS, M.D.
*Assistant Professor of Neurological Surgery and
 Radiology
Neurosurgeon, Department of Neurological Surgery
Medical and Health Care Division
University of Pittsburgh
Pittsburgh, Pennsylvania*

FOREWORD

Dr. Latchaw's previous effort in this area, *Computed Tomography of the Head, Neck, and Spine* (as the first edition was titled) was the definitive work to date on that subject. Knowing him well, I was captivated by his ongoing comments about producing the next edition. Magnetic resonance imaging has made such a massive impact on imaging practice in this area that it has become dominant, whereas computed tomography has faded somewhat, burgeoning, however, in its contribution to the evaluation of the abdomen and pelvis, and thus not losing much luster. However, its use is on the decline in neuroradiology.

Other authors and editors have had the same problem, that is, having to redo a book that was largely CT oriented, after MRI. Most of them have not fared well, either in the text or in the illustrations. They generally have attempted to add to their previous material rather than take on the whole new subject, and thus produce a lesser product, in some ways, than the first attempt. This book, however, is basically all new. The contents are massively MR oriented, with appropriate references to CT as indicated.

The book is profusely illustrated and provides references that are up-to-date to the point of printing. The discussions are excellent. In this day of constantly changing, moving-target technology, one expects that a book of this genre will be largely clinical, because patients and diseases remain stable fixation points. It *is* clinical, but it also is profusely and informatively technologic. There are insights here on contrast material and image quality that have not surfaced elsewhere, and which make the book worth reading for that reason alone. Brilliant explanations of pathophysiologic changes as manifested by images accompany these images and the text describing them.

A major work such as this is a real tour de force. Dr. Latchaw, a brilliant bundle of energy, left the university (academic) setting for a large private group practice adjacent to the Rockies. One would predict that he would have had difficulty in putting everything together. But no. He has prevailed, and brilliantly so. This is a superb effort and stands as the definitive text as well as an encyclopedia on the subject of brain, head, neck, and spine imaging, that is, neuroimaging. These efforts must be viewed to be appreciated. I commend Dr. Latchaw and his co-authors for a major, major contribution. While it may not overshadow Dick's beloved mountains, it is a great start.

DAVID O. DAVIS, M.D.
Professor and Acting Chairman
Department of Radiology
George Washington University Medical Center
Washington, D.C.

PREFACE

In the first edition of this book, entitled *Computed Tomography of the Head, Neck, and Spine,* we stressed the correlation of pathophysiology and CT imaging. We wanted our readers to understand why we see what we see on a CT scan. That approach was highly successful.

As we brought the first book to press, MRI was rapidly emerging. We wished to write as definitive a book on MRI as we had on CT, so we waited until MR contrast agents became available.

Throughout the late 1980s, it became apparent that MRI would become the imaging procedure of choice for many neurological diseases. However, in writing a book on MRI, we also wished to incorporate what we knew from CT. We had learned so much from CT that it was logical to carry it over to MR. For many of the diseases, CT and MR show similar types of findings, albeit with a slightly different appearance. In practice, the two are frequently intertwined: hence this book, which combines the two modalities.

The divisions of this book are similar to those of the first book, except for the addition of a chapter on certain physical principles of MRI. There has been no attempt to introduce a great deal of physics in this book; other books are far more proficient in that undertaking. Rather, the chapter stresses the optimization of the MR scan, demonstrating ways to obtain better contrast-to-noise and signal-to-noise ratios. We again ended the book with such exciting procedures as stereotactic neurosurgery on the MR scanner (just as we have performed on CT scanners). In between, there is a discussion of numerous clinical entities, comparing and contrasting their MR and CT appearances.

We sincerely hope that our readers will conclude that with the publication of the second edition of *MR and CT Imaging of the Head, Neck, and Spine,* we have accomplished our goals.

RICHARD E. LATCHAW, M.D.

ACKNOWLEDGMENTS

It is unnecessary that I say thank you in print to the co-authors of this monumental project. They need only read their colleagues' material to feel the same kind of pride that I do in a project well done. Rather, my thanks go to all of the unsung heros whose names do not appear in the list of contributors: all of those secretaries who labored so hard to get the final product into production. Without their help, a project like this could never have occurred.

There is one individual who deserves the highest level of praise: my wife Joan. Formerly, as my secretary at the University of Pittsburgh, Joan Roberge was of immense help in preparing *Computed Tomography of the Head, Neck, and Spine.*

We then began to tackle the second edition: *MR and CT Imaging of the Head, Neck, and Spine.* She has been my strength throughout its production, and has helped me gather figures, obtain references, and write and edit numerous chapters, and has put up with my continual modifications. During my tenure as Interim Chairman of the Department of Radiology at the University of Pittsburg, she, as Departmental Administrator, protected me, so that I could spend time with my favorite project. I was so enamored of her abilities that I decided to marry her. Now, it's our book.

RICHARD E. LATCHAW, M.D.

CONTENTS

CONTENTS

xix

PART VIII

Sella and Parasellar Regions

Sella and Parasellar Regions: Normal Anatomy

William L. Hirsch, Jr., M.D.

Helen M.N. Roppolo, M.D.

L. Anne Hayman, M.D.

Vincent C. Hinck, M.D.

IMAGING TECHNIQUES

Computed Tomography

Sellar Contents and Suprasellar Cistern

The pituitary gland and sella are optimally imaged using direct coronal computed tomography (CT) with the following scan parameters: 1.5-mm-thick contiguous cuts, 256^2 matrix, 12.8-cm display field of view (FOV), head calibration, soft tissue resolution with a technique of 120 kV, 170 milliamps, and 3-second scan time. Bone windows are usually adequate for evaluation of the sella, but bone algorithms provide superior detail and require little additional reconstruction time using modern scanners. Coronal scanning requires hyperextension of the neck and may be performed either in the prone or supine position, whichever is better tolerated by the patient. If the patient is unable to hyperextend his neck, 1.5-mm axial cuts through the sella and suprasellar cistern are used to generate reformatted sagittal and coronal images.

All patients are scanned initially after intravenous contrast infusion and receive a total of 40 to 45 g of iodine unless contraindicated. Half of the contrast is given as a bolus and the other half is administered as a rapid drip infusion during scanning.

Parasellar Region

Optimal imaging of parasellar lesions requires examination in two planes using both soft tissue and bone algorithms. The following scanning parameters are recommended: 3-mm-thick contiguous sections, 3-mm spacing, 120 kV, 170 milliamps, 3-second scan time, using soft tissue as well as bone algorithms. Coronal sections are made perpendicular to the sellar floor and extend from the orbital apex to the prepontine cistern using a 17-cm FOV. Axial images are made parallel to the hard palate, from the hard palate up to the top of the orbit using a 19-cm display FOV. The wide scan margins around the parasellar region are needed to evaluate for spread of lesions into the surrounding structures, particularly in evaluation of perineural extension.

Magnetic Resonance

Sellar Contents and Suprasellar Cistern

To identify small pituitary lesions with magnetic resonance (MR), contrast resolution must be maximized and voxel volume minimized (in order to eliminate partial volume averaging). The specific pulsing sequences used continue to change as MR technology evolves. At present the following spin-echo (SE) sequences are obtained using a 1.5T magnet and the following parameters:

- *Coronal plane:* TR 600, TE 25, 256^2 acquisition matrix, two excitations, 18-cm FOV, 3-mm-thick sections, 0.5-mm interslice gap, for a total of seven cuts through the sella
- *Sagittal plane:* TR 500, TE 20, 256^2 acquisition matrix, two excitations, 20-cm FOV, 5-mm-thick sections, 1-mm interslice gap

A "square" pulse wave is used to reduce interslice crosstalk. The coronal scans are most important for the detection of small lesions and for evaluation of the cavernous sinuses. The scans are performed before and after intravenous injection of gadolinium (Schering AG) 0.2 mL/kg body weight (each milliliter containing 469.01 mg of gadopentetate dimeglumine). The sagittal plane is used to evaluate the size of the sella and the relationship of large sellar masses to the sphenoid sinus, clivus, and suprasellar structures.

Parasellar Region

When confronted with a parasellar lesion, MR imaging (MRI) is performed to evaluate its relationship to the parasellar segment of the carotid artery, the cavernous sinus, and cranial nerves II, III, IV, V, and VI. To evaluate for possible extracranial extension through nearby skull base foramina, the scan margin must extend sufficiently below the sella.

Currently the following SE sequences are used: axial TR 800, TE 20, 256^2 acquisition matrix, 16-cm FOV, four excitations, 3-mm-thick cuts with 1-mm interslice gap for a total of 16 cuts. Scans are made from the hard palate through the suprasellar cistern. Coronal scans are made from the orbital apex to the prepontine cistern using the same parameters. Scans are performed before and after contrast infusion. The precontrast scans exploit the inherent contrast between fat planes adjacent to the skull base and soft tissue neoplasms. If only contrast studies were performed, these boundaries may be obscured. This is particularly true for densely enhancing tumors (i.e., meningioma) which may become isointense with surrounding fat on postcontrast MR studies. In addition, an axial T2-weighted series is performed using the following parameters: TR 2,500, TE 30/80, 256 × 128 acquisition matrix, 20-cm FOV, two excitations, 5-mm slice thickness, and 1-mm interslice gap.

NORMAL ANATOMY
Bony Sella

The anterior wall and floor of the sella consist of cortical bone which varies from several millimeters to only a few microns in thickness depending on the degree of pneumatization of the underlying sphenoid sinus.[1] Pneumatization of the body of the sphenoid bone begins at age 3 years, but the extent of pneumatization is variable and is sometimes even absent in adult life (Fig 22–1,A–C).[2]

If the sphenoid sinus is well pneumatized the parasellar carotid artery can be expected to impress a groove in its posterosuperior wall. The bone between artery and sinus is very thin or even incomplete in one third of people. In these the carotid artery is covered only by sinus mucosa and is therefore vulnerable to injury during transsphenoidal surgery.[2] If the sphenoid sinus is incompletely pneumatized, transsphenoidal surgery is more difficult. Infection of the sphenoid sinus is another relative contraindication to transsphenoidal surgery.[3]

The configuration of the sellar floor is quite variable. Localized defects or depressions are sometimes encountered (see Fig 22–1,A). Attempts have been made to correlate dips in the sellar floor with location of microadenomas, but such correlation has proved to be very poor. It is best to disregard the shape of the floor when evaluating for pituitary adenomas.[1, 4]

Coronal CT with bone algorithms is ideal for evaluation of the bony sella and skull base. Hyperostosis, erosion, and remodeling are better demonstrated by CT than by MRI,[5] but MRI is good for demonstrating replacement of normal bone marrow. This may occur in neoplastic infiltration of marrow cavities.

Dural Relationships

In life, the bony sella is invested with dura. As the dura passes anteriorly from the dorsum it divides into an outer layer which lines the floor and an inner layer which forms the roof of the pituitary fossa. The latter is the diaphragma sellae, which is perforated, usually in the center, by a foramen for passage of the pituitary infundibulum. This foramen varies in size from small (just large enough to allow passage of the pituitary infundibulum) to large with only a narrow rim of surrounding dura (Fig 22–2,A and B).[1, 6]

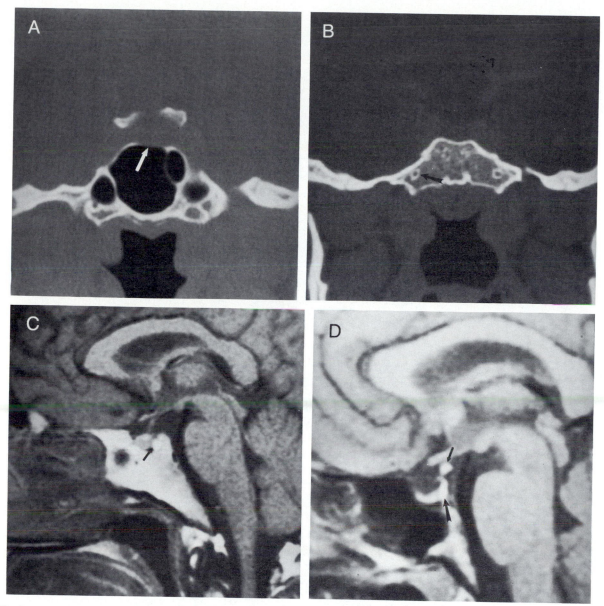

FIG 22–1.
Normal variants of sella. **A,** CT, bone windows of a well-pneumatized sphenoid sinus. Focal thinning of the floor *(arrow)* is normal. **B,** coronal CT (bone algorithm) of a nonpneumatized sphenoid bone. Transsphenoidal surgery is difficult in this situation. Incidentally, Vidian's canal is well seen *(arrow)*. **C,** sagittal spin-echo (SE) (TR 500, TE 20) MRI of a nonpneumatized sphenoid sinus. The sphenoid bone marrow has high signal on short TR images. There is a normal high signal in the posterior pituitary gland *(arrow)*. **D,** sagittal SE (TR 500, TE 20) MRI. Prominent fat in the dorsum sella *(small arrow)* mimics ectopic posterior pituitary tissue. Note the normal posterior pituitary lobe *(large arrow)*.

On MRI the diaphragma sellae is sometimes seen as a thin band between the pituitary fossa and the suprasellar cistern on proton-density (long TR, short TE SE) images. When visible, this structure helps to differentiate suprasellar from intrasellar pathology. The diaphragma sella is not visualized by CT (Fig 22–3,B).[7, 8]

Lateral to the sella the dura splits into two layers, one forming the medial wall of the cavernous sinus and the other the lateral wall and roof of the cavernous sinus. Between these dural reflections lie numerous venous channels (Figs 22–2,D and 22–3,A).[6] Winslow coined the term *cavernous sinus* in 1732 because he thought it was a trabecu-

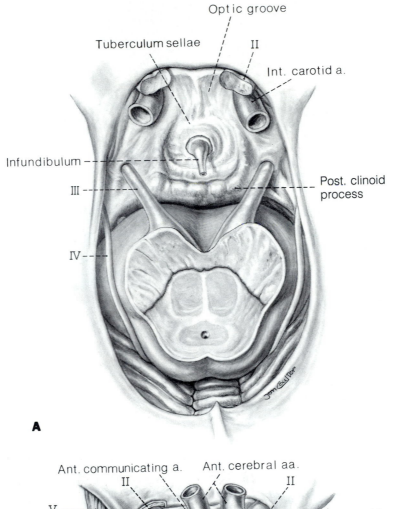

Optic groove
Tuberculum sellae
II
Int. carotid a.
Infundibulum
III
IV
Post. clinoid process

A

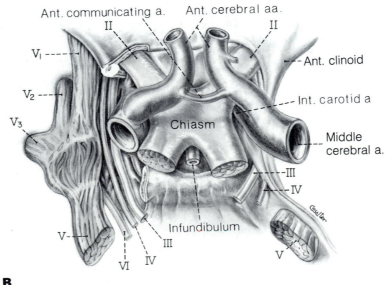

Ant. communicating a.
II
Ant. cerebral aa.
II
V₁
Ant. clinoid
V₂
Int. carotid a
V₃
Chiasm
Middle cerebral a.
III
IV
V
III
Infundibulum
VI
IV
V

B

FIG 22–2.

Sellar anatomy. **A,** sella viewed from above. The diaphragma sellae is a sheet of dura connecting the tuberculum sellae anteriorly with the posterior clinoids. There is a foramen for passage of the infundibulum. The tentorium blends into the superolateral border of the cavernous sinus. **B,** sella and suprasellar cistern viewed from above. The dura of the left cavernous sinus has been removed. The A1 segments and the anterior communicating artery course just superior to the optic chiasm. The origin of the recurrent artery of Heubner from the right anterior cerebral artery is shown.

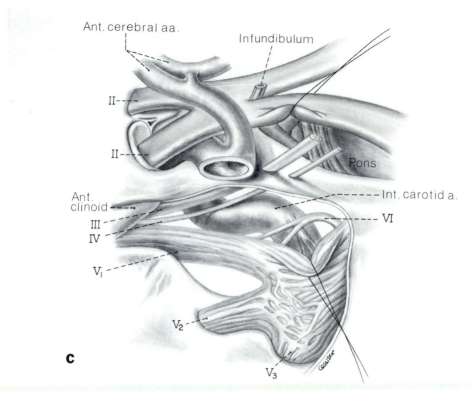

Ant. cerebral aa.

Infundibulum

II

II

Pons

Ant. clinoid

Int. carotid a.

III

IV

VI

V₁

V₂

V₃

C

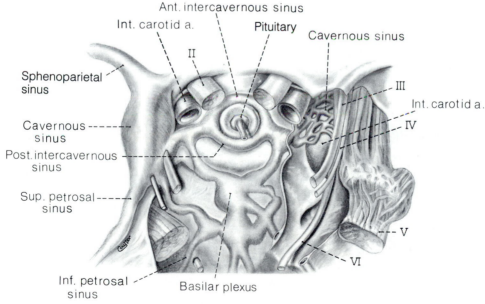

Ant. intercavernous sinus

Int. carotid a.

Pituitary

Cavernous sinus

II

Sphenoparietal sinus

III

Int. carotid a.

Cavernous sinus

IV

Post. intercavernous sinus

Sup. petrosal sinus

V

VI

Inf. petrosal sinus

Basilar plexus

D

FIG 22–2 (cont.).
C, lateral view of sella. The lateral dura of the cavernous sinus has been removed. Cranial nerve V₃ exits Meckel's cave and immediately passes through the foramen ovale to the masticator space; it never enters the cavernous sinus. Cranial nerve V₂ courses through the most inferior aspect of the cavernous sinus, then exits through the foramen rotundum into the pterygopalatine fossa. Cranial nerves V₁, VI, IV, and III all run in the cavernous sinus and exit through the superior orbital fissure into the orbit. **D,** venous anatomy viewed from above. The dural covering on the right has been removed to expose the venous anatomy within the cavernous sinus.

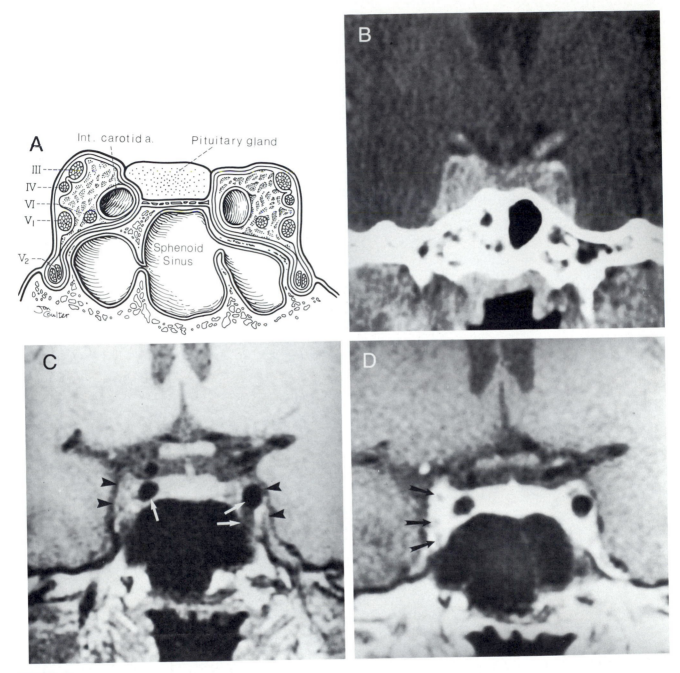

FIG 22–3.
Normal sella and cavernous sinus. **A,** coronal section of the pituitary gland and cavernous sinus. Note that cranial nerves III, IV, and V₁ run adjacent to the lateral wall of the cavernous sinus; cranial nerve VI runs medially within the venous plexus. **B,** enhanced coronal CT. Intravascular contrast causes enhancement of the cavernous venous plexus. Extravasated contrast enhances the pituitary gland because its vessels lack an effective blood-brain barrier. The thin pituitary capsule (medial wall of cavernous sinus) between the pituitary and cavernous sinus is not visualized. **C,** unenhanced spin-echo (SE) (TR 500, TE 20) coronal image. The cavernous sinus *(arrowheads)* has a speckled signal pattern which makes the confident identification of the cranial nerves seen in **A** difficult. The characteristic absence of signal can be seen in the intracavernous carotid arteries. **D,** enhanced SE (TR 500, TE 20) coronal MRI with gadolinium enhancement. As with CT there is uniform enhancement of the venous plexus of the cavernous sinus and pituitary gland. Cranial nerves III, V₁, and V₂ *(arrows)* can be identified on the patient's right side. See **A.**

lated venous space which resembled the corpus cavernosum of the penis.[9, 10] Other investigators claim that the cavernous sinus is really a plexus of small veins.[6, 11] The paired cavernous sinuses connect with each other through variable intrasellar channels (which may be anterior or posterior to the pituitary gland) as well as extrasellar communications (see Fig 22–2,D). These anastomotic channels are usually small, but they occasionally bleed severely during transsphenoidal surgery. The cavernous sinus drains the superior and inferior ophthalmic veins, middle and inferior cerebral veins, and the sphenoparietal sinus. They, in turn, drain into the basilar plexus, the transverse sinus (via the superior petrosal sinus), the jugular bulb (via the inferior petrosal sinus), and the pterygoid plexus (via a vein passing through the foramen ovale) (Fig 22–2,D).[12]

On contrast CT, the veins of the cavernous sinus blend together. A similar effect is seen on gadolinium-enhanced MRI (Fig 22–3,B and D). On unenhanced MRI the cavernous sinus has a speckled appearance, probably related to flow-rate differentials within the venous plexus (Fig 22–3,C). Small globules of fat are also found normally within the cavernous sinuses and are visible on both CT and MR images.[13]

The internal carotid artery passes between the dural leaves of the cavernous sinus giving off small branches to supply the tentorium, pituitary capsule, and gasserian ganglion. These intracavernous branches are not seen on CT or MR images and are

only rarely demonstrated by angiography. The ophthalmic artery usually arises from the carotid artery after it has pierced the dura and entered the cranial cavity, but it originates from the intracavernous portion of the carotid artery in 8% of anatomic dissections.[1, 11] This variation, difficult to recognize angiographically or by other imaging modalities, is nonetheless important when aneurysms are discovered arising at the origin of the ophthalmic artery since it makes it difficult to determine preoperatively whether or not the cavernous sinus will have to be entered in order to clip the aneurysm's neck. The carotid artery is fixed at its exit from the cavernous sinus by a tight dural band but its intracavernous course is variable. Usually it is separated from the pituitary gland by a distance of about 1 mm, but in one third of autopsy specimens the artery is more medial and actually indents the pituitary gland (Fig 22–4).[14, 15] Occasionally, both carotid arteries course medially and may be separated from each other by as little as 4 mm (Fig 22–5). Transsphenoidal surgery in such cases may be proscribed. MRI is ideal for demonstrating intercarotid distance.

In addition to the venous plexus and the carotid artery, two other structures run within the dural envelope of the cavernous sinus. These are (a) the plexus of sympathetic nerves which accompa-

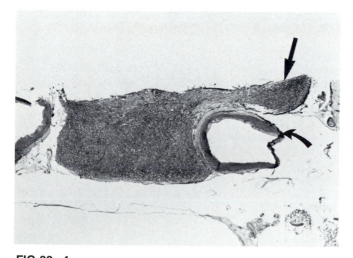

FIG 22–4.
Coronal histologic section of an autopsy specimen shows a normal variation in the position of the cavernous carotid artery *(curved arrow)*. A tonguelike extension of pituitary tissue *(straight arrow)* extends over the carotid.

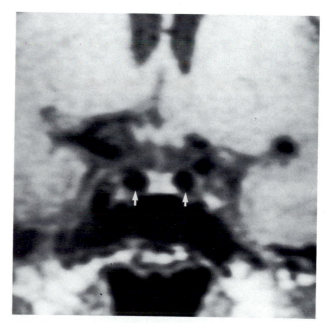

FIG 22–5.
Coronal SE (TR 600, TE 20) MRI through the floor of the pituitary fossa. Note the normal, but unusually medial position of both of the cavernous carotid arteries *(arrows)*.

nies the cavernous carotid artery and (b) cranial nerve VI which penetrates the posterior wall of the cavernous sinus at Dorello's canal, courses superiorly and laterally through the sinus, and exits through the superior orbital fissure (Fig 22–2,C and D).[1, 16, 17]

The lateral wall of the cavernous sinus consists of a tough outer layer and a thin inner reticular layer. The inner layer is formed by the sheaths of cranial nerves III, IV, and V_1 (see Fig 22–3,A).[18] These nerves converge anteriorly, pass through the superior orbital fissure, and supply motor fibers to the extraocular muscles and sensory fibers to the cornea, upper face, and scalp. The su-

perior ophthalmic vein also courses through the superior orbital fissure to drain into the cavernous sinus.

Just posterior to the cavernous sinus is a dural reflection, Meckel's cave (Fig 22–6,C). After exiting from the ventral surface of the pons, the axons of the fifth nerve enter Meckel's cave and synapse in the gasserian ganglion. Cranial nerve V_3 does not enter the cavernous sinus, but courses laterally instead to exit through the foramen ovale. Cranial nerve V_2 courses through only a small portion of the inferior aspect of the cavernous sinus before exiting through the foramen rotundum. Cranial nerve V_1 traverses the entire length of the cavern-

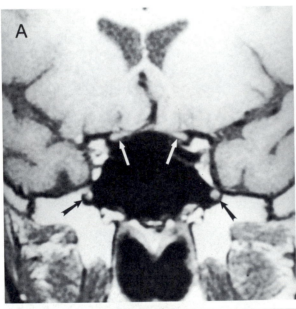

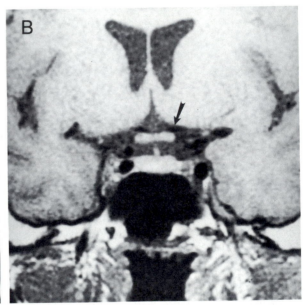

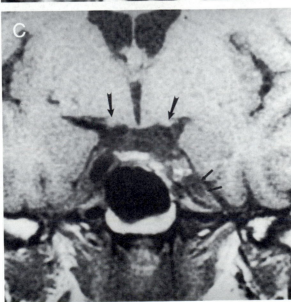

FIG 22–6.
Serial coronal scans. **A,** coronal SE (TR 800, TE 20) MRI at the level of the optic canals. The optic nerve *(white arrows)* passes through the canal medial to the anterior clinoid. The clinoid has a high signal because it contains marrow fat. It blends with fat in the superior orbital fissure. Note cranial nerve V_2 as it passes through the foramen rotundum bilaterally *(black arrows).* **B,** coronal SE (TR 800, TE 20) MRI at the level of the infundibulum. The optic nerves join to form the chiasm, which is located just anterior to the infundibular stalk. The A1 segment of the carotid artery lies immediately superior to the chiasm *(arrow)* and appears as a signal void. **C,** coronal SE (TR 800, TE 20) MRI at the level of the dorsum sellae. The optic tracts *(large arrows)* are visualized. The hypothalamus can be seen between these tracts as it forms the roof of the suprasellar cistern and the floor of the third ventricle. Meckel's cave, which contains the ganglion of cranial nerve V, is well seen on the patient's left *(small arrows).*

ous sinus to exit through the superior orbital fissure (see Fig 22–2,C).[1, 16, 18]

On careful inspection of unenhanced coronal MR images, cranial nerves III, V_1, V_2, and VI are difficult to recognize as they run in the lateral wall of the cavernous sinus (see Fig 22–3,C). They are more readily seen on CT or MR images following contrast enhancement (see Fig 22–3,D).[13, 16] The cavernous sinuses should be symmetric in size. The lateral walls may be flat or slightly convex laterally. On CT, the lateral wall is defined between the enhancing cavernous sinus medially and the temporal lobe laterally.[19] On MRI, the lateral wall and adjacent cerebrospinal fluid (CSF) are defined as a band of low signal (see Fig 22–3,C). The medial wall of the cavernous sinus, which is much thinner, is not demonstrated on CT and is rarely shown on MRI.[5, 14] On either CT or MRI masses within the cavernous sinus are usually recognized by unilateral sinus enlargement; small masses which do not change the contour of cavernous sinus are more difficult to discern.

Suprasellar Cistern (Neural and Vascular Contents)

Above the pituitary fossa lies an expansion of the subarachnoid space, the suprasellar cistern.

This cistern contains the optic nerves, chiasm, and tracts, the circle of Willis, and the pituitary infundibulum. Familiarity with its complex anatomy is helpful in identifying suprasellar pathology by either CT or MRI.

Coronal Plane

The optic nerve leaves the orbit through the optic canal medial to the anterior clinoid process (see Fig 22–6). Intracranially, it courses medially and posteriorly to join its contralateral companion forming the optic chiasm in the suprasellar cistern. The vertical dimension of the optic chiasm is variable but is generally less than 0.6 mm. The pituitary infundibulum runs anteriorly and inferiorly from the hypothalamus to the posterior lobe of the pituitary gland. It is located immediately behind the chiasm. The A1 segments of the anterior cerebral arteries and the anterior communicating artery are usually located just above the chiasm. The optic tracts extend posteriorly and laterally from the chiasm to the lateral geniculate nuclei.

Axial Plane

It is helpful to think of the suprasellar cistern as shaped like a six-pointed star (Fig 22–7). The anterior point of the star indicates the location of the interhemispheric fissure containing the ante-

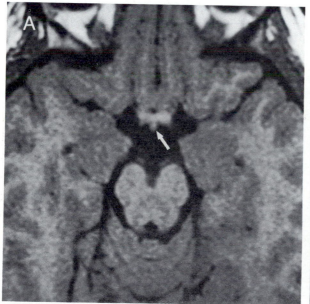 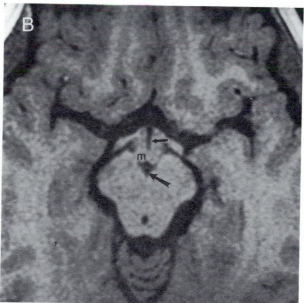

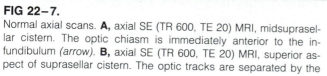

FIG 22–7.
Normal axial scans. **A,** axial SE (TR 600, TE 20) MRI, midsuprasellar cistern. The optic chiasm is immediately anterior to the infundibulum *(arrow).* **B,** axial SE (TR 600, TE 20) MRI, superior aspect of suprasellar cistern. The optic tracks are separated by the slitlike infundibular recess *(small arrow).* The mammillary bodies *(m)* are located just anterior to the interpeduncular cistern *(large arrow).*

rior cerebral arteries; the anterolateral points indicate the sylvian fissures which contain the proximal middle cerebral vessels; the posterolateral points of the star enter the perimesencephalic cisterns which contain the proximal parts of the anterior choroidal, posterior cerebral, and superior cerebellar arteries as well as the basal vein of Rosenthal. The posterior point defines the interpeduncular cistern. Lower axial sections show the optic nerves entering the orbit and joining one another at the chiasm anterior to the infundibulum. An axial section through the midportion of the cistern shows the optic nerves, tracks, and chiasm. On axial sections through the superior aspect of the cistern, the diverging optic tracks are seen. On this same section one finds the slitlike infundibular recess of the third ventricle. The mammillary bodies and the interpeduncular cistern can also be identified on superior axial sections. These anatomic details are visible on both CT and MRI, but the superior contrast resolution of MRI makes it the preferred modality for studying these structures. Short TR SE images are to be preferred over long TR sequences because they are less subject to CSF flow artifacts.

Sagittal Plane

The chiasm is usually centered directly over the pituitary gland (see Fig 22–1,C). In 5% to 10% of people the intracranial segment of the optic nerve is short and the chiasm is centered directly over the tuberculum sellae (the prefixed chiasm). In 15% of cases the intracranial optic nerves are longer than usual and the chiasm overlies the dorsum sellae (the postfixed chiasm). These normal anatomic variations become important when an anterior subfrontal surgical approach to the sella or suprasellar cistern is contemplated. With this approach, access to the sella may be blocked by short optic nerves (prefixed chiasm) or by a large tuberculum. In such cases resection of the tuberculum will usually provide adequate exposure.[20]

On parasagittal scans there may be partial volume averaging of the pituitary gland and the cavernous carotid artery (Fig 22–8). This should not be mistaken for intrasellar pathology. Occasionally, intrasellar herniation of the optic nerve, optic chiasm, and optic tract can occur. Kaufman et al.[21] have shown that there is no correlation between this finding and visual disturbances in the patient.

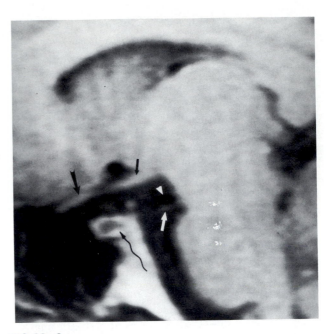

FIG 22–8.
Parasagittal scan. Sagittal spin-echo (TR 600, TE 20) MR scan shows the optic nerve *(large black arrow)*, optic tract *(small black arrow)*, cranial nerve III *(small white arrow)*, and the signal void of the posterior communicating artery *(white arrowhead)* just above cranial nerve III. The low signal in the pituitary fossa *(wavy arrow)* is due to partial volume averaging of the signal from the adjacent carotid artery.

Hypothalamus

The roof of the suprasellar cistern is formed by the hypothalamus. This small structure is important in such varied functions as temperature regulation, water balance, feeding and drinking behavior, and sexual activity.[22]

The hypothalamus is a thin layer of tissue which comprises the floor and adjacent lateral walls of the third ventricle (separating the ventricle from the suprasellar cistern) (Fig 22–6,C). Accordingly, the inferior surface of the hypothalamus is exposed to the CSF of the suprasellar cistern and consists of a ridge of gray matter which extends from the lamina terminalis and optic chiasm anteriorly to the posterior margin of the mammillary bodies. This ridge of tissue (excluding the mammillary bodies) is called the tuber cinereum. A swelling on the surface of the tuber cinereum, the median eminence, is continuous with the infundibulum and posterior lobe of the pituitary gland. Collectively, they constitute the neurohypophysis. At the lateral margins of the hypothalamus are the optic tracts and the sulci of the adjacent temporal lobes.[22]

The hypothalamus controls pituitary function through direct neuronal links with the posterior lobe (neurohypophysis) and a vascular link with the anterior lobe (adenohypophysis).[23] The supraoptic and paraventricular nuclei of the hypothalamus consist of neurosecretory cells where antidiuretic hormone (ADH, vasopressin) is produced (Fig 22–9,A). This octapeptide (with a carrier protein or neurophysin) is transported via the unmyelinated axons. The modified axon terminals are located either along the infundibulum or, more commonly, in the posterior lobe of the pituitary. When stimulated, they release ADH into the systemic circulation (via a plexus of veins in the posterior lobe). Oxytocin is a similar octapeptide which is produced and transported in an analogous fashion. This hormone causes uterine contractions during parturition and mammary smooth muscle contraction during milk ejection. Control of the anterior lobe is different (Fig 22–9,B), there being no direct neuronal links from the hypothalamus to the anterior lobe. Instead, releasing factors are produced by hypothalamic cells and delivered to the anterior lobe by the hypophyseal portal system which runs from hypothalamic veins to the vascular sinusoids of the anterior pituitary gland. These hypothalamic factors may inhibit tonic hormone release, as in the case of prolactin, or may stimulate hormone release and production as with growth hormone (GH), thyroid-stimulating hormone (TSH), and adrenocorticotrophic hormone (ACTH).[24]

The details of production and transport of these hormones may be important in understanding the MR signal characteristics of the posterior

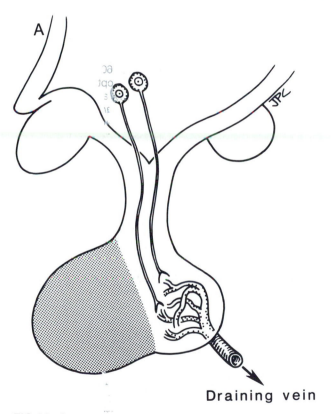

Draining vein

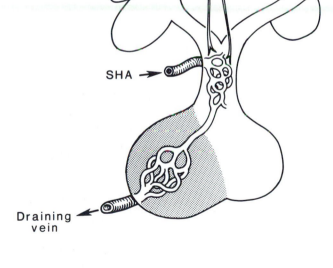

FIG 22–9.
A, neurohypophysis. ADH and oxytocin are synthesized in the neurons of the supraoptic and paraventricular nuclei. These octapeptides are bound to neurophysines (carrier proteins) and transported down the nerve axons in the infundibulum to bulbous axon terminals in the posterior lobe. From here ADH or oxytocin is released directly into systemic veins. Pituicytes, modified glial cells supporting the axon terminals, accumulate intracytoplasmic fat in proportion to their neurosecretory activity. Some investigators contend that this fat gives the posterior lobe its characteristic high signal on T1-weighted images. **B,** adenohypophysis. Releasing factors are synthesized by hypothalamic neurons. From axon terminals in the median eminence they are released into the superior part of the hypothalamic portal system. They are carried by blood flow inferiorly to the vascular sinusoids of the anterior pituitary where they stimulate (in the case of GH, ACTH, TSH) or inhibit (in the case of prolactin) the release of systemically active anterior pituitary hormones. SHA = superior hypophyseal artery. (Diagrams based on Kelly W, Kucharczyk W, Kucharczyk J, et al.: *AJNR* 1988; 9:453–460.)

lobe of the pituitary gland. (See the following section on the pituitary gland.)

Pituitary Gland

The pituitary gland consists of two embryologically distinct structures which have close functional and anatomic relationships: the adenohypophysis (anterior lobe) and the neurohypophysis (posterior lobe). The adenohypophysis arises from Rathke's pouch, an upgrowth of rudimentary ectoderm from the primitive mouth. The neurohypophysis arises as a downgrowth of neuroectoderm from the diencephalon. The adenohypophysis and neurohypophysis are separated by the pars intermedia, a thin layer of tissue which has numerous, usually small, colloid-containing cysts.[25] Each of these areas is discussed separately in the sections which follow.

Anterior Lobe

The adenohypophysis occupies the anterior two thirds of the sella. It is composed of glandular cells responsible for the production of numerous hormones including growth hormone, thyroid-stimulating hormone, follicle-stimulating hormone, luteinizing hormone, ACTH, and prolactin. On enhanced CT the anterior lobe is normally of inhomogeneous density. Histologic correlations demonstrate that CT-dense areas consist of tightly packed cells often containing numerous intracellular secretory granules. CT-lucent areas consist of less tightly packed cells which have fewer intracellular granules (Fig 22–10).[26] On enhanced CT, differences in vascularity also produce variations of density. For instance, there is a collection of venous sinusoids on the superior aspect of the midanterior lobe. On dynamic bolus-contrasted CT, this capillary bed enhances more than the adjacent pituitary tissue. Displacement of this vascular tuft is a secondary sign for diagnosing pituitary masses (tuft sign).[27] CT-lucent areas are also frequently seen separating the anterior lobe from the adjacent cavernous sinus. Histologically, these hypodense areas represent adipose or connective tissue.

Tissue variations within the anterior lobe are probably less noticeable on MRI because of the thicker cuts (3 mm as opposed to 1.5 mm) which result in obscurement due to partial-volume averaging (see Fig 22–3C,D). The anterior lobe typically is isointense with brain on both short and long TR SE images.

The size and shape of the anterior lobe vary with age, sex, and stage of the menstrual cycle. Young women generally have the largest pituitary glands, which normally may be up to 9 mm in

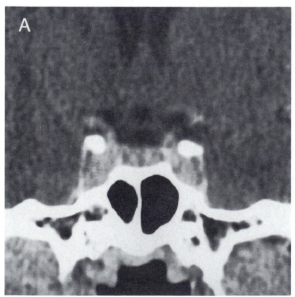
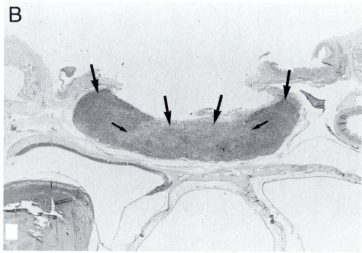

FIG 22–10.
Normal inhomogeneity of the anterior lobe. **A,** contrast-enhanced coronal CT through the anterior lobe of the pituitary gland shows vertical bands of hypointense signal. **B,** coronal histologic section (hematoxylin-eosin) shows the inhomogeneity of the anterior lobe. Strongly staining areas *(large arrows)* consist of tightly compacted heavily granulated cells. Weakly stained areas *(small arrows)* consist of loosely compacted mildly granulated cells. Note the similarity to **A.**

height (average 4.2 mm in women and 3.5 mm in men). The upper margin of the gland may be concave, flat, or symmetrically convex (Fig 22–11). Asymmetric upward convexities are abnormal and indicate an underlying pituitary mass.[28, 29]

Pars Intermedia

The pars intermedia is an inconspicuous tissue layer separating the adenohypophysis from the neurohypophysis. It is nonfunctional but important from an imaging standpoint, because it normally contains small vesicles which represent the embryologic remnants of the posterior wall of Rathke's pouch.[25] Histologically, these vesicles are true cysts with an epithelial lining and they contain variable numbers of goblet cells. In aggregate, these tiny cysts can appear as a CT-lucent area (Fig 22–12).[26] Normally, they are not recognized on MRI. Occasionally they enlarge and compress adjacent structures.

Posterior Lobe

The neurohypophysis occupies the posterior one third of the sella. It consists of the bulbous terminal axons of hypothalamic neurons and pituicytes (modified glial cells). On axial enhanced CT the posterior lobe is visualized in one third of normal subjects. It is less dense than the anterior lobe, probably because of its less cellular compactness.

The posterior lobe is distinctive in that it often

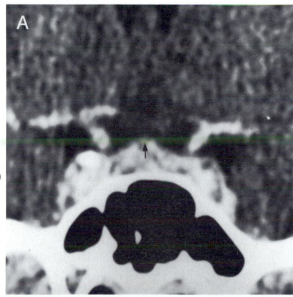

FIG 22–11.
Normal pituitary. Fifteen-year-old girl imaged following minor head trauma. Extensive endocrinologic testing showed no abnormality. **A,** contrast coronal CT shows symmetric convex superior surface of the gland *(arrow).* The density variations in the anterior lobe are normal. **B** and **C,** spin-echo coronal and sagittal MRI (TR 600, TE 20) in the same patient. The superior surface of the gland *(arrows)* almost touches the optic chiasm.

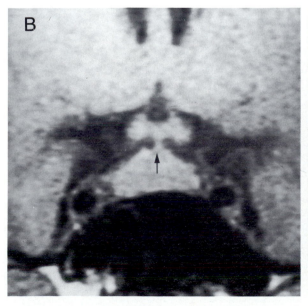

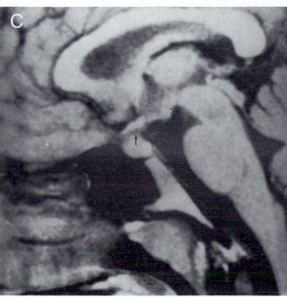

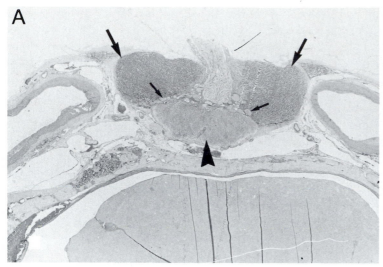

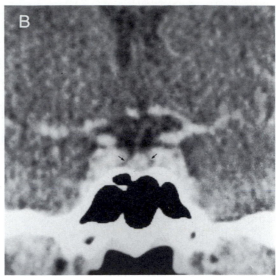

FIG 22–12.
Pars intermedia. **A,** coronal histologic section (hematoxylin-eosin) at the level of the infundibulum. The posterior lobe *(arrowhead)* is separated from the posterolateral extensions of the anterior lobe *(large arrows)* by the pars intermedia *(small arrows)* which con- tains numerous tiny colloid cysts. **B,** corresponding enhanced CT. The pars intermedia *(arrows)* is less dense than the surrounding tissue. This lucent band may be unilateral if the pars intermedia is asymmetric.

has very high signal on short TR MR images (see Fig 22–1,C and D).[23] This high signal has been attributed to the neurosecretory substances formed by the hypothalamus. Others ascribe it to lipid found within modified astrocytes (pituicytes) which are associated with the terminal axons.[24] In either case, on short TR images the posterior lobe has high signal in most infants and adults.[30, 31] This high signal is absent in about 10% to 50% of the healthy population.[23, 32] Brooks and co-workers[32] compared the size and signal intensity of the posterior lobe in 36 patients who had at least two MR scans and concluded that temporal variations in the size and signal intensity of the posterior lobe were common. It is also absent in conditions which disturb hypothalamic secretion or axonal transport to the neurohypophysis, such as physical compression of the infundibulum by a suprasellar mass or infiltration of the hypothalamus or infundibulum as by hypothalamic glioma, optic glioma, germinoma, or histiocytosis X. Gudinchet et al.[31] reported loss of bright signal in the posterior lobe in all of 13 children with diabetes insipidus.

Physical disruption of axonal transport may lead to high signal in the infundibulum itself, as has been observed with large macroadenomas that compress the infundibulum and after hypophysectomy.[33] These findings support the hypothesis that the bright signal may be due to accumulation of neurosecretory material proximal to the block in the axonal transport system.[23, 33]

Rarely, the posterior lobe is located with a small fossula in the posterior wall of the bony sellae. Very rarely, high signal attributable to the posterior pituitary is seen in the suprasellar cistern. This has been described as a normal variant,[32] but it is also seen in pituitary dwarfs.[34]

After gadolinium enhancement, the posterior lobe blends with the anterior lobe or may even be less intense. This reflects the greater enhancement of the anterior lobe and is analogous to the density pattern seen on enhanced CT scans.[35] The border between the posterior lobe and the pars intermedia may be convex, flat, or concave. The posterior lobe is occasionally off the midline, and then the infundibulum may be deviated as well.

REFERENCES

1. Rhoton AL, Harris FS, Renn WH: Microsurgical anatomy of the sellar region and cavernous sinus. *Clin Neurosurg* 1971; 24:54–85.
2. Johnson DM, Hopkins RJ, Hanafee WN, et al: The unprotected parasphenoidal carotid artery studied by high-resolution computed tomography. *Radiology* 1985; 155:137–141.
3. Dolinskas CA, Simeone FA: Transsphenoidal hypophysectomy: postsurgical CT findings. *AJNR* 1985; 6:45–50.

4. Dubois PJ, Orr DP, Hoy RJ, et al: Normal sellar variations in frontal tomograms. *Radiology* 1979; 131:105–110.
5. Hirsch WL, Hryshko FG, Sekhar LN, et al: Comparison of MR imaging, CT, and angiography in the evaluation of the enlarged cavernous sinus. *AJNR* 1988; 9:907–915.
6. Taptas JN: The so-called cavernous sinus. A review of the controversy and its implications for neurosurgeons. *Neurosurgery* 1982; 11:712–717.
7. Daniels DL, Pojunas KW, Kilgore DP, et al: MR of the diaphragma sellae. *AJNR* 1986; 7:765–769.
8. Sage MR, Blumbergs PC, Mulligan BP, et al: The diaphragma sellae: Its relationship to the configuration of the pituitary gland. *Radiology* 1982; 145:703–708.
9. Bedford MA: The cavernous sinus. *Br J Ophthalmol* 1966; 50:41–46.
10. Parkinson D, West M: Lesions of the cavernous plexus region, in Youmans JR (ed), *Neurological Surgery,* ed 2. Philadelphia, WB Saunders Co, 1982, pp 3004–3023.
11. Parkinson D: Surgical anatomy of the cavernous sinus, in Wilkins RH, Rengachary SS (eds): *Neurosurgery.* New York, McGraw-Hill Book Co., 1984; pp 1478–1483.
12. Kaplan HA, Browder J, Krieger AJ: Intracavernous connections of the cavernous sinuses. *J Neurosurg* 1976; 45:166–168.
13. Daniels DL, Pech P, Mark L, et al: Magnetic resonance imaging of the cavernous sinus. *AJNR* 1985; 6:187–192.
14. Scotti G, Yu CY, Dillon WP, et al: MR imaging of cavernous sinus involvement by pituitary adenomas. *AJNR* 1988; 9:657–664.
15. Sekhar LN, Burgess J, Akin O: An anatomical study of the cavernous sinus emphasizing operative approaches and the related vascular and neural reconstruction. *Neurosurgery* 1987; 21:806–816.
16. Tshuha M, Aoki H, Okamura T: Roentgenological investigation of cavernous sinus structure with special reference to paracavernous cranial nerves. *Neuroradiology* 1987; 29:462–467.
17. Sekhar LN, Moller AR: Operative management of tumors involving the cavernous sinus. *J Neurosurg* 1986; 64:879–889.
18. Umansky F, Nathan H: The lateral wall of the cavernous sinus. *J Neurosurg* 1982; 56:228–234.
19. Moore T, Ganti SR, Mowad M, et al: CT and angiography of primary extradural juxtasellar tumors. *AJNR* 1985; 145:491–496.
20. Patterson RH: Subfrontal approach to the pituitary gland, in Wilkins RH, Rengachary SS (eds): *Neurosurgery,* New York, McGraw-Hill Book Co, 1985, pp 902–904.
21. Kaufman B, Tomsak RL, Kaufman BA, et al: Herniation of the suprasellar visual system and third ventricle into empty sellae: Morphologic and clinical considerations. *AJNR* 1989; 10:65–76.
22. Nolte J: *The Human Brain: Introduction to Its Functional Anatomy.* St Louis, CV Mosby Co, 1981.
23. Columbo N, Berry I, Kucharczyk J, et al: Posterior pituitary gland: Appearance on MR images in normal and pathologic states. *Radiology* 1987; 165:481–485.
24. Kucharczyk J, Kucharczyk W, Berry I, et al: Histochemical characterization and functional significance of the hyperintense signal on MR images of the posterior pituitary. *AJNR* 1988; 9:1079–1083.
25. Tinall GT, Barrow DL: *Disorders of the Pituitary.* St Louis, CV Mosby Co, 1986, pp 1–22.
26. Roppolo HMN, Latchaw RE: The normal pituitary gland. Part II: Microscopic anatomy—CT correlation. *AJNR* 1983; 4:937.
27. Bonneville JF, Cattin F, Moussa-Bacha K, et al: Dynamic computed tomography of the pituitary gland: The tuft sign. *Radiology* 1983; 149:145–148.
28. Peyster RG, Hoover ED, Viscarello RR, et al: CT appearance of the adolescent and preadolescent pituitary gland. *AJNR* 1983; 4:411–414.
29. Wolpert SM, Molitich ME, Goldman JA, et al: Size, shape and appearance of the normal female pituitary gland. *AJR* 1984; 143:37–38.
30. Wolpert SM, Osborne M, Anderson M, et al: The bright pituitary gland—A normal MR appearance in infancy. *AJNR* 1988; 9:1–3.
31. Gudinchet F, Brunelle F, Barth MO, et al: MR imaging of the posterior hypophysis in children. *AJNR* 1989; 10:511–514.
32. Brooks BS, Gammal TE, Allison JD, et al: Frequency and variation of the posterior pituitary bright signal on MR images. *AJNR* 1989; 10:943–948.
33. El Gammal T, Brooks BS, Hoffman WH: MR imaging of the ectopic bright signal of posterior pituitary regeneration. *AJNR* 1989; 10:323–328.
34. Kelly WM, Kucharczyk W, Kucharczyk J, et al: Posterior pituitary ectopia: An MR feature of pituitary dwarfism. *AJNR* 1988; 9:435–460.
35. Bonneville JF, Cattin F, Portha C, et al: Computed tomographic demonstration of the posterior pituitary. *AJNR* 1985; 6:889–892.

23

Sella and Parasellar Regions: Pathology

William L. Hirsch, Jr., M.D.

Helen M.N. Roppolo, M.D.

L. Anne Hayman, M.D.

Vincent C. Hinck, M.D.

PITUITARY ADENOMAS

Classification

Pituitary adenomas arise from the glandular cells of the anterior pituitary gland. They are common (accounting for at least 15% of intracranial neoplasms) and are a frequent incidental finding at autopsy, a fact that illustrates their highly variable natural history. There are three ways of classifying pituitary adenomas, and each gives an insight into the nature and behavior of these neoplasms. The following is a review of the radiologic, functional, and pathologic/histologic classification systems.[1]

Radiologic Classification

Pituitary adenomas greater than 1 cm in size are called macroadenomas (see Figs 23–1 to 23–7), while smaller neoplasms are microadenomas (see Figs 23–8 to 23–13). Microadenomas are usually confined to the sella, but macroadenomas may extend superiorly into the suprasellar cistern, inferiorly into the sphenoid sinus, or laterally into the cavernous sinuses. Detection of the adenoma and assessment of the surrounding structures are the primary goals of imaging. Although the distinction between microadenomas and macroadenomas is made frequently, it is largely artificial. Histologically the tumors are inseparable, and there is no way to distinguish which adenomas will remain small throughout life and which will not.[2]

Functional Classification

The majority of clinically evident pituitary adenomas (70%) are endocrine active (functional) and produce an excessive amount of a specific pituitary hormone. Hypersecretion of pituitary hormones causes clinical symptoms even while the adenoma is still quite small. For example, adrenocorticotropic hormone (ACTH)-producing adenomas cause hypercortisolism (Cushing's syndrome) and almost always are microadenomas at presentation. On the other hand, endocrine-inactive (nonfunctional) tumors are macroadenomas at presentation because they manifest themselves only by compressing surrounding structures; suprasellar extension compresses the optic chiasm to produce visual deficits, while lateral extension into the cavernous sinus may result in diplopia due to compression of cranial nerves III, IV, or VI. Some macroadenomas present with headaches without focal neurologic deficit.

Histologic Classification

To understand the behavior of neoplasms of the anterior pituitary, it is best to consider them as part of a single continuum of pathology. The benign end of this behavioral spectrum is represented by pituitary adenomas that are derived from cells of the adenohypophysis. They are slow growing and are well demarcated but not encapsulated. They are surrounded by compressed nontu-

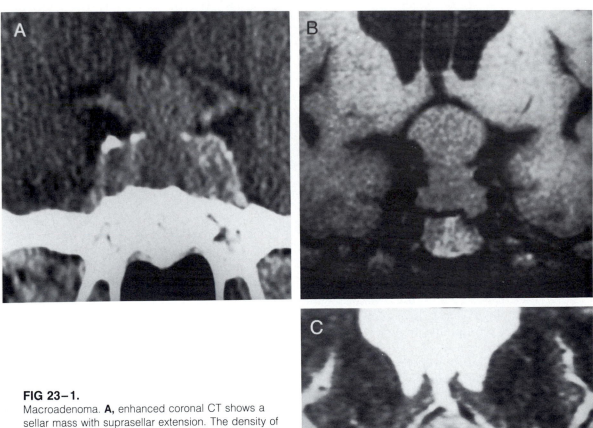

FIG 23–1.
Macroadenoma. **A,** enhanced coronal CT shows a
sellar mass with suprasellar extension. The density of
the enhancing tumor is almost the same as the adjacent
cavernous sinus. **B,** coronal SE (TR 600, TE 20) MRI
shows the macroadenoma to be isointense to gray
matter. The tumor is constricted at the diaphragma
sellae. **C,** coronal SE (TR 2,500, TE 100) image. The
suprasellar portion of the tumor is hyperintense relative
to gray matter.

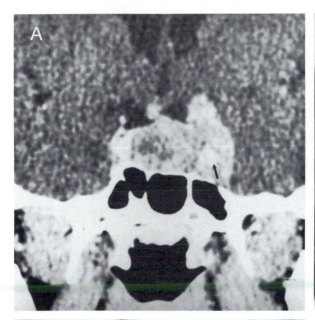

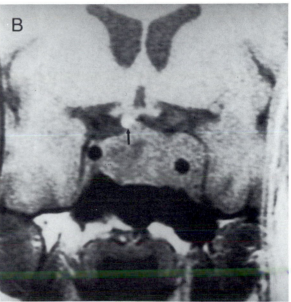

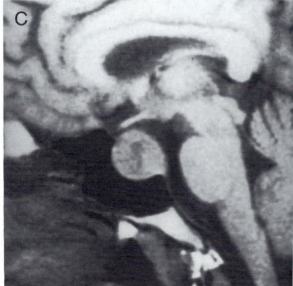

FIG 23–2.

Macroadenoma with cavernous sinus involvement. **A,** bolus-enhanced coronal CT reveals a sellar mass with central lucency. The left cavernous sinus is enlarged. Thanks to bolus contrast administration the carotid artery can be distinguished from the surrounding tumor *(arrow)*. Complete engulfment of the carotid is the only reliable criteria of cavernous sinus invasion. **B,** coronal SE (TR 600, TE 20) MRI confirms that the left cavernous carotid is engulfed by tumor. The infundibulum is compressed by the tumor and there is high signal intensity in the distal stalk *(arrow)*. This may reflect mechanical interruption of axonal transport due to compression by the mass. **C,** sagittal SE (TR 600, TE 20) MRI shows expansion of the sella by the adenoma. The hyperintense signal usually seen in the posterior pituitary is absent.

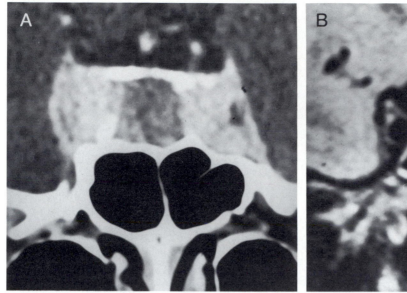

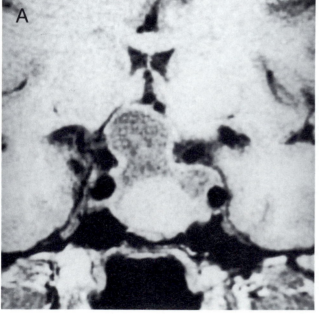

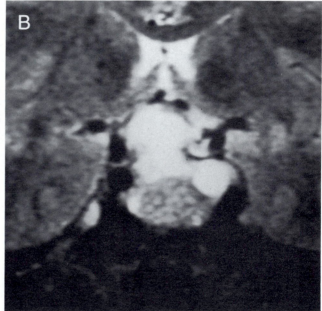

FIG 23–3.
Pitfall, inappropriate scan angle. **A,** enhanced CT. There appears to be enlargement of the cavernous sinus bilaterally. **B,** coronal SE (TR 2,000, TE 80) MRI 10 days later (no treatment) shows an intra-sellar mass but normal-appearing cavernous sinuses. The CT impression of cavernous enlargement is due to the inappropriate scan angle, which is closer to the axial than the coronal plane.

FIG 23–4.
Macroadenoma with cavitation/necrosis. **A** and **B,** coronal SE (TR 800, TE 20 and TR 2,500, TE 100) MRI. The intrasellar portion of the mass is isointense to gray matter on all pulsing sequences. The suprasellar portion of the mass is cavitated and has low signal on short TR and high signal on long TR sequences. The tumor encroaches on the left cavernous carotid, but this is not diagnostic of cavernous sinus invasion; the pituitary capsule is stretched but may be intact.

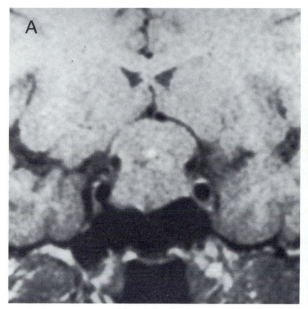

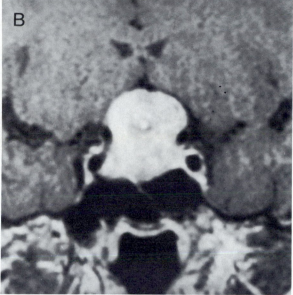

FIG 23–5.
Undifferentiated macroadenoma. **A,** coronal SE (TR 700, TE 25) MRI shows a large sellar and suprasellar mass. The central focus of high signal was also present in T2-weighted images, which sug- gests that it may be a focal hemorrhage. **B,** postcontrast, there is mottled enhancement of the mass.

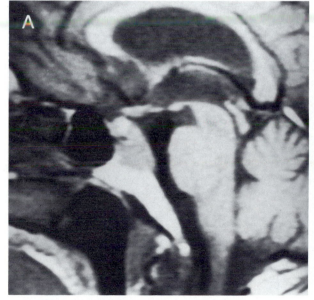

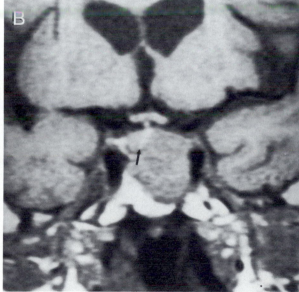

FIG 23–6.
Atypical macroadenoma without sellar enlargement. **A,** sagittal SE (TR 600, TE 20) MRI shows a mass inferior and posterior to a nor- mal-sized sella. **B,** coronal SE (TR 600, TE 20) MRI. The mass dis- places the pituitary gland to the right. The higher signal band *(ar- row)* represents the compressed posterior lobe. This macro- adenoma is unusual in that it has not expanded the sella; instead it has eroded the clivus.

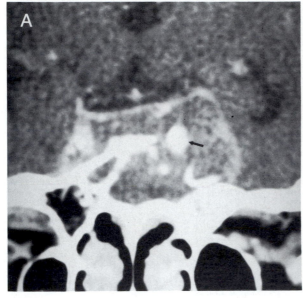
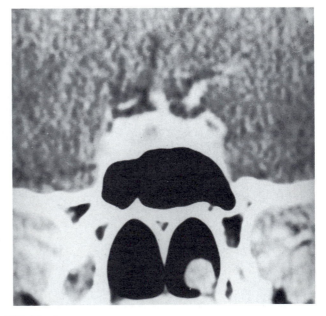

FIG 23–7.
Macroadenoma with bone destruction. **A,** enhanced coronal CT shows the large sellar mass invading the right cavernous sinus and the sphenoid air cells. The calcified carotid artery *(arrow)* is engulfed by tumor. **B,** bone windows show destruction, not remodeling of the floor of the sella.

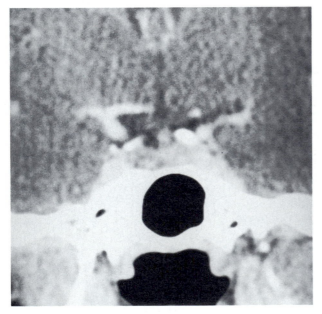

FIG 23–8.
Microadenoma. Coronal enhanced CT shows prolactin-secreting adenoma in the right side of the gland with low-density periphery and central high density. There are no secondary signs of adenoma due to mass effect.

FIG 23–9.
Microadenoma. Coronal enhanced CT shows a low-density prolactinoma on the right. There is asymmetrical bulging of the right surface of the gland and displacement of the infundibulum to the left.

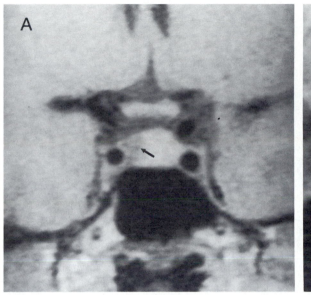

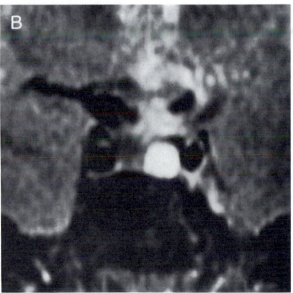

FIG 23–10.
Microadenoma. **A,** coronal SE (TR 600, TE 20) MRI shows a small mass on the right *(arrow)* that is lower in signal than is the rest of the pituitary. **B,** coronal SE (TR 3,000, TE 100) MRI reveals high T2 signal within this prolactinoma.

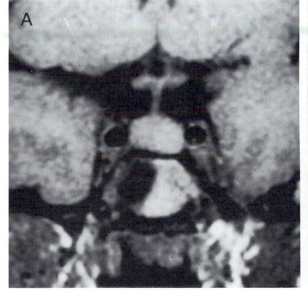

FIG 23–11.
Atypical microadenoma. **A,** coronal SE (TR 600, TE 25) MRI shows a slight asymmetry in the pituitary and higher signal on the left. It is difficult to localize this prolactin-secreting adenoma on the short TR images. **B,** coronal SE (TR 2,500, TE 100) MRI clearly shows a high-signal adenoma on the left. Most microadenomas are better demonstrated on T1-weighted images.

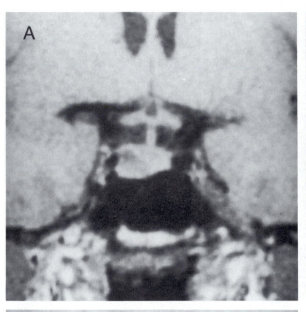

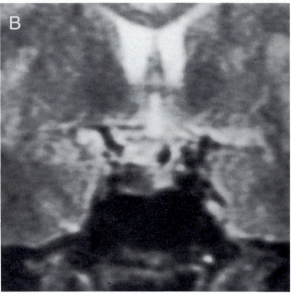

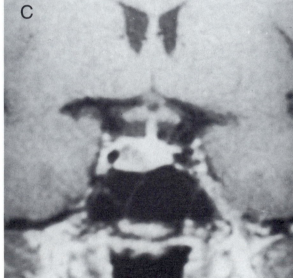

FIG 23–12.
Microadenoma. **A,** coronal SE (TR 600, TE 25) image shows a low-intensity prolactinoma on the right. **B,** coronal SE (TR 2,500, TE 100) MRI. This adenoma has low T2 signal. **C,** following intravenous gadolinium DTPA administration the adenoma enhances less than normal pituitary tissue does. This is typical soon after contrast administration. On delayed scans (30 minutes or more after injection) an adenoma may enhance more than normal pituitary due to delayed washout of the gadolinium from the adenoma, which typically is less vascular than a normal pituitary is.

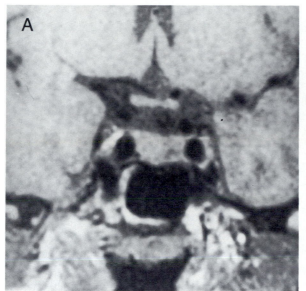 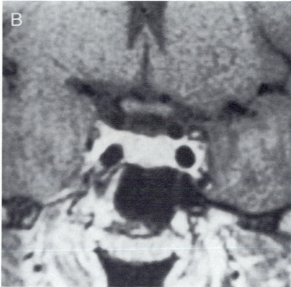

FIG 23–13.
Microadenoma obscured following contrast enhancement. **A,** coronal SE (TR 500, TE 20) MRI suggests a microadenoma on the left.

B, following intravenous gadolinium DTPA administration the microadenoma is less conspicuous than on the unenhanced scan.

morous tissue. The opposite end of the behavioral spectrum is represented by the rare pituitary carcinoma. The latter may infiltrate dura, bone, and surrounding neural structures, but its cells are histologically indistinguishable from the benign adenoma. Because of this, distant metastases (either hematogenous or cerebrospinal fluid [CSF] borne) are required to make the diagnosis of pituitary carcinoma. "Invasive" pituitary adenomas represent the intermediate part of the pathologic spectrum. These infiltrate surrounding structures including bone and dura but grow more slowly than do pituitary carcinomas and, by definition, never metastasize. Of prolactinomas, 33% of the microadenomas and 67% of the macroadenomas will be "invasive." This helps explain the 50% recurrence of hyperprolactinemia following surgical removal of prolactin-producing microadenomas.[2]

Although histologic characteristics cannot predict behavior, they do separate adenomas on the basis of endocrinologic activity. When using immunoperoxidase techniques, antibodies to specific pituitary hormones selectively stain adenoma cells. In this way, prolactin-secreting adenomas may be differentiated on a histologic basis from adenomas producing other hormones. Similar functional distinctions can be made on the basis of the ultrastructural features of adenoma cells seen with the electron microscope.[2]

Prolactin-Secreting Adenomas

In the normal state, the anterior lobe continually produces prolactin. Control is exerted by hypothalamic neurons, which secrete prolactin-inhibiting factor (dopamine or a closely related neurotransmitter) into the hypophyseal portal system. Prolactin-secreting adenomas become at least partially independent of this inhibitory control. In premenopausal women, excess secretion of prolactin causes oligomenorrhea, amenorrhea, and/or galactorrhea. These symptoms are usually noticed, and hence in this group of patients, the tumors are usually microadenomas at the time of presentation. In men, excess prolactin secretion results in gynecomastia, loss of libido, or impotence, symptoms that are frequently ignored. As a result, prolactinomas in men are often macroadenomas at the time of presentation. It is important to note that an elevated serum prolactin level does not guarantee the presence of a prolactin-secreting adenoma. Damage to the hypothalamus or compression of the pituitary stalk by any suprasellar mass may interfere with the production or transport of prolactin-inhibiting factor from the hypothalamus, thereby indirectly causing moderate elevation of serum prolactin levels. Patient's taking phenothiazines may also have moderate elevations of the serum prolactin concentration. However, a marked elevation in prolactin content (greater than 200 ng/mL) almost always indicates the presence of a pituitary adenoma.[3]

Macroadenomas

Large adenomas are easily detected by computed tomography (CT). The adenoma will be identified because of mass distortion of the normal anatomy of the pituitary gland (Fig 23–1,A). Most CT evaluations of pituitary adenomas are done with contrast only; bolus contrast administration is particularly helpful (Fig 23–2). Most macroadenomas are isodense with the surrounding pituitary gland and cavernous sinuses. Lucent areas are found within 10% to 30% of macroadenomas (Fig 23–2). The hypodense areas represent necrosis or fluid-containing cavities within the tumor. Calcification is rare.

MRI is preferred to CT in evaluating macroadenomas because of superior demonstration of tumor extent, specifically suprasellar and intracavernous (Fig 23–3). On unenhanced MRI, most macroadenomas are isointense with brain on both long and short repetition time (TR) spin-echo sequences. The normal gland therefore may be indistinguishable from the macroadenoma. Areas of necrosis within the tumor have variable signal characteristics but are most often bright on long TR, long echo time (TE) spin-echo images (Fig 23–4,C).[4, 5] Following contrast, macroadenomas generally enhance irregularly, depending on tumor vascularity and necrosis (Fig 23–5). Normal anterior pituitary tissue is usually compressed and obscured by the adenoma. The high-signal posterior lobe may or may not be visualized (Figs 23–2,C and 23–6,B). The ability to image the sagittal plane gives MRI an advantage over CT in evaluating superior extension of macroadenomas. Lateral extension into the cavernous sinus is also common but more difficult to evaluate. The pituitary capsule, which blends imperceptibly with the medial wall of the cavernous sinus, is normally invisible, so it is frequently impossible to tell whether the cavernous sinus is simply displaced or actually invaded by a pituitary mass. Only if the carotid artery is completely engulfed by tumor can cavernous sinus invasion be diagnosed with certainty (see Fig 23–2).[6] Enlargement of the sella and gross invasion of the sphenoid sinus and clivus are well demonstrated with MRI, particularly on sagittal images (Fig 23–6). However, CT remains superior in documenting the bone changes associated with macroadenomas (Fig 23–7).

Microadenomas

CT and MRI are able to demonstrate all macroadenomas because of the morphologic changes in surrounding anatomy that accompany tumor, not because of unique signal characteristics. In fact, as noted above, the MRI signal characteristics and CT density of macroadenomas are frequently indistinguishable from normal pituitary tissue. The problem in recognizing microadenomas is that the majority do not significantly distort the surrounding morphology but must be recognized on the basis of density or signal differences from the surrounding gland. These may be minimal. Opinions vary widely on the ability of CT to identify prolactin-secreting microadenomas, with figures ranging between 50% and 90% accuracy.[4, 7] Our own experience suggests that many small adenomas are not visible by CT or MRI and that careful correlation between imaging, endocrinologic, and clinical data is needed for establishing the diagnosis.

Most commonly on enhanced CT, the microadenoma appears as a focal hypodense lesion within the pituitary gland that causes no significant mass effect (Fig 23–8). Indirect signs including focal convexity of the superior surface of the pituitary gland or a bowed infundibulum are helpful in localizing and/or confirming the presence of an adenoma (Fig 23–9). However, the absence of these signs is meaningless because they occur in only about one third of cases. Focal thinning or sloping of the floor of the sella is frequently observed adjacent to microadenomas but is an unreliable (and frequently false) localizing sign that is best disregarded because wide variations in the thickness and contour of the sellar floor occur normally.[7, 8] On MRI microadenomas may have any combination of signal characteristics (Figs 23–10 to 23–12), but typically they are hypointense on short TR and hyperintense on long TR spin-echo sequences. Short TR sequences demonstrate anatomic details such as focal convexities of the superior surface of the gland and infundibular stretching, secondary signs of adenoma. Gadolinium enhancement may increase the conspicuity of microadenomas because they usually enhance less than the normal gland (Fig 23–12,C). However, enhancement may also obscure microadenomas, particularly if the images are improperly windowed (Fig 23–13). It is helpful to view the images on the scanner console so that the gland may be examined at various window settings. Enhancement of the adenoma on delayed postcontrast scans is variable; some adenomas become more intense than surrounding normal pituitary tissue.[9, 10] A large prospective study is needed to determine whether enhanced CT or MRI is more sensitive in the detection of microadenomas.[11]

Management of Prolactinomas

The natural history of pituitary adenomas is quite variable, especially considering the 20% incidence of asymptomatic adenomas discovered at autopsy. Some apparent prolactinomas less than 1 cm in diameter grow very slowly or not at all and never become macroadenomas. This fact along with the mild nature of the symptoms caused by an elevated prolactin level prompts some endocrinologists to advocate no therapy for small prolactinomas in women who do not want to become pregnant.

Patients who wish to become pregnant may be treated medically or surgically. Bromocriptine and pergolide are dopamine agonists that effectively lower serum prolactin levels in over 90% of prolactin-secreting adenomas. They act by mimicking hypothalamic secretion of prolactin-inhibiting factor (dopamine), to which the adenoma is at least partially responsive. While pharmacologic therapy frequently eliminates galactorrhea and restores normal menses, it is not curative. When suppressive therapy is discontinued, hyperprolactinemia returns in most cases.[12]

Some patients with pituitary adenomas choose surgery because it can be curative. Eighty-five percent of surgically treated microadenomas have a positive clinical response (normal prolactin level, return of menses, and absence of galactorrhea). However, hyperprolactinemia returns in 50% of patients after 4 years, thus suggesting a high incidence of recurrence.[13] Therefore, the possibility of cure must be weighed against the 0.5% mortality and the complications of trans-sphenoidal resection, which include diabetes insipidus, postoperative hypopituitarism, CSF leak, and visual disturbance.

Adrenocorticotropic Hormone–Secreting Adenomas (Cushing's Disease)

Cushing's syndrome is caused by excess serum cortisol. The three basic causes of hypercortisolism are pituitary adenomas (60% of cases), adrenal tumors (25% of cases), and ectopic production of ACTH (15% of cases), often from a hormonally active carcinoma of the lung. The clinical features of Cushing's syndrome are nonspecific. They include obesity, hypertension, weakness, depression and increased susceptibility to infection. Early cases are difficult to diagnose, but the well-developed syndrome is usually easily recognized. Untreated Cushing's syndrome is a serious medical problem with a 50% 5-year mortality due to complications of hypertension or infection.[14]

Almost all adrenal tumors that cause Cushing's syndrome are large and easily identified by abdominal imaging.[15] Identifying a pituitary adenoma as a cause for Cushing's syndrome is more difficult. ACTH-producing adenomas are almost always microadenomas at the time of presentation and frequently measure only 2 to 3 mm in diameter.[16] CT enhancement characteristics are often similar to those of the surrounding gland (Fig 23–14,A). Fifty percent to 70% of surgically confirmed ACTH adenomas have normal enhanced high-resolution CT scans.[4, 17] MRI is probably more sensitive than CT in detecting these microadenomas. As with prolactinomas, ACTH-producing microadenomas may have any combination of signal characteristics but most commonly are less intense than normal pituitary tissue on short TR images and hyperintense on long TR spin-echo sequences. One report suggests that the use of gadolinium increases the sensitivity of MRI to 80%.[10] The enhancement characteristics of the adenomas were variable. Most enhanced less than surrounding pituitary tissue initially, but some enhanced to a greater degree than surrounding normal tissue on delayed scans. If the high sensitivity of enhanced MRI is confirmed, it will represent an important advance enabling preoperative localization of most ACTH-producing microadenomas, a goal not realized by CT. In only a minority is Cushing's disease caused by macroadenomas that are easily recognized by both MRI and CT.

Definitive therapy is required in all cases because of the high mortality when Cushing's disease remains untreated. Trans-sphenoidal resection of ACTH-producing microadenomas is effective with a 75% to 90% cure rate. Radiation therapy is used as an adjunct to surgery in patients with recurrent tumors or with macroadenomas that cannot be completely resected.[18, 19]

Bilateral adrenalectomy has been used to control hypercortisolism in patients with Cushing's disease, but in the absence of feedback inhibition from high cortisol levels, the ACTH-producing ad-

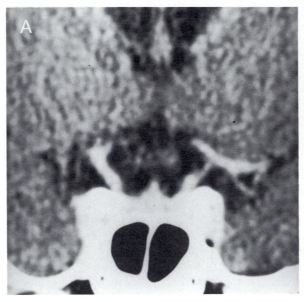
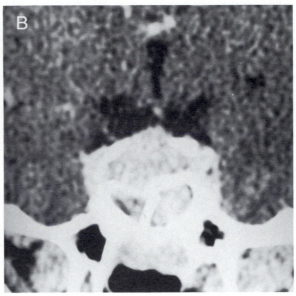

FIG 23–14.
Nelson's syndrome in a 10-year-old boy with Cushing's syndrome. **A,** preoperative coronal enhanced CT failed to show the adenoma found at trans-sphenoidal resection. Many ACTH-secreting adenomas are invisible to CT. Hypercortisolism persisted despite surgery; bilateral adrenalectomy was performed. **B,** coronal enhanced CT 2 years after adrenalectomy. There is a large sellar mass with extension into the sphenoid sinus and suprasellar cistern. Recurrent ACTH-producing adenoma was confirmed surgically.

enoma tends to grow aggressively (Fig 23–14,B). ACTH levels in this situation can be very high, and because of structural similarities between ACTH and melanocyte-stimulating hormone, cutaneous hyperpigmentation results. This syndrome was described by Nelson et al.[20] Pituitary imaging in Nelson's syndrome will usually reveal a large macroadenoma, often associated with bone erosion and extension into the cavernous sinus and suprasellar cistern. The prognosis for patients with these aggressive lesions is poor. Surgery and radiotherapy together are curative in only 30% of cases.[19] The incidence of Nelson's syndrome will decline with decreasing use of bilateral adrenalectomy to treat hypercortisolism.

Growth Hormone–Secreting Adenomas

Acromegaly (from the Greek *akron* [extremity] and *megas* [large]) results from excess secretion of growth hormone (GH). Almost all cases are caused by pituitary adenomas that secrete excessive GH alone (70%) or in combination with prolactin (30% of cases). Clinical features are distinctive and include enlargement of the face and hands as well as thickening of the skin. Characteristic radiographic findings are those of a sellar mass as well as enlargement of paranasal sinuses, enlargement of the extraocular muscles, overgrowth of the tufts of the distal phalanges, and accelerated degenerative arthritis. If hypersecretion of GH occurs in childhood before closure of the epiphyseal plates, long bone growth is stimulated. This results in gigantism. If left untreated these individuals will ultimately develop the typical features of acromegaly as well.[21] At presentation, the majority of GH-secreting tumors are microadenomas (Fig 23–15). High-resolution, enhanced, coronal CT will detect between 50% and 80% of these microadenomas, which appear as focal hypodense lesions.[22] Large GH-producing adenomas are indistinguishable from other macroadenomas (Fig 23–16).

Acromegaly is a debilitating disease. Structural changes in the cardiovascular system result in severe atherosclerosis, hypertension, and eventual cardiac failure; excessive GH levels result in glucose intolerance and diabetes mellitus; and bone overgrowth produces severe debilitating arthritis. Early definitive treatment is important in order to avoid these complications. Trans-sphenoidal surgery is the primary therapeutic approach and has a 90% cure rate for GH-secreting microadenomas. Radiation therapy is used as an adjunct to surgery of macroadenomas where complete excision is difficult to achieve. Bromocriptine, which elevates GH levels in normal individuals, paradoxically lowers serum levels in acromegaly; this drug is

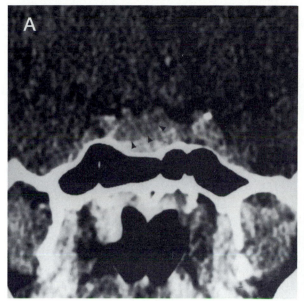

FIG 23–15.
Acromegaly. **A,** enhanced coronal CT. The adenoma *(arrowheads)* is subtle but slightly less dense than the remainder of the gland. **B,** coronal SE (TR 900, TE 28, 0.3 Tesla) MRI shows that the mass in the right side of the gland is displacing the infundibulum to the left.

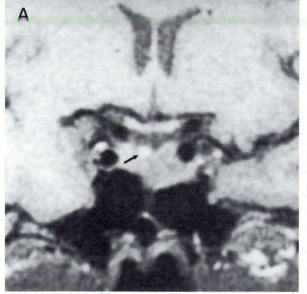
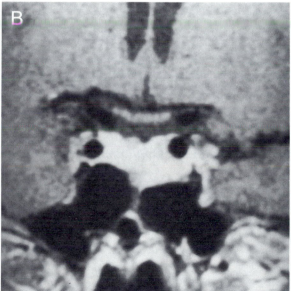

FIG 23–16.
Acromegaly in a 45-year-old woman with typical facial, hand, and foot changes. **A,** coronal SE (TR 600, TE 25) images show a mass in the left side of the pituitary. The high-signal region on the superior surface of the gland *(arrow)* is the insertion of the pituitary stalk. **B,** enhanced coronal SE (TR 600, TE 25) MRI. There is uniform enhancement of the tumor. The high signal at the insertion of the stalk is obscured by the enhanced pituitary tissue.

used in patients unresponsive to medical and surgical management.[21]

Thyroid-Stimulating Hormone–Secreting Adenomas

Pituitary adenomas secreting thyroid-stimulating hormone (TSH) are extremely rare. The patients are hyperthyroid due to excessive stimulation of the thyroid gland by the elevated TSH levels. Rigid endocrinologic criteria must be met before a definite diagnosis of TSH-secreting adenoma is made since both hyperthyroidism and pituitary adenoma are common and may coexist without being related.[23] No specific imaging features of TSH-secreting adenomas have been established.

There has been a misconception that TSH-secreting adenomas arise in patients with hypothyroidism.[24] The reasoning goes that in the face of thyroid gland failure, the hypothalamus is stimulated to increase production of thyroid-releasing hormone (TRH). The elevated TRH levels supposedly foster the development of a TSH-producing adenoma. This has not been substantiated. Instead, the elevated TRH levels cause hyperplasia and enlargement of the anterior lobe (see the section on pituitary gland hyperplasia). Confusion arises because the hyperplastic gland may enlarge the sella and closely mimic the appearance of a macroadenoma.[25]

Follicle-Stimulating Hormone– and Luteinizing Hormone–Secreting Adenomas

Another rare form of pituitary adenoma produces gonadotropin: follicle-stimulating hormone (FSH) or luteinizing hormone (LH). Elevated levels of LH and FSH produce minimal clinical symptomatology, and as a result, these adenomas are usually large at presentation.[23]

Nonfunctional Adenomas

Twenty-five percent of pituitary adenomas have no recognized endocrine function. They represent a heterogeneous group. One fourth are oncocytomas, which have a characteristic electron microscopic appearance; their cytoplasm is packed with mitochondria. The other three quarters have a nonspecific pathologic appearance. They may secrete undetectable quantities or inactive subunits of normal pituitary hormones.[26] These various types of nonfunctional adenomas are indistinguishable by imaging. They produce symptoms by mass effect on adjacent structures. Intrasellar expansion

may compress the normal gland and cause pituitary insufficiency. Compression or invasion of the cavernous sinuses may result in extraocular muscle palsy with resultant diplopia. Suprasellar extension causes visual field deficits or decreased visual acuity by compressing the optic nerves, chiasm, or tracts.

PITUITARY APOPLEXY

Pituitary apoplexy is a dramatic but uncommon clinical syndrome. Fifteen percent of macroadenomas have hemorrhage within them at surgery, but fewer than 1% will present with an apoplectic episode (Fig 23–17). Apoplexy is characterized by a sudden onset of headache, extraocular muscle palsy, visual loss, and/or pituitary insufficiency. The syndrome typically develops because a pituitary macroadenoma undergoes infarction and hemorrhage. This in turn causes rapid expansion of the tumor with compression of adjacent structures. Necrotic or hemorrhagic material may be expelled into the subarachnoid space and produce signs and symptoms identical to those of subarachnoid hemorrhage.[27] In fact, hemorrhagic necrosis in an unsuspected pituitary adenoma should be considered

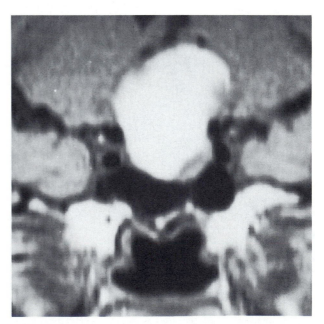

FIG 23–17.
Hemorrhagic macroadenoma in a 52-year-old man with a 2-year history of blurred vision but no acute neurologic symptoms. Coronal SE (TR 500, TE 28, 0.3 Tesla) MRI shows high signal within a large pituitary mass that is compressing the chiasm. At surgery several milliliters of "bloody fluid" was drained from the mass.

in patients with subarachnoid hemorrhage but normal angiographic findings (i.e., no aneurysm or arteriovenous malformation [AVM]).[28, 29] Treatment of macroadenomas with radiation or bromocriptine increases the likelihood of an apoplectic event by facilitating tumor necrosis. About one half of cases of pituitary apoplexy present fulminantly with less than a 24-hour history. The remainder have a subacute presentation extending over a few days to weeks.[27]

Although apoplexy may occur in small adenomas or even within a normal pituitary gland,[29, 30] it is usually associated with macroadenomas. Plain skull films will usually show an enlarged sella, while CT usually shows a macroadenoma of mottled density (Figs 23–18,A and 23–19,A). Unequivocal hyperdense hemorrhage is seen only occasionally.[27] MRI may also fail to demonstrate acute hemorrhage unless specific pulsing sequences (such as low–flip angle, gradient-recalled echo sequences) sensitive to acute hemorrhage are used. In subacute cases MRI is sensitive to the presence of methemoglobin, which will appear bright on both short and long TR spin-echo sequences (Figs 23–17 to 23–19).

Patients with pituitary apoplexy who have severe neurologic or visual defects require prompt surgical decompression. The trans-sphenoidal approach is currently favored. Apoplexy frequently causes pituitary insufficiency. Glucocorticoid replacement in these patients can be lifesaving.[27]

ADENOMAS FOLLOWING MEDICAL THERAPY

Prolactinomas and, to a lesser degree, GH-secreting adenomas can be effectively treated pharmacologically. In the case of prolactinomas, bromocriptine and pergolide often lower serum prolactin levels and provide symptomatic relief including resumption of normal menses and return of fertility. Histologic studies indicate that these drugs reduce the number of cytoplasmic organelles and the cytoplasmic volume of the adenoma cells. Imaging studies will reveal a decrease in size of the adenoma in about two thirds of cases. GH-secreting tumors may also respond to bromocriptine or analogues of somatostatin with reduction of adenoma size in over half of the cases. Medical therapy may shrink adenomas to the point that they disappear on imaging studies. Also, drug therapy may alter the MRI characteristics of some adenomas. Therefore, CT or MRI examinations should be carried out before therapy is instituted so that the response can be documented. Medical control is not reserved for microadenomas but can be essential in treating macroadenomas that are incur-

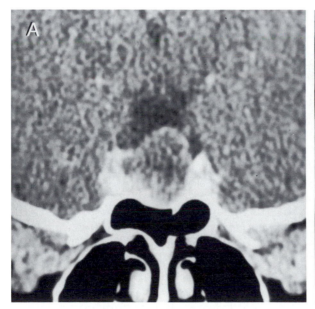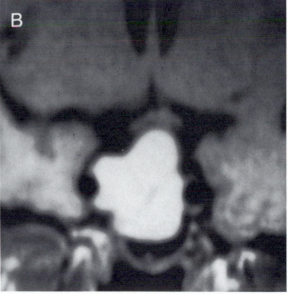

FIG 23–18.
Pituitary apoplexy in a 31-year-old with a sudden onset of severe headache 3 days before the CT scan. **A,** enhanced coronal CT shows the mass to be isodense with brain. No acute hemorrhage is detected. **B,** a coronal SE (TR 500, TE 28, 0.3 Tesla) image shows a high-signal pituitary mass. The mass looks similar to that in Figure 23–17, but the clinical symptoms were much more severe.

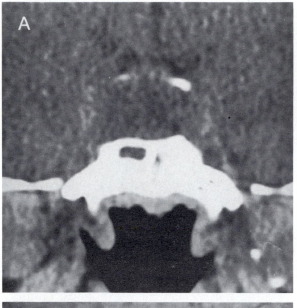

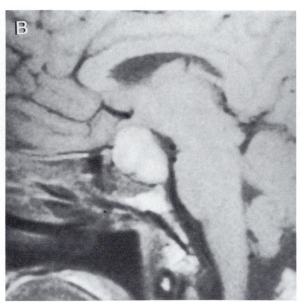

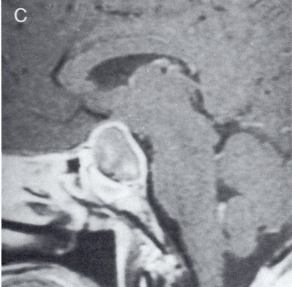

FIG 23–19.
Hemorrhagic macroadenoma in a 30-year-old man with headache for 3 days. **A,** coronal CT shows a large pituitary mass. No unusual increased density is evident. **B,** sagittal SE (TR 600, TE 20) MRI shows high signal within the mass. **C,** gadolinium-enhanced sagittal SE (TR 600, TE 20) images show rim enhancement of the mass. The high signal seen on the unenhanced scan is obscured when the image is windowed to show the peripheral enhancement.

able by surgery or radiation therapy. Although these drugs reduce the size of pituitary adenomas, they are not tumoricidal. Discontinuance of therapy may result in return of abnormal function and tumor regrowth.[31–33]

THE POSTOPERATIVE SELLA

The most common surgical approach to sellar masses is trans-sphenoidal. The transcranial approach is reserved for those tumors with marked suprasellar extension, hourglass constriction by the diaphragma sellae, a large suprasellar component with normal or only slightly enlarged sella, and in suprasellar tumors that are found to be tough or fibrous in consistency and difficult to remove with the trans-sphenoidal approach.[34–36]

Immediate postoperative scans show opacification of the sphenoid and ethmoid sinuses that may persist for up to 2 months. The sella itself will contain a confusing mixture of air, blood, and fat or soft-tissue packing as well as normal residual pituitary tissue (Fig 23–20). Little can be gained from analyzing the intrasellar contents at this time. These scans are used to evaluate extrasellar complications of surgery such as subarachnoid hemorrhage, hydrocephalus, or infarction.[37, 38]

In contrast, scans obtained 3 months after surgery are extremely useful as a baseline. Opacifica-

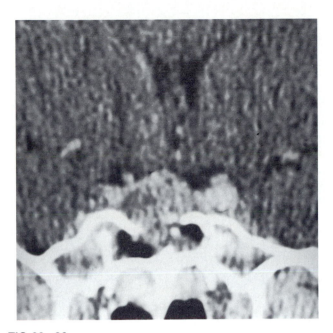

FIG 23–20.
Immediate postoperative trans-sphenoidal resection: enhanced coronal CT 6 days after trans-sphenoidal surgery. The lucency in the right gland has little meaning; it may be postoperative edema or packing. Soft-tissue density in the sphenoid sinus may persist for up to 2 months (same patient as in Fig 23–15).

tion of the ethmoid and sphenoid sinuses (which is expected immediately after surgery) should clear within 2 months, so persistent opacification should suggest chronic sinusitis, usually secondary to surgical damage of the ostia. Clear nasal discharge from sinusitis may mimic a CSF leak. If the latter is suspected, radionuclide cisternography should be performed. If the radionuclide scan confirms a CSF leak, contrast cisternography may demonstrate its source.

Following trans-sphenoidal resection of microadenomas the majority of patients have a normal-appearing pituitary gland. However, one third of these harbor residual tumor as evidenced by eventual recurrence of endocrinologic abnormalities. Herniation of the suprasellar subarachnoid space into the pituitary fossa is also common postoperatively (Fig 23–21). However partial herniation does not exclude residual, endocrine-active tumor (Fig 23–22). CT density and MRI signal characteristics of the postoperative sellar contents vary with the operation and the packing used to fill in the operative cavity (Figs 23–23 to 23–25). Fat will be lucent on CT and have high signal on short TR spin-echo sequences. The fat packing may be replaced by fibrous tissue over time, or it may persist indefinitely. Focal enhancement in the postop-

erative sella may represent recurrent or residual tumor, but it may also represent muscle packing and associated surrounding inflammatory response. Persistent displacement of the infundibulum postoperatively indicates residual tumor in about two thirds of cases, but in the absence of residual tumor, retraction by scar may actually be responsible.[37–39] Imaging is less sensitive and less specific than hormonal assays for detecting residual, functional adenoma, but when dealing with nonfunctional adenomas, progressive enlargement on serial studies is the only sure way of identifying tumor recurrence.

PITUITARY ABSCESS

Pituitary abscesses are rare. They may arise de novo but much more often develop in a sellar mass such as adenoma, craniopharyngioma, or Rathke's cleft cyst. Pituitary abscesses can be surprisingly indolent, the duration of symptoms ranging from days to months.

Imaging studies are nonspecific, particularly since most cases are associated with pre-existing sellar tumor (Figs 23–26 and 23–27). A central lucency surrounded by a rim of contrast is considered typical but is more common with uninfected cavitated or hemorrhagic adenomas. Bone destruction may be present, particularly in cases of sphenoid sinus infection invading the sella. It is difficult to make a correct preoperative diagnosis on the basis of imaging alone. Clinical clues such as fever and headache out of proportion to the size of the mass are most helpful. Early treatment with antibiotics, stress doses of hydrocortisone (to prevent pituitary insufficiency), and trans-sphenoidal drainage help decrease the high mortality and morbidity of this lesion.[39, 40]

LYMPHOID ADENOHYPOPHYSITIS

As its name implies, the disease is characterized by abnormal infiltration of lymphocytes into the anterior lobe of the pituitary gland (adenohypophysis). It occurs only in women and, in the vast majority of cases, occurs within 1 year of an uncomplicated labor and delivery. The presenting symptoms are usually those of pituitary insufficiency, and the condition can be fatal if replacement therapy is not instituted. The disease is believed to be autoimmune; there often are elevated

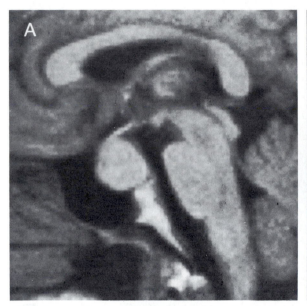

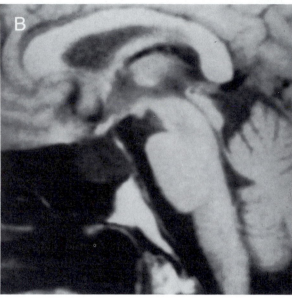

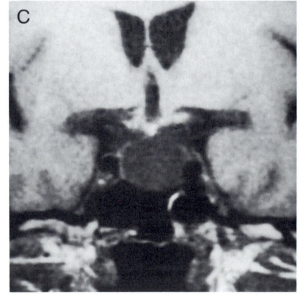

FIG 23–21.
Postoperative study. **A,** sagittal SE (TR 500, TE 17) MRI. Preoperative scanning shows a macroadenoma. **B** and **C,** sagittal and coronal SE (TR 600, TE 20) images obtained 6 months after trans-sphenoidal resection show CSF filling the enlarged sella. The stalk has been amputated and the posterior lobe removed. There is no evidence of residual or recurrent tumor.

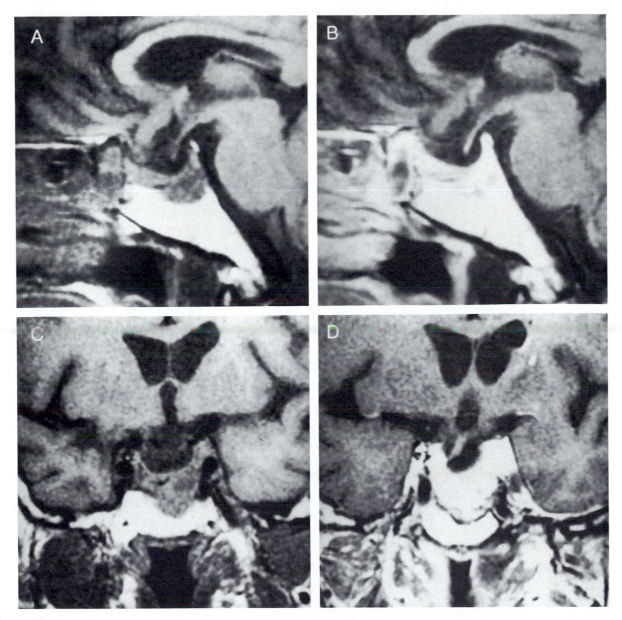

FIG 23–22.
Recurrent adenoma in a 60-year-old man after resection and radiation therapy for a macroadenoma. **A** and **B,** sagittal SE (TR 500, TE 20) MRI before and after contrast. There is partial herniation of the suprasellar cistern into the enlarged sella. The sella is lined with a rind of enhancing tumor that is eroding the clivus. After contrast it is difficult to differentiate enhancing tumor from fat in the marrow of the clivus, which shows the value of unenhanced images in some cases. **C** and **D,** coronal SE (TR 600, TE 25) MRI before and after contrast. The infundibulum extends into the partially empty sella. In most cases of residual or recurrent disease the tumor mass itself occupies the sella, and the infundibulum does not extend as inferior as in this case.

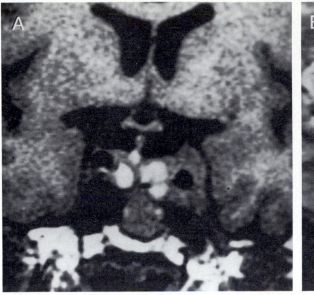

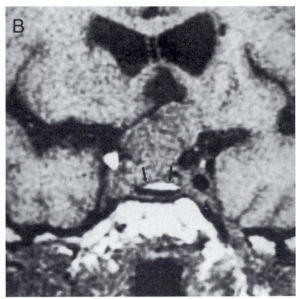

FIG 23–23.
Postoperative sella. A macroadenoma was removed 1 year earlier. **A,** coronal SE (TR 600, TE 20) MRI shows high signal within the residual pituitary tissue. This could be due to fat packing, hemorrhage, or proteinaceous fluid in a necrotic cavity. **B,** coronal SE (TR 2,500, TE 100) MRI. The high-signal foci persist on "T2-weighted" images, which suggests that they do not represent fat. There is residual tumor in the left cavernous sinus that has high signal on a T2 basis (same patient as in Fig 23–2).

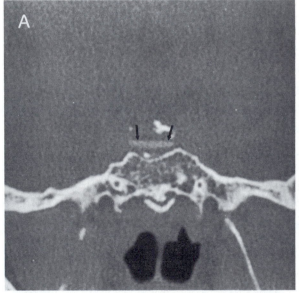

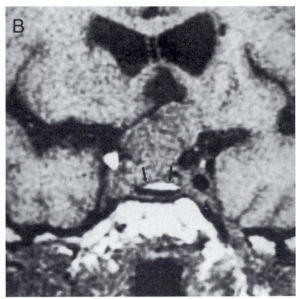

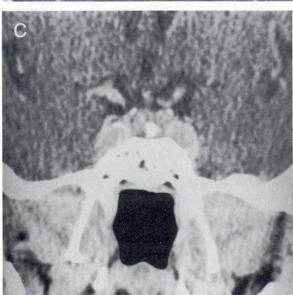

FIG 23–24.
Varied postoperative appearances. **A** and **B,** coronal CT (bone algorithm) and MRI (TR 600, TE 20) show prosthetic material *(arrows)* laid in the floor of the sella following transcranial resection of a pituitary adenoma. The transcranial approach was chosen because of a large suprasellar component and little pneumatization of the sphenoid bone. There is a large amount of residual or recurrent tumor. Incidentally, there is occlusion of the right cavernous carotid. **C,** coronal enhanced CT from a different patient shows calcification in the sella following trans-sphenoidal resection and radiation therapy for a pituitary adenoma. The nature of the calcification in this case is unknown. Pituitary adenomas rarely calcify.

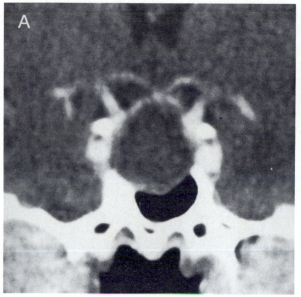

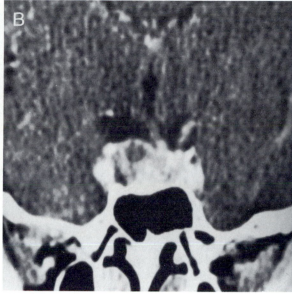

FIG 23–25.
Cavitated macroadenoma in a 37-year-old man treated 6 years ago with radiation therapy for a sellar mass (no biopsy). **A,** enhanced CT shows a peripherally enhancing mass in the sella and suprasellar cisterns. The floor of the sella appears to be absent. At surgery 8 cc of "old blood" was drained from this mass. The wall contained adenoma cells. **B,** coronal enhanced CT 1 year later. The tumor is smaller but is still evidenced by low density and mass effect. The sellar floor has reconstituted.

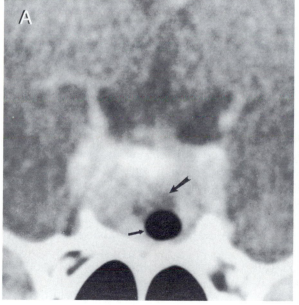

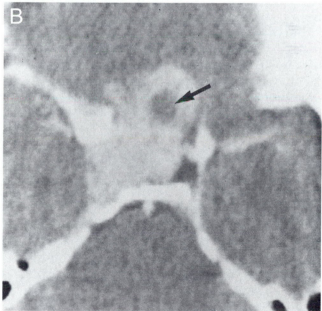

FIG 23–26.
Pituitary abscess. **A,** coronal enhanced CT shows a sellar mass with central lucency *(large arrow).* There is also a bubble of gas *(small arrow).* At surgery an abscess within a recurrent pituitary adenoma was found. **B,** an axial enhanced CT scan from a differ-ent patient demonstrates a mass with central lucency *(arrow)* and peripheral enhancement. At surgery this was an abscess within an adenoma.

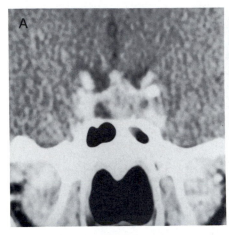 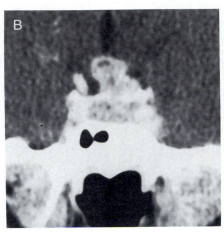 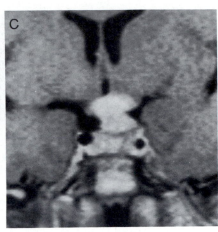

FIG 23–27.

Chronic pituitary/hypothalamic granuloma in a 57-year-old woman with panhypopituitarism. **A,** an initial coronal CT scan shows an enhancing sellar mass that has a low-density component on the right. The infundibulum is thickened. The patient underwent trans-sphenoidal resection. A sterile granuloma with chronic inflammatory cells was found. **B,** enhanced coronal CT scan 2 years later. The patient returned with new visual complaints. The granuloma had recurred and now extends into the suprasellar cistern and compresses the chiasm. **C,** enhanced coronal MRI (TR 700, TE 26) shows abnormal enhancement of the optic chiasm and infundibulum, which are involved by the inflammatory process. Repeat trans-sphenoidal surgery again revealed granulation tissue with acute and chronic inflammation. Cultures were negative.

serum levels of antibodies to prolactin-secreting cells. Imaging studies show an enhancing sellar mass, often with suprasellar extension, that is indistinguishable from a pituitary adenoma. When this disease is suspected because of the clinical setting, surgery may be averted. Serial imaging should be performed to ensure that the lesion is unchanging or regressing.[41, 42] Spontaneous recovery of anterior pituitary function has been reported but is uncommon.[43]

PRIMARY EMPTY-SELLA SYNDROME

A primary empty sella results from the protrusion of an arachnoid diverticulum from the suprasellar cistern into the pituitary fossa. If the infundibular foramen in the diaphragma sellae is large, cisternal herniation is facilitated. The pituitary gland per se is flattened against the floor of the sella. In autopsy series, about 5% of patients without known pituitary symptoms have an empty sella.[44]

Clinical studies suggest that diverse factors may account for the development of the empty sella. Seventy-five percent of cases occur in obese, hypertensive middle-aged women. A high incidence of empty sella in pseudotumor cerebri has led some authors to suggest that chronic increased intracranial pressure is a contributing factor. Mild disturbances of pituitary function occur in one

third of patients, but clinically significant endocrinopathy is rare. Occasionally, CSF rhinorrhea is associated with an empty sella and requires trans-sphenoidal repair. Very rarely visual disturbances may result from the optic chiasm sagging into a primary empty sella. Repositioning of the chiasm in the suprasellar cistern (chiasmapexy) has been reported to improve vision in this unusual situation, but that is controversial.[45, 46] The primary empty-sella syndrome discussed above is distinct from a secondary empty sella. The latter occurs in the setting of pre-existing intrasellar pathology, usually a macroadenoma. Following surgery or radiation therapy, marked shrinkage of tumor occurs, and the extra volume within the enlarged sella is filled by downward herniation of the suprasellar cistern (see Fig 23–21). Spontaneous necrosis and shrinkage of a macroadenoma may also produce this appearance.[47]

Imaging studies of a primary empty sella show the pituitary to be flattened against the floor and walls of the sella. The infundibulum may be displaced slightly posteriorly but still extends well into the pituitary fossa to insert on the posterior lobe, which is flattened against the dorsum sellae. Visualization of the infundibulum extending into the sella ("infundibulum sign") helps to exclude a cystic or cavitated mass, which would elevate the infundibulum out of the sella.[48] The infundibulum enhances readily with contrast, so it can be demonstrated in almost all cases on coronal CT. Coronal

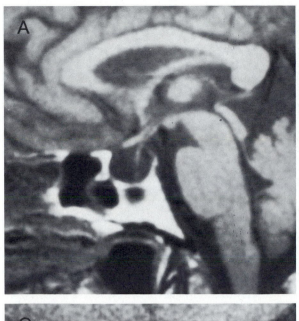

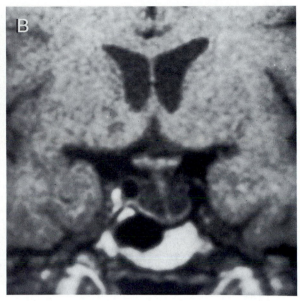

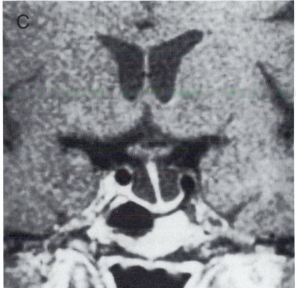

FIG 23–28.
Empty sella. **A,** sagittal SE (TR 500, TE 20) MRI shows an enlarged sella. The infundibulum extends into the sella. The high signal normally seen in the posterior lobe is absent. **B** and **C,** coronal SE (TR 600, TE 25) MRI before and after contrast. The infundibulum inserts into the residual pituitary tissue, which is flattened against the floor of the sella. Both the stalk and the pituitary tissue enhance following contrast. There is no evidence of a pituitary mass (compare with Fig 23–22).

and sagittal MRI will also reliably demonstrate the infundibulum and the flattened pituitary gland (Fig 23–28). The high signal normally seen in the posterior lobe may be absent, perhaps due to compression from the adjacent arachnoid diverticulum. The infundibulum sign will usually differentiate an empty sella from an intrasellar arachnoid cyst, cavitated pituitary adenoma, intrasellar craniopharyngioma, and Rathke's cleft cyst. Occasionally, however, the infundibulum will extend into the sella despite the presence of residual or recurrent tumor (see Fig 23–22,C and D). In ambiguous cases contrast cisternography will confirm extension of the subarachnoid space into the sella.

PITUITARY GLAND HYPERPLASIA

Pituitary hyperplasia during and shortly after pregnancy is physiologically normal. Pathologic hyperplasia results from excessive stimulation of the gland due to primary end organ failure and is seen in hypothyroidism or rarely in primary hypogonadism.

Imaging will reveal an enlarged pituitary gland with a convex superior margin (Fig 23–29). The hyperplastic tissue enhances uniformly (Fig 23–30). This is helpful in differentiating hyperplasia from pituitary adenoma; most adenomas have more heterogenous enhancement (see Figs 23–1

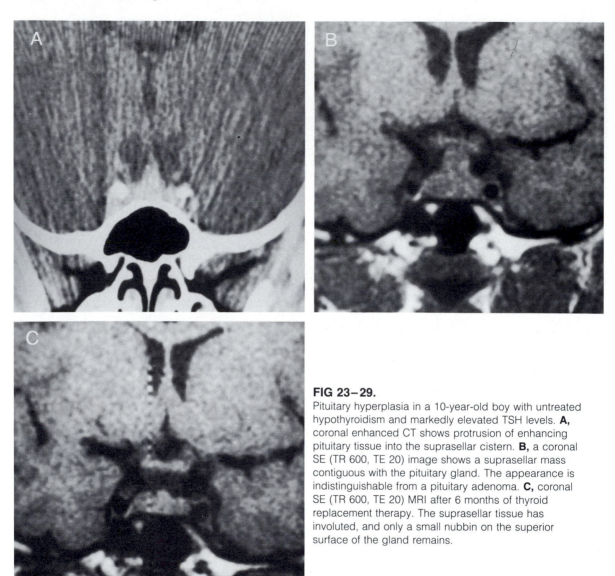

FIG 23–29.
Pituitary hyperplasia in a 10-year-old boy with untreated hypothyroidism and markedly elevated TSH levels. **A,** coronal enhanced CT shows protrusion of enhancing pituitary tissue into the suprasellar cistern. **B,** a coronal SE (TR 600, TE 20) image shows a suprasellar mass contiguous with the pituitary gland. The appearance is indistinguishable from a pituitary adenoma. **C,** coronal SE (TR 600, TE 20) MRI after 6 months of thyroid replacement therapy. The suprasellar tissue has involuted, and only a small nubbin on the superior surface of the gland remains.

to 23–6). In long-standing cases remodeling and enlargement of the sella may occur. Hyperplasia resolves when hormonal balance is restored either spontaneously or through replacement therapy (Figs 23–29,D and 23–30,D).[24]

NONNEOPLASTIC INTRASELLAR CYSTS

Imaging procedures occasionally demonstrate well-defined "cystic" lesions within the sella. If endocrine function is normal and there is no compression of extrasellar structures, these may be ignored. Symptomatic intrasellar cysts do occur, usually in women who present with irregular menses or galactorrhea. Dynamic endocrinologic tests help to distinguish a cavitated prolactinoma from an intrasellar cyst. Intrasellar cysts have been divided into four groups: arachnoid, pars intermedia, Rathke's cleft cysts, and miscellaneous cysts.[49]

Purely intrasellar arachnoid cysts are uncommon and must be differentiated from suprasellar arachnoid cysts that have extended into the sella. The latter occur in infancy, whereas purely intrasellar arachnoid cysts have been reported only in adults (mean age at presentation of 42 years). They are the only cranial arachnoid cysts that occur extradurally, although some are more properly called arachnoid diverticula because of a pinhole communication that connects the cyst and subarachnoid

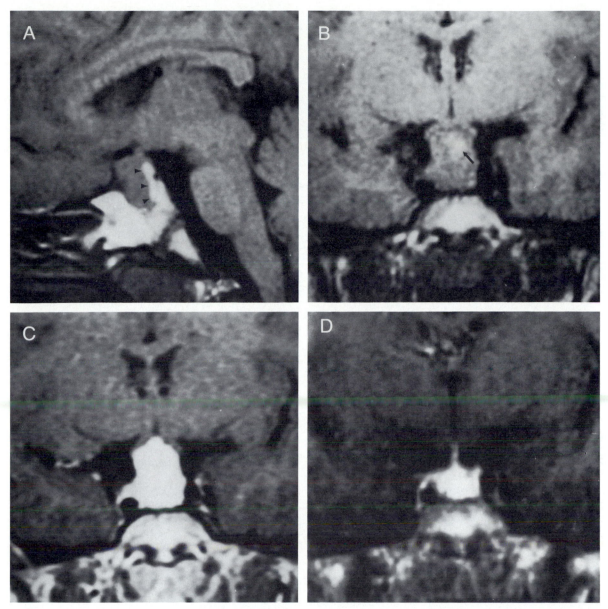

FIG 23–30.
Pituitary hyperplasia in a 5-year-old girl with hypothyroidism secondary to autoimmune thyroiditis. **A,** sagittal SE (TR 500, TE 20) MRI. There is enlargement of the anterior lobe with suprasellar extension. The high-signal posterior lobe *(arrowheads)* is flattened posteriorly. **B,** coronal SE (TR 600, TE 25) MRI. There is a marked enlargement of the pituitary with suprasellar extension. Note the high-signal posterior lobe *(arrow).* This lesion looks like a macroadenoma. **C,** following intravenous gadolinium administration, there is uniform enhancement of the hyperplastic pituitary tissue. **D,** coronal SE (TR 600, TE 25) MRI after 4 months of thyroid replacement therapy. There has been a dramatic reduction in the size of the pituitary.

space. The lesions are well-defined lucencies on CT and display neither contrast enhancement nor calcification. They may not fill on contrast cisternography because of the smallness of their communication with the subarachnoid space. On MRI, the cyst would be expected to have signal similar to CSF. At surgery the cyst contains clear fluid, has a fibrous tissue wall, and has a pinhole communica-

tion with subarachnoid space as indicated above. The surgical site is packed with muscle or fat to prevent recurrence.[49]

Cysts of the pars intermedia or colloid cysts arise from a thin tissue layer between the anterior and posterior lobes that embryologically arises from the posterior wall of Rathke's pouch (see Figs 22–12,A and 23–31). These cysts are small (less

FIG 23–31.
Colloid cyst. A coronal histologic section (hematoxylin-eosin) demonstrates a colloid cyst *(short thick arrow)* centrally in the gland, surrounded by densely compacted acidophilic tissue *(long thick arrows)* and an unsuspected chromophobe adenoma *(long thin arrow)*. Colloid cysts are a normal finding seen at almost all autopsies, although they are usually smaller than the cyst shown in this specimen. While almost universally present, demonstration of distinct colloid cysts with CT or MRI is unusual.

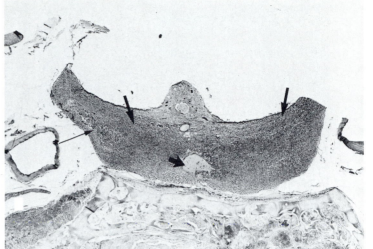

than 3 mm), contain clear fluid, and have a fibrous tissue wall. Some authors include these cysts as a subset of Rathke's cleft cysts, which are discussed below.[50]

Rathke's cleft cysts are moderate in size and measure 3 to 10 mm. As their name implies they are derived from remnants of Rathke's pouch. This upgrowth of oral ectoderm is the embryologic precursor of the anterior lobe, pars intermedia, and pars tuberalis (which is a thin layer of anterior pituitary cells surrounding the infundibulum and extending for a short distance above the diaphragma sellae). The walls of these cysts are lined by epithelial cells that may be cuboidal, columnar, or pseudostratified columnar cells. Mucin-secreting goblet cells may also be encountered. Depending on the activity of the goblet cells and the rate of epithelial desquamation, the material within the cyst may range from serous to mucoid. This variation of content is reflected in CT density and MRI signal characteristics. CT shows a noncalcified, nonenhancing, well-circumscribed lesion that may have low to intermediate density (Fig 23–32). The MRI signal characteristics of these lesions are

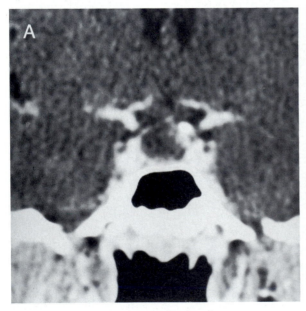 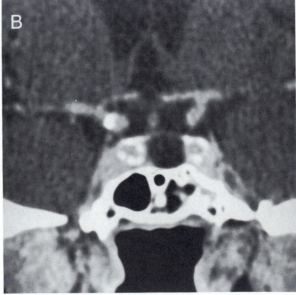

FIG 23–32.
Rathke's cleft cyst. **A,** coronal CT of a 12-year-old who had transsphenoidal removal of a 1-cm Rathke's cleft cyst. The cyst is nonenhancing and of CSF density. It would be difficult to distinguish this lesion from an intrasellar craniopharyngioma or a necrotic adenoma. **B,** coronal CT of a 1-cm "pituitary cyst" (not proven) discovered incidentally in a 60-year-old patient with dementia. This lesion was asymptomatic and is being managed by obtaining occasional follow-up examinations to ensure that it is unchanging.

highly variable. Most commonly cyst contents will be similar in signal to CSF, but with greater mucoid content, they may have high signal on short TR and low or high signal on long TR spin-echo sequences. The signal variability is analogous to that seen in colloid cysts of the third ventricle.[50, 51]

There is a subset of Rathke's cleft cysts that are complex and have areas of wall thickening and contrast enhancement. The contents of these cysts have various CT densities and MRI signal characteristics. This lesion probably represents a transitional form between a simple Rathke's cyst and craniopharyngioma and has been called a benign cystic craniopharyngioma.[50] This overlap is not surprising because childhood craniopharyngiomas are thought to be derived from remnants of Rathke's cleft.[52] Rare etiologies for intrasellar "cysts" include cysticercosis, epidermoid, and pituitary abscess. However, keep in mind that the most common cystic-appearing mass within the sella will be a cavitated pituitary adenoma.

METASTASIS TO THE PITUITARY

Metastatic tumors to the pituitary gland generally occur in patients with advanced, widely disseminated, malignant disease. At autopsy, 1% to 5% of cancer patients will have metastases to the pituitary. These patients generally die before the pituitary lesion becomes symptomatic. Metastases sometimes spread between the sella and suprasellar regions via the infundibulum, in which case a dumbbell-shaped mass may result.

There are no radiographic signs peculiar to metastatic lesions. Bone destruction is suggestive but may also be seen in other lesions such as aggressive pituitary adenomas, pituitary abscess, and chordoma. Enhancement is usually dense and homogenous (Fig 23–33), although cavitation may occur and result in rim enhancement instead. By MRI these lesions are indistinguishable from invasive adenomas. In addition to hematogenous spread, the sella may become involved by direct extension by nasopharyngeal and sphenoid sinus neoplasms.

TUMORS OF THE NEUROHYPOPHYSIS

There is a highly specific neoplasm that arises in the neurohypophysis, probably from the pituicytes. Variously called choristoma, myoblastoma, and pituicytoma the term *parasellar granular cell tumor* is now preferred by pathologists. Microscopic granular cell tumors are commonly seen in the pituitary gland at autopsy, but the large symptomatic variety is very rare. This neoplasm is more common extra-

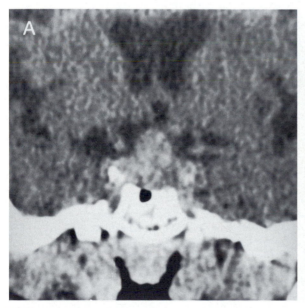
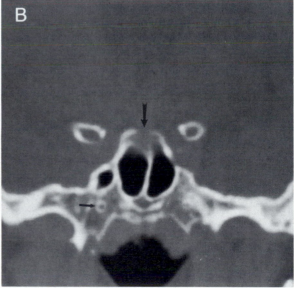

FIG 23–33.
Pituitary metastasis. **A,** coronal CT of a pituitary metastasis that has enlarged the sella and extended into the suprasellar cistern. The primary lesion was breast carcinoma. **B,** bone windows show erosion of the tuberculum sellae *(large arrow)*. Bone erosion is characteristic of metastatic lesions but not specific. It may also be seen in invasive adenomas. Incidentally, Vidian's canal is nicely demonstrated *(small arrow)*.

cranially and occurs in the tongue, along the gastrointestinal tract, and in the omentum, retroperitoneum, bladder, larynx, and breast.[53] CT shows a densely enhancing noncalcified suprasellar mass that may extend along the infundibulum into the sella. Angiography usually reveals a vascular blush. The MRI findings have not been established. Diagnosis is made by biopsy. These are vascular, tough, nonsuckable tumors that are difficult to resect completely. Fortunately, after subtotal removal they grow very slowly, often not recurring for decades. Postoperative radiotherapy is not of proven benefit.[54]

PARASELLAR PATHOLOGY

In the past, masses of the cavernous sinus were rarely treated surgically because of potential bleeding from the cavernous venous plexus, injury to the internal carotid artery, or damage to cranial nerves III, IV, and VI. New surgical approaches, utilization of the operative microscope, and intraoperative monitoring of cranial nerve function have facilitated surgical management of these lesions.[55]

Cavernous sinus neoplasms must be differentiated from aneurysms, their treatment being radically different. Once aneurysm is excluded, it becomes important to determine the relationship of the intracavernous mass to the adjacent carotid ar-

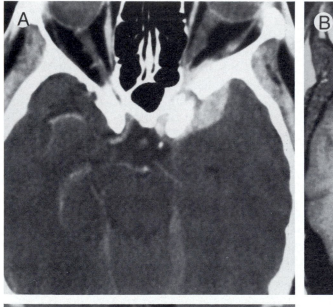

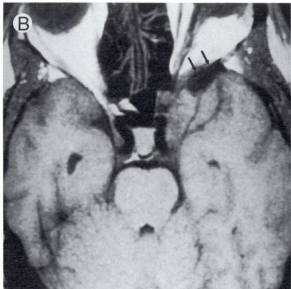

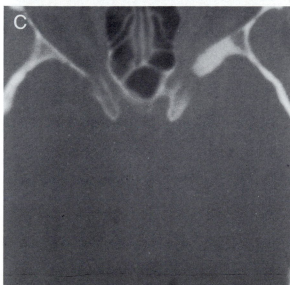

FIG 23–34.
Cavernous meningioma. **A,** axial CT shows an enhancing mass involving the left cavernous sinus, left orbital apex, and the greater wing of the left sphenoid bone. **B,** axial SE (TR 600, TE 20) MRI. The meningioma is isointense with gray matter. The thickened hyperostotic bone is well demonstrated *(arrows).* **C,** bone windows better demonstrate hyperostosis, which is found in two thirds of parasellar meningiomas.

tery and cranial nerves. CT and MRI are complimentary in evaluating these masses. Frequently both are needed for optimal assessment.[55]

Meningioma

Meningiomas arise from arachnoid cap cells found in the outer layer of the arachnoid membrane. About 15% of meningiomas occur in the parasellar region. They present with extraocular muscle palsies due to compression of the nerves running in the lateral wall of the cavernous sinus. Lesions that arise more anteriorly along the greater wing of this sphenoid bone may involve the back wall of the orbit and present with exophthalmos or decreased visual acuity secondary to optic nerve

compression. Meningiomas are generally benign tumors but are locally aggressive and invade dura, bone, and the adjacent paranasal sinuses. CT reveals a well-circumscribed or slightly lobulated hyperdense mass prior to contrast infusion (Fig 23–34). It may contain calcium. With contrast there is dense enhancement, sometimes making differentiation from aneurysm difficult (Fig 23–35) unless dynamic CT scanning with bolus contrast injection is employed. Cavitation and adjacent brain edema are uncommon with parasellar meningiomas. Adjacent hyperostosis occurs in two thirds of patients and helps differentiate meningiomas from other parasellar masses (Fig 23–34,B and C). It is impossible to differentiate reactive hyperostosis from what represents actual bone invasion.

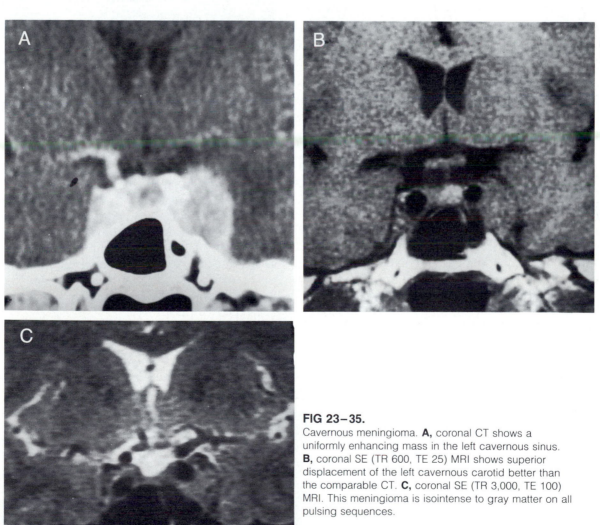

FIG 23–35.
Cavernous meningioma. **A,** coronal CT shows a uniformly enhancing mass in the left cavernous sinus. **B,** coronal SE (TR 600, TE 25) MRI shows superior displacement of the left cavernous carotid better than the comparable CT. **C,** coronal SE (TR 3,000, TE 100) MRI. This meningioma is isointense to gray matter on all pulsing sequences.

Therefore, when possible, hyperostotic bone is removed at surgery to reduce the chance of recurrence.

On unenhanced MRI, meningiomas are typically isointense or hypointense relative to brain on short TR spin-echo sequences, whereas on long TR images two thirds are isointense and one third hyperintense. Because they may lack distinctive signal characteristics, MRI recognition of parasellar meningiomas depends on the distortion of surrounding anatomy (Fig 23–35). There is bulging of the lateral wall of the cavernous sinus in most cases.[55] The cavernous carotid artery may be displaced (Fig 23–35) or completely engulfed by the meningioma; when the latter occurs, the carotid lumen may be narrowed (Fig 23–36). Arterial narrowing is well demonstrated by MRI and is rarely seen in cavernous neoplasms other than meningioma. Parasellar meningiomas spread along dural pathways, anteriorly into the orbital apex, and posteriorly along the tentorium cerebelli and clivus. With intraorbital extension, the fat in the superior orbital fissure is replaced (see Fig 23–34,A). Assessment of the optic nerve at the level of the optic canal and chiasm is particularly important in preoperative evaluation of these lesions. Meningiomas that extend into the sella can usually be distinguished from the pituitary gland by slight differences in signal characteristics (Fig 23–36).[56–58] Following gadolinium infusion meningiomas enhance intensely on short TR spin-echo sequences (Fig 23–37). They are indistinguishable in signal from the cavernous sinus per se but usually enhance more than the adjacent pituitary gland. Intraorbital extension is difficult to recognize on postcontrast studies because enhancing tumor is similar in signal to orbital fat. The need to differentiate enhancing tumor from normal adjacent fat underscores the importance of precontrast short TR spin-echo sequences in evaluating parasellar masses. This is not an issue with CT where enhanced scans are usually sufficient. However, enhanced MRI may also be important. Lesion conspicuity is increased on postcontrast MRI. The margins between enhancing tumor and adjacent neural tissue (optic nerve, brain) or other soft tissue at the skull base are better defined following contrast injection. Therefore, both precontrast and postcontrast short TR as well as long TR spin-echo sequences are required for optimal evaluation of parasellar lesions. While MRI is best for the evaluation of surrounding soft tissues, CT with bone algorithms remains the primary modality for the evaluation of calcifica-

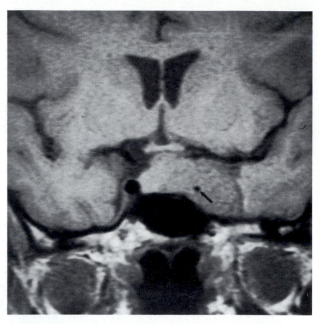

FIG 23–36.
Cavernous meningioma: coronal SE (TR 600, TE 20) MRI. The mass engulfs the left cavernous carotid and narrows the vascular lumen *(arrow)*. Vascular compromise is typical of meningioma but rare with other parasellar neoplasms.

tion and bone changes that are sometimes associated with parasellar and other skull base neoplasms. Angiography has no essential role in determining the extent of parasellar meningiomas, but for some surgeons it remains important as a qualitative indicator of tumor vascularity.[57] Balloon test occlusion of the carotid artery has been advocated for testing the feasibility of carotid artery sacrifice during tumor extirpation.[59] This is particularly important when the meningioma encases the carotid artery.

Nerve Sheath Tumor

Nerve sheath tumors arise from Schwann cells that ensheathe the axons of the cranial nerves peripheral to the pia. (Other terms for this neoplasm include neuroma, neurinoma, and neurilemoma.) Parasellar nerve sheath tumors occur from the fifth nerve ("trigeminal neuroma") or uncommonly from the third nerve. Fifth nerve sheath tumors may involve any portion of the nerve from its exit at the belly of the pons to its peripheral branches and spread by growing along the nerve. Tumors arising within the trigeminal ganglion obliterate rather than displace Meckel's cave.[60] Extracranial spread is easily demonstrated. Involvement of the mandibular division of the nerve may expand the fora-

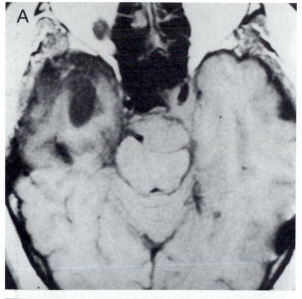

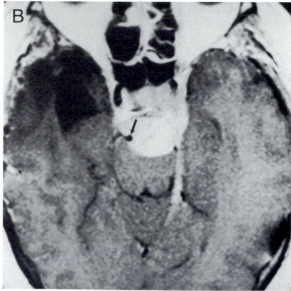

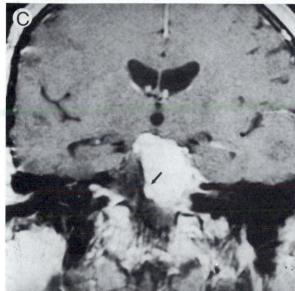

FIG 23–37.
Recurrent cavernous meningioma in a 56-year-old woman after resection of a right cavernous meningioma. She now has left-sided ophthalmoplegia. **A,** axial SE (TR 550, TE 20) MRI shows an isointense mass involving the left cavernous sinus and prepontine cistern. There is encephalomalacia of the right temporal lobe from previous surgery. **B,** postcontrast MRI shows dense although somewhat uneven enhancement of the mass. The basilar artery *(arrow)* is partially encased by the neoplasm. **C,** coronal postcontrast MRI (TR 800, TE 20). The anterior inferior cerebellar artery *(arrow)* courses through the mass.

men ovale (Fig 23–38), involve the masticator space, or enlarge the mandibular foramen and the canal of the inferior alveolar nerve. Involvement of the maxillary division of the trigeminal nerve may result in expansion of the cavernous sinus, enlargement of the foramen rotundum, or obliteration of the fat in the pterygopalatine fossa (Fig 23–39). Spread along the first or ophthalmic division of the trigeminal nerve results in expansion of the superior orbital fissure, displacement of fat at the orbital apex, and sometimes expansion of the infraorbital canal that conducts a branch of the nerve to the face.

Enhanced CT shows dense contrast enhancement that may be uniform or irregular (see Figs 23–50 and 23–51). To study the extent of the lesion and expansion of the exit foramina 1.5- to 3.0-mm axial and coronal CT sections with bone algorithms are required. If the masticator space is involved, cuts should be extended inferiorly to include the mandibular foramen and canal.

On MRI nerve sheath tumors are isointense or hypointense relative to brain on short TR spin-echo sequences, similar to a cavernous meningioma. On long TR sequences nerve sheath tumors tend to have high signal intensity that is often irregular (see Fig 23–38). There is intense enhancement following contrast injection. Nerve sheath tumors frequently displace the carotid artery but seldom produce the luminal narrowing characteris-

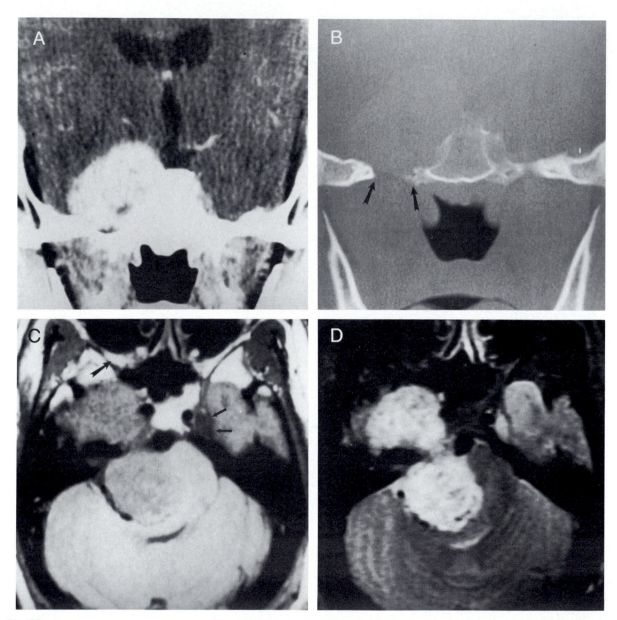

FIG 23–38.
Fifth nerve sheath tumor. **A,** coronal CT shows a densely enhancing right parasellar mass. **B,** a bone algorithm shows no hyperostosis. There is enlargement of the foramen ovale on the right *(arrows).* **C,** axial SE (TR 800, TE 20) MRI. The mass is isointense to gray matter. Meckel's cave is normal on the left *(arrows)* and re-placed by tumor on the right. The fat signal in the pterygopalatine fossa is normal *(long arrow),* which indicates that the tumor has not spread along the maxillary division of the nerve. **D,** axial SE (TR 2,500, TE 75) MRI. The tumor has high signal and is inhomogeneous.

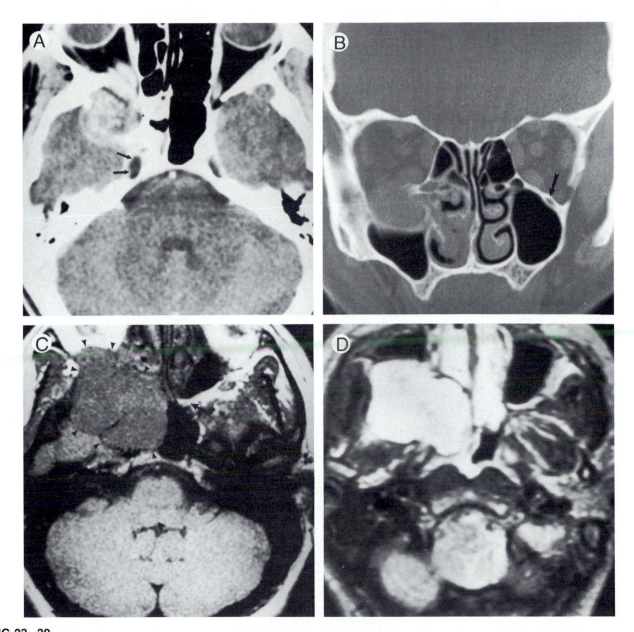

FIG 23–39.
Nerve sheath tumor. **A,** axial CT shows an irregularly enhancing mass involving the right cavernous sinus. Meckel's cave is not involved *(arrows)*. **B,** a coronal CT bone algorithm shows enlargement of the infraorbital canal; for comparison see the normal canal on the left *(arrow)*. The tumor has spread along the infraorbital nerve, a branch of the maxillary division of the trigeminal nerve. **C,** axial SE (TR 600, TE 20) MRI. The left pterygopalatine fossa is normal *(arrow)* but on the right it is replaced by a large tumor mass *(arrowheads)*. **D,** axial SE (TR 2,500, TE 100) MRI shows that the mass has intense T2 signal.

tic of meningiomas. While MRI is inferior to CT in demonstrating expansion of the cranial nerve foramina, it is competitive with CT in demonstrating extracranial extension. In particular, unenhanced short TR spin-echo images are helpful in identifying the fat that surrounds most cranial nerves where they exit from the skull (specifically cranial nerves III, IV, V_1, and VI are surrounded by the fat in the superior orbital fissure; V_2 by fat in the pterygopalatine fossa; V_3 by fat below the foramen ovale in the superior aspect of the masticator space; and VII by fat in the stylomastoid foramen).

Parasellar Metastasis

Metastasis to the parasellar region usually involve the cavernous sinus and may result from hematogenous, direct, or perineural spread (Figs 23–40 and 23–41). Symptoms usually consist of an acute painful rapidly progressive ophthalmoplegia.[61]

Imaging studies show expansion of the cavern-

ous sinus on the side of the ophthalmoplegia (Fig 23–40). CT will show a uniform enhancing mass indistinguishable from most other cavernous sinus neoplasms. About half of metastatic lesions will have adjacent bone destruction. This may help differentiate metastasis from benign cavernous neoplasms such as nerve sheath tumor or meningioma that tend to produce bony remodeling or hyperostosis rather than frank destruction.[61] MRI characteristics of metastasis are nonspecific. Lymphoma may also occur in the cavernous sinus directly or may spread to it from an adjacent nasopharyngeal focus.

Tolosa-Hunt Syndrome

Tolosa and Hunt described an inflammatory granuloma of the anterior cavernous sinus or orbital apex that produced orbital pain and extraocular muscle palsy due to dysfunction of cranial nerves III, IV, or VI. This disorder is a variant of orbital pseudotumor. Systemic steroid therapy re-

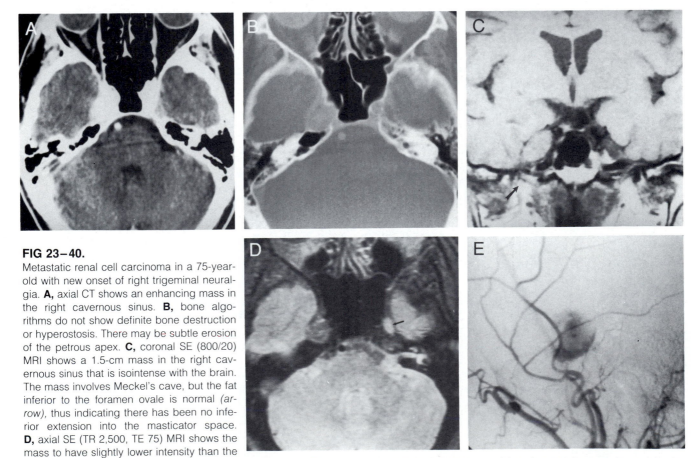

FIG 23–40.
Metastatic renal cell carcinoma in a 75-year-old with new onset of right trigeminal neuralgia. **A,** axial CT shows an enhancing mass in the right cavernous sinus. **B,** bone algorithms do not show definite bone destruction or hyperostosis. There may be subtle erosion of the petrous apex. **C,** coronal SE (800/20) MRI shows a 1.5-cm mass in the right cavernous sinus that is isointense with the brain. The mass involves Meckel's cave, but the fat inferior to the foramen ovale is normal *(arrow)*, thus indicating there has been no inferior extension into the masticator space. **D,** axial SE (TR 2,500, TE 75) MRI shows the mass to have slightly lower intensity than the surrounding brain. The left Meckel's cave is normal *(arrow)*. **E,** a lateral view of a right external carotid angiogram shows a dense vascular blush, typical for metastatic deposits from renal cell carcinoma.

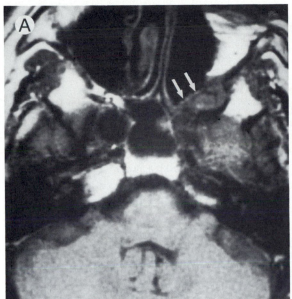
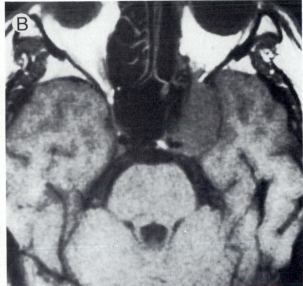

FIG 23–41.
Adenoid cystic carcinoma with perineural spread. **A,** axial SE (TR 600, TE 25) MRI shows replacement of the normal fat in the left pterygopalatine fossa with soft tissue *(arrows).* **B,** a more superior cut shows a mass in the left cavernous sinus from spread along V₂.

sults in dramatic improvement, often within 24 hours of administration. This dramatic response to steroids is usually diagnostic of the condition. Occasionally orbital lymphoma, which will mimic orbital pseudotumor clinically, pathologically, and radiographically, also responds temporarily to steroid administration.

Imaging studies have normal findings in most cases. Occasionally the cavernous sinus is enlarged by an enhancing mass, and/or soft tissue infiltrates the fat at the orbital apex. In these exceptional cases where imaging results are positive, the prompt clinical response to steroids followed by eventual reversion of the cavernous sinus and orbital apex to normal will permit differentiation from other cavernous sinus masses (particularly orbital lymphoma).[62, 63]

Cavernous Sinus Thrombosis

Another syndrome presenting with painful ophthalmoplegia is cavernous sinus thrombosis. Unlike Tolosa-Hunt syndrome, patients with cavernous sinus thrombosis are usually in a toxic condition and have fever, rapidly progressive proptosis, exophthalmos, and extraocular muscle palsy. Symptoms are unilateral initially, but the contralateral eye may become involved due to spread of the thrombotic process across intercavernous communications to involve the contralateral sinus. Throm-

bosis of the ophthalmic vein is responsible for the exophthalmos and conjunctival edema (chemosis). The disorder is usually caused by a septic venous thrombophlebitis originating from an infection in the face, nose, orbit, nasopharynx, or paranasal sinuses. On enhanced CT there may be irregular filling defects within the cavernous sinus, but these are difficult to differentiate from normal inhomogeneity of enhancement or from small bits of fat that normally occur in the cavernous sinus. There may be abnormal prominence of the superior ophthalmic vein and exophthalmos with periorbital edema. Opacity of sphenoid, ethmoid, and occasionally mastoid air cells may indicate the source of septic thrombophlebitis.[64] The MRI findings in cavernous sinus thrombosis remain to be established.

Early diagnosis and prompt aggressive antibiotic therapy are indicated. Even with optimum treatment, mortality from this disorder is about 30%. Because venous infarction of the brain may accompany cavernous sinus thrombosis, the desirability of anticoagulation is controversial. It might increase the incidence of hemorrhage into areas of infarction.[65]

Carotid Cavernous Fistula

There are two types of carotid cavernous fistulas: direct and indirect. The most common are the high-flow, high-pressure shunts that develop directly between the intracavernous portion of the carotid artery and the surrounding cavernous sinus (direct fistulas). These are due to spontaneous rupture of intracavernous aneurysms or to trauma through laceration of the intracavernous carotid artery. The patient experiences rapid onset of pulsating exophthalmos, a prominent bruit over the affected eye, marked venous congestion, conjunctival edema (chemosis), and impaired eye movement due to extraocular muscle swelling or cranial nerve palsy. When the venous drainage of the fistula is primarily forward through the superior ophthalmic veins, symptoms may be bilateral thanks to the intercavernous communications. Rarely eye symptoms are absent because drainage is primarily posterior to the clival venous plexus and petrosal sinuses.

Diagnosis and evaluation are primarily made by angiography, which shows early opacification of the cavernous sinus. CT shows enlargement of the sinus in long-standing cases. Secondary CT signs are similar to those of cavernous sinus thrombosis and include enlargement of the superior ophthalmic vein, exophthalmos, and increased densities in the orbital fat ("dirty fat") due to venous congestion (see Fig 28–11).

The high-pressure variety of fistula requires treatment to relieve the severe proptosis, extraocular muscle palsy, and retinal ischemia that can result from the elevated venous pressure. Treatment of these high-flow fistulas was revolutionized in the 1970s with the development of detachable balloons that are placed transarterially into the fistula to seal the leak.[66]

Indirect fistulas are low-flow, low-pressure shunts that develop spontaneously, usually in middle age. These occur between the cavernous sinus and dural branches of the external and/or internal carotid artery (Fig 23–42). Clinically they present with eye findings that have developed insidiously.

The natural history of the low-flow fistula is more benign than with direct fistulas; spontaneous reduction or complete closure of the fistula occurs in many cases. However, these fistulas, which are really dural AVMs involving the cavernous sinus, may produce ocular symptoms and subarachnoid or parenchymal hemorrhage. Symptomatic indirect fistulas can be treated transarterially by using particulate emboli.[67]

Intracavernous Carotid Artery Aneurysms

Aneurysms of the cavernous carotid artery constitute from 3% to 11% of all intracranial aneurysms.

Their etiology may be post-traumatic, iatrogenic (a complication of trans-sphenoidal surgery),[68] mycotic (a complication of septic cavernous sinus thrombosis), or spontaneous. The latter is most common, but its pathophysiology is poorly understood. Most intracranial aneurysms arise at apices of large vessel bifurcations. The cavernous carotid has no such bifurcations, so these aneurysms may arise at the origin of the small intracavernous branches or, more likely, at points of congenital weakness of the internal elastic lamina within the parasellar carotid artery.[69] The symptoms produced by cavernous carotid aneurysms may be compressive or vascular. Large aneurysms growing laterally impinge on the parasellar cranial nerves to produce extraocular muscle palsy and facial pain (Figs 23–43 and 23–44). Anterior growth of an aneurysm will impinge on the superior orbital fissure, compress cranial nerves, and produce exophthalmos or glaucoma due to compression of the superior ophthalmic vein. Superior and medial extension may compress the pituitary infundibulum and result in hyperprolactinemia due to disinhibition of prolactin secretion (Fig 23–45).[70] Vascular symptoms include distal embolization from thrombi formed within the aneurysm and subarachnoid hemorrhage, which can occur if a portion of the aneurysm protrudes through the dural envelope of the cavernous sinus. Epistaxis and hemorrhagic otitis develop rarely and occur when an aneurysm erodes into the sphenoid sinus or petrous bone, respectively.

Images of cavernous carotid aneurysms vary with their size and degree of intraluminal thrombosis. On enhanced CT scans small aneurysms will blend imperceptibly with the surrounding cavernous sinus. Although the lumen of a small aneurysm will be apparent on MRI, it may not be recognized on tomographic scans due to the normal variability and tortuosity of the cavernous carotid artery. These small aneurysms are usually incidental discoveries on angiography done for other reasons.

CT of larger aneurysms will show a uniformly enhancing mass indistinguishable from cavernous sinus neoplasms (see Figs 23–43 and 23–44). Dynamic bolus contrast CT is diagnostic in these cases because the aneurysm's lumen is distinguished from the surrounding cavernous sinus.[71] By MRI, patent aneurysms will appear as a signal void with evanescent internal echos within the lumen due to slow or turbulent flow within the aneurysm.[72] Occasionally it may be difficult to distinguish a patent lumen from a thrombus within the aneurysm because of the internal signal (see Fig

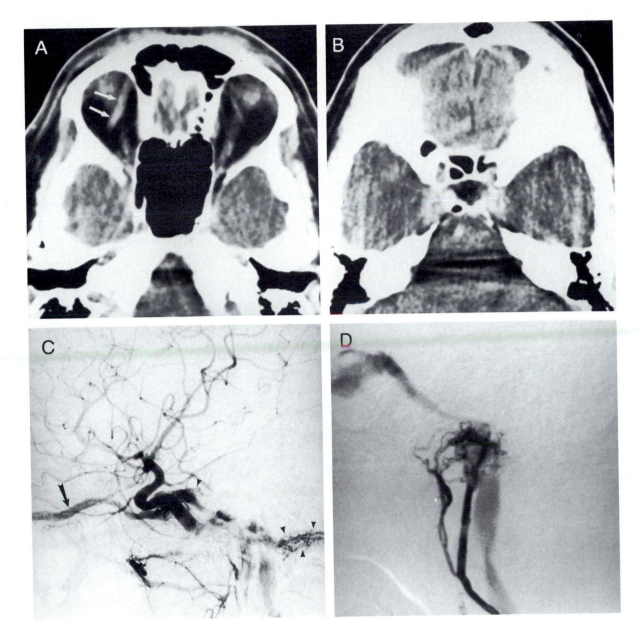

FIG 23–42.
Indirect carotid cavernous fistula. **A,** axial enhanced CT. The right superior ophthalmic vein *(arrows)* is larger than the left. **B,** no definite abnormality of the ipsilateral cavernous sinus is apparent. **C,** Right common carotid injection, lateral view. There is opacification of the right cavernous sinus and superior ophthalmic vein *(arrow)* during the arterial phase. The dural AVM is extensive *(arrowheads)*. **D,** a selective right external carotid injection, lateral view, shows that the dominant supply to the fistulas is from the external circulation.

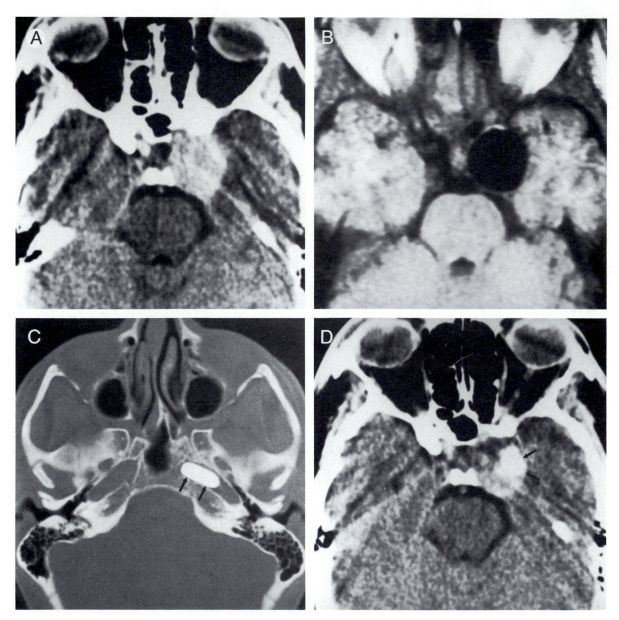

FIG 23–43.
Parasellar aneurysm in a 30-year-old woman with headaches and double vision for several years. **A,** axial CT shows an enhancing parasellar mass. Initially, this was felt to be a parasellar meningioma. **B,** axial SE (TR 800, TE 20) MRI. The flowing blood in the patent lumen produces almost no signal. **C,** a contrast-filled balloon *(arrows)* was placed proximal to the aneurysm to occlude the parent artery. **D,** unenhanced CT following embolization shows a dense clot forming within the lumen of the aneurysm *(arrows)*. Follow-up angiography confirmed complete thrombosis.

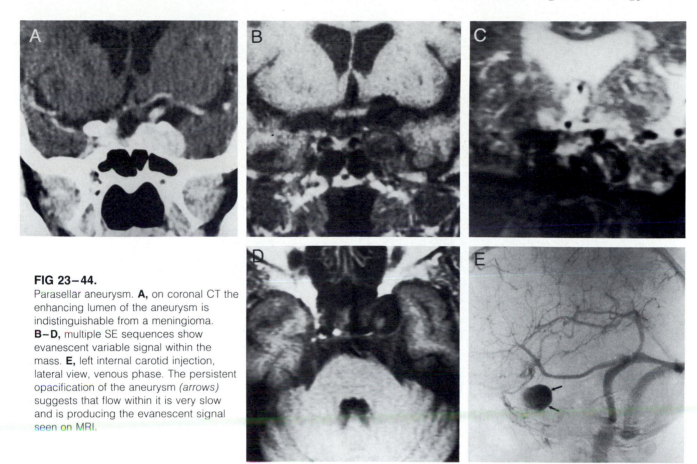

FIG 23–44.
Parasellar aneurysm. **A,** on coronal CT the enhancing lumen of the aneurysm is indistinguishable from a meningioma. **B–D,** multiple SE sequences show evanescent variable signal within the mass. **E,** left internal carotid injection, lateral view, venous phase. The persistent opacification of the aneurysm *(arrows)* suggests that flow within it is very slow and is producing the evanescent signal seen on MRI.

23–44,B–D). In such cases, comparison with angiography or dynamic CT will differentiate a thrombus from the lumen.

Completely thrombosed aneurysms pose a diagnostic challenge for all modalities. CT shows a ring enhancing mass with a hypodense center (Fig 23–46). Rim calcification may be a helpful clue that this mass is an aneurysm. MRI characteristics of thrombosed aneurysms vary greatly depending upon the age of the clot within the aneurysm. A subacute clot is bright on all pulsing sequences, while an old thrombus may be isointense. Peripheral hemosiderin deposition will appear as a rim of low signal on long TR spin-echo sequences and may help differentiate a clotted aneurysm from other parasellar masses.[73]

The indications for treatment of cavernous carotid artery aneurysms are controversial. Small, incidentally discovered aneurysms can probably be neglected because intracranial subarachnoid rupture is rare and intracavernous rupture with formation of a carotid cavernous fistula is also uncommon. There is a tendency to be more aggressive with larger aneurysms that produce ophthalmople-gia or incapacitating trigeminal neuralgia[74]; giant aneurysms tend to grow[75] despite their thick wall and threaten fatal subarachnoid hemorrhage. Treatment options include surgery and endovascular balloon embolization. Balloon therapy generally consists of occlusion of the ipsilateral carotid artery, proximal to the aneurysm. (see Fig 23–43,C and D) Balloons may also be placed within the lumen of the aneurysm to preserve the parent vessel. The latter procedure is hazardous if the aneurysm is partially thrombosed due to the risk of distal embolization of a fresh mural thrombus extruded during balloon inflation. Embolization procedures generally produce symptomatic improvement, probably because of reduced pulsation and diminished mass effect from eventual retraction of the clotted aneurysm. Combining several series, the overall mortality of proximal endovascular balloon embolization is 2%, which is considerably lower than that of surgery.[76–79]

Cavernous carotid aneurysms that occur as a complication of surgery or trauma are distinct and require aggressive management. These aneurysms tend to present with life-threatening epistaxis and,

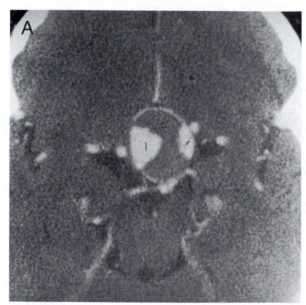

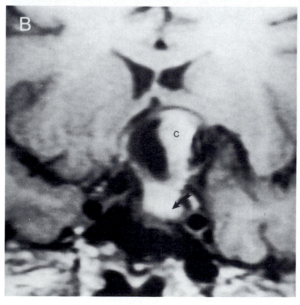

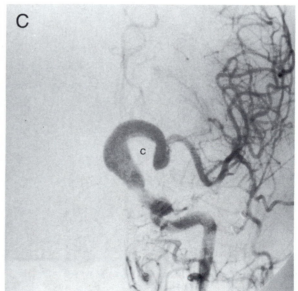

FIG 23–45.
Sellar and suprasellar aneurysm. **A,** axial CT through the suprasellar cistern shows the contrast-enhancing lumen *(1)* and nonenhancing clot *(c)* within this partially thrombosed aneurysm. **B,** coronal SE (TR 600, TE 20) MRI shows the patent lumen as a signal void and the clot *(c)* as high signal. Note the intrasellar extension of the clotted portion of the aneurysm *(arrow).* **C,** anteroposterior (AP) view of a left common carotid injection shows the patent lumen of the aneurysm. The clotted portions *(c),* including the intrasellar component, do not fill.

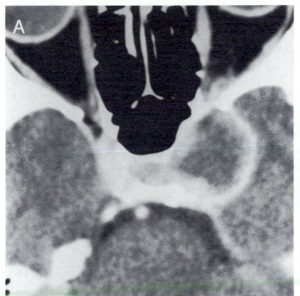

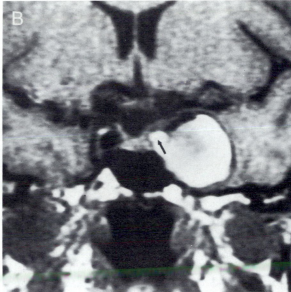

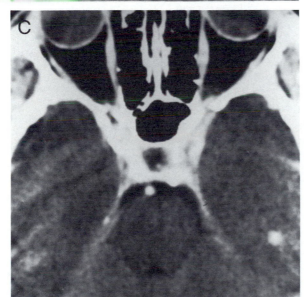

FIG 23—46.
Spontaneous thrombosis of a parasellar aneurysm in a
49-year-old woman with a 2-week history of periorbital
pain and sixth nerve palsy. **A,** axial CT shows a ring
enhancing parasellar mass. **B,** coronal SE (TR 800, TE
20) MRI. The thrombus within the aneurysm and
adjacent carotid artery lumen *(arrow)* has high signal
due to methemoglobin. **C,** axial CT 3 months later
shows remarkable shrinking of the clotted aneurysm.
The patient's sixth nerve palsy resolved spontaneously.
The degree of shrinkage following thrombosis of large
aneurysms is quite variable.

once they have bled, tend to have recurrent, massive, life-threatening hemorrhages. These aneurysms are often small and irregular and requiring angiography for definitive evaluation (Fig 23–47). Treatment requires isolating the diseased segment with endovascular balloons and/or surgery.[80] The mortality rate of these aneurysms is about 50%. Most patients with mycotic intracavernous aneurysms will die of the accompanying cavernous sinus infection, so the initial treatment is systemic antibiotics.

SUPRASELLAR PATHOLOGY

Meningioma

Suprasellar meningiomas most frequently arise from the tuberculum sellae. The most common presenting symptoms are those of headache and visual loss due to compression of the optic nerves or chiasm. CT features are typical of meningioma elsewhere, with dense enhancement, smooth margination, hyperostosis, and occasionally calcification (Fig 23–48). MRI characteristics are also similar to other meningiomas. Pituitary macroadenomas with suprasellar extension may have a similar CT and MRI appearance to tuberculum meningiomas. Distinction of these lesions is important because tuberculum meningiomas will be approached by craniotomy whereas macroadenomas often are treated with partial trans-sphenoidal resection and radiation therapy. Features suggesting meningioma include (1) hyperostosis rather than bone erosion, (2) no expansion of the sella, (3) broad-based attachment to the tuberculum sellae, (4) mass centered anteriorly over the tuberculum rather than over the sella, and (5) visualization of the diaphragma sellae in normal position. Angiography may not be definitive in these cases because of the qualitative overlap of the vascularity of adenomas and meningiomas. Suprasellar meningiomas may also arise from the diaphragma sellae, the clinoid processes, or the optic nerve sheaths.[81]

Craniopharyngioma

Craniopharyngiomas account for 2% to 4% of all tumors affecting the brain. They occur at all ages but have a peak incidence in children under 15 years old. Histologic differences between adult and childhood craniopharyngiomas suggest that they have different origins. The childhood form is believed to derive from ectoblastic remnants of Rathke's pouch, whereas the adult variety is thought to arise from metaplasia of nests of squamous epithelium (epithelial nests of Erdheim)

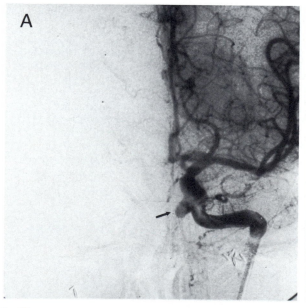 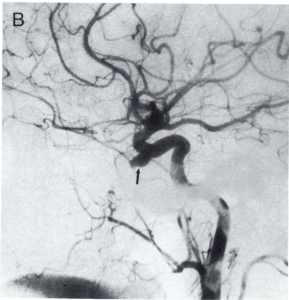

FIG 23–47.
Iatrogenic parasellar aneurysm. During a transethmoidal approach to an ACTH-producing adenoma there was bleeding from the left cavernous sinus region that was difficult to control. The angiogram was performed several months postoperatively after multiple episodes of massive epistaxis. **A** and **B,** AP and lateral carotid angiograms show a lobulated aneurysm arising from the medial aspect of the cavernous carotid *(arrow).* These aneurysms must be treated aggressively by trapping the diseased segment either surgically or transarterially.

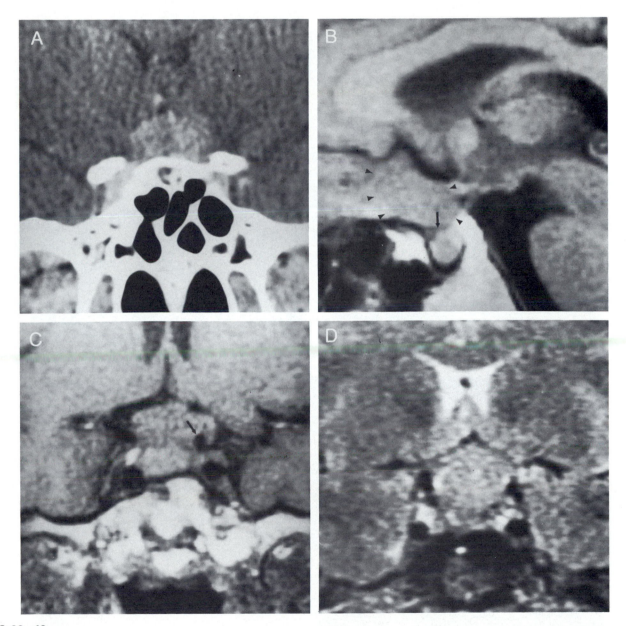

FIG 23–48.

Tuberculum sellae meningioma. **A,** coronal CT shows an enhancing suprasellar mass with broad attachment to the tuberculum sellae. **B,** sagittal SE (TR 600, TE 20) MRI. The meningioma *(arrowheads)* is isointense with brain. Features that distinguish it from a pituitary macroadenoma include the normal size of the sella, the separation of the tumor from the pituitary by the diaphragma sellae *(arrow),* and the broad base attachment to the tuberculum and pla-num sphenoidale. The tumor is also centered more anteriorly than most macroadenomas. **C,** coronal SE (TR 600, TE 20) MRI. The mass partially engulfs the supraclinoid left internal carotid *(arrow)*—an important preoperative observation. The separation of the mass from the pituitary is less apparent than on the sagittal view. **D,** coronal SE (TR 2,500, TE 100) MRI. The meningioma is isointense and somewhat difficult to recognize on long TR images.

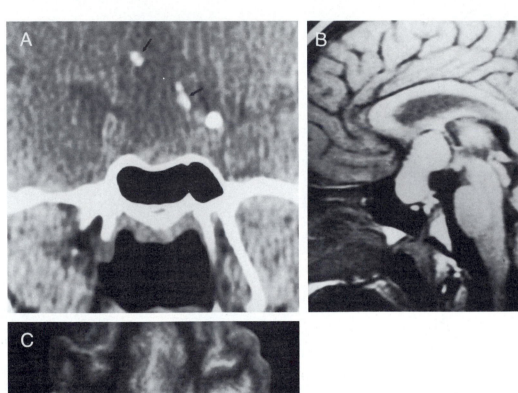

FIG 23–49.
Craniopharyngioma in an 18-year-old with delayed onset of
puberty. **A,** coronal noncontrast CT shows a large suprasellar mass
with calcification *(arrows)*. **B,** sagittal SE (TR 500, TE 20) MRI
shows a high-signal mass expanding the sella and extending into
the suprasellar cistern. The intrasellar component is more apparent
than on the CT scan. **C,** axial SE (TR 2,500, TE 80) MRI. The mass
also has intense T2 signal.

normally found on the anterior surface of the infundibulum and pars tuberalis of the pituitary gland.[52]

Twenty percent of craniopharyngiomas originate in the sella turcica, while the remaining 80% originate above the diaphragma sellae. They vary greatly in size, but about 60% are large enough at presentation to obstruct the foramen of Monro. Children tolerate visual loss without complaint and hence usually present with hydrocephalus, whereas adults will present earlier with visual symptoms. Endocrine dysfunction occurs in 70% to 90% of patients due to compression of the pituitary infundibulum and hypothalamus. Craniopharyngiomas typically consist of both solid and liquid components. The cavitated or "cystic" components arise from desquamation of the epithelial layer that makes up the wall of these lesions. Frequently the colloid component is densely calcified.[52]

The appearance of craniopharyngiomas is highly variable, and the imaging features overlap those of most other suprasellar masses. The cavitated portions of the tumor may range from low to high density on CT (Fig 23–49). Low density is attributed to a high cholesterol content within the cyst, whereas high density is the result of high protein content.[82–84] The MRI characteristics of craniopharyngiomas also vary widely. Most lesions will have high signal on long TR spin-echo images (Figs 23–49 to 23–51). On short TR spin-echo sequences, however, half of the lesions will be hyperintense (Figs 23–49 and 23–51), and half will be isointense or hypointense to surrounding brain (Fig 23–50). One exceptional craniopharyngioma has been reported that was hypointense on long TR spin-echo sequences and contained an ossifying matrix.[85] Enhancement characteristics of these lesions are also highly variable and range from dense enhancement of solid components and ring enhancement around cavitated components (Fig 23–52) to a total absence of enhancement. Calcification occurs in 70% to 90% of childhood craniopharyngiomas and 30% to 50% of the adult form. The high sensitivity of CT in detecting calcification makes it more specific than MRI in the diagnosis of craniopharyngioma preoperatively (see Fig 23–49). However, MRI is superior in defining tumor extent, relationship to surrounding structures, and evaluation of recurrent tumor.[85]

Craniopharyngiomas are usually considered to be extra-axial neoplasms, but they may indent the brain and incite an intense glial reaction. They may also be adherent to the arteries of the circle of Willis (see Fig 23–51). The treatment of choice is complete surgical removal, but understandably, this is difficult. Operative mortality ranges from 5%

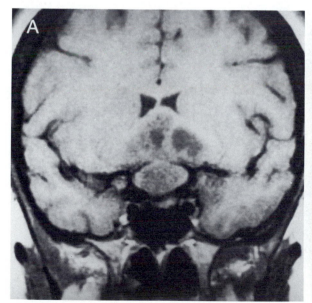
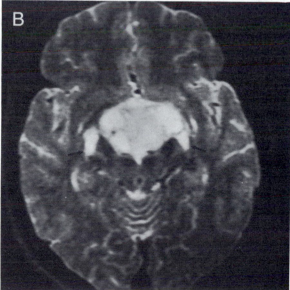

FIG 23–50.
Craniopharyngioma in a 47-year-old accountant with decreasing ability to calculate and visual difficulties for 2 months. **A,** coronal SE (TR 800, TE 20) MRI shows a complex suprasellar mass. It is difficult to tell whether this is intra-axial or extra-axial. The optic chiasm appears large. This lesion is indistinguishable from a suprasellar glioma. **B,** axial SE (TR 2,500, TE 100) MRI. The mass has heterogeneous but primarily high signal on a T2 basis. High signal extending along the optic tracts bilaterally *(arrows)* presumably represents edema due to compression by the adjacent craniopharyngioma.

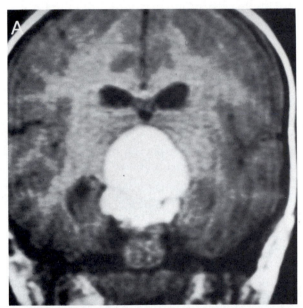

FIG 23–51.
Craniopharyngioma. **A,** coronal SE (TR 400, TE 20) MRI. There is a large suprasellar mass, high signal on a T1 basis. **B,** axial SE (TR 3,000, TE 80) MRI. The mass also has high signal on a T2 basis. The vertebral artery *(arrow)* is enveloped by tumor. **C,** axial SE (TR 500, TE 30) MRI after intravenous gadolinium administration. Enhancement, if present, is obscured by the intrinsic high signal of the lesion.

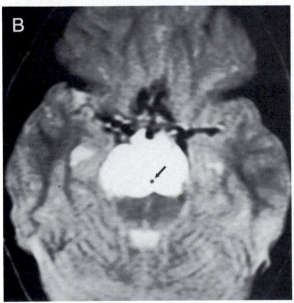

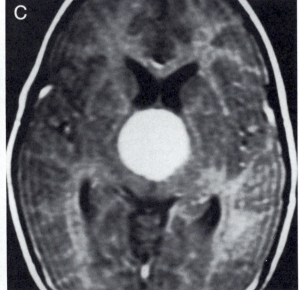

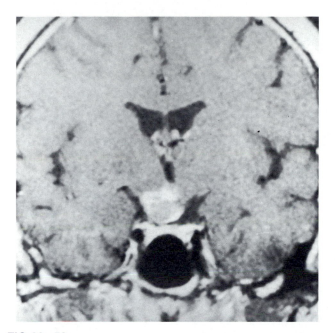

FIG 23–52.
Craniopharyngioma. Enhanced coronal SE (TR 600, TE 25) MRI shows irregular enhancement in a recurrent craniopharyngioma.

to 10%. Adjunctive radiation therapy may be used if complete resection is impractical. If the tumor is going to recur, it will generally do so within 3 years of surgery.[52]

Epidermoid

Epidermoid and dermoid tumors arise from epithelial cells misplaced in the calvarium, meninges, ventricles, or brain parenchyma. One theory is that epithelium is trapped during embryogenesis due to incomplete cleavage of neural and cutaneous ectoderm. Others argue that these tumors arise from pleuripotential stem cells that undergo improper differentiation to epithelial cells. Whatever their origin, epidermoids consist solely of squamous epithelium that, through maturation and desquamation, forms a central tumor core of keratin and cholesterol crystals surrounded by a fibrous capsule of connective tissue. These tumors grow in a linear fashion similar to all epithelial tissue. They are ten times more frequent than dermoids.[86]

Epidermoids can be intradural or extradural in location. They arise either in the midline or slightly off midline, as compared with dermoids, which are characteristically midline in location. Epidermoids have irregular, nodular, or rounded margins; their surface morphology is likened to a cluster of grapes (Fig 23–53). The tumor often insinuates itself into adjacent fissures of the brain, which makes complete surgical removal difficult. If even a small part of the capsule is not removed, the lesion will recur.[86] The CT density of epidermoids is usually similar to that of CSF (Figs 23–53 and 23–54). Rarely they approach the density of brain tissue. The variability is a result of differences in cholesterol and protein concentrations within the lesions. Enhancement is unusual and, if present, will only involve the peripheral capsule of the tumor. Rimlike capsular calcification may also occur. Intrathecal contrast will surround the tumor and demonstrate its nodular appearance (Fig 23–54).[87, 88] MRI signal characteristics like CT densities are also generally similar to those of CSF (on all pulsing sequences). Only rarely will epidermoids have high signal on short TR SE images.[89] Sometimes there are cleavage planes within the mass that allow differentiation from an arachnoid cyst (Fig 23–53). An interesting problem is presented by CT or MRI scans following resection of an epidermoid. These lesions, which are longstanding, remodel the surrounding brain. On postoperative studies the molded tumor cavity is filled with CSF, so the postoperative scan resembles the preoperative study. Detection of recurrent tumor depends on the appearance of new or increased mass effect and, when present, internal echos. Contrast cisternography is helpful in ambiguous cases (Fig 23–54). Rarely the capsule of an epidermoid may rupture and release the proteinaceous or cholesterol contents into the subarachnoid space to produce aseptic meningitis.[86]

Dermoid

Like epidermoid tumors, dermoids are derived entirely from ectoderm. Epidermoids consist purely of squamous epithelium, but dermoids also contain sebaceous glands, sweat glands, and hair follicles. These additional elements are of ectodermal origin but normally lie within mesodermal connective tissue (the dermis). The squamous epithelial cells undergo continuous division. In epidermoids the desquamated debris is a solid, flaky, dry material that contains a large amount of cholesterol and keratin. Dermoid cysts contain more fluid than do epidermoids because of the secretions of the sweat and sebaceous glands they contain. The fluid consists of an oily mixture of lipid metabolites and has CT density and MRI signal characteristics similar to fat (Fig 23–55). This explains the

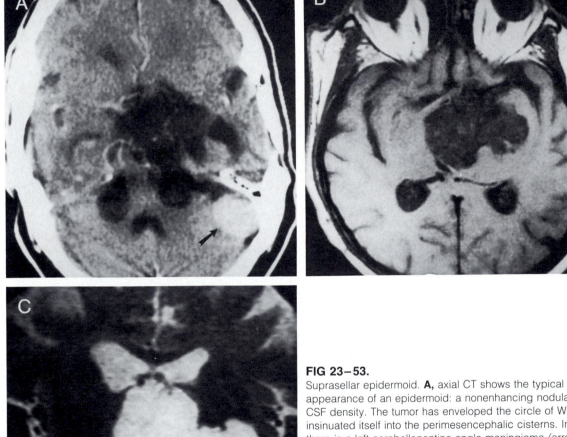

FIG 23–53.
Suprasellar epidermoid. **A,** axial CT shows the typical
appearance of an epidermoid: a nonenhancing nodular mass of
CSF density. The tumor has enveloped the circle of Willis and
insinuated itself into the perimesencephalic cisterns. Incidentally,
there is a left cerebellopontine angle meningioma *(arrow).* **B,** axial
SE (TR 600, TE 25) MRI. The tumor has some internal irregularity
giving rise to internal echoes that allow differentiation from CSF.
C, coronal SE (TR 3,000, TE 100) MRI. The signal characteristics
of the epidermoid are indistinguishable from CSF.

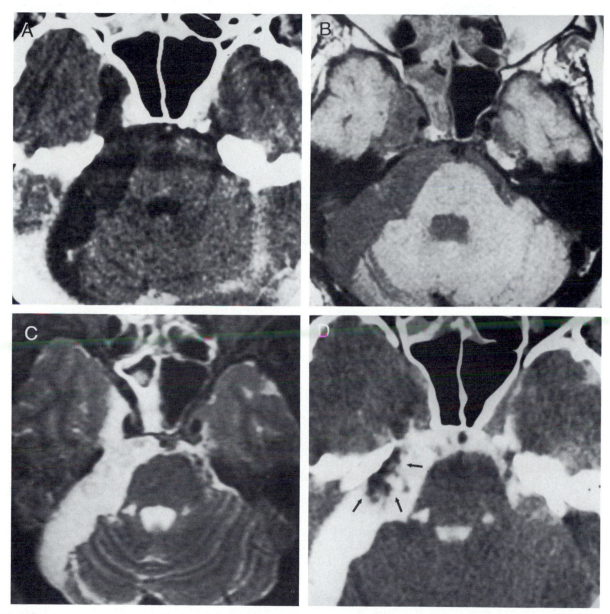

FIG 23-54.
Parasellar and cerebellopontine angle (CPA) epidermoid in a middle-aged man after partial resection of a right CPA epidermoid. **A,** axial CT shows a CSF-density lesion involving the right CPA and the right cavernous sinus. **B** and **C,** axial SE MRI scans (TR 800, TE 25 and TR 3,000, TE 100) show the lesion to have signal characteristics similar to CSF. **D,** cisternography is the only method that differentiates the irregular residual epidermoid tumor *(arrows)* from the surrounding CSF-filled cavity. The tumor had extended into the right cavernous sinus. This component of the tumor could not be removed from the retromastoid approach and required an infratemporal approach.

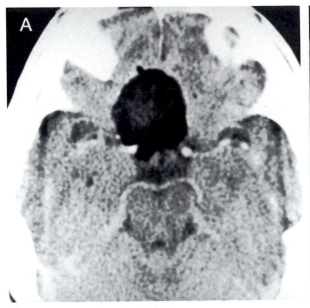
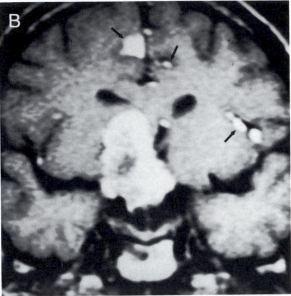

FIG 23–55.
Ruptured suprasellar dermoid. **A,** axial CT shows a low-density mass in the suprasellar cistern. The central portion of the mass has soft-tissue density. There is no definite enhancement. **B,** coronal SE (TR 600, TE 20) MRI. The peripheral component of the tumor has high signal. The dermoid has ruptured, and there are droplets of oily material *(arrows)* in the interhemispheric and left sylvian fissures.

low density and high T1 signal that is characteristic of dermoids even though they lack mesodermal fat (as is contained in lipomas or true teratomas).[90] Because of their greater complexity, the capsules of dermoids are thicker and more frequently calcify than do those of epidermoids. The relative lack of contrast enhancement in dermoids and epidermoids may be helpful for differentiating them from the more common craniopharyngiomas.[86]

Teratoma

Teratomas are similar to dermoids except that they contain elements of all three germ cell layers. Seventy percent of teratomas occur in the region of the pineal gland, but about 20% are suprasellar. CT density and MRI signal characteristics are highly variable, and there is often inhomogeneous enhancement within the lesion. Teratomas are difficult to differentiate from dermoids. Occasionally, they undergo malignant degeneration.

Lipoma

Lipomas are rare in the suprasellar cistern. Most are discovered incidentally, but they have been reported to compress the pituitary infundibulum or hypothalamus and cause endocrine dysfunction. They are of maldevelopmental origin and may involve the leptomeninges as well as the underlying neural tissue. They consist of adipocytes with variable amounts of vascular, fibroblastic, osseous, or cartilaginous elements.[26] It is thought that

> they grow as part of the general growth of the body . . . clinical progress, therefore, in the case of intracranial lipoma is hardly ever secondary to tumor growth and much more frequently due to involvement of surrounding structures into regressive changes within the lipoma tissue.[91]

Surgery is seldom helpful in alleviating symptoms.

CT shows a nonenhancing mass near the midline that is of low density (−100 Hounsfield units) and may have a calcified shell. It may be difficult to differentiate a lipoma from a dermoid cyst or teratoma. The later lesions are usually more complex and enhance following contrast. On MRI scans the fat within a lipoma will have high signal on a T1 basis and will "fade" or become isointense on "T2-weighted" images. In small lipomas the T2 signal characteristics are difficult to define because of CSF flow artifacts within the suprasellar cistern and chemical shift effect. Also, it can be difficult to differentiate lipoma from ectopic posterior pituitary tissue (see below) on short TR spin-echo sequences. In questionable cases CT will be definitive and demonstrate fat density (Fig 23–56).

Germinoma

Germinomas are neoplasms derived from germinal tissue that normally differentiates to form sperm cells or ova. They usually occur in the ovaries and testes of adolescents and young adults but may also occur intracranially. The neoplasm is nonneuroectodermal and probably derives from displaced primitive germ cells that fail to migrate to the gonads during embryogenesis. Most commonly intracranial germinomas develop in the region of the pineal gland, but about 20% occur in the suprasellar cistern, the floor of the third ventricle, or the basal ganglia. This neoplasm is slightly more prevalent in Japan where it constitutes 4% of brain tumors. Symptoms are often insidious, develop over months or years, and reflect involvement of the hypothalamus and optic chiasm. Diabetes insipidus, visual field defects, pituitary dysfunction, and decreased mentation are common. Late in the course the tumor may produce hydrocephalus due to obstruction at the foramen of Monro.[92]

The tumors are usually large at presentation.

They may appear well demarcated from surrounding structures (Fig 23–57) but are infiltrating and spread along the walls of the third ventricle and into the optic tracts (Fig 23–58). CT shows a moderate to densely enhancing mass without calcification. Bone erosion and expansion of the sella may occur. MRI experience is limited, but reports show these lesions to be isointense or slightly hypointense on short TR and hyperintense on long TR spin-echo images. The appearance both on CT and MRI is nonspecific. These lesions are difficult to differentiate from hypothalamic or optic chiasm gliomas, histiocytosis X, and inflammatory granulomas.[81]

Germinomas are nonencapsulated infiltrating neoplasms that cannot be excised completely. The role of surgery is to debulk the lesions, to decompress the optic nerves, tracts, and chiasm, and to obtain a histologic diagnosis. Pure germ cell tumors are among the most radiosensitive tumors and have a 50% to 80% 5-year survival rate with radiotherapy alone. Because of a high incidence of CSF seeding, complete cerebrospinal axis radiation is frequently advocated. If the tumor is of mixed histology (i.e., contains elements of other germ cell lines such as embryonal carcinoma or choriocarcinoma), it will be less sensitive to radiotherapy. Adjuvant chemotherapy is then recommended.[93]

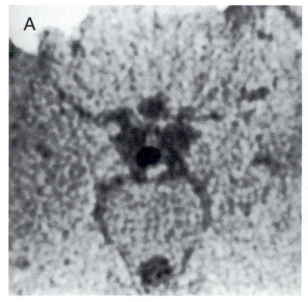

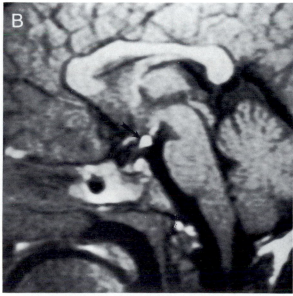

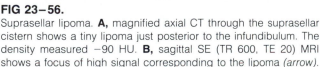

FIG 23–56.
Suprasellar lipoma. **A,** magnified axial CT through the suprasellar cistern shows a tiny lipoma just posterior to the infundibulum. The density measured −90 HU. **B,** sagittal SE (TR 600, TE 20) MRI shows a focus of high signal corresponding to the lipoma *(arrow).*

This must be differentiated from fat in the dorsum sellae and from "ectopic" posterior pituitary signal described in pituitary dwarfism. In this case the posterior pituitary is well demonstrated in its normal location within the sella.

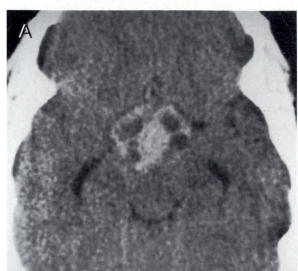
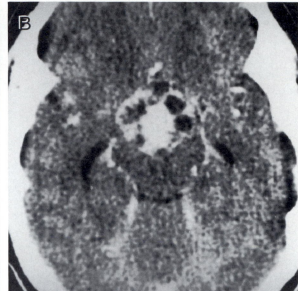

FIG 23–57.
Suprasellar germinoma. **A,** unenhanced CT shows an inhomogeneous mass in the suprasellar cistern that has hyperdense components. **B,** after contrast there is enhancement of the more cellular portions of the tumor.

Suprasellar Metastasis

Metastases to the suprasellar region are of three varieties: hematogenous, CSF borne, or from direct extension of an adjacent neoplasm, frequently along the infundibulum. Even small lesions may produce profound clinical problems including diabetes insipidus, panhypopituitarism, and visual deficit. Biopsy of these lesions carries a risk of substantial morbidity; fortunately, a known diagnosis of a primary neoplasm elsewhere is frequently present.[94]

Suprasellar metastases have a nonspecific imaging appearance (Figs 23–59 and 23–60). They are usually densely enhancing noncalcified lesions. MRI is more precise than CT in defining what structures are involved in the lesion. On an imaging basis alone it is difficult to differentiate metastatic lesions from inflammatory granulomas, histiocytosis X, germinomas, and enhancing suprasellar gliomas.

Suprasellar Gliomas

The term *suprasellar glioma* includes a diverse group of neoplasms that differ in their behavior and response to therapy but overlap in their imaging and pathologic appearance.[95] As a result lesions that look the same by imaging studies may have very different clinical courses.

Most patients present at 2 to 20 years of age

(mean, 6 years); one third have neurofibromatosis. The most common symptom is visual disturbance, usually diminished acuity but occasionally a field cut. The degree of visual disturbance correlates poorly with the size or extent of the tumor.[96] CT and MRI show a variable-sized suprasellar mass; in 80% there is enhancement following intravenous contrast administration.[95] Calcification is rare in optic gliomas and, if present, suggests that the mass may be a craniopharyngioma. Tubular thickening of the intraorbital optic nerves in addition to the suprasellar mass is the most characteristic finding and effectively excludes other lesions (except meningioma, which is usually seen in an older age group). The lesion may also extend posteriorly to involve the optic tracts and optic radiations (Fig 23–61). Globular chiasmal gliomas that lack optic nerve enlargement are difficult to differentiate from other suprasellar masses (e.g., craniopharyngioma) and may require biopsy for diagnosis.[95]

Long term follow-up studies of the treatment and outcome for chiasmal gliomas are conflicting.[97, 98] Some indicate that these gliomas are indolent and rarely progress or require treatment. Others indicate that radiation therapy significantly reduces morbidity and mortality. There is general consensus on the following:

1. The role of surgery is to take biopsy samples from lesions in which there is serious question as to the correct diagnosis. Major operations to re-

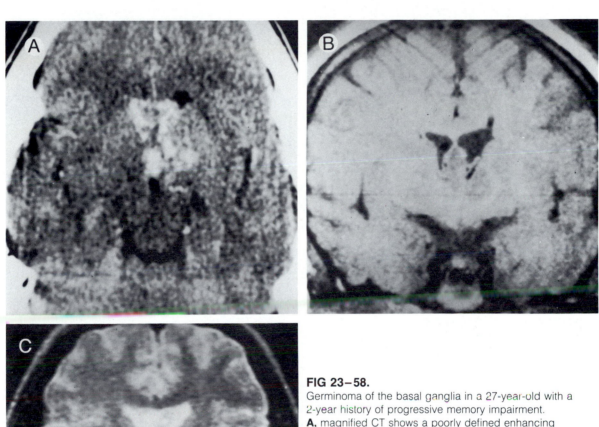

FIG 23–58.
Germinoma of the basal ganglia in a 27-year-old with a
2-year history of progressive memory impairment.
A, magnified CT shows a poorly defined enhancing
mass surrounding the lateral and third ventricles near
the foramen of Monro. **B,** coronal SE (TR 700, TE 20)
MRI shows abnormal signal in the left corpus striatum
(the caudate and lentiform nuclei are interconnected by
bands of gray matter passing through the anterior limb
of the internal capsule; the striated appearance gives
the nuclei collectively the name corpus striatum). The
fornix is grossly enlarged bilaterally. **C,** axial SE (TR
2,500, TE 100) MRI. The abnormal tissue has high
signal intensity on a T2 basis.

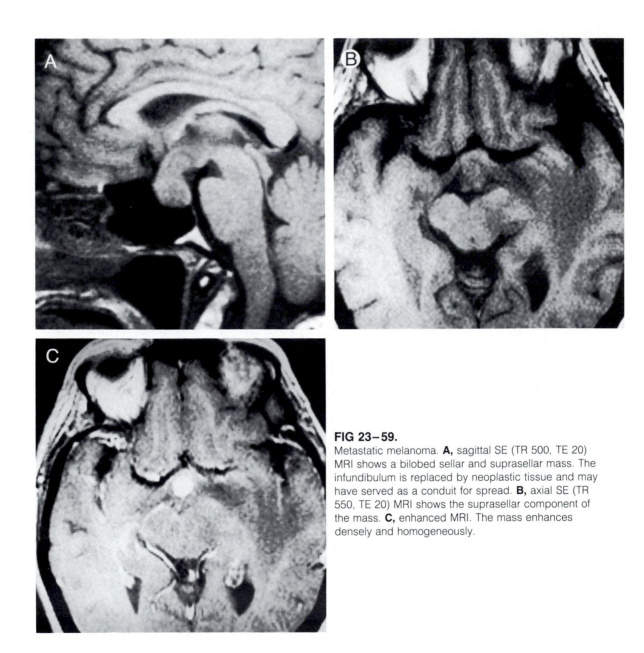

FIG 23–59.
Metastatic melanoma. **A,** sagittal SE (TR 500, TE 20) MRI shows a bilobed sellar and suprasellar mass. The infundibulum is replaced by neoplastic tissue and may have served as a conduit for spread. **B,** axial SE (TR 550, TE 20) MRI shows the suprasellar component of the mass. **C,** enhanced MRI. The mass enhances densely and homogeneously.

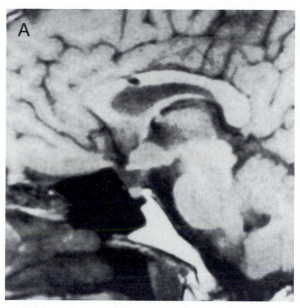

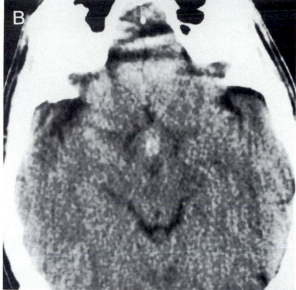

FIG 23–60.
Atypical suprasellar metastasis: Posterior fossa primitive neuroec-todermal tumor resected 5 years earlier. The patient received che-motherapy and craniospinal irradiation. This lesion was followed for several years with only minimal growth. **A,** sagittal (TR 800, TE 20) SE MRI shows a suprasellar mass that did not enhance follow-ing contrast. The lack of enhancement is atypical. **B,** an unen-hanced CT scan shows calcification within the mass. Calcification in a metastatic lesion is unusual.

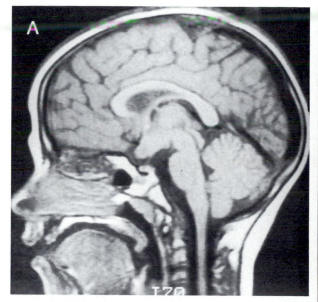

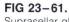

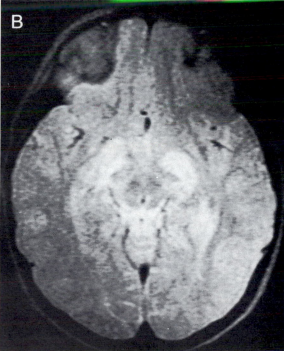

FIG 23–61.
Suprasellar glioma. **A,** sagittal SE (TR 500, TE 20) MRI shows enlargement of the optic chiasm and extension into the hypothalamus. **B,** axial SE (TR 2,500, TE 100) MRI shows abnormally high signal in the optic tracts and lateral geniculate nuclei.

move large portions of the tumor are not helpful.

2. If the lesion is going to enlarge, it will usually do so within a few years of diagnosis. Therefore, patients must be watched closely shortly after diagnosis and vigilance gradually relaxed once an indolent course is established. However, late malignant degeneration may occur.

3. Radiation therapy is indicated if there is growth of the lesion on serial imaging studies or if there is deterioration of vision as determined by formal testing. The use of radiation before documented growth or progression of symptoms remains controversial.

4. Radiation therapy may cause shrinkage of tumor (evidenced by imaging studies), but symptomatic improvement may not accompany the decrease in tumor size.

Large suprasellar gliomas in infants are a distinct subgroup of chiasmal region gliomas. This group consists of children under 2 years of age with large (greater than 3 cm) suprasellar gliomas (Fig 23–62). Visual disturbance (sometimes hard to detect in young children) and abnormal rotary nystagmoid eye movements are the most common presenting symptoms. Fifty percent of the infants also manifest the "diencephalic syndrome" (severe emaciation in a child who appears inappropriately happy or even euphoric). This syndrome is almost always due to a suprasellar glioma. CT and MRI show a large suprasellar mass; frequently there is extensive infiltration of the basal ganglia and temporal lobes. Contrast enhancement is usually intense, but calcification is rare. These tumors are cytologically low-grade benign fibrillary astrocytomas. However, despite the benign histology, the prognosis is poor with less than 50% 5-year survival rates even with radiation therapy. The patients have extensive neurologic disability. At autopsy there is typically extensive infiltration of the thalamus and temporal lobes in addition to a large component of exophytic tumor involving the suprasellar cistern.[99]

Suprasellar Arachnoid Cysts

Arachnoid cysts account for 1% of intracranial masses. Fifteen percent occur in the suprasellar cistern and present in infancy with obstructive hydrocephalus. If the hydrocephalus is mild, symptoms may be intermittent. Patients who are undetected until the second or third decade of life may present with seizures or hypothalamic dysfunction.

The correct radiographic and surgical approach depends upon an understanding of how these cysts are formed. The underlying defect is believed to be a lack of fenestration in the membrane of Liliequist that may be congenital or acquired (due to adhesive arachnoiditis). Radiographically the membrane of Liliequist can only be visualized in normal patients by pneumoencephalography. It separates the interpeduncular and chiasmatic regions of the suprasellar cistern by attaching to the dorsum sellae, oculomotor nerves, hypothalamus, and ventral midbrain. If it forms a barrier to the flow of CSF from the posterior fossa to the suprasellar cistern, an upward bulging diverticulum will form. In extreme cases the diverticulum may invaginate through the floor of the hypothalamus into the third ventricle and even obstruct the foramen of Monro. The diverticulum may lose its original connection with the subarachnoid space and become a true cyst. The hypothalamus and ependymal lining of the third ventricle are part of the dome of the cyst, so transventricular biopsy may lead to a pathologic misdiagnosis of ependymal cyst unless the inner wall of the cyst (arachnoid) is carefully marked by the surgeon. Postoperative diabetes insipidus and hypothalamic dysfunction may occur if portions of the hypothalamus are removed in such a biopsy, although compression of the hypothalamus alone may lead to endocrine dysfunction.[100, 101]

These lesions are rounded, well-demarcated, thin-walled, homogeneous CSF density (or intensity) uncalcified masses. They do not enhance following contrast. They may be confused with the suprasellar epidermoid tumor unless intrathecal contrast medium (via the ventricular or subarachnoid route) is used to distinguish the smooth inner walls of the arachnoid membrane from the irregular, lobulated interstices of the epidermoid. Because the lesions are frequently associated with marked hydrocephalus, there may be some reluctance to administer intrathecal contrast via lumbar puncture, although this has been performed safely. Differentiation of suprasellar arachnoid cysts, ependymal cysts of the third ventricle, enlargement of the third ventricle, and parasitic cysts may be difficult by imaging studies.[100]

Histiocytosis X

Histiocytosis is a chronic disease that chiefly affects the reticuloendothelial system. The basic disorder is a proliferation of histiocytes of un-

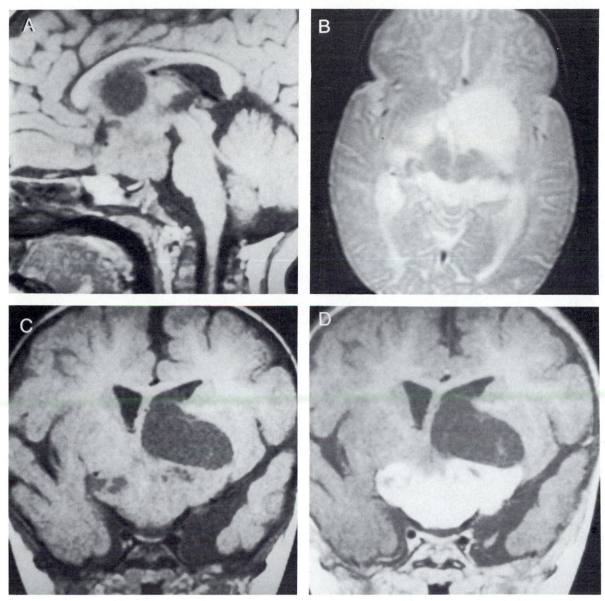

FIG 23–62.
Large suprasellar glioma in an infant 9 months old. **A,** sagittal SE (TR 500, TE 20) MRI shows a large suprasellar mass. **B,** axial SE (TR 2,875, TE 80) MRI shows the mass to have high T2 signal. **C,** coronal SE (TR 600, TE 25) MRI. The mass involves the optic chi-asm, hypothalamus, and thalami. There is a large low-signal component that probably represents cavitation. **D,** following intravenous gadolinium DTPA administration there is dense enhancement.

known etiology. There is a broad spectrum of disease ranging from easily controlled solitary benign *eosinophilic granuloma* of bone in children and adults to a malignant systemic disease of infants, *Letterer-Siwe disease,* which is fatal. The former does not involve brain parenchyma, while in the latter there may be diffuse infiltration of the leptomeninges by histiocytes. The intermediate form of histiocytosis X is *Hand-Schuller-Christian disease.* It is characterized by multiple eosinophilic

granulomas that most frequently involve the orbit, the skull base, and the hypothalamus. Hypothalamic granulomas may extend down the infundibulum and infiltrate the posterior lobe of the pituitary. Hypothalamic involvement is manifested as anterior and posterior pituitary dysfunction, but diabetes insipidus is typically the most apparent endocrine disturbance.[26]

CT and MRI will show the thickening of the hypothalamus and enlargement of the pituitary infundibulum (Fig 23–63). The abnormal tissue will enhance following contrast administration, and the high signal normally seen in the posterior lobe of the pituitary may be absent. Histiocytosis cannot be differentiated from other suprasellar granulomas unless the characteristic osteolytic skeletal lesions are discovered.

Sarcoidosis

Sarcoidosis is a disease of unknown etiology that is characterized by noncaseating granulomas in many tissues in the body. Neurologic abnormalities occur in 5% of patients. Lesions are located diffusely in the leptomeninges and are prominent at the base of the brain, particularly in the suprasellar region. They also occur on the ependymal surface of the ventricles and may produce hydrocephalus. Clinically patients present with multiple cranial neuropathies, most frequently facial palsy. Suprasellar lesions may infiltrate the optic nerve and alter vision. Infiltration of the hypothalamus results in endocrine dysfunction.

Imaging studies may or may not show enhancement of the leptomeninges and ependyma. Suprasellar granulomas enhance and may produce thickening of the hypothalamus and lamina termi-

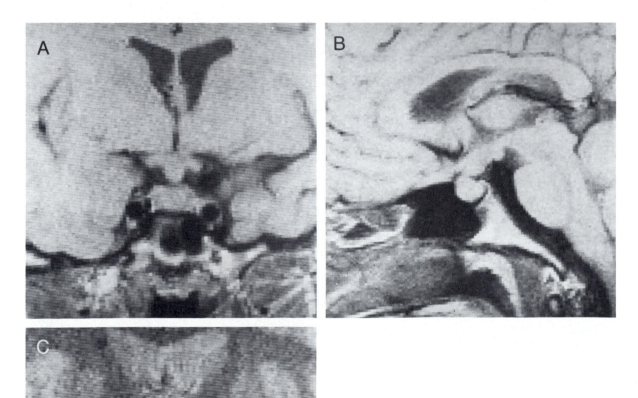

FIG 23–63.
Hypothalamic histiocytosis X in a 16-year-old with diabetes insipidus. Previously there was eosinophilic granuloma of bone. **A** and **B,** coronal and sagittal SE (TR 500, TE 40, 0.35 Tesla) MRI. The hypothalamus and infundibulum are thickened. **C,** coronal SE (TR 2,000, TE 80) MRI shows abnormal high signal in the hypothalamus *(arrows).*

nalis (Fig 23–64). The accompanying mass may partially obliterate the third ventricle.

About 60% of patients with central nervous system (CNS) sarcoid will have clinical manifestations of systemic sarcoidosis. In the remaining patients the CNS masses may be the first manifestation of the disease. Diagnosis is made by leptomeningeal biopsy. The CNS granulomas may regress following steroid therapy, which often must be continued for several months.[102, 103]

Hypothalamic Hamartomas

Hypothalamic hamartomas are congenital malformations that consist of a mass of neuronal tissue usually attached to the tuber cinereum or the mammillary bodies by a thick pedicle. Clinical symptoms are noted before the age of 6 years in almost all cases and consist of precocious puberty (75% of cases), generalized seizures, and gelastic epilepsy (the latter consists of bouts of laughter followed by facial grimacing that often occur 20 to 30 times a day). There is no definite sex predilection.[104] Rarely hypothalamic hamartomas are associated with multiple congenital anomalies including absent olfactory bulbs, absent pituitary, imperforate anus, syndactyly, and short metacarpals (Hall-Pallister syndrome).[26]

Because of the specific clinical presentation, a differential diagnosis is not usually a problem. CT will reveal a noncalcified, nonenhancing mass in the suprasellar cistern that is smooth or slightly lobulated and may range in size from 0.5 to 3.5 cm in diameter (Fig 23–65).[104] Contrast cisternography improves the sensitivity of CT in detecting small lesions. Often imaging in both the axial and coronal plane is helpful. MRI will show a mass that lies posterior to the infundibulum and projects from the hypothalamus into the interpeduncular and suprasellar cisterns. Reported cases show hamartomas to be indistinguishable from gray matter on short TR spin-echo sequences and hyperintense relative to gray matter on long TR images (Fig 23–65). Aside from the mass, per se, the radiologist can encounter an advanced bone age in these patients.[105]

Treatment is directed at controlling the hormonal imbalance produced by this lesion. Chemical inhibition of gonadotropin production may delay secondary sexual maturation and prevent premature epiphyseal closure.[105] The lesions grow very slowly and rarely cause compressive symptoms. In general, surgical intervention is discouraged. The lesions can only be partially resected due to their attachment to the hypothalamus. Partial removal has no effect on precocious puberty but occasionally leads to a reduction in the number of seizures.[106]

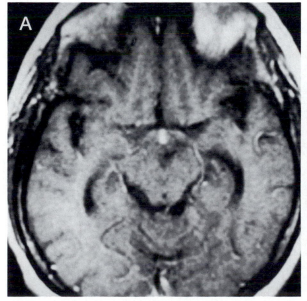 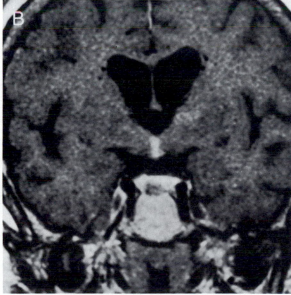

FIG 23–64.
Sarcoidosis in a 50-year-old woman; leptomeningeal biopsy shows noncaseating granulomas. The patient is in clinical remission following steroid therapy. **A** and **B,** postcontrast axial (TR 600, TE 30) and coronal (TR 650, TE 25) SE scans show abnormal enhancement in the hypothalamus.

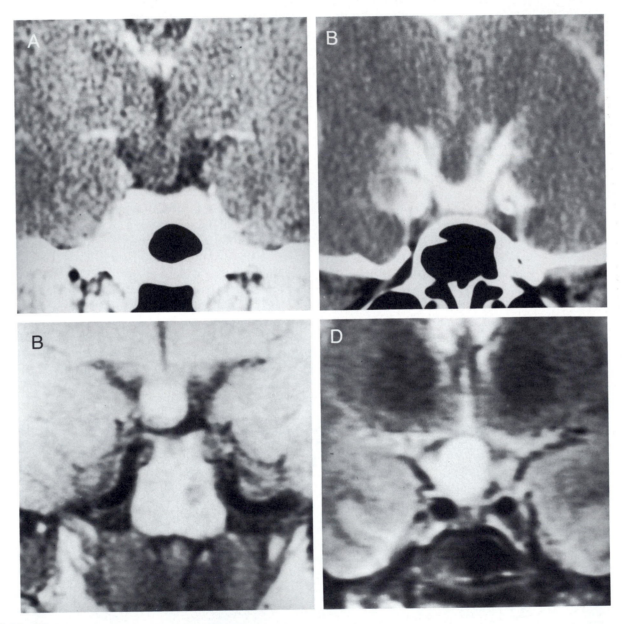

FIG 23–65.
Hypothalamic hamartoma (unproven). **A,** coronal CT shows a non-enhancing suprasellar mass that is not calcified. **B,** coronal CT after intrathecal contrast administration shows that the mass is polypoid and attached to the hypothalamus by a thick pedicle. **C,** coronal SE (TR 600, TE 20) MRI. The mass is isointense on a T1 basis. **D,** the mass is hyperintense on "T2-weighted" (TR 3,000, TE 75) SE sequences.

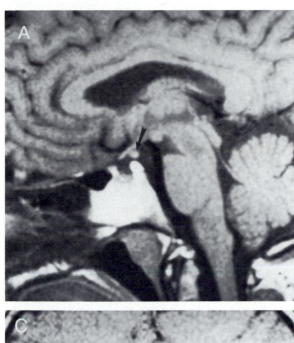

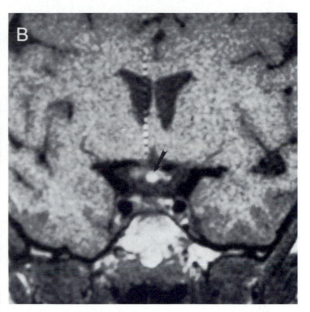

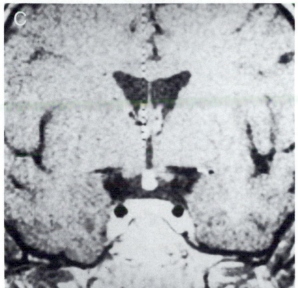

FIG 23–66.
Pituitary dwarfism (ectopic posterior pituitary) in a 29-year-old woman with a history of hypogonadism, hypothyroidism, and growth hormonal deficiency since 12 years of age. She has normal posterior pituitary function. **A** and **B,** sagittal and coronal SE (TR 600, TE 25) MRI. The infundibulum is not visualized. There is a high-signal bud at the tuber cinereum *(arrow)*. This is presumed to represent posterior pituitary tissue in an ectopic location. The pituitary gland (anterior lobe) is very small. **C,** on an immediate postcontrast scan the suprasellar nodule enhances.

Idiopathic Hypopituitarism (Pituitary Dwarfism)

Ten percent of cases of growth retardation are due to an idiopathic deficiency of human growth hormone (HGH). Affected children are usually recognized at 1 to 3 years of age because they show low height, subnormal growth velocity, truncal obesity, and delayed bone age. The diagnosis is based on low baseline serum GH levels that fail to increase appropriately (<5 ng/mL) to insulin-induced hypoglycemia or to an infusion of L-arginine. Imaging usually shows a normal or small sella and a small pituitary gland (<2 mm in height). The infundibulum may appear normal but more often is attenuated or invisible. Short TR spin-echo images reveal a 3- to 8-mm high-signal nodule at the median eminence and an absence of the high-signal posterior lobe in its usual location (Fig 23–66). This nodule may represent ectopic posterior pituitary tissue. These patients have preserved synthesis and regulation of antidiuretic hormone. Pituitary dwarfism is associated with perinatal hypoxia. Difficult deliveries, breech presentations or low Apgar scores are seen in over 50% of affected children. The frequent abnormalities of the infundibulum suggest that the cause of the disorder is an injury to the pituitary stalk or the hypophyseal portal system at the time of delivery.[107, 108]

REFERENCES

1. Kovacs K, Horvath E, Asa SL: Classification and pathology of pituitary tumors, in Wilkins RH, Rengachary SS (eds): *Neurosurgery.* New York, McGraw-Hill International Book Co, 1985, pp 834–842.
2. Scheithauer BW, Kovacs KT, Laws ER, et al: Pathology of invasive pituitary tumors with special reference to functional classification. *J Neurosurg* 1986; 65:733–744.
3. Tindall GT, Barrow DL (eds): *Disorders of the Pituitary.* St Louis, CV Mosby Co, 1986, pp 123–143.
4. Davis PC, Hoffman JC, Tindall GT, et al: CT-surgical correlation in pituitary adenomas: Evaluation in 113 patients. *AJNR* 1985; 6:711–716.
5. Davis PC, Hoffman JC, Spencer T, et al: MR imaging of pituitary adenoma: CT, clinical, and surgical correlation. *AJR* 1987; 148:797–802.
6. Scotti G, Yu CY, Dillon WP, et al: MR imaging of cavernous sinus involvement by pituitary adenomas. *AJNR* 1988; 9:657–664.
7. Marcovitz S, Wee R, Chan J, et al: Diagnostic accuracy of preoperative CT scanning of pituitary prolactinomas. *AJNR* 1988; 9:13–17.
8. Dubois PJ, Orr DP, Hoy RJ, et al: Normal sellar variations in frontal tomograms. *Radiology* 1979; 131:105–110.
9. Kucharczyk W, Davis D, Kelly WM, et al: Pituitary adenomas: High resolution MR imaging at 1.5T. *Radiology* 1986; 161:761–765.
10. Dwyer AJ, Frank JA, Doppman JL, et al: Pituitary adenomas in patients with Cushing disease: Initial experience with Gd-DTPA–enhanced MR imaging. *Radiology* 1987; 163:421–426.
11. Haughton VM, Leighton M: MRI of intrasellar and parasellar lesions. *MRI Decisions* 1988; 2:17–27.
12. Tindall GT, Barrow DL (eds): *Disorders of the Pituitary.* St Louis, CV Mosby Co, 1986, pp 253–280.
13. Nelson PB, Goodman M, Maroon JC, et al: Factors in predicting outcome from operation in patients with prolactin-secreting pituitary adenomas. *Neurosurgery* 1983; 13:634–640.
14. Saris, Patronas NJ, Doppman JL, et al: Cushing syndrome: Pituitary CT scanning. *Radiology* 1987; 162:775–777.
15. Dunnick NR: The adrenal gland, in Taveras JM, Ferrucci JT (eds): *Radiology Diagnosis—Imaging—Intervention,* vol 4. Philadelphia, JB Lippincott, 1988, pp 1–10.
16. Pojunas KW, Daniel DL, Williams AL, et al: Pituitary and adrenal CT of Cushing Syndrome. *AJNR* 1986; 7:271–274.
17. Marcovitz S, Wee R, Chan J, et al: The diagnostic accuracy of preoperative CT scanning in the evaluation of pituitary ACTH-secreting adenomas. *AJNR* 1987; 8:641–644.
18. Tagliaferri M, Berselli ME, Loli P: Trans-sphenoidal microsurgery for Cushing's disease. *Acta Endocrinol* 1986; 113:5–11.
19. Tindall GT, Barrow DL (eds): *Disorders of the Pituitary.* St Louis, CV Mosby Co, 1986, pp 231–252.
20. Nelson DH, Meaken JW, Thorn GW: ACTH-producing pituitary tumors following adrenalectomy for Cushing's syndrome. *Ann Inter Med* 1960; 52:560.
21. Louis ER: Acromegaly and gigantism in neurosurgery, in Wilkins RH, Rengachary SS (eds): *Neurosurgery.* New York, McGraw-Hill International Book Co, 1985, pp 864–867.
22. Marcovitz S, Wee R, Chan J, et al: Diagnostic accuracy of preoperative CT scanning of pituitary somatotroph adenomas. *AJNR* 1988; 9:19–22.
23. Tindall GT, Barrow DL (eds): *Disorders of the Pituitary.* St Louis, CV Mosby Co, 1986, p 301.
24. Danziger J, Wallace S, Handel S, et al: The sella turcica in primary end organ failure. *Radiology* 1979; 131:111–115.
25. Floyd JL, Dorwart RH, Nelson MJ, et al: Pituitary hyperplasia secondary to thyroid failure: CT appearance. *AJNR* 1984; 5:469–471.
26. Russel DS, Rubinstein LJ: *Pathology of Tumors of the Nervous System,* ed 5. Baltimore, Williams & Wilkins, 1989.
27. Ebersold L, et al: Pituitary apoplexy treated by trans-sphenoidal surgery. *J Neurosurg* 1983; 58:315–320.
28. Bjerre P, Videbaek H, Lindholm J: Subarachnoid hemorrhage with normal cerebral angiography: A prospective study on sellar abnormalities and pituitary function. *Neurosurgery* 1986; 19:1012–1015.
29. Bjerre P, Lindholm J: Pituitary apoplexy with sterile meningitis. *Acta Neurol Scand* 1986; 74:304–307.
30. Jeffcoate WJ, Birch CR: Apoplexy in small pituitary tumors. *J Neurol Neurosurg Psychiatry* 1986; 49:1077–1078.
31. Bonneville JF, Poulignot D, Cattin F, et al: Computed tomographic demonstration of the effects of bromocriptine on pituitary microadenoma size. *Radiology* 1982; 143:451–455.
32. Horowitz BL, Hamilton DJ, Sommers CJ, et al: Effect of bromocriptine and pergolide on pituitary tumor size and serum prolactin. *AJNR* 1983; 4:415–417.
33. Weissbuch SS: Explanation and implications of MR signal changes within pituitary adenomas after bromocriptine therapy. *AJNR* 1986; 7:214–216.
34. Guidetti B, Fraioli B, Cantore GP: Results of surgical management of 319 pituitary adenomas. *Acta Neurochir* 1987; 85:117–124.

35. Ciric I, Mikhael M, Stafford T, et al: Transsphenoidal microsurgery of pituitary macroadenomas with long-term follow-up results. *J Neurosurg* 1983; 59:395–401.

36. Snow RB, Lavyne MH, Lee BC, et al: Craniotomy versus transsphenoidal excision of large pituitary tumors: The usefulness of magnetic resonance imaging in guiding the operative approach. *Neurosurgery* 1986; 19:59–64.

37. Dolinskas CA, Simeone FA: Transsphenoidal hypophysectomy. *AJNR* 1985; 6:45–50.

38. Kaplan HC, Baker HL, Houser OW, et al: CT of the sella turcica after transsphenoidal resection of pituitary adenomas. *AJNR* 1985; 6:723–732.

39. Nelson PB, Haverkos H, Martinez AJ, et al: Abscess formation within pituitary tumors. *Neurosurgery* 1983; 12:331–334.

40. Enzmann DR, Sieling RJ: CT of pituitary abscess. *AJNR* 1983; 4:79–80.

41. Quencer RM: Lymphocytic adenohypophysitis: Autoimmune disorder of the pituitary gland. *AJNR* 1980; 1:343–345.

42. Meichner RH, Riggio S, Manz H, et al: Lymphocytic adenohypophysitis causing pituitary mass. *Neurology* 1987; 37:158–161.

43. McGrail KM, Beyerl BD, Black P, et al: Lymphocytic adenohypophysitis of pregnancy with complete recovery. *Neurosurgery* 1987; 20:791–793.

44. Carmel P: Empty sella syndrome, in Wilkins RH, Rengachary SS (eds): *Neurosurgery*. New York, McGraw-Hill International Book Co, 1985, pp 884–888.

45. Welch K. Stears JC: Chiasmapexy for the correction of traction on the optic nerves and chiasm associated with their descent into an empty sella turcica: Case report. *J Neurosurg* 1973; 39:674

46. Kaufman B, Tomsak RL, Kaufman BA, et al: Herniation of the suprasellar visual system and third ventricle into empty sellae: Morphologic and clinical considerations. *AJNR* 1989; 10:65–76.

47. Pituitary tumors and the empty sella (review). *Lancet* 1986; 1:1370–1372.

48. Haugton VM, Rosenbaum AE, Williams AL, et al: Recognizing the empty sella by CT: The infundibulum sign. *AJNR* 1980; 1:527–529.

49. Baskin DS, Wilson CB: Transsphenoidal treatment of non-neoplastic intrasellar cysts. *J Neurosurg* 1984; 60:8–13.

50. Kucharcyzk W, Peck W, Kelly W, et al: Rathke cleft cysts: CT, MR imaging and pathologic features. *Radiology* 1987; 165:491–495.

51. Nemoto Y, Inoue Y, Fukuda T, et al: MR appearance of Rathke's cleft cysts. *Neuroradiology* 1988; 30:155–159.

52. Carmel P: Craniopharyngiomas, in Wilkins RH, Rengachary SS (eds): New York, *Neurosurgery*.

New York, McGraw-Hill International Book Co, 1985, pp 905–916.

53. Korbrine AD, Ross E: Granular cell myoblastomas of the pituitary region. *Surg Neurol* 1973; 1:275–279.

54. Becker DH, Wilson CB: Symptomatic parasellar granular cell tumors. *Neurosurgery* 1981; 8:173–180.

55. Hirsch WL, Hryshko FG, Sekhar LN, et al: Comparative assessment of MR, CT and angiography in the evaluation of the enlarged cavernous sinus. *AJNR* 1988; 9:907–915.

56. Bradac GB, Riva A, Schorner W, et al: Cavernous sinus meningiomas: An MRI study. *Neuroradiology* 1987; 29:578–581.

57. Yeakley JW, Kulkarni M, McArdle CB, et al: High-resolution MR imaging of juxtasellar meningiomas with CT and angiographic correlation. *AJNR* 1988; 9:279–285.

58. Young SC, Grossman RI, Goldberg HI, et al: MR of vascular encasement in parasellar masses: Comparison with angiography and CT. *AJNR* 1988; 9:35–38.

59. Erba SM, Horton JA, Latchaw RE, et al: Balloon test occlusion of the internal carotid artery with stable xenon/CT cerebral blood flow imaging. *AJNR* 1988; 9:533–538.

60. Beck DW, Menezes AH: Lesions in Meckel's cave: Variable presentation and pathology. *J Neurosurg* 1987; 67:684–689.

61. Post MJ, Mendez DR, Kline LB, et al: Metastatic disease to the cavernous sinus: Clinical syndrome and CT diagnosis. *J Comput Assist Tomogr* 1985; 9:115–120.

62. Kwan ES, Wolpert SM, Hedges TR, et al: Tolosa-Hunt syndrome revisited: Not necessarily a diagnosis of exclusion. *AJNR* 1987; 8:1067–1072.

63. Hunt WE: Tolosa-Hunt syndrome: One cause of painful ophthalmoplegia. *J Neurosurg* 1976; 44:544–549.

64. Ahmadi J, Keane JR, Segall HD, et al: CT observations pertinent to septic cavernous sinus thrombosis. *AJNR* 1985; 6:755–758.

65. Southwick F, Swartz M: Inflammatory thrombosis of major dural venous sinuses and cortical veins, in Wilkins RH, Rengachary SS (eds): *Neurosurgery*. New York, McGraw-Hill International Book Co, 1985, pp 1956–1961.

66. DeBrun GM: Treatment of traumatic carotid cavernous fistula using detachable balloon catheters. *AJNR* 1983; 4:355.

67. Halbach VV, Higashida RT, Hieshima GB, et al: Dural fistulas involving the transverse and sigmoid sinuses: Results of treatment in 28 patients. *Radiology* 1987; 163:443–446.

68. Chambers EF, Rosenbaum AE, Norman O, et al: Traumatic aneurysm of cavernous internal carotid

artery, secondary epistaxis. *Am J Neuroradiol* 1981; 2:405–409.

69. Stehbens WE: *Pathology of the Cerebral Blood Vessels*. St Louis, CV Mosby Co, 1972, pp 351–470.

70. Mindel JS, Sachoey VP, Kline LB, et al: Bilateral intracavernous carotid aneurysms mimicking a prolactin-secreting pituitary tumor. *Surg Neurol* 1983; 19:163–167.

71. Pinto PS, Cohen WA, Kricheff I: Giant intracranial aneurysms: Rapid sequential computed tomography. *AJNR* 1982; 3:495–499.

72. Olsen WL, Brant-Zawadzki M, Hodes J, et al: Giant intracranial aneurysms: MR imaging. *Radiology* 1987; 163:431–435.

73. Kwan ES, Wolpert SM, Scott RM, et al: MR evaluation of neurovascular lesions after endovascular occlusion with detachable balloons. *AJNR* 1988; 9:523–531.

74. Mullan S: Carotid cavernous fistulas and intracavernous aneurysms, in Wilkins RH, Rengachary SS (eds): *Neurosurgery*. New York, McGraw-Hill International Book Co, 1985, pp 1483–1494.

75. Schubiger O, Valavanis A, Wichmann W: Growth-mechanism of giant intracranial aneurysms: Demonstration by CT and MR imaging. *Neuroradiology* 1987; 29:266–271.

76. Fox AJ, Vinuela F, Pelz DM, et al: Use of detachable balloons for proximal artery occlusion in the treatment of unclippable cerebral aneurysms. *J Neurosurg* 1987; 66:40–46.

77. Scialfa G, Vaghi A, Valsecchi F, et al: Neuroradiological treatment of carotid and vertebral fistulas and intracavernous aneurysms. *Neuroradiology* 1982; 24:13–25.

78. Raymond J, Theron J: Intracavernous aneurysms: Treatment by proximal balloon occlusion of the internal carotid artery. *AJNR* 1986; 7:1087–1092.

79. Berenstein A, Ransohoff J, Cupersmith M, et al: Transvascular treatment of giant aneurysms of the cavernous carotid and vertebral arteries. *Surg Neurol* 1984; 21:3–12.

80. Liu MY, Shih CJ, Wang YC, et al: Traumatic intracavernous carotid aneurysm with massive epistaxis. *Neurosurgery* 1985; 17:569–573.

81. Karnaze MG, Sartor K, Winthrop JD, et al: Suprasellar lesions: Evaluation with MR imaging. *Radiology* 1986; 161:77–82.

82. Fahlbusch R, Grumme THE, Aulich A, et al: Suprasellar tumors in the CT scan, in Lanksch W, Kazner E (eds): *Cranial Computerized Tomography*. Berlin, Springer-Verlag Publishing Co, 1986, pp 114–127.

83. Braun IF, Pinto RS, Epstein F: Dense cystic craniopharyngiomas. *AJNR* 1982; 3:139.

84. Davis KR, Roberson GH, Taveras JM, et al: Diagnosis of epidermoid tumor by computed tomography: Analysis and evaluation of findings. *Radiology* 1976; 119:347.

85. Pusey E, Kortman KE, Flannigan BD, et al: MR of craniopharyngiomas: Tumor delineation and characterization. *AJNR* 1987; 8:439–444.

86. Baxter JW, Netsky MG: Epidermoid and dermoid tumors, in Wilkins RH, Rengachary SS (eds): *Neurosurgery*. New York, McGraw-Hill International Book Co, 1985, pp 655–661.

87. Naidich TP, Pinto RS, Kushner MJ, et al: Evaluation of sellar and parasellar masses by computed tomography. *Radiology* 1976; 120:91.

88. Zimmerman RA, Bilaniuk LT: Cranial computed tomography of epidermoid and congenital fatty tumors of maldevelopmental origin. *CT Comput Tomogr* 1979; 3:40–50.

89. Houston LW, Hinke ML: Neuroradiology case of the day. *AJR* 1986; 146:1094–1097.

90. Smith AS: Myth of the mesoderm. *AJNR* 1989; 10:449.

91. Kazner E, Stochdorph O, Wende S, et al: Intracranial lipoma: Diagnostic and therapeutic considerations. *J Neurosurg* 1980; 52:234–245.

92. Walsh JW: Suprasellar germinomas, in Wilkins RH, Rengachary SS (eds): *Neurosurgery*. New York, McGraw-Hill International Book Co, 1985, pp 921–925.

93. Naidich T, Cacayorin E, Stewart WA, et al: Radiologic-pathologic correlation conference: SUNY upstate medical center. *AJR* 1986; 146:1246–1252.

94. Chakers DW: Computed tomography demonstration of a hypothalamic metastasis. *Neuroradiology* 1983; 25:103–104.

95. Fletcher WA, Ines RK, Hoyt W: Chiasmal gliomas: Appearance and long-term changes demonstrated by computerized tomography. *J Neurosurg* 1986; 65:154–159.

96. Housepian EM, Marquardt MD, Behrens M: Optic gliomas, in Wilkens RH, Rengachary SS (eds): *Neurosurgery*. New York, McGraw-Hill International Book Co, 1985, pp 916–921.

97. Ines RK, Hoyt WF: Childhood chiasmal gliomas: Update on the fate of patients in the 1969 San Francisco study. *Prog Exp Tumor Res* 1987; 30:108–112.

98. Weiss L, Sagerman RH, King GA, et al: Controversy in the management of optic nerve glioma. *Cancer* 1987; 59:1000–1004.

99. Davis PC, Hoffman JC, Weidenheim KM: Large hypothalamic and optic chiasm gliomas in infants: Difficulties in distinction. *AJNR* 1984; 5:579–585.

100. Gentry LR, Smoker WRK, Turski PA, et al: Suprasellar arachnoid cysts: I. CT recognition. *AJNR* 1986; 7:79–86.

101. Fox JL, Al-Mefty O: Suprasellar arachnoid cysts:

An extension of the membrane of Liliequist. *Neurosurgery* 1980; 7:615–618.

102. Reed LD, Abbas S, Markivee CR, et al: Neurosarcodosis responding to steroids. *AJR* 1986; 146:819–821.

103. Greco A, Steiner R: Magnetic resonance imaging in neurosarcodosis. *Magn Reson Imaging* 1987; 5:15–21.

104. Diebler C, Ponsot G: Hamartomas of the tuber cinereum. *Neuroradiology* 1983; 25:93–101.

105. Hahn FJ, Leibrock LG, Huseman CA, et al: The MR appearance of hypothalamic hamartoma. *Neuroradiology* 1988; 30:65–68.

106. Sato M, Ushio Y, Arita N, et al: Hypothalamic hamartoma: Report of two cases. *Neurosurgery* 1985; 16:198–206.

107. Kelly WM, Kucharczyk W, Kucharczyk J, et al: Posterior pituitary ectopia: An MR feature of pituitary dwarfism. *AJNR* 1988; 9:453–460.

108. Inoue Y, Nemoto Y, Fujita K, et al: Pituitary dwarfism: CT evaluation of the pituitary gland. *Radiology* 1986; 159:171–173.

PART IX

Cerebral Congenital Anomalies

24

Congenital Anomalies of the Brain

Richard E. Latchaw, M.D.

Jeffery P. Hogg, M.D.

Michael J. Painter, M.D.

A number of classifications of congenital abnormalities of the central nervous system (CNS) have been suggested such as the one by DeMyer (Table 24–1).[1, 2] While there is a significant body of accumulated knowledge regarding both normal embryogenesis and abnormal embryonic development, this knowledge and its associated classification systems are of limited value in the assessment of an individual case at presentation. A radiologist is a specialist in visual images and bases his differential diagnosis on specific visual findings or image patterns. Therefore, we have produced the classification of congenital cerebral abnormalities presented in Table 24–2, which organizes the abnormalities upon the presence of specific visually determined features. This classification allows the radiologist and clinician to establish the most appropriate differential diagnosis, given the pattern of findings on the magnetic resonance (MR) or computed tomographic (CT) images.

The most striking visual finding is used as the basis of organization. For example, dilatation of the third and lateral ventricles is the most dramatic aspect of aqueductal stenosis, and therefore the entity is listed with those conditions in which the most prominent finding is that of third and lateral ventricular dilatation. While schizencephaly may be associated with enlarged ventricles, the most dramatic radiographic finding is the presence of the hemispheric clefts. This entity is therefore listed under abnormalities presenting with lateral hemispheric defects within the category of craniocerebral malformations.

It is obvious that a particular anomaly could be placed into a number of categories. For example, the Chiari malformations, particularly Chiari II and Chiari III, obviously have gross distortion of multiple portions of the brain and therefore could be categorized with the craniocerebral malformations. However, the most dramatic finding in the Chiari II and III malformations at the time of *initial presentation* is the pronounced dilatation of the third and lateral ventricles. The Chiari II and III malformations are therefore listed under abnormalities presenting with increased ventricular size as a basis for differential diagnosis. The Chiari I malformation, however, may present with little or no ventricular dilatation, and is therefore listed under the cerebellar craniocerebral malformations, again for purposes of differential diagnosis.

Categories I through V are discussed at length in this chapter. The congenital tumors listed in category VI are discussed in Chapters 16 and 18 of this volume. Arachnoid cysts are discussed briefly in this chapter and more extensively in Chapter 17. The Sturge-Weber syndrome is discussed in Chapter 18 with the other phakomatoses, while the rest of the vascular lesions are dealt with in Chapter 11. Craniopharyngioma and Rathke's pouch cyst are discussed in Chapter 23.

TABLE 24–1.

Classification of Cerebral Malformations According to Developmental Stages*

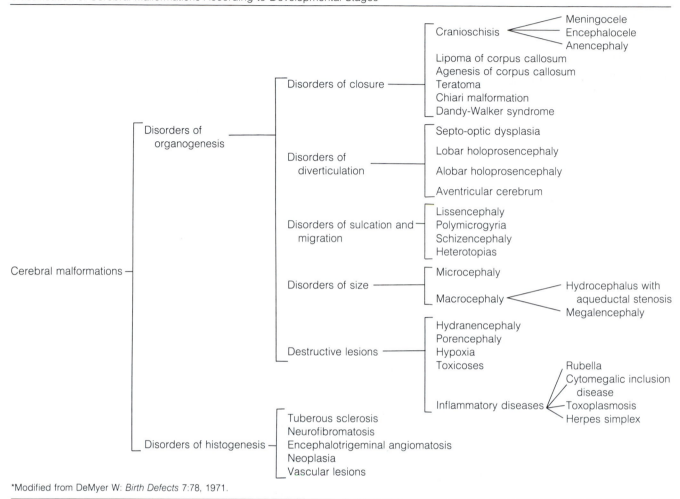

*Modified from DeMyer W: *Birth Defects* 7:78, 1971.

Patients with potential cerebral anomalies may be imaged either with MR imaging (MRI) or CT. While CT scanning has been available for a longer period of time and is clearly superior for detection of abnormal calcification, MRI is the procedure of choice.[3] MRI is better than CT for anatomic definition. Multiple high-quality projections of the brain are obtained routinely with MRI, whereas routine CT in sedated children is largely limited to the axial plane. Sagittal and coronal reformatting of axial CT images is possible but add technical time to the study and are of relatively poor quality when compared with MRI. The high-resolution sagittal and coronal MR images have proved well suited to the evaluation of midline defects and congenital anomalies.[4–6] MRI enjoys special advantage over CT in evaluation of the pediatric posterior fossa, site of the preponderance of pediatric tumors, as well as Dandy-Walker and Chiari malformations, in that troublesome beam-hardening artifact, which limits CT study of the posterior fossa, is not a feature of MR. Sagittal MRI allows the easy definition of the flow void of the normal aqueduct, or the lack thereof in aqueductal stenosis.[7] The kink of the cervicomedullary junction in the Chiari II malformation is easy to evaluate with sagittal MRI.[8] MRI also allows for definition of the surface of the brain in far better fashion than CT, again because beam-hardening artifact from the calvarial inner table with CT partially obscures adjacent cortical surface detail.[9] This is important in evaluating the lissencephaly syndromes.[10, 11]

MRI is better than CT in the differentiation and characterization of cerebral tissues. White matter is far better differentiated from gray matter, important for the appropriate evaluation of migra-

TABLE 24–2.

A Morphologic Approach to Brain Abnormalities During Development

I. Normal developmental midline variants
  A. Cavum septum pellucidum
  B. Cavum vergae
  C. Cavum velum interpositum
II. Increased ventricular size
  A. Third and/or lateral ventricles
    1. Aqueductal stenosis
    2. Chiari malformations
    3. Inflammatory obstruction
    4. Volume loss
  B. All ventricles
    1. Posterior fossa cysts
      a. Dandy-Walker complex
      b. Arachnoid cyst
      c. Prominent cisterna magna
      d. Trapped fourth ventricle
    2. Inflammatory obstruction
    3. Volume loss
III. Craniocerebral malformations
  A. Midline cerebral hemispheric abnormalities
    1. Holoprosencephaly
    2. Septo-optic dysplasia
    3. Agenesis of the corpus callosum
  B. Lateral cerebral hemispheric abnormalities
    1. Focal hypoplasia/aplasia
    2. Destructive lesions
      a. Agenetic porencephaly
        (1) Unilateral: porencephaly
        (2) Bilateral: schizencephaly
      b. Encephaloclastic porencephaly
      c. Perinatal/postnatal focal cavitation
    3. Heterotopic gray matter
  C. Cerebral cortical abnormalities
    1. Lissencephaly (agyria, pachygyria)
    2. Polymicrogyria
  D. Global hemispheric abnormalities
    1. Anencephaly
    2. Hydranencephaly
    3. Multicystic encephalomalacia
  E. Cerebellum
    1. Chiari I malformation
    2. Hypoplasia/aplasia
      a. Vermis
        (1) Dandy-Walker complex
        (2) Joubert syndrome
      b. Hemisphere
      c. Entire cerebellum
        (1) Hypoplasia
        (2) Aplasia: Chiari IV malformation
  F. Cranium and meninges
    1. Cranial dermal sinus
    2. Meningocele
    3. Encephalocele
    4. Craniosynostosis
IV. Global brain size
  A. Micrencephaly
  B. Megalencephaly
V. Brain maturation
VI. Neoplasms
  A. Teratomatous tumors: teratoma, germinoma, dermoid, epidermoid
  B. Hamartomas
  C. Lipoma
  D. Craniopharyngioma
  E. Neuroectodermal tumors
VII. Cysts
  A. Rathke's pouch cyst
  B. Neuroepithelial cyst
  C. Arachnoid cyst
VIII. Abnormal vasculature
  A. Arteriovenous malformation (including vein of Galen aneurysm)
  B. Encephalotrigeminal angiomatosis (Sturge-Weber syndrome)
  C. Aneurysm

tional disorders.[9, 12] Ectopic gray matter has a pathognomonic appearance on MRI, with relaxation parameters equal to superficial gray matter, allowing distinction from neoplastic tissue.[13–15] Different protein concentrations leading to different relaxation parameters allow distinction of a neoplastic cyst from an arachnoid cyst.[16, 17] Hamartomatous changes in the brain in patients with tuberous sclerosis or neurofibromatosis are far easier to see with MRI than with CT.[18] However, CT is certainly better for parenchymal calcifications.[3, 19] If it is important to determine the presence of subtle calcification, as in patients with postinflammatory changes, certain metabolic disorders, or in subtle cases of tuberous sclerosis, CT scanning is necessary.

For definition of the anatomic abnormalities of congenital malformations, and the characterization of accompanying tissue changes, MRI is the technique of choice.[8, 18, 20, 21] In this chapter the majority of illustrations are MR images. Reference to CT scans will be made, however, because of the extensive experience with this modality.

DEVELOPMENTAL VARIANTS

Three developmental variants that were frequently imaged with pneumoencephalography and that are now seen with CT and MR scanning are the cavum septum pellucidum (Fig 24–1), cavum vergae (see Fig 24–1), and cavum velum interpositum (Fig 24–2). The cavum septum pellucidum is a cerebrospinal fluid (CSF) collection located between the leaves of the septum pellucidum. The cavum generally communicates with one or both of

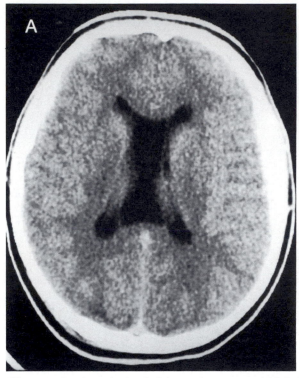

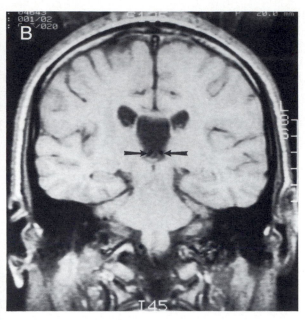

FIG 24–1.
Cavum septum pellucidum and cavum vergae. **A,** the axial CT scan demonstrates both a cavum septum pellucidum and a cavum vergae. **B,** a coronal MR scan (TR 700, TE 20) in a different patient is at the level of the cavum vergae which is located above the internal cerebral veins *(arrows)*. This distinguishes a cavum vergae from a cavum velum interpositum, through which course the internal cerebral veins.

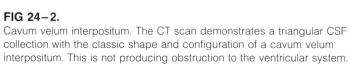

FIG 24–2.
Cavum velum interpositum. The CT scan demonstrates a triangular CSF collection with the classic shape and configuration of a cavum velum interpositum. This is not producing obstruction to the ventricular system.

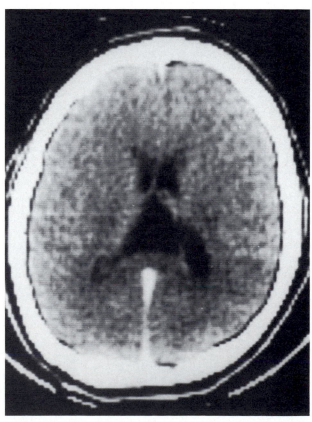

the lateral ventricles, so that it fills with air at the time of pneumoencephalography. It is commonly seen on the CT or MR scan of an infant. Autopsy studies have demonstrated a cavum septum pellucidum in 82% of neonates, with a progressive decrease in incidence with increasing age.[22] Ten percent of young infants have a cavum septum pellucidum on CT scan, but only 5% have this variant by age 2 years, paralleling the decreased autopsy incidence.[22] The cavum septum pellucidum may be large, laterally displacing normal-sized frontal horns. This is not a pathologic condition, the key being the lack of ventricular dilatation. Rarely, a cyst of the septum pellucidum may exist and lack communication with the ventricular system, produce obstruction of the foramina of Monro, and dilatation of the lateral ventricles.[23]

The cavum vergae is less frequent than the cavum septum pellucidum, being found in only 30% of newborns at autopsy.[22] While the cavum vergae may be an isolated variant, it is more commonly found in association with a cavum septum pellucidum (see Fig 24–1), with which it typically communicates. The cavum vergae has a flask shape on axial scans (Fig 24–1,A) in contradistinction to the triangular or trapezoidal shape of a cavum velum interpositum (see Fig 24–2).

The velum interpositum is the subarachnoid cistern lying above the third ventricle and below the corpus callosum that contains the internal cerebral veins and the posteromedial choroidal arteries. The cavum velum interpositum is a collection of CSF within this cistern. Air typically fills this cavum from the ambient and quadrigeminal cisterns rather than from the ventricles during pneumoencephalography. Coronal MRI demonstrates the internal cerebral veins within this cavum, whereas the internal cerebral veins are below a cavum vergae (Fig 24–1,B). A cavum velum interpositum may be large but there are no symptoms of mass effect, and of itself is of little significance. Rarely, a cyst of the cavum velum may arise, producing symptoms of mass effect.

INCREASED VENTRICULAR SIZE

Third and/or Lateral Ventricles

Aqueductal Stenosis

Russell described four types of congenital stenosis of the cerebral aqueduct: simple stenosis, gliosis, septum formation, and a forking deformity.[24] The first is a true stenosis without evidence of gli-

osis to suggest a postinflammatory etiology of the narrowed diameter. The presence of gliosis suggests an inflammatory etiology such as intrauterine mumps, influenza, parainfluenza 2, reovirus, or toxoplasma infection.[25] In the third type there is a neuroglial septum or web[24] which is sometimes treated by surgical perforation.[7] Forking of the aqueduct is characterized by two small channels separated by normal tissue. This form of aqueductal malformation has been described in patients with the Chiari II malformation, and is attributed to the compressive effects of the hydrocephalus.[7] The aqueduct was not seen or only faintly seen on sagittal MR images in 17 of 24 Chiari II patients in a recent study.[8]

Whatever the form of aqueductal stenosis, the resulting CT scan appearance is the same. There is dilatation of the third and lateral ventricles, with a small fourth ventricle. Such a disparity in ventricular size strongly suggests the presence of an aqueductal block. An enhanced CT scan fails to show evidence of neoplasm or other enhancing lesion in the region of the aqueduct.

MRI normally demonstrates a flow void in the aqueduct on short TR scans because of rapidly moving CSF, and uninterrupted hyperintensity on long TR/TE sequences. This flow void is commonly but not always interrupted or absent with aqueductal stenosis or obstruction (Fig 24–3).[7] Distal aqueductal obstruction from a membrane may produce a dilated proximal portion of the aqueduct in which there is a flow void on the short TR scan or on both it and the long TR/TE sequence secondary to CSF turbulence. Signal void in the third ventricle of a hydrocephalic patient on the long TR/TE scan may also be secondary to CSF turbulence.[26]

The MR flow void within the aqueduct is usually but not always missing with juxta-aqueductal pathology such as tumor. Tectal enlargement (the mean normal collicular thickness on midline sagittal T1-weighted images is 5 mm with a range of 2–7 mm) is seen with primary and secondary neoplasms, granulomatous disease, and hamartomas. Tectal enlargement is not seen in aqueductal stenosis due to a web or gliosis from an inflammatory cause. Many nondevelopmental lesions produce an abnormal signal on T2-weighted images. It is therefore important to obtain multiple views of the aqueduct, tentorial incisura, and posterior fossa with both T1-weighted and T2-weighted sequences when an aqueductal obstruction is suspected.

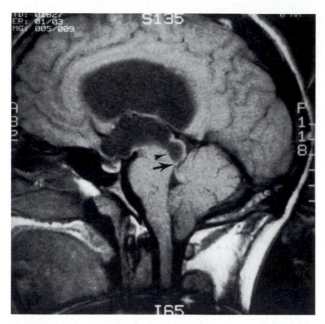

FIG 24–3.
Aqueductal stenosis. Sagittal MR scan (TR 700, TE 20) demonstrating a web in the distal aqueduct *(arrow)* producing a short length of obstruction. The proximal aqueduct *(arrowhead)* is dilated, as are the third and lateral ventricles, while the fourth ventricle is small. Note the inferior displacement of the cerebellar tonsils.

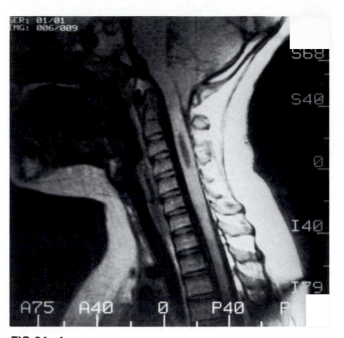

FIG 24–4.
Chiari I malformation and syringohydromyelia. Sagittal MR scan (TR 600, TE 20) showing the tips of the cerebellar tonsils extending down to the base of the odontoid. There is a cystic cavity within the cervical cord at the C3–4 level.

Chiari Malformations

Chiari originally described four malformations of the hindbrain. Type IV is severe cerebellar hypoplasia or aplasia, and is discussed later in this chapter. In the Chiari III malformation, the medulla, fourth ventricle, and cerebellum are displaced caudally into an upper cervical and occipital encephalocele; encephaloceles are also discussed later in this chapter. The Chiari II malformation commonly presents in infancy and is almost always associated with spinal or cranial dysraphism, or both. The Chiari I malformation is the mildest form and is frequently asymptomatic or presents with symptoms in adulthood.

Chiari I Malformation.—The Chiari I malformation is a dysplasia of the craniocervical junction. Logue and Edwards found craniovertebral junction anomalies, including atlantoaxial assimilation, high odontoid, short clivus, and Klippel-Feil deformity, in 37% of cases.[27, 28] Other authors have found basilar impression (25%–50%), assimilation of the atlas (10%), Klippel-Feil deformity (10%), and incomplete ossification of the C1 ring (5%).[18, 29] Syringohydromyelia (Fig 24–4) is present in 20% to 70% of cases, depending upon the series.[18, 29, 30] A low position of the medulla with a cervicomedul-

lary "kink" was said to be absent in the original series of Chiari I malformations described by Chiari.[31] However, it has been found in 12% of patients at the time of surgery,[32] and in 71% of all Chiari I patients imaged with MRI (and in 90% of those patients who also had syringohydromyelia).[30] Such a high percentage in patients imaged with MRI is probably due in part to the definition of a "kink" (anteroposterior angulation only or an overlap of the medulla and cervical cord) and in part to the ability to image the craniocervical junction in sagittal view in a noninvasive way. Meningomyelocele and encephalocele are almost never present with the Chiari I malformation. Hydrocephalus is present in 3%.[27, 28]

The diagnostic method of choice for the diagnosis of the Chiari I malformation is MRI.[30] T1-weighted images in the sagittal and coronal planes allow direct visualization of the cerebellar tonsils. MRI has demonstrated that the tonsils may normally project below the foramen magnum to a slight degree. In a recent study of 200 normal subjects and 25 patients with the Chiari I malformation, the cerebellar tonsils were found to lie from 8 mm above to 5 mm below the foramen magnum, with a mean position of 1 mm above the foramen. Utilizing 2 mm below the foramen magnum as the threshold for normality, there was a 100% prediction of symptomatic patients, with a specificity of 98.5% and a false-positive rate of 1.5% and no false-negatives.[33]

The caudally displaced tonsils may be either enlarged and rounded (Fig 24–5) or pointed (Fig 24–6). The pointed shape of the cerebellar tonsils and the compactness of tissue within the foramen magnum were considered in the past to be valuable predictors of symptomatology when the measurement of the tonsillar tips was equivocal.[29, 33] In the same study of 200 normal subjects and 25 patients with a Chiari I malformation cited previously, all patients with protrusion of the tonsils greater than 1 mm demonstrated narrowing or loss of the CSF spaces within the foramen magnum. Pointed tonsils were seen in both symptomatic and asymptomatic patients. Therefore, configuration of tissue and effacement of CSF in the foramen magnum may be misleading.[33]

The medulla is either normal in location or mildly displaced inferiorly; an anteroposterior kink of the cervicomedullary junction may be present in up to 90% of cases.[30] The fourth ventricle varies from a normal position to mild inferior displacement. There is usually no hydrocephalus or very mild ventricular enlargement secondary to the slight elongation of the fourth ventricle and aqueduct, with the tissue compaction at the foramen magnum preventing free flow of CSF.

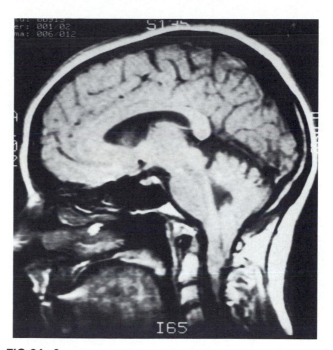

FIG 24–6.
Chiari I malformation with pointed tonsils. Sagittal MRI (TR 700, TE 20) demonstrates the tip of the cerebellar tonsils extending down to below the base of the odontoid. The tonsils are pointed in configuration and the foramen magnum appears "tight," but there is no hydrocephalus. There is a small "bump" at the junction of the tonsils with the upper cervical cord.

CT scanning of the foramen magnum region is less precise for demonstration of the tonsillar tips than is MRI. Spatial and contrast resolution is limited, and while direct coronal imaging may be possible, direct sagittal imaging is not possible in most adults and reformatted imaging is suboptimal. CT scanning in the axial and coronal projections following the instillation of a water-soluble contrast medium into the thecal sac will facilitate demonstration of the position of the tonsils (Fig 24–7). Five cubic centimeters of 140 mgI/mL nonionic contrast material is used in this procedure, which may be performed on an outpatient basis.

Just as there is a spectrum of what anatomically constitutes the Chiari I malformation and its distinction from the Chiari II malformation, there is a spectrum of symptomatology with the Chiari I malformation. The abnormal tonsillar position may be an incidental finding in an asymptomatic patient, or the symptoms may be more referable to the cervical spinal cord than to the cervicomedullary junction. Other patients may present with vague posterior fossa signs and symptoms suggesting intrinsic cerebellar or brain stem disease.[33] The symptomatology and the age of presentation frequently suggest a presumptive diagnosis of multi-

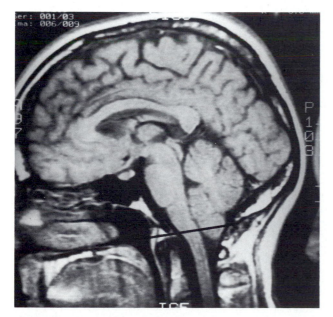

FIG 24–5.
Chiari I malformation with enlarged rounded tonsils. Sagittal MRI (TR 600, TE 20) demonstrates rounded and enlarged cerebellar tonsils extending 5 mm below a line drawn from the hard palate to the posteroinferior bony margin of the foramen magnum.

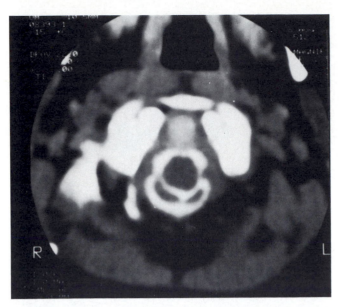

FIG 24–7.
Chiari I malformation with low cerebellar tonsils demonstrated on CT scanning with intrathecal contrast material. Five cubic centimeters of 140 mgI/mL water-soluble contrast material was injected intrathecally in the lumbar region and run into the cervical region for scanning of the cervicomedullary junction. The cerebellar tonsils are seen behind the medulla on this scan just below the foramen magnum. The tips of the tonsils extended down to the base of the odontoid. There appears to be sufficient room for the neural structures within the foramen magnum.

ple sclerosis.[18, 33] The clinician and the radiologist must have a high degree of suspicion for the presence of the Chiari I malformation so that appropriate imaging studies are performed, particularly MRI. The correct diagnosis may result in occipital and high cervical decompression which may relieve the symptomatology.

Chiari II Malformation.—The Chiari II malformation is a complex malformation affecting calvarium, dura, cerebellum, mesencephalon, diencephalon, and telencephalon. The vast majority of patients present in the newborn period. Over 99% of patients with myelomeningocele or encephalocele have a Chiari II malformation with hydrocephalus.[34, 35] Given a Chiari II malformation, most patients have spinal or cranial dysraphism. However, cases diagnosed as the Chiari II malformation in the older child or adult without dysraphism have occurred. Obviously, in cases without the complete spectrum of changes classically seen in the Chiari II malformation, there is a spectrum of hindbrain abnormalities between the Chiari II and Chiari I malformations, with the particular designation dependent upon the degree of dis-

placement of cerebellar tonsils, brain stem, cerebellar vermis, and fourth ventricle.

No theory of pathogenesis has been universally accepted to explain this malformation. Numerous authors have attempted to link the malformation to spinal dysraphism, including myelomeningocele and tethering of the spinal cord. However, some patients have a Chiari II malformation without dysraphism, and the earliest embryologic evidence of the malformation is at 10 weeks of gestation, far later than the earliest evidence of spina bifida.[34] Others have proposed intrauterine hydrocephalus as the underlying and unifying mechanism of the Chiari malformation and myelomeningocele. However, there are many observations that contradict this theory.[1]

There is a small posterior fossa, with a low insertion of the tentorium on the petrous bones (Fig 24–8) and just above the foramen magnum. The foramen magnum is enlarged, whereas the diameter of the C1 segment is small and its posterior arch is incomplete in 70% of patients.[34] The medulla is inferiorly displaced, and there is kinking of the cervicomedullary junction (Figs 24–8 and 24–9). The spinal cord is displaced inferiorly, and the upper cervical nerve roots are directed superiorly.[34] The cerebellar tonsils are displaced inferiorly to a marked degree, as low as the upper thoracic spine. Behind the cerebellar tonsils, the cerebellar vermis is displaced inferiorly. Sagittal MRI has demonstrated abnormal signal in this displaced vermis, consistent with gliotic, hemorrhagic, and ischemic changes.[21, 34] These inferiorly displaced tissues form layers, so that in the upper cervical region there is, from anterior to posterior, spinal cord, medulla, cerebellar tonsils, and vermis. The fourth ventricle is elongated and displaced inferiorly (Figs 24–9, 24–10), and there may be a fourth ventricular diverticulum which forms an additional layer behind the cerebellar vermis.[8, 34]

Syringohydromyelia is present in 40% to 95% of patients depending upon the study.[34, 35] MRI now reveals the high incidence of this cystic abnormality of the spinal cord, even without cord enlargement.[8]

Medullary compression within the first 6 months of life may present as vocal cord paralysis, strider, apnea, and feeding problems, and may be life-threatening. Neurologic presentations after 6 months of age tend to be limb pareses and spasticity, and eye movement disorders.[36, 37] If the medullary kink is at the C3–4 disc space level or lower, there is a significant chance of the patient

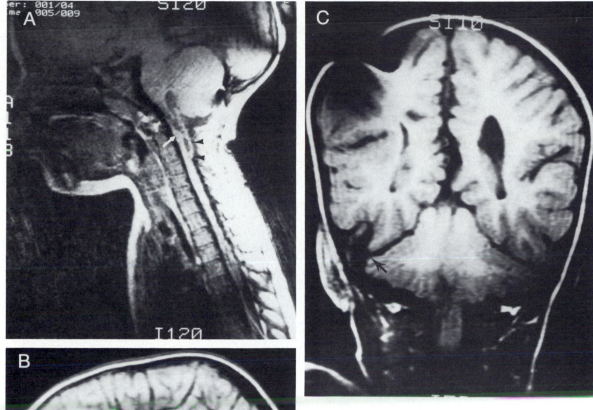

FIG 24–8.
Chiari II malformation. **A,** T1-weighted sagittal MRI at the craniocervical junction (TR 600, TE 20) shows an overlap of medulla and upper cervical spinal cord *(arrow)* in the upper cervical spine. It is difficult to distinguish medulla from spinal cord. There is inferior displacement of cerebellar tonsils *(arrowheads),* with the tips extending down to the C3 level. **B,** sagittal imaging of the head (TR 700, TE 20) demonstrates the beaked colliculi *(arrow),* the enlarged massa intermedia *(arrowhead),* and hypoplasia of the body of the corpus callosum with aplasia of the splenium. **C,** coronal imaging (TR 700, TE 20) shows the low position of the tentorium on the right petrous bone *(arrow),* and the towering of the cerebellum through the widened tentorial incisura. The falx is hypoplastic and the interhemispheric fissure is wavy.

developing symptomatic brain stem or corticospinal tract dysfunction.[21] Compression at the craniovertebral junction is in part due to the anatomic relationships of the neural tissues to the overlying bony structures. The subarachnoid space at the craniovertebral junction is effaced, and has been observed to increase with age; thus, as the child grows, the likelihood of neural compression decreases somewhat.[21] In addition, MR studies with surgical correlation have demonstrated a trans-verse dural band attached to the laminae of the C1 arch posteriorly.[21, 34] Basilar impression and C1 assimilation to the occiput, common features in the Chiari I malformation, are not observed in Chiari II.[34]

Even though the cerebellum is abnormally small in Chiari II patients,[38] there is little room for the cerebellum within the small posterior fossa. The cerebellum wraps around the medulla and pons, and extends superiorly through the capa-

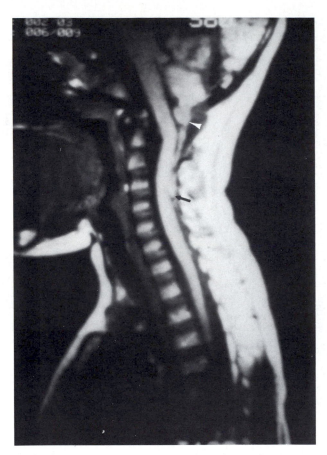

FIG 24–9.
Chiari II malformation with cervicomedullary "kink." The T1-weighted MR sagittal view demonstrates an overlap of the inferiorly displaced medulla and upper cervical spinal cord at the C2 level. It is difficult to distinguish displaced medulla from compressed cervical cord. The tips of the cerebellar tonsils *(arrow)* extend down to C4, the cerebellar vermis *(arrowhead)* extends through the foramen magnum, and the fourth ventricle is markedly elongated and caudally displaced into the lower posterior fossa and upper spinal canal. (Courtesy of Dr. Sylvester Chuang, Toronto.)

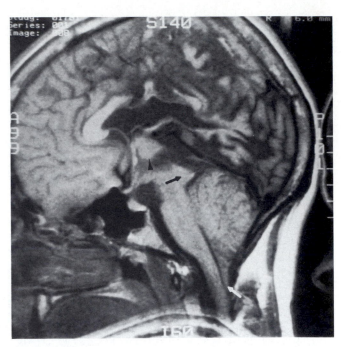

FIG 24–10.
Chiari II malformation with elongated fourth ventricle. The sagittal MR scan (TR 600, TE 20) demonstrates the inferior displacement of the cerebellar tonsils *(white arrow)*, the markedly flattened and elongated fourth ventricle, the "beaking" of the colliculi *(black arrow)*, and the enlarged massa intermedia *(arrowhead)*. The midportion of the body of the corpus callosum is markedly hypoplastic and the splenium is small. There is marked hypoplasia of the medial parietal gyri and subcortical white matter.

cious tentorial incisura ("bullet-nosed cerebellum") (Figs 24–8, 24–11, and 24–12). The quadrigeminal plate is either bulbous or beaked, with the tip of the beak inserting into a notch in the superior vermis (Figs 24–8, 24–10, and 24–13).[8] The deformed colliculi are partially or totally fused. These changes are more apparent after a shunting procedure has relieved the impaction. The aqueduct of Sylvius, underlying the deformed colliculi, is severely shortened and its lumen becomes irregular and tortuous ("forked").[39]

Hydrocephalus is an important feature of the Chiari II malformation, requiring early shunting in the majority of patients. The cause of the hydrocephalus remains controversial. The aqueduct may be intrinsically abnormal, as described previous-

ly.[39] Some argue that the herniation of the medial temporal and occipital lobes over the edges of the widened tentorial hiatus produces hydrocephalus by compressing and deforming the mesencephalon.[35, 40] The fourth ventricle is elongated craniocaudally and narrowed transversely and the caudal aspect may be either effaced or dilated to form a diverticulum.[8, 34] There is evidence of a significant incidence of fourth ventricular outlet obstruction in Chiari II patients.[41] Hydrocephalus, therefore, may be a result of any or all of these abnormalities.

The third ventricle appears to be disproportionately smaller than the lateral ventricles because of compression by enlarged thalami and a large massa intermedia (Figs 24–8, 24–10, and 24–14).[8, 20, 42] There may also be an enlarged suprapineal recess that herniates through the tentorial incisura into the posterior fossa. An accessory commissure (Meynert's commissure) lies between the anterior commissure and the chiasm, and was frequently demonstrable by thin-section sagittal tomography during pneumoencephalography when this procedure was performed.

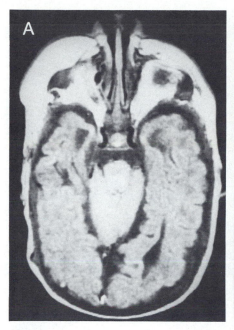
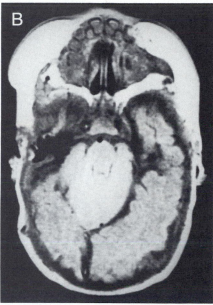
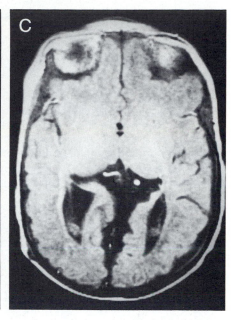

FIG 24–11.
Chiari II malformation with circummedullary cerebellum and en-larged retrothalamic cisterns. **A,B,** axial MR images (TR 600, TE 20) demonstrate the cerebellum wrapping around the medulla and lower pons. **C,** at a higher level there is confluence of the cisterns of the quadrigeminal plate, vein of Galen, velum interpositum, and superior cerebellar vermis with the enlarged wings of the ambient cisterns to produce a diamond-shaped CSF space.

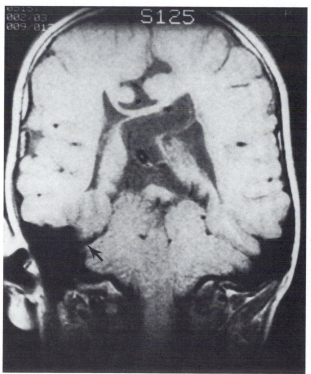

FIG 24–12.
Chiari II malformation with towering cerebellum and gyral interdigitation. The coronal T1-weighted MR scan (TR 700, TE 20) demonstrates the low position of the tentorium *(arrow)* relative to the right petrous bone. There is an enlarged tentorial incisura, with towering of the cerebellar hemispheres into the supratentorial compartment. The superior cerebellar cisterns and the cisterns of the great vein of Galen and the quadrigeminal plate are enlarged. A hypoplastic falx allows the interdigitation of the gyri and the wavy interhemispheric fissure.

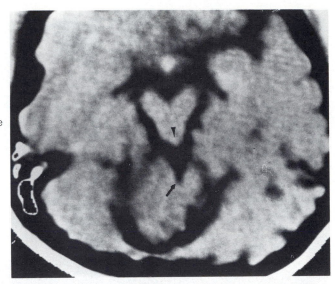

FIG 24–13.
Chiari II malformation. An axial slice through the quadrigeminal plate and superior cerebellar vermis, depicted with a reversed window, nicely demonstrates the combined collicular fusion and mesencephalic beaking *(arrowhead)* and the notch in the superior cerebellar vermis *(arrow)*.

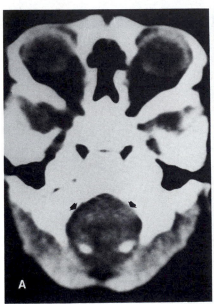

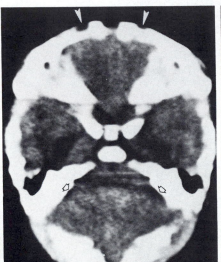

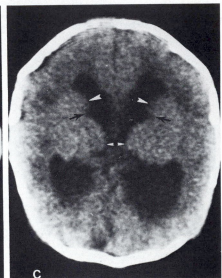

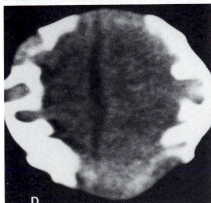

FIG 24–14.
Chiari II malformation. Bony changes include enlargement of the foramen magnum (**A,** *black arrows*), scalloping of the petrous bones (**B,** *open arrows*), and craniolacunia (lückenschädel) (**B,** *white arrowheads;* **D).** Ventricular changes include lack of visualization of the fourth ventricle (**B),** and the "figure-3" configuration of the frontal horns and third ventricle (**C).** This figure-3 configuration in **C** is produced by enlargement of the caudate nuclei *(large white arrowheads),* enlargement of the thalami *(small white arrowheads),* a relatively small third ventricle secondary to the thalamic enlargement, and "pointing" of the frontal horns *(black arrows).*

The frontal horns of the lateral ventricles appear to be smaller than the bodies because of enlarged caudate nuclei. These caudate impressions produce "pointing" along the lateral margins of the frontal horns.[34] When combined with the prominent concavity of the third ventricle produced by the thalami, a "figure-3" configuration is produced (see Fig 24–14). There is also pointing of the floors of the lateral ventricles, seen in the coronal projection.[8] The septum pellucidum may be totally or partially absent.

The posterior portions of the lateral ventricles appear to be disproportionately enlarged (see Fig 24–14). This may well be due to the absence of the splenium of the corpus callosum. While this structure is said to be missing in 12% to 16% of pa-

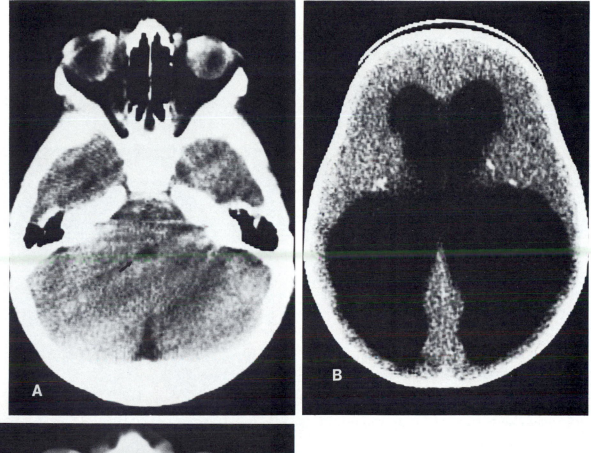

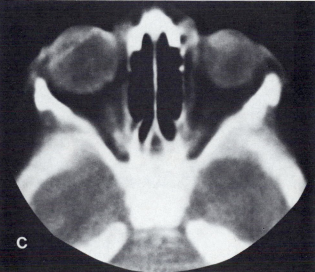

FIG 24–15.
Congenital rubella. This 15-month-old child had an enlarging head and positive titers for rubella. There is a small fourth ventricle (**A**, *arrow*), while there is marked enlargement of the third and lateral ventricles **(B)**, indicative of an aqueductal obstruction by inflammatory tissue. Periventricular calcifications are present **(B)**, indicating foci of inflammation. The left globe is small **(C)**, and there is a prominent lens.

tients,[8, 35] MRI has demonstrated hypoplasia of the splenium in a large proportion of patients (see Figs 24–8 and 24–10). A lack of development of the white matter tracts in the medial portions of the parietal lobes (see Fig 24–10) may allow the disproportionate enlargement of the posterior horns. Following ventricular shunting, confluence of the cisterns of the vein of Galen, velum interpositum, superior vermis, and ambient wings produce a prominent diamond-shaped CSF space (see Figs 24–11 and 24–12). Again, this may be due to the relative hypoplasia of the medial portions of the parietal lobes and hypoplasia of the splenium.

Additional abnormalities include hypoplasia and fenestration of the falx (see Fig 24–8), allowing for interdigitation of the medial portions of the cerebral hemispheres in up to 100% of patients (see Fig 24–12).[43] This produces a wavy appearance of the interhemispheric fissure.

Craniolacunia *(lückenschädel)* is present in at least 85% of patients with the Chiari II malformation (see Fig 24–14). These bony impressions have a gyral appearance, but are not secondary to increased intracranial pressure. Whether or not there is hydrocephalus, these digital markings regress by 6 months of age. They are differentiated from digital impressions secondary to increased intracranial pressure by the sharpness of the margins of the craniolacuniae early after birth, by being present on both inner and outer tables of the calvarium, and by their natural regression.

Migrational anomalies of the cerebral hemispheres are said to be present in up to 92% of patients,[35] reflecting the diffuse insult to the brain in early gestation. It must be emphasized that the Chiari II malformation is not just an abnormality of the hindbrain; this is a diffuse abnormality involving many aspects of the neural tube.

Inflammatory Obstruction

Intrauterine inflammatory disease, whether bacterial, viral, or protozoal, may produce scarring which can obstruct the foramen of Monro leading to lateral ventricular enlargement, or obstruct the aqueduct to produce lateral and third ventricular dilatation.[24, 44] Intrauterine infectious diseases affecting the brain have been denoted by the mnemonic TORCHS (*t*oxoplasmosis, *o*ther, *r*ubella, *c*ytomegalovirus [CMV], *h*erpes, *s*yphilis). Any of these disease entities may produce calcifications that are punctate, nodular, or confluent and that may be located in cortical, subcortical, or periventricular regions or a combination of these locations

(Figs 24–15 to 24–19).[45] Acquired immunodeficiency syndrome (AIDS) secondary to the human immunodeficiency virus (HIV) should be added to the list of congenital infectious diseases affecting the brain.[46] One could add the A of AIDS to the TORCHS mnemonic and drop the nonspecific O to make STARCH. Congenital HIV infection produces a diffuse hazy calcification of the brain on CT examination in contradistinction to the adult form of AIDS encephalopathy in which calcification does not occur (see Chapter 12).

Ventricular enlargement may be secondary to obstruction (see Fig 24–15), but tissue destruction and loss may also be present including multicystic encephalopathy (see Fig 24–16). Both toxoplasmosis and CMV infection produce periventricular calcifications. In general, toxoplasmosis also has more

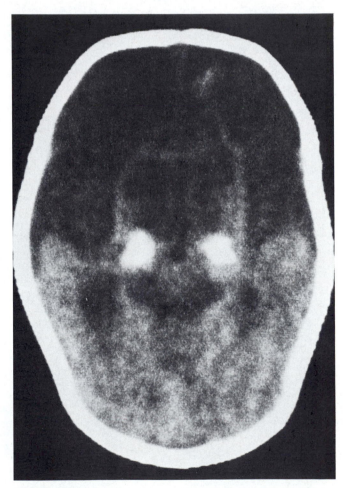

FIG 24–16.
Congenital herpes encephalitis. This 4-month-old child had cutaneous herpes and was born of a mother with genital herpes. The scan demonstrates extensive cystic encephalomalacia involving both frontal lobes, dilatations of the frontal horns, and thalamic calcifications bilaterally.

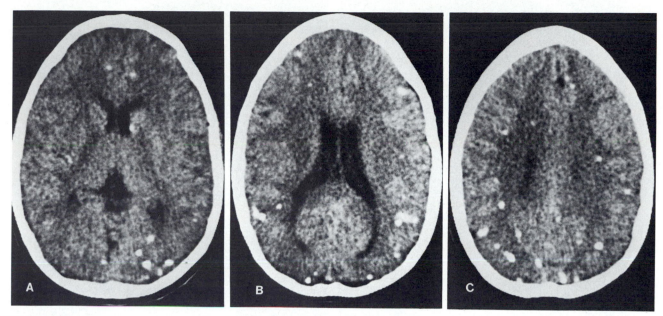

FIG 24–17.
Congenital toxoplasmosis. **A–C,** the CT scan demonstrates multiple parenchymal calcifications throughout both cerebral hemispheres. A few periventricular calcifications (**A** and **B**) are also present. The patient had high toxoplasmosis titers and the findings of chorioretinitis typical of toxoplasmosis.

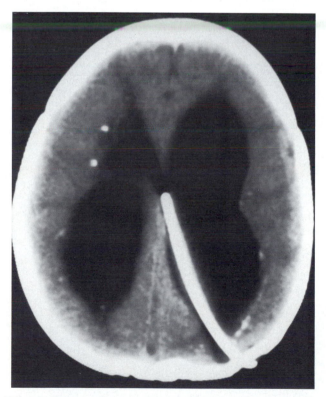

FIG 24–18.
Congenital cytomegalovirus (CMV) infection with Chiari malformation. This nonenhanced CT scan demonstrates periventricular calcifications, and the patient had high CMV titers. She also had a myelomeningocele and the Chiari II malformation accounting for the ventricular dilatation.

diffuse calcifications (see Fig 24–17) while CMV is limited to the periventricular regions (see Fig 24–18).[45] Further, if ventricular obstruction and an enlarged head is present, it is usually due to toxoplasmosis producing aqueductal obstruction[47, 48] rather than CMV, which usually leads to atrophy and microcephaly; however, aqueductal obstruction occasionally can occur with CMV. The presence of multiple calcifications requires evaluation for intrauterine infection, including serologic tests for syphilis, toxoplasmosis, rubella, herpes, and CMV; evaluation of the retinas for the chorioretinitis of toxoplasmosis and the optic atrophy of rubella (see Figs 24–15, 24–19); and evaluation of the urine for CMV.

Congenital infection is only one of a number of etiologies leading to cerebral calcifications. Table 24–3, without attempting to be exhaustive, lists other causes, including trauma and infarction; metabolic causes such as hypothyroidism, pseudohypoparathyroidism, and pseudopseudohypoparathyroidism, Fahr's disease, Cockayne's syndrome, mitochondrial encephalopathies including the MELAS (*m*itochondrial myopathy, *e*ncephalopathy, *l*actic *a*cidosis, and *s*trokelike episodes) and MERRLA (*m*yoclonus, *e*pilepsy, *r*agged *r*ed fibers, and *l*actic *a*cidosis) syndromes; and the phakomatoses (especially Sturge-Weber syndrome and tuberous sclerosis).[49–60]

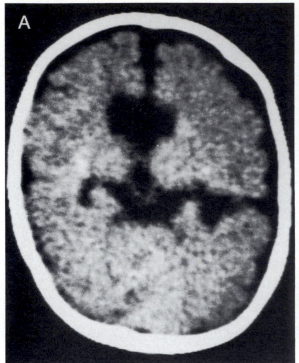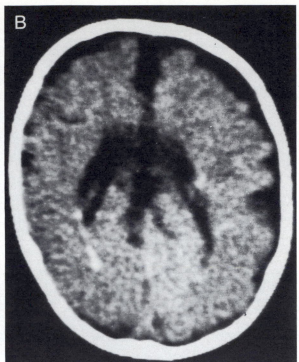

FIG 24–19.
Congenital rubella infection with schizencephaly. **A** and **B,** the nonenhanced CT scan demonstrates multiple periventricular calcifications. The patient had optic atrophy and high rubella titers on serologic testing. There is also schizencephaly of the left hemisphere, with a cortical defect extending from the left parietal surface to the left ventricular atrium, along with a missing septum pellucidum **(A)** and an unusual configuration of the bodies of the lateral ventricles **(B).** The diffuse volume loss is secondary to the intrauterine rubella infection.

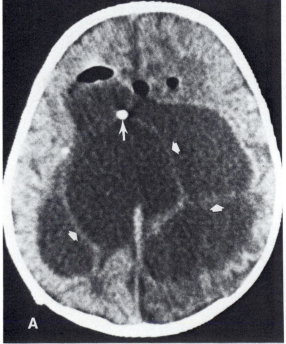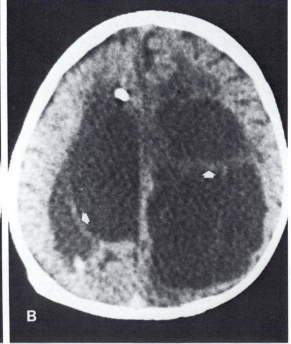

FIG 24–20.
Postinflammatory intraventricular membranes. Perinatal infection has produced multiple intraventricular adhesions (**A** and **B,** *small arrows*), which obstruct portions of the lateral ventricles. A single shunt tube (**A,** *large arrow*) is ineffectual at decompressing the entire ventricular system.

TABLE 24–3.
Etiologies of Intracranial Calcifications

I. Inflammatory
   A. Intrauterine infection: TORCHS (?STARCH)
      1. Syphilis
      2. Toxoplasmosis
      3. Acquired immunodeficiency syndrome (AIDS)
      4. Other
      5. Rubella
      6. Cytomegalovirus (CMV)
      7. Herpesvirus
   B. Neonatal infection
II. Metabolic/hereditary
   A. Hypoparathyroidism
      1. Hypoparathyroidism
      2. Pseudohypoparathyroidism
      3. Pseudopseudohypoparathyroidism
   B. Hypothyroidism
   C. Fahr's disease
   D. Cockayne's syndrome
   E. Mitochondrial encephalopathies
      1. MELAS syndrome
      2. MERRLA syndrome
III. Vascular
   A. Arteriovenous malformation
   B. Infarction
IV. Trauma
   A. Extracerebral organized hemorrhage
   B. Posttraumatic encephalomalacia
V. Phakomatoses
   A. Sturge-Weber syndrome
   B. Tuberous sclerosis
   C. Neurofibromatosis
VI. Tumors
   A. Glial
      1. Astrocytoma
      2. Oligodendroglioma
   B. Primitive neuroectodermal tumor (PNET)
      1. Medulloblastoma
      2. Pineocytoma/pineoblastoma
      3. Glial form
   C. Others; see Chapter 18

TORCHS = *toxoplasmosis, other, rubella, cytomegalovirus; herpes, syphillis;* STARCH = *syphilis, toxoplasmosis, AIDS, rubella, cytomegalovirus, herpes;* MELAS = *mitochondrial myopathy, encephalopathy, lactic acidosis, strokelike episodes;* MERRLA = *myoclonus, epilepsy, ragged red fibers, lactic acidosis.*

Intraventricular membranes may be congenital in origin as a result of intrauterine inflammatory disease (Fig 24–20).[61] Such membranes may be extremely difficult to see on the CT scan because they are so thin relative to the large volume of CSF. It is important to detect the membranes, because multiple loculations within the ventricular system will require several shunts for ventricular decompression. When membranes are visualized, ventriculography with a water-soluble contrast agent is of great value in determining the degree of communication of the various compartments.

Volume Loss

Atrophic processes involving primarily the cerebrum will lead to dilatation of the lateral ventricles only or both the third and lateral ventricles. A common etiology is that of perinatal hypoxic-ischemic events, with the scan demonstrating ventricular enlargement with multiple areas of encephalomalacia. There may or may not be enlargement of cortical sulci in the neonatal period. Other congenital etiologies of diffuse atrophy include intrauterine infection and the intrauterine exposure to toxins.

All Ventricles

Posterior Fossa Cysts

Many terms have been used for the variety of posterior fossa cysts, including *Dandy-Walker malformation, Dandy-Walker variant,*[62] *mega cisterna magna,*[63] *arachnoid cyst,* and *Blake's pouch,*[62, 64] among others. All of the abnormalities are based upon maldevelopment of the cerebellar vermis or hemispheres; maldevelopment of the fourth ventricle, the tela choroidea, and its perforation (the foramen of Magendie); and the surrounding meningeal coverings including the cisterna magna, tentorium, and falx cerebelli. In-depth discussions of the embryology of this region are provided by Raybaud[65] and by Barkovich et al.[66]

Raybaud has classified the posterior fossa cysts using a combination of anatomic configuration and CSF flow patterns.[65] In his schema, the fundamental lesion in both the classic Dandy-Walker malformation and the Dandy-Walker variant is vermian agenesis. In the classic Dandy-Walker malformation, the foramen of Magendie is imperforate, and there is no communication between the fourth ventricle–cyst complex and the perimedullary CSF spaces. There is always hydrocephalus. In the Dandy-Walker variant, the foramen of Magendie is open and there is communication between the fourth ventricle–cyst and the perimedullary CSF spaces. The degree of expansion within the posterior fossa is less than with the classic malformation, and hydrocephalus only occurs in approximately one third of patients.

The two Dandy-Walker malformations are distinguished from the group of arachnoid pouches by Raybaud.[65] Here, as in the Dandy-Walker malformations, the tela choroidea evaginates posteriorly, but the inferior vermis is intact. Three subcategories of arachnoid pouches are described. In the first, there is free communication between the pouch or cyst and both the fourth ventricle and the subarachnoid spaces. In the second, there is communication only with the fourth ventricle but not with the perimedullary CSF spaces, conforming to what Blake originally described (Blake's pouch). Finally, if there is no communication between the cystic space and the fourth ventricle or the other CSF spaces, the enclosed cyst is called an *arachnoid cyst*. Hydrocephalus is present in the majority of cases with arachnoid pouches.

Barkovich and colleagues have attempted to classify posterior fossa "cysts" primarily by their anatomic appearance on MRI, dividing them into three categories.[66] They believe that the variety of posterior fossa expansions in communication with the fourth ventricle are all part of a continuum which they call the *Dandy-Walker complex*. Hence, all cases previously called the classic Dandy-Walker malformation, the Dandy-Walker variant, and the mega cisterna magna are part of this spectrum. They divide this category into two types. In type A, the inferior vermis is either markedly hypoplastic or less hypoplastic but rotated, both of which result in a wide-open communication between the fourth ventricle and the cystic expansion. In type B, the inferior vermis is less hypoplastic and/or less malrotated, resulting in interposition of a portion of the vermis between the fourth ventricle and the enlarged cyst/cisterna magna. Almost all patients with type A have hydrocephalus, and half of the type B patients have hydrocephalus. There is an increased size of the posterior fossa in all patients.

The second category of Barkovich et al. includes patients with discrete posterior fossa CSF collections that do not communicate directly with the fourth ventricle. There is no vermian or cerebellar hemispheric dysgenesis, but displacement by mass effect may be present. This category is analogous to cases described as noncommunicating arachnoid cysts.

Finally, the term *prominent cisterna magna* is used for an acquired condition producing atrophy of the cerebellar vermis and hemispheres, resulting in an increased size of CSF spaces but no posterior fossa expansion and no hydrocephalus. Communication among all the CSF spaces is normal.[66]

According to Barkovich et al.,[66] the distinctions among the various entities described in their Dandy-Walker complex do not really matter clinically. If hydrocephalus or focal mass effect is present, shunting of either the ventricles or the cyst or both will be performed. If a closed noncommunicating cyst is present, the cyst will either be shunted or resected.

The key to this terminologic dilemma is the role of CSF dynamics. While Raybaud has attempted to classify the cysts in part on the basis of CSF flow dynamics, Barkovich and co-workers have attempted to unify a number of entities precisely upon the effect those dynamics have on the rest of the ventricular system and on underlying neural tissue. The following description will follow the classification of Barkovich et al. All of these entities are to be distinguished from an acquired trapped fourth ventricle, secondary to inflammatory obstruction of the foramina of Luschka and Magendie.

Dandy-Walker Complex

Type A.—There is partial or complete absence of the inferior vermis; with lesser degrees of hypoplasia there may be rotation of the inferior vermis so that there is a widely patent communication between the posterior fossa cystic expansion and

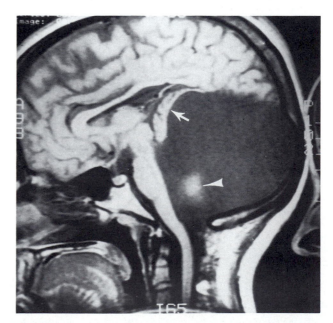

FIG 24–21.
Dandy-Walker complex (type A or "classic"). The sagittal MR scan (TR 700, TE 20) demonstrates a huge posterior fossa cystic expansion. The remaining superior cerebellar vermis *(arrow)* is markedly displaced anteriorly and superiorly while there is a remnant of cerebellar tissue inferiorly *(arrowhead)*. There is upward displacement of the tentorium and torcula, anterior displacement of the brain stem, and posterior and inferior bowing of the occipital bone by this large expansion.

the fourth ventricle.[66] The superior vermis is commonly present, although it may be displaced superiorly.[67] This feature is best appreciated on sagittal MRI (Fig 24–21).[68] While the cystic expansion is in continuity with the fourth ventricle, communication with other CSF spaces is not present, and hydrocephalus is almost always present.[65, 66, 69–71] The cerebellar hemispheres are hypoplastic and displaced anteriorly (Fig 24–22). There is a high torcula and tentorium, and dolichocephaly is common secondary to the bulging occiput.[67] However, there is a great deal of variability in the size of the cyst, the degree of hydrocephalus, and the position of the tentorium and torcula.[65, 72, 73]

Type B.—In this type, the inferior vermis is interposed between the cyst and the fourth ventricle. It may be hypoplastic, with or without rotation (Figs 24–23 and 24–24), or intact (Fig 24–25).[66] Cases with inferior vermian hypoplasia have previously been called the Dandy-Walker variant or a mega cisterna magna. The case in Figure 24–25 with anterior displacement of an intact vermis

would probably have been previously labeled as a communicating form of arachnoid cyst, a mega cisterna magna, or an arachnoid pouch (type proportional to the forms of communication between it and the surrounding CSF spaces). The cerebellar hemispheres may be normal or slightly hypoplastic. Hydrocephalus is present in approximately one half of these cases.[66]

Common Findings in the Dandy-Walker Complex.—Cerebral angiography of patients with the Dandy-Walker complex typically demonstrates hypoplasia of the posteroinferior cerebellar arteries. The degree of hypoplasia is proportional to the degree of hypoplasia of the inferior vermis and cerebellar hemispheres.[74,75] Use of water-soluble contrast material placed either into the lateral ventricles or the posterior fossa cyst, either by direct puncture or by a shunt tube within the CSF space, may be of value in determining the degree of communication between the ventricular system and the posterior fossa cyst. An evaluation of these flow dynamics may be useful in determining the need

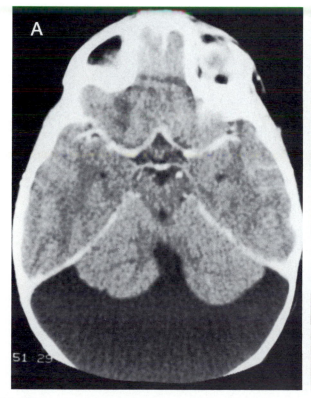 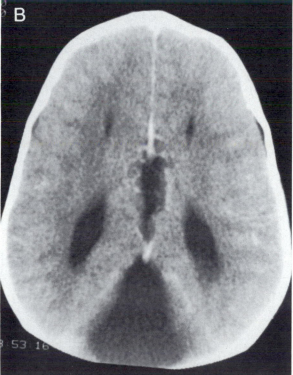

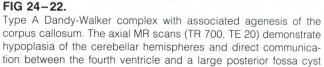

FIG 24–22.
Type A Dandy-Walker complex with associated agenesis of the corpus callosum. The axial MR scans (TR 700, TE 20) demonstrate hypoplasia of the cerebellar hemispheres and direct communication between the fourth ventricle and a large posterior fossa cyst

(A). A higher cut demonstrates parallel lateral ventricles and displacement of the third ventricle superiorly through a partially agenetic corpus callosum **(B)**.

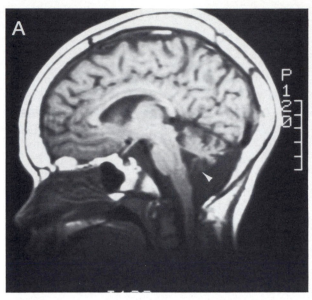

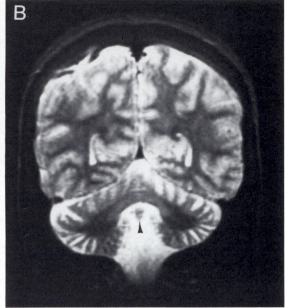

FIG 24–23.
Dandy-Walker complex, type B. **A,** the sagittal short TR MR scan (TR 600, TE 20) shows a hypoplastic but intact inferior vermis *(arrowhead)* interposed between a normal-sized fourth ventricle and a prominent retrocerebellar CSF space. There is mild expansion of the inner table of the occipital bone. **B,** the long TR/TE coro-nal study (TR 2,500, TE 80) shows the intact but hypoplastic inferior vermis *(arrowhead)* and mild hypoplasia involving the medial portions of the cerebellar hemispheres. This case would previously have been called a Dandy-Walker variant or a mega cisterna magna.

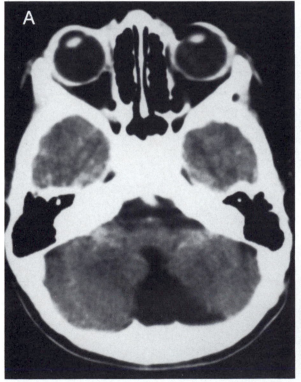

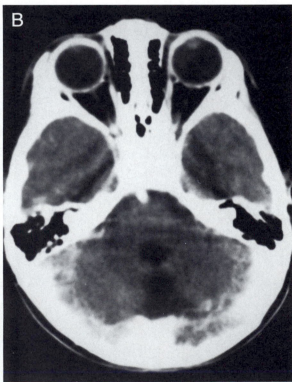

FIG 24–24.
Dandy-Walker complex, type B. Axial CT scans through the posterior fossa show a communication between a normal-sized fourth ventricle and a prominent CSF space **(A).** A cut a few millimeters higher **(B)** demonstrates a hypoplastic but intact inferior vermis be-tween the two CSF-containing structures. This case would previously have been called either a Dandy-Walker variant or a mega cisterna magna if the inferior vermian hypoplasia had not been appreciated.

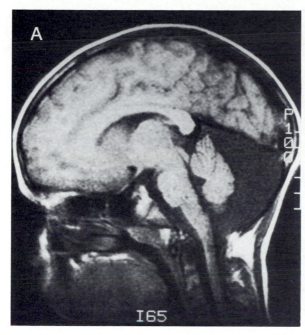
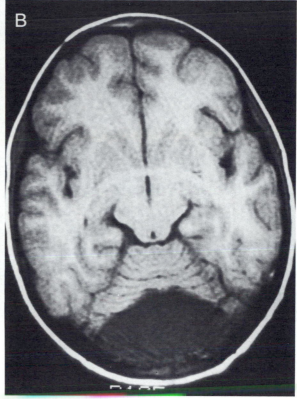

FIG 24–25.
Dandy-Walker complex, type B. Sagittal **(A)** and coronal **(B)** MR scans (TR 700, TE 20) demonstrate a large CSF space in the retrocerebellar region, anteriorly displacing the cerebellar vermis **(A)** and splaying the cerebellar tissue **(B)**. The inferior vermis is intact and the sagittal view clearly demonstrates communication between the normal-sized fourth ventricle and the CSF space. This is a part of the spectrum of the Dandy-Walker complex. It might previously have been called an arachnoid cyst (of the communicating form) in view of the anterior displacement of intact cerebellar tissue or some type of arachnoid pouch. No hydrocephalus is present, but there is posterior bowing of the occipital bone, and symptoms were due to pressure on posterior fossa structures.

for shunting of only the cyst or of shunting of both the cyst and the ventricular system.

The Dandy-Walker complex is often accompanied by other CNS malformations, including agenesis of the corpus callosum (15%) (see Fig 24–22),[70, 75] the lissencephaly syndromes and/or migrational heterotopias (25%–35%),[70, 76] holoprosencephaly,[76] and meningoceles and encephaloceles.[76, 77] Other non-CNS abnormalities have been described including malrotations of the gut, complex cardiac malformations, polycystic kidneys, and orofacial anomalies.[76, 77] While the Dandy-Walker malformation has been reported in siblings, there is no clear pattern of hereditary transmission.[78]

Arachnoid Cyst.—A true arachnoid cyst has no communication with the fourth ventricle or with the surrounding subarachnoid spaces.[66] Such a concept eliminates the terminology of a "communicating arachnoid cyst," which makes no sense; such a cystic CSF space would be part of the Dandy-Walker complex. The arachnoid cyst typically produces mass effect on the surrounding neural tissues (Fig 24–26), and there may be secondary hydrocephalus. While Barkovich et al. state that there is no hypoplasia of the vermis or cerebellar hemispheres with this category of their classification,[66] arachnoid cysts in other intracranial locations are accompanied by hypoplasia of the underlying tissues secondary to their origin in early gestational life (see Fig 24–72), and similar findings would be expected with a posterior fossa arachnoid cyst. The key finding is the lack of communication with other CSF spaces, generally requiring cyst shunting or resection if it is producing local mass effect or hydrocephalus.

Prominent Cisterna Magna.—This is an acquired condition in which there is hypoplasia of the cerebellar vermis and cerebellar hemispheres. The cerebellar folia are normally formed but there is increased CSF space between them, along with increased CSF cisterns and an increased size of the cisterna magna. Hydrocephalus is not present,

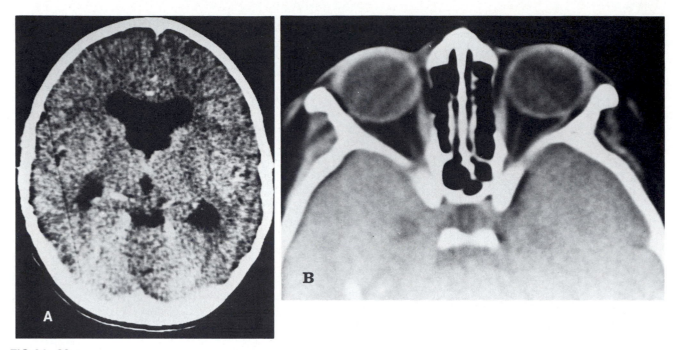

FIG 24–26.
Septo-optic dysplasia with hypoplastic optic nerves. **A,** the axial scan of the brain demonstrates a missing septum pellucidum and "squaring" of the frontal horns. **B,** the axial scan of the orbits demonstrates small optic nerves bilaterally.

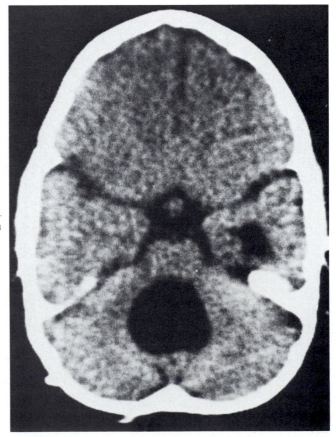

FIG 24–27.
Isolated fourth ventricle. This child had neonatal intraventricular hemorrhage producing adhesions throughout the ventricular system and a need for ventricular shunting. The left temporal horn is dilated. In addition, there is pronounced dilatation of the fourth ventricle as a result of adhesion within the aqueduct and involving the foramina of the fourth ventricle. Such adhesions isolate the fourth ventricle and prevent its decompression from ventricular shunting.

and the patient has symptoms referable to loss of previously functional cerebellar tissue.[66]

Trapped Fourth Ventricle.—Another acquired condition is the trapped fourth ventricle secondary to adhesions of the outlets of the fourth ventricle and ependymitis producing aqueductal block (Fig 24–27). Even if the lateral ventricles are shunted, the blocked aqueduct prevents decompression. The cerebellum is not hypoplastic, nor is there enlargement of the posterior fossa.[79]

Inflammatory Obstruction

Obstruction to the flow of CSF over the cerebral convexities will produce dilatation of the entire ventricular system. In such cases, there is communication between the ventricular system and the subarachnoid space of the spinal canal, thereby acquiring the term *communicating hydrocephalus* (extraventricular obstructive hydrocephalus). Such convexity obstruction may be from intrauterine or neonatal inflammatory disease (Fig 24–28). Other causes include intrauterine subarachnoid hemorrhage producing arachnoid scarring, and congenital hypoplasia or absence of the arachnoid granulations leading to decreased CSF resorption.[80] It should be emphasized that many cases of communicating hydrocephalus (approximately 60%) do not have dilatation of the fourth ventricle associated with dilatation of the third and lateral ventricles; a diagnosis of communicating hydrocephalus rather than obstructive hydrocephalus cannot be based solely on the presence of dilatation of the fourth ventricle. Radioisotope cisternography allows evaluation of CSF flow dynamics and may prove useful in this setting.

Volume Loss

The various causes of atrophy have been previously discussed. To produce dilatation of the entire ventricular system, atrophy will involve both the cerebrum and cerebellum.

CRANIOCEREBRAL MALFORMATIONS

Midline Cerebral Hemispheric Abnormalities

The common denominator of holoprosencephaly, septo-optic dysplasia, and agenesis of the corpus callosum is dysplasia of midline structures. In holoprosencephaly it is lack of segmentation into normal hemispheres and lobes. Septo-optic dysplasia can be thought of as a type of holoprosenceph-

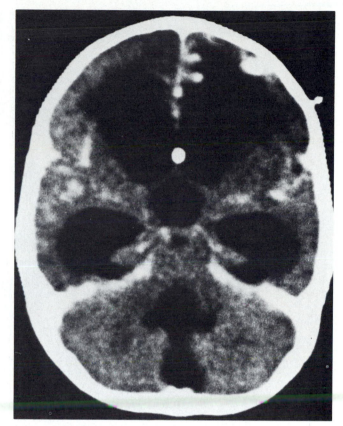

FIG 24–28.
Neonatal meningitis producing communicating hydrocephalus. *Haemophilus influenzae* meningitis has produced a communicating form of hydrocephalus, as denoted by enlargement of the lateral, third, and fourth ventricles. There is enhancement of inflammatory tissue within the subarachnoid spaces of multiple supratentorial cisterns and sulci.

aly, with incomplete development of the intraventricular septum, optic chiasm, and optic nerves. Agenesis of the corpus callosum is a partial or complete maldevelopment of the corpus callosum.

Holoprosencephaly

The holoprosencephalies are a spectrum of congenital abnormalities in which there is incomplete cleavage of the prosencephalon transversely into the normal diencephalon and telencephalon, and lack of complete cleavage of the telencephalon into cerebral hemispheres and lobes. The malformation is divided into three varieties with a descending degree of severity: alobar, semilobar, and lobar holoprosencephaly.[81–87]

In alobar holoprosencephaly, there is a small cerebrum without division into lobes or hemispheres. There is a monoventricular cavity, and the thin cerebral parenchyma is located primarily anteriorly and laterally (Fig 24–29). This ventricular

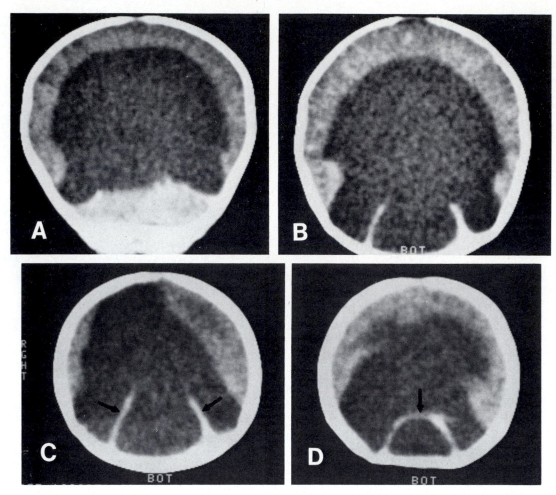

FIG 24–29.
Alobar holoprosencephaly. **A,** the lowest cut demonstrates brain covering a monoventricle anteriorly and laterally. Cerebellar tissue is seen posteriorly. **B,** a slightly higher cut demonstrates communication of the supratentorial monoventricle with a cyst located within the posterior fossa. Cerebellar hypoplasia and posterior fossa cysts have been reported with holoprosencephaly. **C** and **D,** the higher cuts demonstrate the high position of the tentorium *(arrows)* resulting from the expansion of the posterior fossa cyst. There is no evidence of an interhemispheric fissure or falx. (Courtesy of Charles Fitz, M.D., Toronto.)

cavity may extend superiorly and posteriorly as a dorsal cyst (Fig 24–30), or even posteriorly and inferiorly into the posterior fossa (see Fig 24–29). The basal ganglia and thalami are fused in the midline (Figs 24–30 and 24–31). The interhemispheric fissure, falx cerebri, and corpus callosum are not formed (Figs 24–29 to 24–31), nor are the olfactory bulbs and nerves.[82–85, 88, 89] Coronal MRI is excellent for demonstrating the thalamic fusion, the lack of the interhemispheric fissure, and the crossing of gray and white matter across the midline (Fig 26–30,A).

In semilobar holoprosencephaly, there is partial separation into two cerebral hemispheres, with some portion of the interhemispheric fissure usually seen (Figs 24–32 and 24–33). There is also some attempt at formation of ventricular horns (see Fig 24–33). While still a monoventricle, there may be more of a "shield" configuration than with the alobar variety (see Fig 24–32), or there may be a horizontal ventricle, concave anteriorly, simulating an open-mouth smile (see Fig 24–33). The corpus callosum is unformed, and while the thalami remain fused (see Fig 24–32), there is a rudimentary third ventricle.[82, 89] A dorsal cyst may be present (see Fig 24–32). An incomplete sylvian fissure may be present indicating incomplete separation of the temporal lobe from the frontal and parietal lobes.

In lobar holoprosencephaly, separation into two cerebral hemispheres is nearly complete. The subtle findings of an incomplete interhemispheric fissure, a shallow falx, or some areas of continuity of gray and white matter across the midline may be

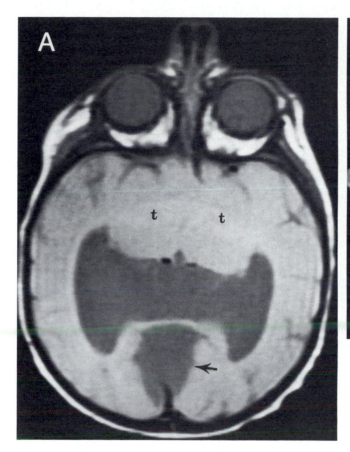

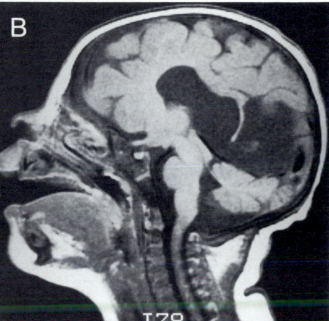

FIG 24–30.
Alobar holoprosencephaly with dorsal cyst. **A,** the axial MR scan
(TR 600, TE 20) demonstrates fused thalami *(t),* fused lateral
ventricles in the shape of a dumbbell, and the inferior portion of a
doral cyst *(arrow).* **B,** the sagittal view (TR 700, TE 20) better
demonstrates the relationship of the dorsal cyst to the ventricular
system. Even though the cyst is supratentorial, it compresses the
cerebellum. **C,** the coronal view (TR 700, TE 20) nicely
demonstrates the continuity of white and gray matter across the
midline, the continuity of the ventricular system, and the fused
thalami. The findings duplicate the pathologic specimen seen in
Figure 24–31.

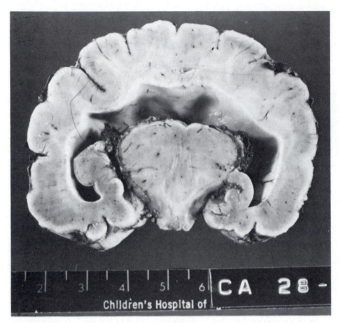

FIG 24–31.
Alobar holoprosencephaly. This pathologic specimen demonstrates the classic findings of alobar holoprosencephaly, including fusion of the thalami, a monoventricle, and the lack of interhemispheric and sylvian fissures.

difficult or impossible to perceive on axial CT scans before or even after shunting (Figs 24–34 and 24–35). Coronal MRI is the procedure of choice to demonstrate the subtle abnormalities. The thalami may still have some degree of fusion (see Fig 24–35) or may be completely separate. Subtle changes of incomplete cleavage of the sylvian fissure may be present (see Fig 24–35).[89] There may be hypoplasia of the corpus callosum with relative "squaring" of the closely approximated frontal horns and flattening of the ventricular roofs, along with absence of the septum pellucidum (see Fig 24–35).[83, 89] These last-named findings are similar to those of septo-optic dysplasia, indicating the close association of the milder forms of holoprosencephaly and septo-optic dysplasia. These mild ventricular changes may be difficult to perceive on axial CT scans which may only demonstrate mild ventricular enlargement.

Anomalies of the face parallel the degree of cerebral dysplasia.[90] The common denominator is hypotelorism. In alobar holoprosencephaly, facial deformities include cyclopia, ethmocephaly, cebocephaly, median cleft lip and palate, and bilateral cleft lip and palate. Semilobar holoprosencephaly is accompanied by median cleft lip and palate and bilateral cleft lip (see Fig 24–32), while lobar hol-

oprosencephaly may have only mild facial deformities such as mild hypotelorism or single upper central incisor.[91] Facial deformities, however, do not always accompany holoprosencephaly. Seventeen percent of patients with alobar holoprosencephaly have been found to have no obvious facial deformities, and a larger percentage of patients with less severe forms of holoprosencephaly have normal facies.[81, 89, 92, 93]

The prognosis is extremely poor for alobar holoprosencephaly, and most patients do not survive infancy.[88] The semilobar malformation is associated with marked mental retardation, while the lobar variety is accompanied by lesser degrees of psychomotor retardation, and the patient may fall in the normal cognitive range.[81, 87]

The etiology of the holoprosencephalies is unknown, but the condition appears to occur between the fourth and eighth weeks of intrauterine life.[1, 81] There is an association with several chromosomal syndromes, including trisomy 13–15 and trisomy 18. Autosomal dominant and autosomal recessive forms have been reported.[87, 92] There is also an association with the Dandy-Walker malformation and schizencephaly.[76, 94] The causes in most human cases remain unknown.[87]

The differential diagnosis of holoprosencephaly with dorsal cyst includes hydranencephaly, severe hydrocephalus, and agenesis of the corpus callosum with interhemispheric cyst.[89] In hydranencephaly, the cortex and white matter of the anterior and middle cerebral artery distributions is absent and replaced by a large fluid-filled cavity (see Figs 24–42 and 24–43), but the falx is present and the thalami are separated, in contradistinction to alobar holoprosencephaly which has an absent falx and interhemispheric fissure, fused thalami, and residual cerebral tissue displaced anteriorly and inferiorly by the dorsal cyst. Obstructive hydrocephalus may be so severe that the intraventricular septum is severely thinned or absent, allowing communication between the two ventricles. However, there is usually persistence of the normal ventricular outline, albeit enlarged, not the round monoventricle found in alobar holoprosencephaly nor the "shield" or "smile" configurations seen in the semilobar form. Agenesis of the corpus callosum may be associated with a large interhemispheric cyst, in some ways simulating the dorsal cyst of holoprosencephaly. However, the cyst with corpus callosal agenesis is between two separated hemispheres, and a falx is present.[89]

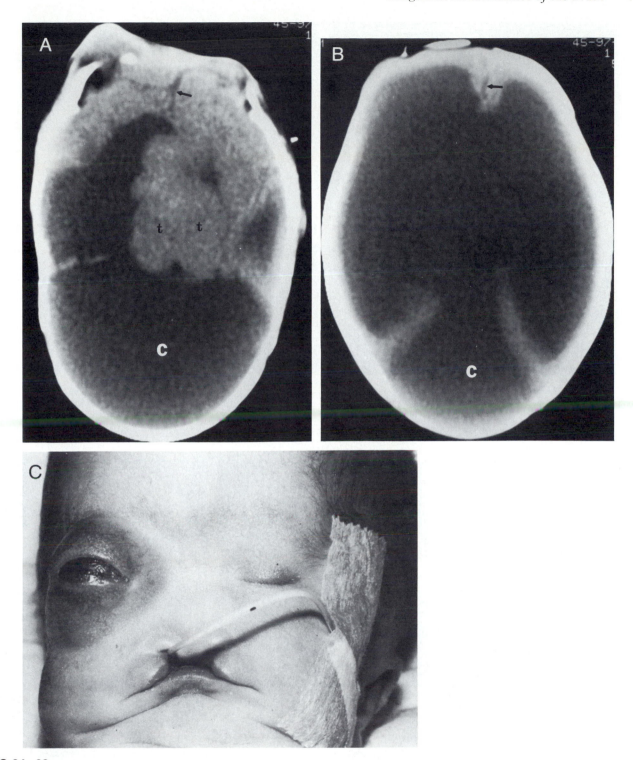

FIG 24–32.
Semilobar holoprosencephaly with abnormal facies. **A,** the axial CT scan demonstrates fused thalami *(t),* and a rudimentary interhemispheric fissure anteriorly *(arrow).* There is a large dorsal cyst extending posteriorly and inferiorly *(C).* A portion of the dilated ventricular system is seen anteriorly on the right. **B,** a higher cut again demonstrates the rudimentary interhemispheric fissure anteriorly *(arrow)* and the dorsal cyst*(C)* extending from the fused lateral ventricles which have minimal separation anteriorly. This is semilobar rather than lobar holoprosencephaly in view of the presence of a portion of the interhemispheric fissure and slight separation of the lateral ventricles anteriorly. **C,** this child has gross facial deformities, including bilateral cleft lip and palate and shallow, malformed orbits and anterior cranial fossae **(A** and **C).**

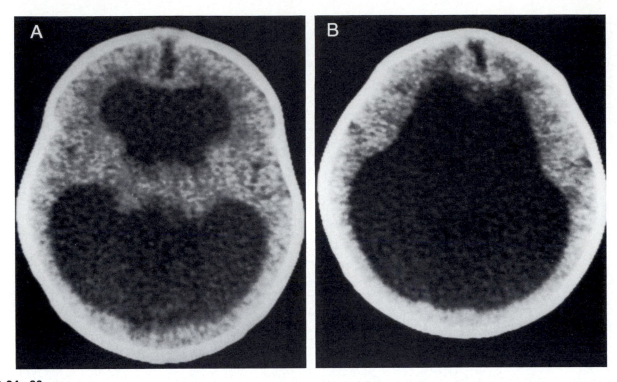

FIG 24–33.
Semilobar holoprosencephaly. The CT scans demonstrate a portion of the interhemispheric fissure anteriorly along with attempted formation of the frontal horns. The more posterior portion of the lateral ventricles unite in a "smile" configuration **(A)** while at a higher level the confluent ventricles form a "shield" **(B).**

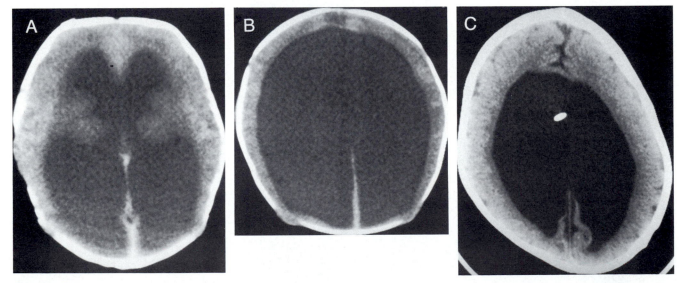

FIG 24–34.
Lobar holoprosencephaly. **A,** a CT scan through the lower portions of the lateral ventricles demonstrates pronounced ventricular enlargement, particularly posteriorly. The interventricular septum is missing. **B,** more superiorly the confluence of the ventricles is seen, and they have a rounded configuration. **C,** it is not until after the ventricles have been shunted that the interhemispheric fissure can be defined and is seen to be normal. The ventricles have an unusual configuration, however, for simple hydrocephalus. Other cuts fail to demonstrate sylvian fissures.

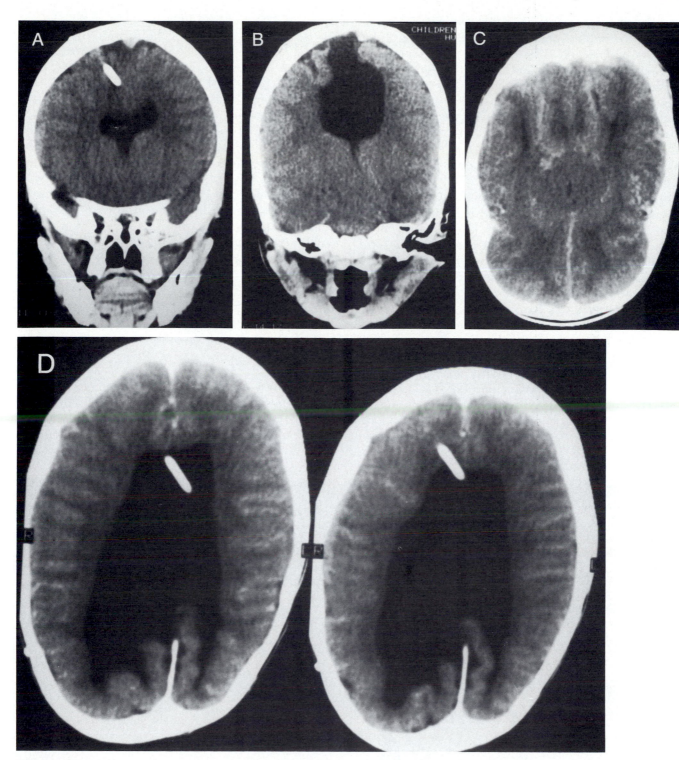

FIG 24–35.
Lobar holoprosencephaly. **A,** a coronal CT scan through the frontal horns demonstrates "squaring" of the frontal horns and a missing interventricular septum. **B,** more posteriorly there is confluence of the lateral ventricles and a rudimentary dorsal cyst. No sylvian fissures are defined. **C,** an axial scan following contrast enhancement fails to show sylvian fissures, and the thalami appear to be partially fused with a small third ventricle in the midline. **D,** higher cuts of this enhanced scan demonstrate an intact falx but unusual configuration to the ventricular system. This case probably represents a point in the continuum between the semilobar and lobar varieties, with an intact interhemispheric fissure, but partially fused thalami and no sylvian fissures.

Septo-optic Dysplasia (deMorsier Syndrome)

Septo-optic dysplasia consists of agenesis of the septum pellucidum (50% of patients); hypoplasia of the optic discs, nerves, and chiasm; and hypoplasia of the pituitary infundibulum.[95, 96] The diagnosis is generally made on a clinical basis in young children (mean 2.5 years) after finding hypoplastic discs, impaired vision, and nystagmus.[95, 97] The presentation of pituitary dysfunction is usually later (mean 5 years of age).[95] Pituitary insufficiency is isolated to decreased growth hormone in 75% of patients, but other hormones such as adrenocorticotropic hormone (ACTH), thyroid-stimulating hormone (TSH), and antidiuretic hormone may be deficient; more than two hormone deficiencies are present in one third of cases.[95] Neonatal hypoglycemia, seizures, and congenital blindness is also a characteristic presentation.[98]

The diagnosis is based upon funduscopic and endocrinologic criteria, and the anatomic findings on CT or MRI may be subtle; a normal scan does not exclude the diagnosis.[97] Patients are best evaluated with both axial and coronal scan projections, preferably with MRI rather than CT because of its clearly superior ability to provide anatomic delineation of the optic nerves and chiasm, pituitary infundibulum, and septum pellucidum in multiple projections. The septum pellucidum is missing in between 27% and 50% of patients (Figs 24–36 and 24–37).[95, 97, 98] Absence of the septum pellucidum is a rare isolated anomaly without the rest of the syndrome, and may also be seen in holoprosencephaly, agenesis of the corpus callosum, severe hydrocephalus, and schizencephaly. The frontal horns have a square appearance (Fig 24–37) which is believed to be secondary to the absent septum and which is not specific for this syndrome.[99] The roof of the frontal horns is flat (see Figs 24–36 and 24–37), and the fornices have a low position with low attachment to the splenium.[99] The frontal horns are usually dilated to a mild degree and are "pointed" along their inferior margins in approximately 50% of cases (see Fig 24–37),[99] as in the Chiari II malformation. There is a bulbous optic recess of the third ventricle, the "optic ventricle," with a hypoplastic infundibular recess. The optic nerves appear hypoplastic on the scans, generally bilaterally (see Fig 24–36),[95, 98] although care must be exercised in avoiding partial volumes errors.

Agenesis of the Corpus Callosum

Agenesis of the corpus callosum may be either partial or complete. While an early injury to the prosencephalon leads to holoprosencephaly, a more localized insult to the precursor of the corpus

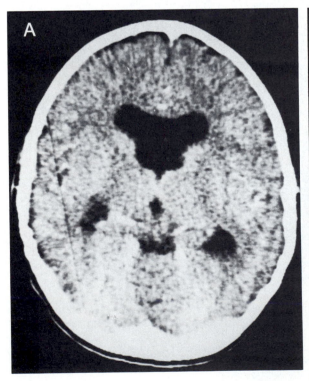
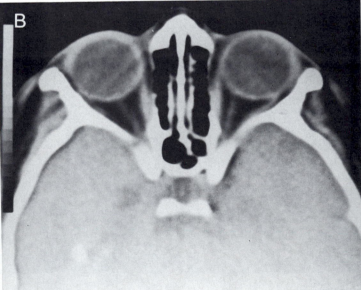

FIG 24–36.
Septo-optic dysplasia with bilateral optic nerve hypoplasia. **A,** the axial CT scan demonstrates a missing septum pellucidum, slight rounding of the frontal horns, and a squaring of the frontal horn configuration. **B,** axial scanning through the orbits demonstrates small optic nerves bilaterally.

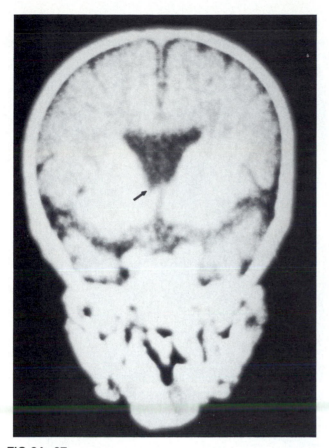

FIG 24–37.
Septo-optic dysplasia. This coronal CT scan shows "pointing" of the inferior aspect of the right frontal horn *(arrow)* and a square configuration to the frontal horns, with a missing septum pellucidum. (Courtesy of Dr. Sylvester Chuang, Toronto.)

callosum, the sulcus medianus telencephali medii, which is a caudal extension of the lamina terminalis, results in malformation of the corpus callosum.[100] The timing of this insult during gestation produces an association with multiple other congenital anomalies. Forty percent to 80% of patients with sphenoethmoidal encephaloceles have agenesis of the corpus callosum (Fig 24–38), and there is a high incidence of facial anomalies associated with both of these entities. The Chiari II malformation is associated with dysgenesis of a portion of the corpus callosum, usually the splenium, in up to 84% of cases.[101] Between 14% and 25% of patients with the Dandy-Walker malformation have corpus callosal agenesis.[102] Other abnormalities associated with callosal dysgenesis are gyral anomalies (32%), ocular anomalies (42%), septo-optic dysplasia, Aicardi's syndrome, trisomy 13–15, and trisomy 18.[103–105] Thirteen percent of patients with callosal agenesis have cardiovascular anomalies.[103] Overall, 62% of patients have other CNS anomalies and 62% have two or more organ systems involved with an anomaly.[103]

The pathologic and scan findings consist of the following:

1. Complete (see Fig 24–38) or partial (Fig 24–39) absence of the corpus callosum. When partial, it almost always affects the posterior portion.[100, 101, 104]

2. Absence of one or more of the hippocampal, anterior, and posterior commissures. These may be present or absent in varying degrees.[100]

3. Lateral deviation of the frontal horns, which have concave medial margins. Because of the lack of formation of the anterior corpus callosum, fibers which would normally cross between hemispheres run longitudinally (the bundles of Probst), producing the impressions on the medial aspects of the frontal horns. Wide separation of the deformed frontal horns produces a "batwing" configuration (see Figs 24–38 and 24–39).

4. Separation and parallelism of the bodies of the lateral ventricles. This may be the only finding on an axial scan to suggest a subtle corpus callosal agenesis (Fig 24–40).

5. Enlarged atria of the lateral ventricles if the splenium is absent (culpocephaly).[100, 104]

6. Radial array of medial hemispheric sulci seen on sagittal views.

7. Hippocampal hypoplasia leading to enlarged temporal horns in "keyhole" configuration in 73% of cases.[106]

8. High position of the third ventricle in 80% of cases which may extend into a large cystic dilatation separating the internal cerebral veins (see Fig 24–40).[104]

9. Large interhemispheric cyst which may be separate from the third ventricle and which may or may not communicate with the lateral ventricles. This cyst may be on both sides of the falx, or favor one side (Fig 24–41).[104]

10. A lipoma may be localized to the region of the genu of the corpus callosum (Fig 24–42), or may extend throughout the region of the corpus callosum (Fig 24–43). Forty percent of patients with an intracranial lipoma have callosal dysgenesis.[107] The lipoma may extend through the choroidal fissures to involve the choroid plexuses of the lateral ventricles.[108]

MRI makes visualization of these abnormalities much easier than CT because both coronal and sagittal views are easily obtainable. Subtle eleva-

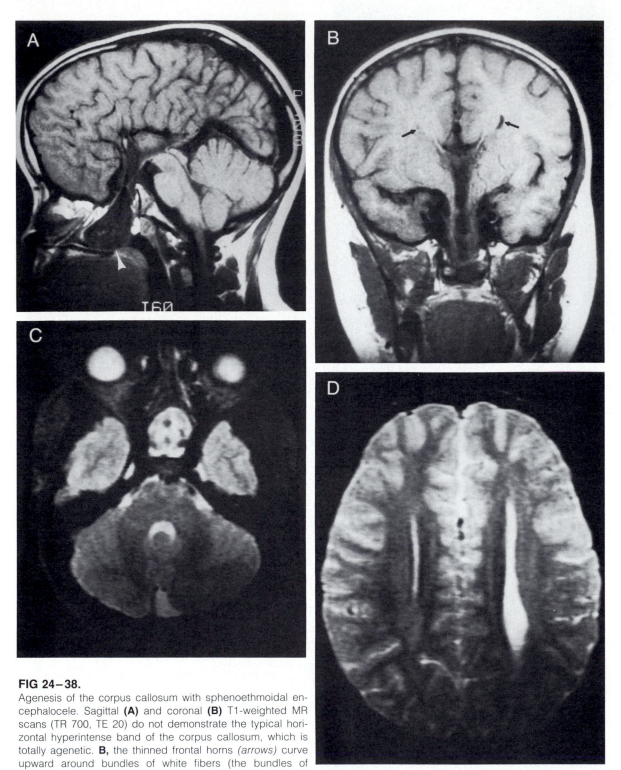

FIG 24–38.
Agenesis of the corpus callosum with sphenoethmoidal encephalocele. Sagittal **(A)** and coronal **(B)** T1-weighted MR scans (TR 700, TE 20) do not demonstrate the typical horizontal hyperintense band of the corpus callosum, which is totally agenetic. **B,** the thinned frontal horns *(arrows)* curve upward around bundles of white fibers (the bundles of Probst). **A,** a sphenoethmoidal encephalocele extends as far as the hard palate *(arrowhead).* **C,** the long TR/TE axial study through the encephalocele (TR 2,500, TE 100) shows neural tissue within the sac. **D,** a higher cut with the same long TR/TE sequence demonstrates parallelism of the lateral ventricles characteristic of corpus callosal agenesis.

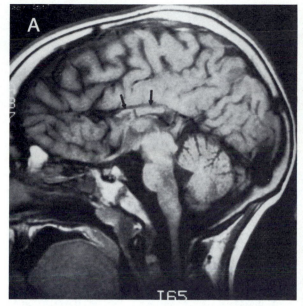

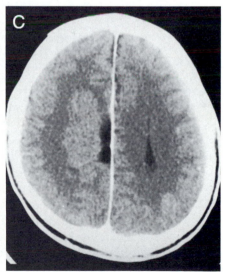

FIG 24–39.
Partial agenesis of the corpus callosum. Sagittal **(A)** and coronal **(B)** MR scans (TR 700, TE 20) demonstrate partial agenesis of the corpus callosum. **A,** a portion of the body is present *(arrows),* while the splenium and genu are missing. **B,** the frontal horns form a "batwing" configuration and the third ventricle is minimally displaced superiorly between the lateral ventricles.

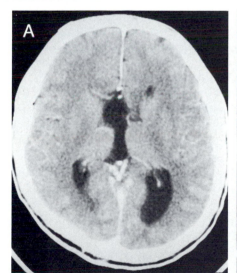

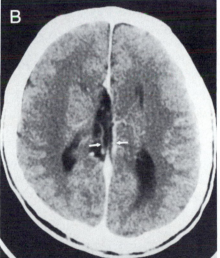

FIG 24–40.
Agenesis of the corpus callosum with elevation of the third ventricle splitting internal cerebral veins. Three axial enhanced CT scans demonstrate the splayed frontal horns and the elevated third ventricle **(A),** which extends superiorly to split the internal cerebral veins **(B,** *arrows).* The CSF collection extends superiorly along the right side of the falx **(C).** The lateral ventricles have a parallel configuration **(B** and **C).**

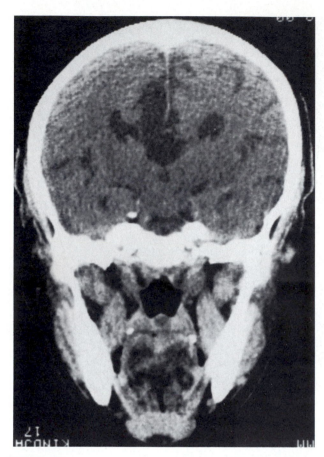

FIG 24–41.
Agenesis of the corpus callosum with interhemispheric cyst. The coronal unenhanced CT scan demonstrates the "batwing" configuration of the frontal horns and a bulbous elevated third ventricle. Above this there is a CSF-containing space which is either an extension of the third ventricle or an interhemispheric cyst extending along the right side of the intact falx.

tion of the third ventricle is easier to see on coronal (Fig 24–39,B) or sagittal views than on axial images, and partial absence of the corpus callosum is easier to see on sagittal than on axial scans (Fig 24–39,A). The absence of one or more of the other commissures, and the presence of both heterotopic gray matter and abnormal gyral formation can be well visualized with MRI but are not easily seen on CT.[103, 105, 109–111]

Agenesis of the corpus callosum itself is usually asymptomatic, with abnormalities demonstrable only on special testing. Symptoms associated with the agenesis syndrome include mental retardation (85%), seizures (42%), and hydrocephalus (23%), among others.[100, 103, 111, 112] Concurrent anomalies account for most of these neurologic disabilities.

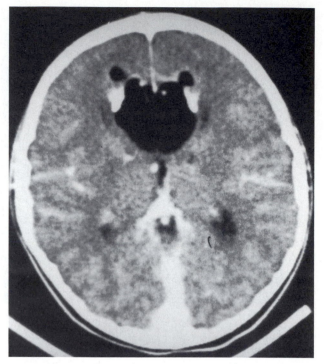

FIG 24–42.
Calcified lipoma of the corpus callosum. The enhanced CT scan demonstrates a classic lipoma with very low attenuation coefficients, in the region of the genu of the corpus callosum. Calcifications are present laterally, and superiorly there are small "daughter" lipomas.

Lateral Cerebral Hemispheric Abnormalities

Focal Hypoplasia and Agenesis

Portions of a cerebral hemisphere may be developmentally small. Normal structural outlines including normal gyral convolutions are present (Fig 24–44) which suggest that the insult occurred sufficiently late in development to allow for the presence of normal structure but resulted in arrested growth. This is not a destructive process, but rather one of growth arrest. Surrounding CSF spaces are enlarged. A variety of etiologic agents probably lead to such growth arrest.

Destructive Lesions

The terminology for the variety of destructive lesions of the prenatal and perinatal brain has been used with imprecision, leading to confusion. In 1859, Heschl coined the term "porencephaly" to denote a cavity within a cerebral hemisphere that communicates with either the ventricular system or the subarachnoid space or with both.[113] However, that term is frequently used to refer to any

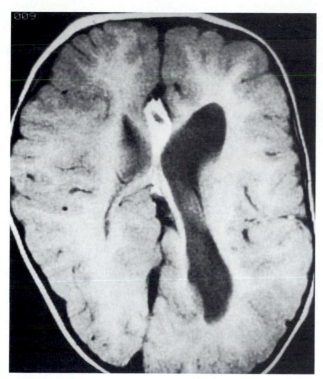

FIG 24–43.
The T1-weighted axial MR scan (TR 700, TE 20) demonstrates an unusual configuration of the posterior portions of the lateral ventricles, with a missing splenium and distal body of the corpus callosum. A lipoma with characteristic high intensity extends from the genu where it is largest in size along the course of the proximal body of the corpus callosum, then to split along the course of the fornices.

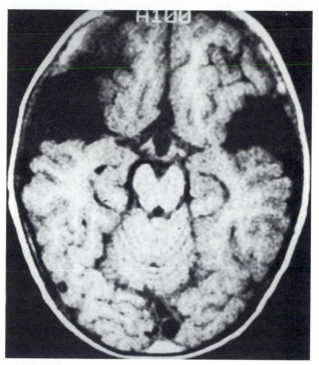

FIG 24–44.
Hypoplasia of the frontal and temporal lobes. The T1-weighted MR axial image (TR 700, TE 20) demonstrates hypoplasia of the anterior temporal lobes and the lateral aspects of the basal portions of the frontal lobes. The frontal opercula are missing. While a similar configuration can be seen in the lissencephaly syndrome, in this case there is normal formation of cortical gyri and sulci and underlying white matter.

type of cystic abnormality of the brain, usually communicating with the ventricular system, originating anywhere from the prenatal period to adulthood. In 1946, Yakovlev and Wadsworth coined the term *schizencephaly*,[114, 115] and classified the process relative to the other destructive processes, termed *agenetic porencephaly* and *encephaloclastic porencephaly*.[116] This classification and these terms refer to the pathologic appearance of the destructive process, not to its etiologic agent. A variety of etiologic insults may lead to a similar result, and the specific etiologic agent in a given case is usually not known. The end result is not only dependent upon the specific etiologic agent, but is also dependent upon the timing, extent, severity, and duration of the insult.

The terminology used in this chapter and an outline of organization of these destructive processes is given in Table 24–4. Agenetic porencephaly represents destruction occurring within the first 6 months of gestation. Such an insult results in cerebral cortical abnormalities and islands

of heterotopia. If the process is unilateral, it is termed *unilateral porencephaly*. If bilateral, the term schizencephaly is used. Encephaloclastic porencephaly occurs within the last trimester. It, too, is unilateral but differs from agenetic porencephaly by its lack of heterotopia and cortical anomalies. In addition, there is a difference in the response to an insult between the pre- and postna-

TABLE 24–4.

Destructive Lesions of the Brain

I. Prenatal
  A. Agenetic porencephalies (early development)
    1. Unilateral porencephaly
    2. Schizencephaly (bilateral)
      (a) With open lips
      (b) With closed lips
  B. Encephaloclastic porencephaly (late development)
  C. Hydranencephaly
II. Perinatal/postnatal
  A. Focal cavitation
  B. Multicystic encephalomalacia

tal brain. Pathologic experience suggests that the developing brain responds with complete resorption of the insulted tissue without gliosis, whereas an insult to the postnatal brain results in incomplete resorption and gliosis.[117] Prenatal encephaloclastic porencephaly, therefore, differs from postnatal cavitation and multicystic encephalomalacia by the attempt at complete resorption of the insulted tissue with minimal or no gliosis.

Hydranencephaly is the end stage of a severe insult occurring either early or late in gestation. The severity of the insult results in essentially total destruction of cerebral tissue in the anterior and middle cerebral artery distributions. If cortical remnants are found to be dysgenetic, the insult can be said to have occurred early in gestation. If no such dysgenesis is found, the insult probably occurred later in gestation. The term *partial hydranencephaly* is imprecise, with the insult actually representing a form of unilateral agenetic or encephaloclastic porencephaly.[116]

Finally, perinatal and postnatal insults result in focal cavitation and multicystic encephalomalacia. In these conditions, there is incomplete resorption of tissue and secondary gliosis. The ventricular walls are generally preserved.[116, 117]

These definitions and observations are from the literature and suffice for classification purposes. Caution is advised, however, regarding attempts at assigning a precise date of insult to a specific destructive lesion. The pathologic distinctions previously discussed are generalizations and are not meant to imply that a precise date of insult can be determined with accuracy. In addition, it is usually quite difficult to precisely date an insult from imaging studies alone without the use of autopsy confirmation.

Before presenting the individual types of destructive lesions, and in order to understand the presence of dysgenetic remnants in early prenatal destructive lesions, it is necessary to summarize our concepts of normal and abnormal neuronal migration.

Normal and Abnormal Migration.—Between the 8th and 16th gestational weeks, neuroblasts that have formed in the periventricular germinal matrix begin moving to the cortical surface.[9, 118, 119] Glial fibers are laid down between the germinal matrix and the cortex with a one-to-one correspondence between a focus in the germinal matrix and a cortical destination. Movement of neuroblasts along these glial fibers occurs primarily during the

8-week interval, with some migration through the 25th week[9, 118]; glial cell migration continues beyond birth. The neuroblasts establish the six-layered cortex, and send out both axons and dendrites. The formation of gyral convolutions is dependent upon the appropriate formation of the cortical layers.

If the neuroblasts are arrested in their move between the germinal matrix and the cortical surface, nests of gray matter may reside in periventricular regions, projecting into the ventricles, or are situated as islands surrounded by white matter and are known as heterotopic gray matter. Lack of cortical layer development and poor organization of neurons leads to both a thickened cortex and incomplete formation of cortical convolutions. If no convolutions are formed, the condition is termed *agyria* or *lissencephaly* (smooth brain). Some formation of wide gyri may occur if the cortical disorganization is less severe; this condition of a few wide gyri is called *pachygyria*. Poor neuronal organization leads to a lack of axonal development, grossly manifested by a thin band of white matter. The junction between the gray and white matter is sharp because of the lack of interdigitation of white matter into cortical convolutions. If neuroblasts reach the cortical surface but later there is laminar necrosis of the fifth layer, numerous small convolutions are formed, termed *polymicrogyria*. The cortical ribbon is thicker than normal, and the zone of white matter thinner than normal, as with agyria and pachygyria.[9]

The cause(s) of migrational disorders is unknown. An intriguing theory is a vascular insult to the germinal matrix before the eighth week of gestation.[9, 120, 121] The periventricular tissues are watershed zones between major vascular distributions and may suffer from low flow during an episode of maternal hypotension. Focal ischemia to the germinal matrix would lead to a loss of normal migration along a glial pathway, resulting in a schizencephalic cleft. More severe ischemia would result in a larger cleft. Because the retinal layers and optic nerves are developing nearby at the same time, ischemia in these nearby regions might result in septo-optic dysplasia.[99, 120, 121]

The ischemia theory can likewise be implicated in the etiology of hydranencephaly. Ischemia not only to watershed zones but to larger portions of the anterior and middle cerebral artery distributions would result in lack of formation of the frontal, parietal, and most of the temporal lobes as is seen with hydranencephaly.

Vascular lesions later in gestation have been documented in twin pregnancies which are monochorionic. Demise of one twin results in the transfer of thromboplastic material to the surviving twin, leading to diffuse intracranial thrombosis and infarction.[122] Some degree of sparing in these distributions would result in an appearance between classic hydranencephaly and severe schizencephaly ("basket brain" of Raybaud).[116] A vascular insult and laminar necrosis of neuroblasts that have migrated to the cortex would lead to lack of appropriate organization and cortical layer development, decreased convolution formation, and thinning of the white matter, all of which are seen with polymicrogyria. Genetic factors may also play an important role, giving susceptibility to environmental factors.[121]

Agenetic Porencephalies.—The agenetic porencephalies occur early in development. This leads to resorption of the insulted tissue, little gliosis, and dysgenetic remnants at the margins of the lesion because of interrupted normal migration.[116]

Unilateral Porencephaly.—Unilateral porencephaly is a prenatal unilateral cystic lesion.[116] It commonly communicates with the ventricular system, but communication with the cortex, or with both, may be evident. Foci of heterotopic gray matter usually line the margins of the cystic lesion. The overlying cortex commonly shows areas of pachygyria or agyria.

Schizencephaly.—The term *schizencephaly* (Gr. *schizein*, to divide + *enkephalos*, brain) denotes a cleft extending from the ventricular margin to the cortical surface. The bilateral and symmetric nature of the clefts, the anomalous development of the overlying cortical surface, the presence of heterotopic gray matter along the clefts, and the absence of the septum pellucidum give evidence for the insult producing schizencephaly to have occurred early in gestational development.

Interruption of the migration of specific neuroblasts along the prescribed glial pathway leads to a cleft extending from the cortex to the ventricular surface. The margins of the cleft are lined by a combination of pia-arachnoid and ependymal elements constituting the "pia-ependymal seam". Polymicrogyria are present along the margins of the schizencephalic cleft, with heterotopic gray matter deep to the cleft.[9, 118–120]

Schizencephaly may be divided into two types. Type I is the more subtle of the two types and consists of close approximation of the margins of the cleft (the lips), with one or more points of fusion of these lips.[9, 119, 120, 123] Foci of polymicrogyria extend along the margins of these lips, not always radiographically visible,[119] and are seen as irregular areas of thickened gray matter.[9, 120, 123] The cleft extends from the cortical surface to the ventricular surface where there is a small outpouching or "dimple" (Figs 24–45 to 24–47). The pia from the cortical surface extends along the cleft to become adherent to the ependymal lining, forming the pia-ependymal seam seen pathologically. A cortical vessel may extend deeply into the cleft (see Fig 24–45), or may be relatively close to the surface (Fig 24–47,A), suggesting only the presence of a deep cortical sulcus on a CT scan.[9, 119, 120, 123] Indeed, the cleft itself may be difficult to visualize by CT scanning, with the diagnosis only suggested by the presence of the ventricular dimple (see Fig 24–46). MR scanning allows much better visualization of the cleft, demonstrating the gray matter extending along the lips from the cortex to the ventricular surface (see Fig 24–45). The presence of associated heterotopic gray matter and the lack of sulcation with pachygyria are much better demonstrated by MRI (Fig 24–48), with its greater ability to differentiate gray and white matter, than by CT.[9, 119] The ventricular septum may be intact or only partially absent in this milder form of schizencephaly.[99] Associated congenital anomalies such as the Dandy-Walker complex, agenesis of the corpus callosum, and holoprosencephaly may be seen (see Fig 24–48).

Type II has wide-open clefts extending between the cortical and ventricular surfaces (Figs 24–48 and 24–49). The ventricular septum is generally absent, denoting the more severe insult in this form.[9, 120] The lateral ventricles are generally enlarged but not on an obstructive basis to produce enlargement of the head. Rather, there is lack of development of cerebral tissue because of the diffuse insult, leading to ventricular enlargement and either a normal-sized head or microencephaly. Those with microencephaly suffer worse clinical impairment with seizures, mental retardation, and developmental delay.[123]

Encephaloclastic Porencephaly.—This is a later form of porencephaly than the agenetic type, and dysgenetic remnants are not found. There is usually an attempt at complete resorption of the in-

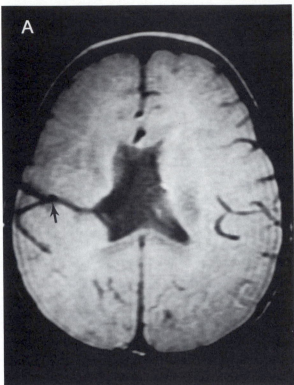

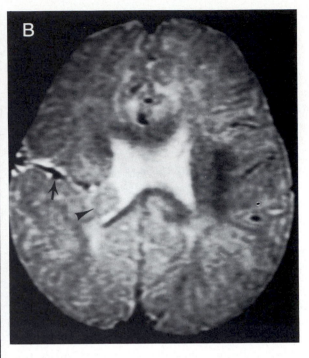

FIG 24–45.
Type I schizencephaly with deep cortical vessels and heterotopic gray matter. **A,** the T1-weighted axial MR scan (TR 600, TE 20) demonstrates a deep cleft extending from the anterior right parietal surface to the right ventricular margin where there is a "dimple." A cortical vessel with rapidly moving blood producing hypointensity *(arrow)* courses deeply into the cleft. **B,** the long TR/TE axial study at a slightly different level (TR 2,000, TE 80) demonstrates the cleft filled with hyperintense CSF and the hypointense cortical vessel *(arrow)*. There is a focal nodule of heterotopic gray matter *(arrowhead)* pressing into the right lateral ventricle. There is poor demarcation of white matter and less sulcation than normal diffusely throughout the brain, indicating lissencephaly.

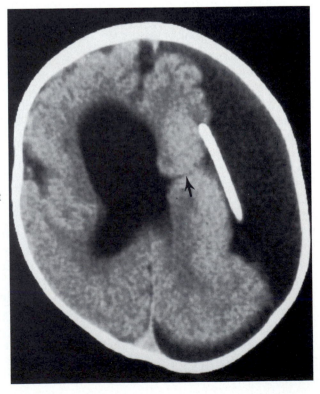

FIG 24–46.
Type I schizencephaly with arachnoid cyst. This axial CT scan demonstrates a large arachnoid cyst over the left cerebral convexity. This cyst has been shunted and there is deformity of the hypoplastic left cerebral hemisphere. There is a thin cleft *(arrow)* extending from the cortical surface to a ventricular dimple. The lateral ventricles have an unusual configuration and there is no interventricular septum.

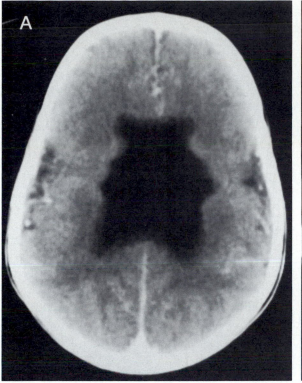 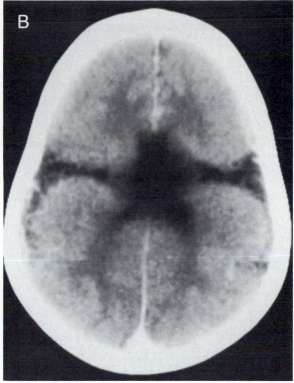

FIG 24–47.
Schizencephaly. **A,** the bilateral ventricular dimples are well visualized, and there is a missing interventricular septum. The frontal horns have a relatively square appearance. **B,** at a slightly different level the bilateral symmetric clefts are visualized. The clefts are intermediate in size.

sulted tissues, with little gliosis, so that differentiation from postnatal focal cavitation may still be possible.[117]

Hydranencephaly.—This is discussed later in this chapter under Global Hemispheric Abnormalities.

Focal Cavitation.—Focal cavitation is the result of a postnatal insult, such as intracranial hemorrhage, ischemia, infection, trauma, and surgery. Complete resorption of tissue or communication of the cavity with the CSF spaces leads to cyst fluid CT density (Fig 24–50) or MR intensity equal to CSF. Cyst isolation, posthemorrhagic cavitation, or incomplete resorption of tissue and breakdown products lead to CT absorption coefficients greater than CSF and shorter T1 and T2 relaxation times.

Secondary volume loss usually results in a shift of the ventricular system toward the side of involvement. Any focal prenatal or perinatal insult to a hemisphere may result in secondary changes of the skull during development, including elevation of the petrous ridge, thickening of the calvarium,

and increased pneumatization of the paranasal sinuses (Dyke-Davidoff-Mason syndrome) (Fig 24–51). Rarely, the cavity may act as a mass and produce thinning of the overlying calvarium, most likely from the "water-hammer" pulsation of fluid within the cyst (Fig 24–52). When the cystic cavity communicates with the ventricular system, there may be a ball-valve action which allows the cavity to enlarge to a size greater than the rest of the ventricular system, resulting in displacement of midline structures to the opposite side and creating an appearance of mass effect rather than volume loss.

An extraaxial cyst such as arachnoid cyst is commonly associated with hypoplasia of the underlying cerebral parenchyma but no increased ventricular size to suggest an early destructive process to the hemisphere. Focal cavitation is commonly associated with ventricular enlargement indicating such a destructive process (see Fig 24–50). Focal cavitation acting as a mass stimulates an extraaxial cyst not communicating with the ventricular system. The key ingredient for therapy is the presence of communication with the ventricular system or subarachnoid CSF spaces. Appropri-

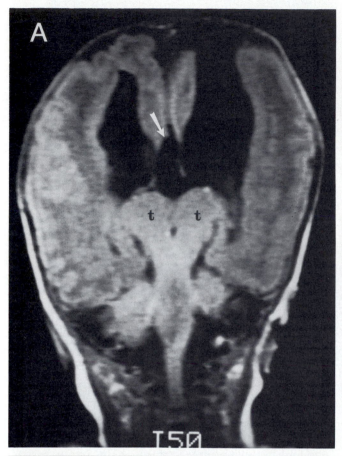

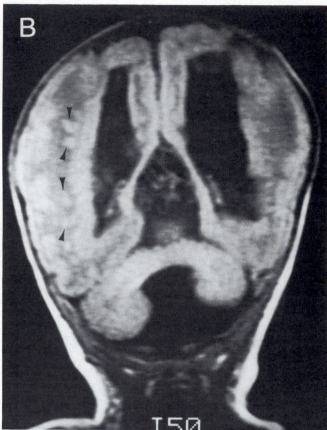

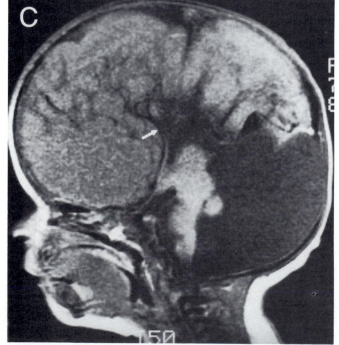

FIG 24–48.
Type II schizencephaly, agenesis of the corpus callosum, holoprosencephaly, and the Dandy-Walker complex. **A,** the coronal MR scan (TR 600, TE 20) demonstrates the wide communication between the roof of the left lateral ventricle and the cortical surface indicative of type II schizencephaly. The third ventricle *(arrow)* is displaced superiorly indicative of agenesis of the corpus callosum. The thalami *(t)* are fused, indicative of holoprosencephaly. **B,** a slightly more posterior cut (TR 600, TE 20) demonstrates a large cyst in the posterior fossa with a wide-open communication between the fourth ventricle and the cyst characteristic of the Dandy-Walker complex, type A. There are multiple foci of heterotopic gray matter *(arrowheads)*. **C,** the sagittal MR scan (TR 600, TE 20) demonstrates posterior positioning of the anterior cerebral artery *(arrow)* characteristic of agenesis of the corpus callosum, and the large posterior fossa cyst. Other cuts showed the lack of formation of the sylvian fissures indicative of holoprosencephaly.

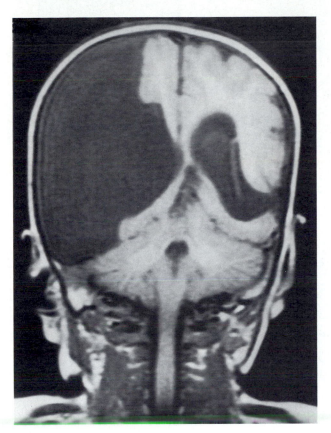

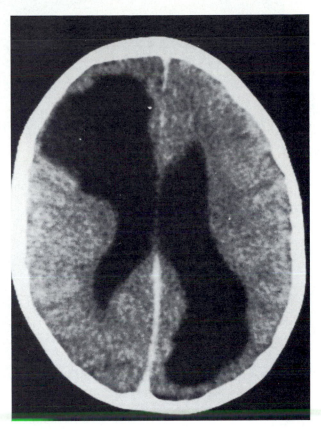

FIG 24–49.
Type II schizencephaly. The coronal T1-weighted MR scan (TR 700, TE 20) demonstrates a wide communication between the right lateral ventricle and the cortical surface indicative of type II schizencephaly. There is a smaller cleft on the left which is of intermediate size.

FIG 24–50.
Bilateral focal cavitation. This 9-year-old boy has had a seizure disorder since birth following perinatal intracerebral hemorrhage. The axial CT scan demonstrates a large area of focal cavitation within the right frontal lobe, communicating with an enlarged ventricle, and a second smaller area of cavitation in the left parieto-occipital region communicating with the enlarged left lateral ventricle.

ate communication may allow for the placement of a single shunt. The placement of a water-soluble contrast material into either the cystic space or ventricular system with CT scanning allows the assessment of this communication.

Multicystic Encephalomalacia.—This is discussed later in this chapter under Global Hemispheric Abnormalities.

Heterotopic Gray Matter

Arrest of the normal migration of neuroblasts from the germinal matrix to the cortex results in foci of heterotopic gray matter. This migrational disorder may present either as an isolated entity or as part of more pervasive congenital anomalies. Patients with only heterotopic gray matter may either be normal or present with seizures and mental retardation.

Radiographically, small accumulations of gray matter may project into the ventricular system and

present a pattern termed "candle dripping" (Fig 24–53). This is a similar pattern to the multiple periventricular tubers of tuberous sclerosis, although the heterotopia do not calcify nor are there cortical tubers. Heterotopic gray matter may also be present in large accumulations producing mass effect (Fig 24–54). In fact, a solitary focus of heterotopic gray matter may be misdiagnosed as a neoplasm, resulting in surgical exploration.[15] MRI allows the appropriate diagnosis. Heterotopic gray matter has T1 and T2 relaxation parameters similar to normal cortex (see Figs 24–53, 24–54), and there is no enhancement with either paramagnetic contrast agents on MRI or iodinated contrast agents on CT (see Fig 24–53).[9, 10, 119]

Cerebral Cortex

As explained earlier under Destructive Lesions, the formation of the gyral convolutions is de-

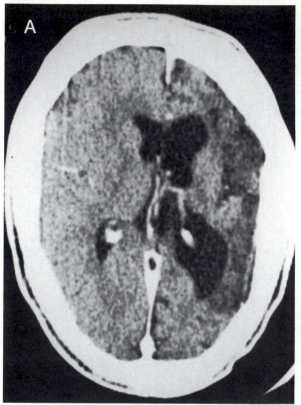 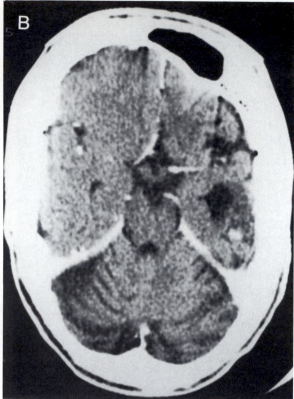

FIG 24–51.
Dyke-Davidoff-Mason syndrome. **A, B,** this 20-year-old male with a intractable seizure disorder has a small left cerebral hemisphere as demonstrated on these two axial CT scans. There are multiple areas of encephalomalacia throughout the left hemisphere, with secondary enlargement of the left lateral ventricle. Thickening of the calvarium and enlargement of the left frontal sinus are indicative of the bony changes that followed the early left hemispheric insult. Volume loss throughout the cerebellum indicates that the insult was of a diffuse nature.

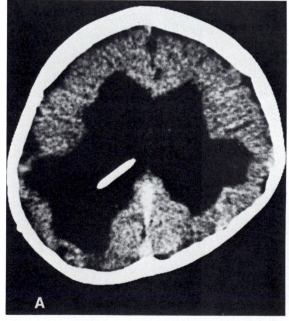 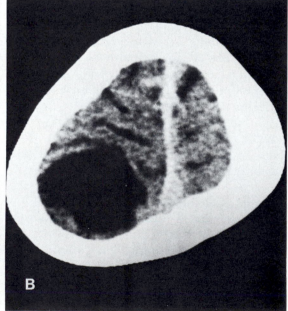

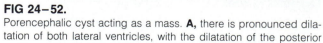

FIG 24–52.
Porencephalic cyst acting as a mass. **A,** there is pronounced dilatation of both lateral ventricles, with the dilatation of the posterior portion of the right lateral ventricle being most dramatic. **B,** this area of porencephaly acts as a mass with pronounced deformity of the overlying skull.

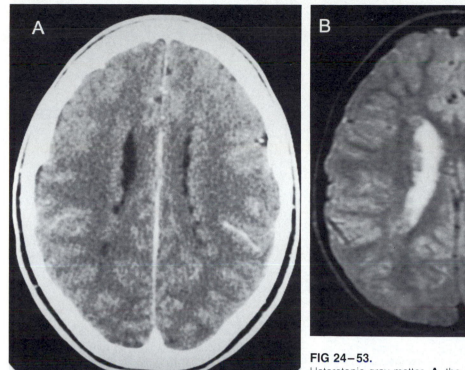

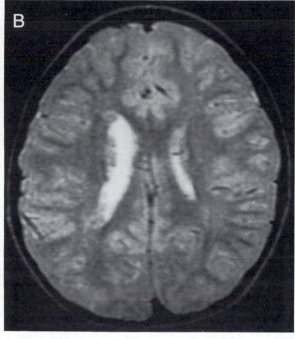

FIG 24–53.
Heterotopic gray matter. **A,** the enhanced CT scan demonstrates multiple projections into the bodies of both lateral ventricles, with these projections having a density equal to cortical gray matter. There is an enhancing vessel coursing deeply in the left parietal region, and there may be a subtle type I schizencephaly. **B,** the axial MR scan (TR 2,500, TE 80) better demonstrates that these periventricular projections have an intensity equal to cortical gray matter. There are no cortical areas of hyperintensity characteristic of tubers, nor are any of the projections calcified, findings typical of tuberous sclerosis.

pendent upon normal cortical organization. Agyria or pachygyria may result from an abnormality in neuronal migration. The term *lissencephaly syndrome* is used to denote the spectrum between agyria and pachygyria (Fig 24–55). Multiple small gyri forming a cobblestone pattern is termed *polymicrogyria*, and probably occurs slightly later in gestation than agyria or pachygyria.[9, 116] In addition, polymicrogyria may occur from a cortical insult, whereas agyria and pachygyria may be secondary to more central ischemia, causing failure of the germinal matrix.[125] Finally, an arrest of normal neuronal migration results in heterotopic gray matter which are nests of neurons presenting as islands within the white matter or remaining in periventricular regions and projecting into the ventricles.[12, 13]

In the lissencephaly syndrome there is a reduced thickness of the white matter while the gray matter on the surface is thick (Fig 24–56). There is a smooth, almost pencil-sharp line between the gray and white matter without the normal interdigitation of white matter into gray matter convolutions (see Fig 24–56).[119, 126] The frontal lobes are

small, and there is a lack of development of the opercula, resulting in wide sylvian fissures and an "hourglass" or figure-of-8 appearance (Fig 24–57).[119] The cortex of the insula is exposed, and middle cerebral artery branches lie within the wide and shallow sylvian fissures without their typical undulating course over the posterior frontal and temporal lobes (see Fig 24–57). Besides the thin white matter, the corpus callosum is underdeveloped, as are white matter tracts, resulting in small cerebral peduncles and a small pons (Figs 24–58 and 24–59).

CT scanning allows recognition of the abnormal formation of the frontal lobes and opercula (see Fig 24–56) and the sharp margination between the gray and white matter (see Fig 24–57). It is more difficult, however, to evaluate the cortical surface with CT than with MRI (see Figs 24–58 and 24–59).[12] Additionally, MRI is far superior at identifying areas of heterotopic gray matter which have signal characteristics identical to cerebral cortex (see Figs 24–53, 24–54, and 24–59).[12, 13, 119]

The lissencephaly syndrome has been divided

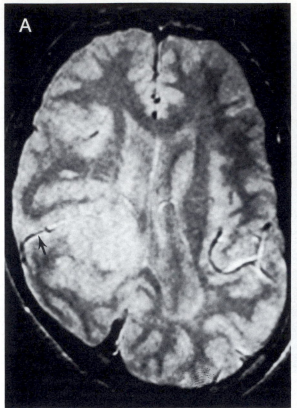

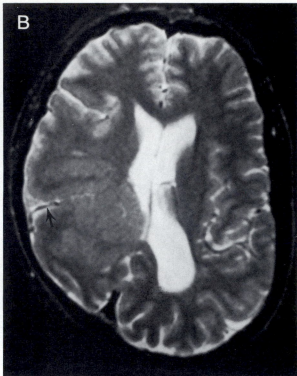

FIG 24–54.
Large area of heterotopic gray matter with probable type I schizencephaly. **A,** the spin-density axial MR scan (TR 2,500, TE 30) demonstrates that the large "mass" indenting the posterior portion of the right lateral ventricle has an intensity equal to cortical gray matter. **B,** this "lesion" maintains its intensity relative to cortical gray matter on the second echo (TR 2,500, TE 80), characteristic findings for a large accumulation of heterotopic gray matter. There is a sulcus containing a cortical vessel **A** and **B,** *(arrows)* coursing deeply toward the heterotopia, characteristic of type I schizencephaly. More anteriorly, in the anterior right parietal and posterior right frontal regions **(A),** there is sharp demarcation between the white matter and the poorly sulcated gray matter, indicative of pachygyria. The right hemisphere is small. Finally, the white matter is thin throughout much of the left hemisphere and there appear to be areas of pachygyria.

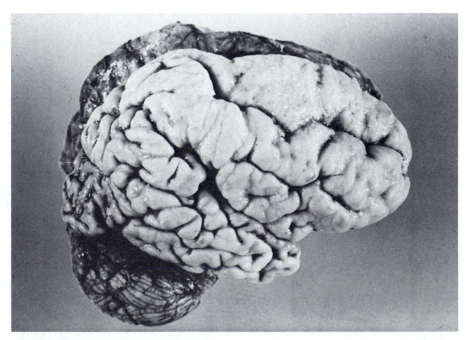

FIG 24–55.
Pachygyria. This photograph of a brain removed at autopsy shows broad gyri over the right convexity. These gyri are smooth, and there is a lack of division by sulci.

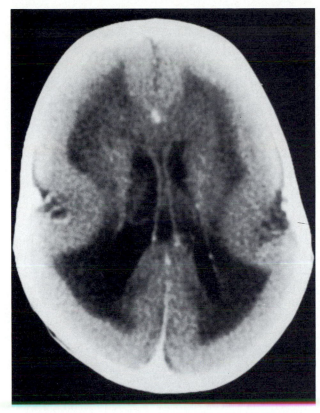

FIG 24–56.
Lissencephaly syndrome (agyria). This axial CT scan demonstrates uniformly smooth but thickened cortex. There is sharp margination between the thickened cortex and the underlying white matter. There are essentially no gyral convolutions (agyria).

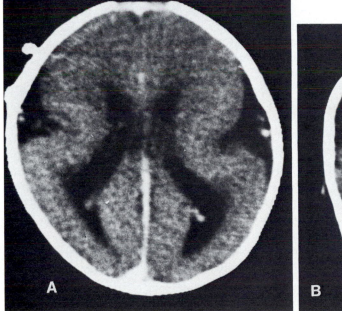

FIG 24–57.
Lissencephaly. This 4-month-old child was scanned because of failure to thrive. The axial **(A)** and coronal **(B)** scans demonstrate small frontal lobes and deep clefts in the regions of the sylvian fissures bilaterally. The clefts are due to lack of development of the temporal and frontal opercula, leaving the insula exposed bilaterally. The surface of the brain is smooth, which gives the name *lissencephaly* ("smooth brain") to the malformation.

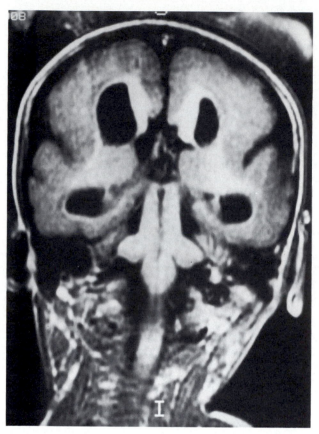

FIG 24–58.
Lissencephaly syndrome demonstrated on coronal MRI. This coronal T1-weighted image (TR 700, TE 20) demonstrates sharp margination between the hyperintense white matter and the lower intense and thickened gray matter. A few areas of pachygyria are present, but the brain is otherwise agyric. The corpus callosum is not definitely identified, and the pons is small.

into three types.[126] Type I, by far the most common, is characterized by mild ventricular enlargement because of hypoplastic cerebral tissues, and microencephaly. In type II, there is hydrocephalus and other severe brain malformations, particularly the Dandy-Walker complex and other malformations of the posterior fossa. While the hydrocephalus may make it more difficult to recognize the lack of formation of the opercula and the smooth surface of the brain, the thin white matter and the sharp margination between gray and white matter is distinctive. Type III is quite rare, and is associated with cerebellar hypoplasia of a severe degree.[116, 126, 127]

Patients with lissencephaly usually have severe mental retardation and seizures, with death usually occurring early.[119, 125, 127] Survival may be more prolonged with pachygyria.[119] Patients with polymicrogyria may present with seizures or motor

retardation.[9] Polymicrogyria is also present in patients with schizencephaly.[9] Heterotopic gray matter may be asymptomatic or present with seizures or motor abnormalities. Some types of lissencephaly have a genetic or chromosomal basis, so early diagnosis allows for appropriate counseling for risk of recurrence, which is 5% to 20% in siblings.[127]

Global Hemispheric Abnormalities

Anencephaly

A defect in the closure of the neural tube results in severe dysraphism denoted by agenesis of the cerebral hemispheres and the overlying meninges and cranium. Disorganized tissue representing brain stem and cerebellum lies upon flattened occipital squama.

The abnormality may be diagnosed in utero by ultrasonography and confirmed by amniocentesis which demonstrates increased amounts of alpha-fetoprotein and acetylcholinesterase in the amniotic fluid.[128] The condition is not compatible with life.

Hydranencephaly

Hydranencephaly consists of the absence of the majority of the cerebral hemispheres except for the occipital lobes, basal portions of the temporal lobes, and thalami. A large membranous sac containing CSF occupies the rest of the intracranial space. The wall of this sac is pia-arachnoid overlying glial fibers, sometimes with small islands of preserved neurons.

CT scans in classic hydranencephaly demonstrate CSF density throughout the supratentorial space (Fig 24–60). Two soft tissue densities at the base of the cerebral hemispheres represent the persisting thalami (Fig 24–60,A) which are fed by perforating branches of the posterior cerebral and basilar arteries. Occipital lobes and the medial-basal portions of the temporal lobes, which are fed by posterior cerebral artery branches, are also visualized (Fig 24–61), along with normal tissue density in the posterior fossa, though often reduced in volume. MRI shows the same findings, with signal intensity of the cystic space typical of CSF.

Hydranencephaly must be differentiated from severe hydrocephalus. Even in the most severe forms of hydrocephalus, there is preservation of some neural parenchyma including gray matter, white matter, and ependyma. The severe intrauterine hydrocephalus severely thins or destroys the intraventricular septum. Reliable differentiation may be difficult on CT scan alone, since the thin

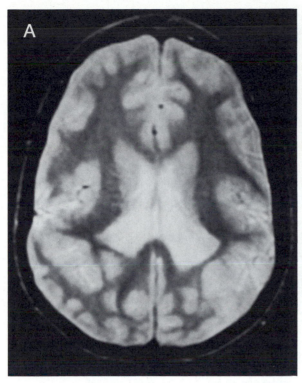

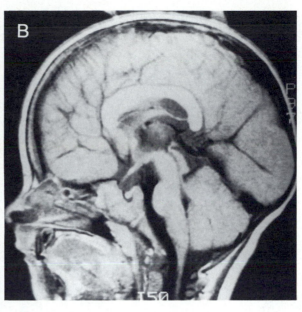

FIG 24–59.
Lissencephaly syndrome on MRI. **A,** the axial scan (TR 2,500, TE 80) demonstrates the sharp margination between thickened gray matter and white matter in the majority of the anterior portions of both cerebral hemispheres. Some convolutions and interdigitations are present (pachygyria) while other areas are totally smooth (agyria). There are a number of foci of heterotopic gray matter in the posterior hemispheres bilaterally. **B,** a midline sagittal view in a different patient (TR 600, TE 20) demonstrates the presence of pachygyria and the relatively small pons.

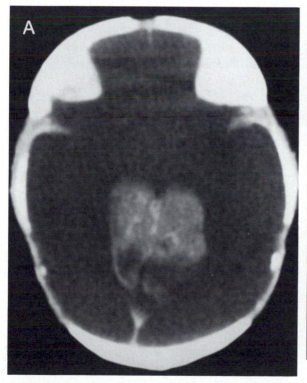

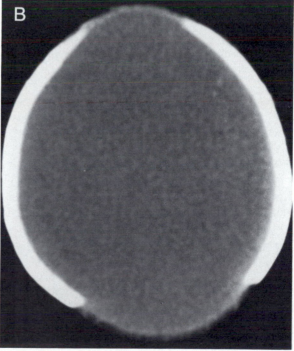

FIG 24–60.
Hydranencephaly. **A,** CT scanning of the cerebral hemispheres demonstrates persisting tissue inferiorly representing remnants of the thalami and medial parietal lobes. **B,** more superiorly there is no remaining cerebral tissue, but only a large CSF space.

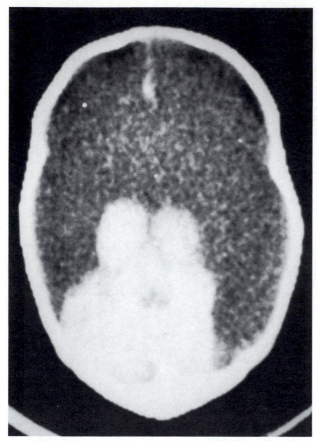

FIG 24–61.
Hydranencephaly. CT scanning through the inferior portions of the cerebral hemispheres demonstrates persisting thalami and more occipital lobe tissue present than in Figure 24–60. (Courtesy of Dr. Sylvester Chuang, Toronto.)

cortical mantle may be volume-averaged with the overlying calvarium. MRI is more efficacious than CT in making this differentiation because of its ability to characterize soft tissues, albeit thinned. The clinical differentiation may be easier, in that hydrocephalic infants have macrocephaly, whereas most hydranencephalic infants are normocephalic. The distinction may be important, in that severe hydrocephalus may be treated with an intraventricular shunt, whereas there is no cerebral tissue to decompress in hydranencephaly. Angiography has been used in this differentiation. In severe hydrocephalus, pial vessels are intact, although stretched and thinned, and there is a subtle capillary blush indicative of metabolically active tissue.[116] In hydranencephaly, vessels in the anterior and middle cerebral artery distributions are either absent or fail to perfuse capillary beds since there is no metabolically active tissue. There is persistence of the posterior cerebral and basilar arteries.

MRI may replace angiography as the definitive differentiating imaging examination.

Occasionally, alobar holoprosencephaly may have such a large dorsal cyst that the inexperienced imager considers hydranencephaly. Alobar holoprosencephaly is characterized by the presence of some cerebral mantle, even in the most severe cases, which should be defined by MRI; the lack of formation of a falx which is present in hydranencephaly; and the development of an azygous anterior cerebral artery coursing far anteriorly because of the lack of separation of the hemispheres; usually the anterior and middle cerebral arteries are absent or extremely thin with classic hydranencephaly.

As previously discussed under Lateral Hemispheric Cerebral Abnormalities, hydranencephaly probably represents the endstage of a number of severe insults at various times during gestation. Some cases of hydranencephaly have been reported in which there is documented CMV or toxoplasmosis intrauterine infections.[116] In one series, 11% of cases of hydranencephaly or severe porencephaly occurred in monozygotic twins. Seventy-five percent of these cases had a dead co-twin. It is hypothesized that thromboplastin is released during the death of the twin and crosses through placental vascular connections to produce vascular occlusions in the surviving twin.[122]

Multicystic Encephalomalacia

Multicystic encephalomalacia is considered to be a result of a perinatal insult. Rather than complete resorption of destroyed tissue, multiple cystic cavities develop, separated by glial tissue.[116] Tissue destruction generally involves the white matter and cortex, with the ventricular wall discernible; ventricular enlargement results from diffuse volume loss.

Diffuse involvement of both cerebral hemispheres with relative sparing of the basal ganglia, brain stem, and cerebellum is usually a result of a diffuse insult such as global hypoxia (see Fig 9–19). A more focal insult results in focal cavitation (see Fig 24–50). Multicystic encephalomalacia has been seen in documented cases of intrauterine infection producing multiple calcifications (see Fig 24–16). Hydranencephaly is a prenatal lesion while multicystic encephalomalacia results from a postnatal insult.[116] They represent portions of a spectrum of global destructive insults, with the resulting loss of tissue dependent upon the timing of the insult, and its severity and duration.

Cerebellum

The most common malformations involving the cerebellum are the Chiari malformations. The Chiari II and III malformations also involve multiple portions of the cerebral hemispheres, whereas the Chiari I malformation is characterized on neuroradiologic examinations primarily by caudal displacement of the cerebellar tonsils. These conditions have been discussed earlier in the chapter.

Hypoplasia of the inferior vermis is the essential finding in the Dandy-Walker complex, as discussed earlier in the chapter. The Joubert syndrome is characterized by nearly total aplasia of the vermis, but without the cystic expansion characteristic of the Dandy-Walker complex. The patients have ataxia, abnormal eye movements, episodic hyperpnea and apnea, and mental retardation.[129-132] Inferior vermian agenesis has also been associated with communicating hydrocephalus and port-wine nevi among family members and has been reported in the Down syndrome (trisome-21).[133]

Hypoplasia (Fig 24–62) or aplasia of one of the cerebellar hemispheres is rare and may be associated with other cerebral anomalies,[1] and with arachnoid cyst. Hypoplasia or aplasia of both cerebellar hemispheres (Fig 24–63) is extremely rare; complete agenesis of the cerebellum (the Chiari IV malformation) is rarer still, but has been reported in association with arthrogryposis multiplex congenita.[134] Figure 24–64 is that of a 67-year-old woman who complained of hearing loss. Scanning and surgery not only demonstrated the presence of an acoustic schwannoma, but also aplasia of the entire cerebellum. Symptoms referable to that aplasia consisted of only a mild degree of midline ataxia.

Cranium and Meninges

Cranial Dermal Sinus, Meningocele, and Encephalocele

Defective closure of the embryologic neural tube may cause an abnormality in the cranium and underlying meninges. There is a spectrum of abnormalities, with the most mild being cranium bifidum occultum, analogous to spina bifida occulta. A cutaneous component is frequently present, such as a dermal sinus leading through the congenital cranial defect, which may be associated with an intracranial dermoid cyst. Herniation of the meninges through the cranial defect is termed a *meningocele*, while herniation of both brain and meninges is, by common usage, called an *encepha-*

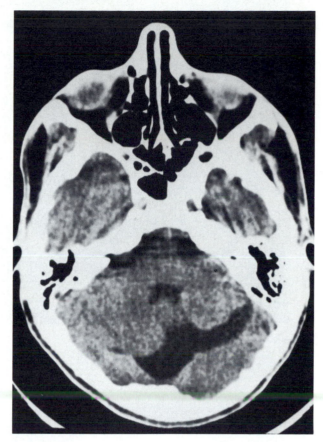

FIG 24–62.
Hypoplasia of the left cerebellar hemisphere. CT scanning demonstrates a small left cerebellar hemisphere but an intact cerebellar vermis. There was no evidence of arachnoid cyst on other views, and this is considered to be a primary cerebellar hemispheric hypoplasia.

locele. The overall incidence of cephaloceles is 1 in 4,000 to 5,000 livebirths, and spinal dysraphism is 6 to 16 times more common than cranial dysraphism.[134]

Occipital encephaloceles account for 71% of cases in the United States. These encephaloceles may be high, above the foramen magnum (Fig 24–65); at the foramen magnum; or involve the upper cervical spine and occipital bone (the Chiari III malformation is a cervico-occipital encephalocele containing the majority of cerebellum). Parietal encephaloceles (Fig 24–66) make up 10% to 14% of cases: 9% are frontal, 9% are nasal (Fig 24–67), and 1% are nasopharyngeal (see Fig 24–38) in location.[135, 136]

Midline encephaloceles result from defects in the developing skull. Basal encephaloceles occur at the junctions of cartilaginous ossification centers, nasal encephaloceles at the junctions of carti-

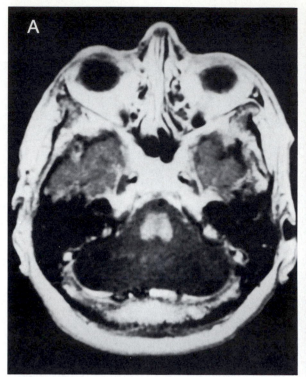

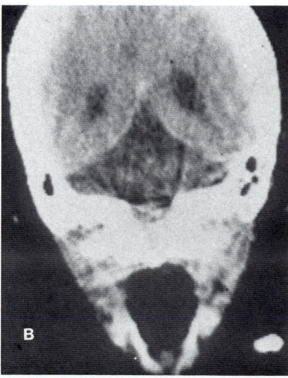

FIG 24–63.
Aplasia of the cerebellar hemispheres. MR scanning (TR 700, TE 20) in axial **(A)** and sagittal **(B)** projections fails to demonstrate any evidence of cerebellar hemispheres. There is a small amount of superior vermis **(B).** There is no posterior fossa expansion nor is there evidence of hypoplastic and displaced cerebellar hemispheres characteristic of the Dandy-Walker complex.

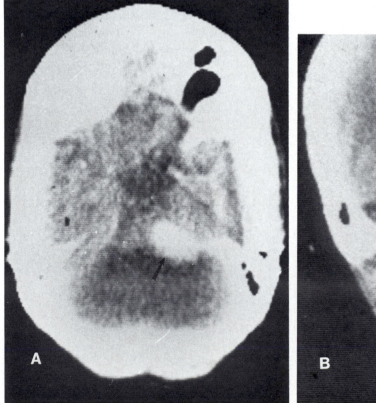

FIG 24–64.
Agenesis of the cerebellum. This 67-year-old woman presented with left-sided hearing loss. **A,** the CT scan demonstrates a well-circumscribed enhancing mass *(arrow)* in the left cerebellopontine angle. There is extensive low density throughout the rest of the posterior fossa behind the brain stem. **B,** the coronal scan demonstrates CSF density throughout the entire posterior fossa below the tentorial leaves. At the time of craniectomy for tumor removal, no cerebellum was seen; the surgeon looked from the edge of the calvarium directly into brain stem and tumor.

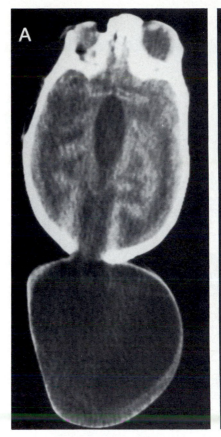
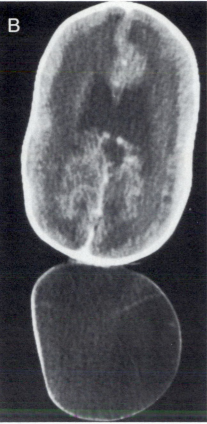

FIG 24–65.
Occipital encephalocele with midline "cystic" anomaly. CT scanning demonstrates a large occipital encephalocele, extension of the cystic space in the region of the tentorium, and a large cystic space where the third ventricle would normally reside **(A)**. The lateral ventricles **(B)** have an unusual configuration with a missing septum pellucidum.

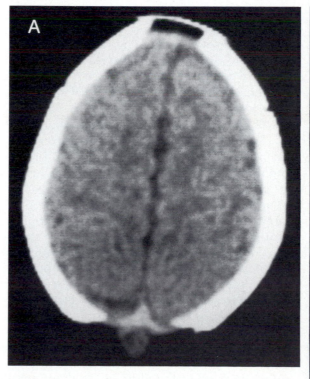
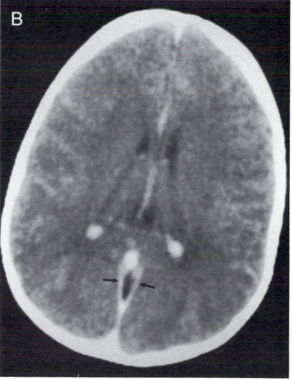

FIG 24–66.
Parietal encephalocele extending through the posterior falx. CT scanning demonstrates separation of the parietal bones and a small midline encephalocele **(A)**. A lower cut **(B)** shows extension of the CSF density between the leaves of the posterior falx *(arrows)*.

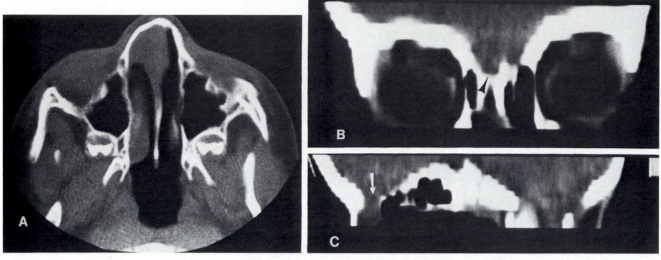

FIG 24–67.
Transethmoidal encephalocele. **A,** the axial scan demonstrates a soft tissue mass in the anterior aspect of the right side of the nose. **B,** a coronal reconstruction shows deformity of the right side of the cribriform plate *(arrowhead).* **C,** a sagittal reconstruction just to the right of the midline shows the bony defect of the cribriform plate *(arrow)* and a soft tissue mass extending inferiorly into the nose.

laginous and membranous centers, and frontal, parietal, and occipital encephaloceles between the paired plates of membranous bone.[134] Lateral encephaloceles can result from constriction of the developing skull by intrauterine amniotic bands.

Sincipital encephaloceles are anterior encephaloceles that are visible externally, usually located near the root of the nose.[134, 137, 138] All encephaloceles in this group have a mass at the glabella, and hypertelorism. The frontal, nasal, and ethmoid bones develop from separate ossification centers, all joining at the foramen cecum, at a point known during embryonic development as the fonticulus frontalis.[139] Encephaloceles in this region are subdivided by their direction of herniation relative to these bony structures, as follows[134, 137]:

1. Interfrontal: There is a defect in the metopic suture, with a large encephalocele containing cerebral tissue ranging from the anterior tip to the anterior half of each cerebral hemisphere. The prognosis for normal development is usually poor.
2. Nasofrontal: The sac extends between the paired frontal bones and the paired nasal bones, separating the deformed orbits.
3. Naso-orbital: The sac courses behind the nasal bones and turns laterally through an osseous defect between the ethmoid bone and the frontal process of the maxilla to lie in the medial orbit.
4. Nasoethmoidal: The mass projects through a defect in the lamina cribrosa of the ethmoid bone, courses between the nasal bones and nasal carti-

lage, to project into the nasal fossa. The patient presents with nasal obstruction.

Basal encephaloceles protrude into the nasal cavity and are not usually visible externally. They are subdivided as follows[138, 141]:

1. Transethmoidal: The defect is in the cribriform plate (see Fig 24–67), with the encephalocele attached to the nasal septum and protruding into one side or the other of the nasal cavity. A large mass may extend through the nares. There is a rare association with optic and cerebral malformations.
2. Transsphenoidal: The sac extends through the sella turcica and sphenoid bone into the nasopharynx (see Fig 24–38). There is a high association with agenesis of the corpus callosum (75%), hypertelorism (90%), and median cleft lip (79%). Optic dysplasias such as cholobomata are common. The sac contains a variable amount of cerebral tissue, with inferior displacement of the third ventricle, pituitary, optic chiasm, and optic nerves.
3. Sphenoethmoidal: The mass extends through the sphenoethmoidal junction to end in the posterior nasal cavity or nasopharynx.

Because nasal polyps and adenoid tissue are rare in infancy, the presence of a nasopharyngeal mass should alert the clinician to the possibility of a basal encephalocele.[135] Snaring of a nasal polyp in infancy should not be done before an encephalocele has been excluded.

The term *nasal glioma* refers to an intra- or extranasal mass containing benign CNS tissue with no apparent connection to the brain. Sometimes (5%–20%) a fibrous stalk connects to skull base lesions, probably representing transethmoidal or sin- cipital encephaloceles that have lost their intracranial connection from overgrowth of the basilar skull defect. In some cases, however, the bony defect persists. Associated facial and other anomalies are rare. The glial tissues of the nasal glioma and

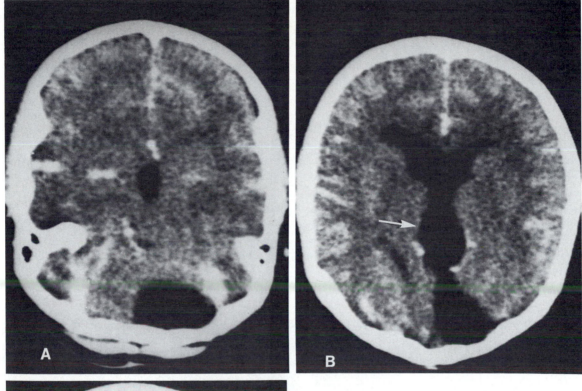

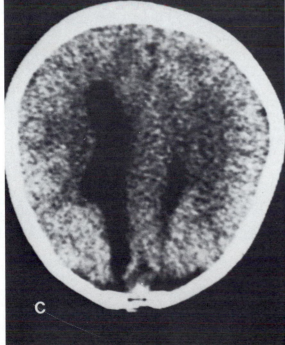

FIG 24–68.
Occipital encephalocele with associated agenesis of the corpus callosum. **A** and **B** demonstrate a large CSF-containing space located in both posterior fossa and supratentorial compartments, just to the left of the midline. The patient had had an occipital encephalocele repaired early in infancy. A tentorial defect must exist to allow the cystic structure to be in both the supratentorial and infratentorial compartments. There is dilatation of the posterior portion of the third ventricle (**B,** *arrow*), which communicates directly with the cystic structure located more posteriorly. Vascular structures are contiguous to this dilated third ventricle, but are laterally displaced. The posterior portion of the corpus callosum is absent. **C,** a higher cut shows separation of the lateral ventricles, characteristic of agenesis of the corpus callosum. The posterior portions of both lateral ventricles extend posteriorly, secondary to the developmental displacement of the brain through the cranial defect.

within the encephalocele are similar, consisting of disorganized nests of astrocytes, with occasional ganglion cells or neurons or both.[140]

MRI is the imaging technique of choice for the evaluation of an encephalocele. The contents of the sac may include CSF, disorganized parenchyma, and even portions of the ventricle (see Fig 24–38). The density within the sac is proportional to the type of tissue present, and is well demonstrated with MRI, which, with its multiple projections and ability to exquisitely define anatomic structures of different densities, is better than CT for evaluating the distorted anatomy of the patient with an encephalocele (see Fig 24–38).

CT is less capable than MRI of defining the different soft tissues within the encephalocele. Water-soluble contrast may have to be placed within the thecal sac and allowed to run into the encephalocele for appropriate evaluation.[142] CT does give excellent evaluation of the bony defect, utilizing sagittal and coronal image reconstructions or, even better, three-dimensional reconstruction. Such three-dimensional images are helpful to the surgeon in repairing the bony defect.[139]

Cerebral angiography is rarely utilized in the evaluation of an encephalocele. It may prove helpful if there is concern about displacement of a dural venous sinus into the sac.[135] However, MRI is usually capable of defining such anatomy.

Imaging procedures are also utilized to demonstrate the presence of associated intracranial anomalies. Encephaloceles are uncommonly associated with the Chiari malformation.[143] Occipital and parietal encephaloceles are associated with holoprosencephaly, and occasionally with the Dandy-Walker complex and aqueductal stenosis. Agenesis of the corpus callosum (Figs 24–38 and 24–68) and other midline abnormalities (see Fig 24–65) are associated with a variety of encephaloceles.[143]

Craniosynostosis

Craniosynostosis is a general term for premature closure of one or multiple cranial sutures. The particular suture or sutures that close prematurely determine the subsequent shape of the head. For example, premature closure of the sagittal suture prevents lateral growth of the cranium, requiring the increasing cerebral volume to be accommodated by an increased growth in the anteroposterior diameter of the head (scaphocephaly). Prema-

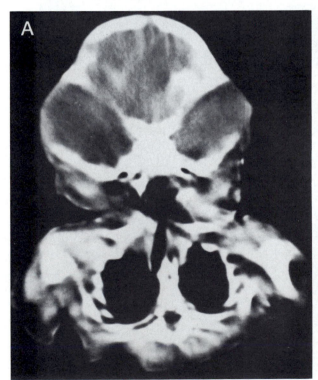
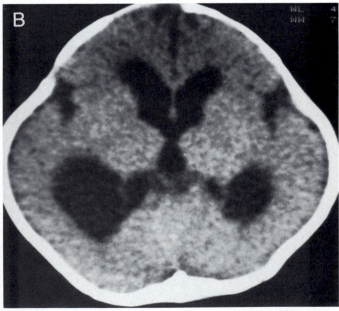

FIG 24–69.
Craniosynostosis: kleeblattschädel (cloverleaf skull). **A,** premature fusion of multiple cranial sutures, including the coronal and lambdoid sutures, has produced gross deformity of the skull. **B,** the anteroposterior diameter of the head is markedly shortened, with shallow orbits and anterior fossae, and midface hypoplasia. The lateral bowing of the temporal regions and high vertex give the name *cloverleaf skull* **(A).** The patient also has a Chiari malformation, with secondary ventricular dilatation. There were multiple other systemic congenital anomalies of the gastrointestinal and genitourinary systems.

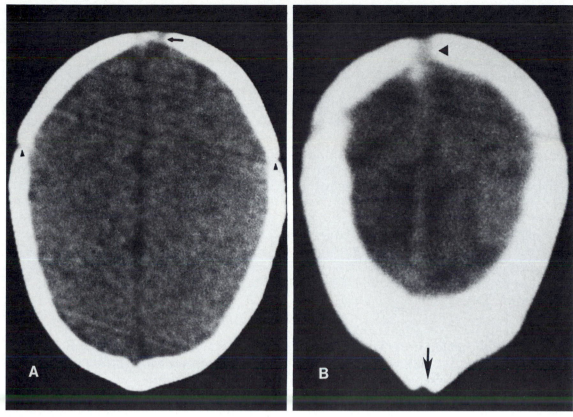

FIG 24–70.
Craniosynostosis: premature fusion of the sagittal suture. The patient was scanned because of elongation of the head in the anteroposterior diameter. **A,** this configuration is seen along with patency of the coronal *(arrowheads)* and distal metopic *(arrow)* sutures. **B,** a higher cut demonstrates patency of the anterior portion of the sagittal suture *(arrowhead),* but a beaked configuration *(arrow)* to the cranium posteriorly. This beaking represents sutural fusion and bony overgrowth.

ture closure of the coronal sutures prevents expansion in the anteroposterior direction, resulting in growth in the lateral and cephalic directions (oxycephaly).

Closure of multiple sutures may produce very unusual configurations of the head such as the kleeblattschädel (cloverleaf skull) (Fig 24–69). Such complex deformities are frequently accompanied by anomalies of the face as seen in Figure 24–69. When oxycephaly is accompanied by a flattening in the anteroposterior diameter of the facial structures, particularly the orbits, bulging of the eyes results. This entire complex of cranial and facial distortions is called Crouzon's disease. The Crouzon malformation may be accompanied by anomalies of the small bones of the hands (Apert's syndrome).

CT scanning has been utilized in the evaluation of the various forms of craniosynostosis.[144] Such scanning requires an extensive use of bone windows to evaluate the status of the cranial su-

tures. One may see a "beaking" when there is sutural fusion and pronounced bony overgrowth (Fig 24–70). Evaluation of the cranium may be difficult, however, requiring multiple cuts to determine sutural patency. Because of the sloping of the skull, a false impression of sutural fusion may occur unless the plane of the cut is at right angles to the portion of the suture in question. Skull films undoubtedly will remain an important radiographic technique for this abnormality, although detection of infantile sutures is difficult on plain films alone. CT and MR scanning are also useful for the detection of underlying cerebral anomalies.

GLOBAL BRAIN SIZE

Microencephaly

Multiple etiologies may lead to a small brain, such as destructive lesions (e.g., infectious lesions of the STARCH group), degenerative and metabolic disorders (e.g., phenylketonuria), chromosomal anomalies, and various cerebral congenital malformations. These malformations include the lissencephaly syndrome, holoprosencephaly, and agenesis of the corpus callosum,[1] all of which have been discussed previously in this chapter.

Megalencephaly

Enlargement of the head (macrocephaly) may occur for many reasons, including hydrocephalus, cerebral edema from a variety of causes, intracranial mass lesion, extracerebral fluid collections, diffuse thickening of the skull, and megalencephaly. The term *megalencephaly* refers to an enlarged brain caused by an increase in the volume of nonedematous cerebral parenchyma.[145]

DeMyer has produced a classification of megalencephaly, basing the classification upon metabolic vs. anatomic causation.[145, 146] The metabolic megalencephalies include cerebral enlargement associated with aminoaciduria; leukodystrophies such as Canavan's and Alexander's diseases and metachromatic leukodystrophy; and lysosomal diseases including Tay-Sachs disease and the mucopolysaccharidoses such as Hunter-Hurler's disease. Chapter 13 discusses these metabolic diseases in detail.

The anatomic megalencephalies are subdi-

vided into those with unilateral and those with bilateral hemispheric enlargement. Patients with unilateral megalencephaly may present with seizure disorders, and there is some evidence, such as pachygyric areas and loss of normal cortical lamination, suggesting that unilateral megalencephaly is a form of neuronal migrational disorder.[9, 119, 147] The unilateral megalencephalies are further subdivided into those without and those with somatic hemihypertrophy. In the latter category are syndromes such as the Klippel-Trenaunay-Weber syndrome which presents with hemangiomatosis of an extremity in addition to unilateral megalencephaly,[145] the Proteus syndrome,[145] and a few rare cases of neurofibromatosis.[147] Bilateral megalencephaly occurs in patients with gigantism, such as cerebral gigantism of Sottas, and pituitary gigantism; patients with neurocutaneous syndromes, such as neurofibromatosis (Fig 24–71) and tuberous sclerosis[148, 149]; and patients with dwarfism such as achrondroplasia.[145, 150, 151] There is controversy regarding the role of ventricular dilatation vs. nonhydrocephalic parenchymal enlargement with achrondroplasia.[150, 151] It has been suggested that while megalencephaly may be present at birth in achrondroplasia, progressive CSF obstruction at the base of the skull and at the foramen magnum leads to progressive hydrocephalus in later life.[151]

The most common condition, however, is the

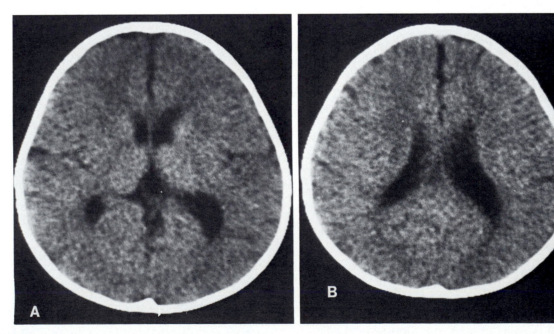

FIG 24–71.
Megalencephaly associated with neurofibromatosis. This 21-month-old child had a head circumference greater than 3 SD of the mean for his age. He had peripheral stigmata of neurofibroma-

tosis. In an absolute sense, the lateral ventricles **(A, B)** are slightly larger than normal for this age, but are proportional to the size of the rest of the brain, characteristic of megalencephaly.

brain that is mildly enlarged during early childhood but that decreases its growth rate in later childhood to remain at the upper limits of normal. The father usually has a relatively large head, as do other family members, and there are no other syndromes. Scanning demonstrates a normal-appearing brain or, in some cases, the ventricular system may appear to be mildly enlarged for age (Fig 24–71). However, the ventricles are normal or only slightly large relative to the amount of cerebral parenchyma present. It is important to emphasize in such cases that the overall cranial enlargement is not due to hydrocephalus, mass lesion, leukodystrophy, etc.[145]

BRAIN MATURATION

Abnormalities of brain maturation may have a variety of etiologies, both genetic and acquired. Patients are studied early in infancy or childhood because of developmental delay or progressive neurologic symptoms, looking for any evidence of a congenital cerebral anomaly, abnormality of brain maturation, etc. It is therefore appropriate that this topic be briefly discussed in this chapter.

MRI allows us to image the myelination process, whereas CT simply does not have the ability to resolve subtle soft tissue differences within and between the white and gray matter to allow a determination of the stage of myelination or any abnormality in that process in other than the most overt case. While only a few MR studies of a large population of infants have been conducted on MR units with high contrast resolution, those early studies demonstrate that the MR changes in myelination parallel the known histochemical processes.[5, 152–157]

Myelin is composed of a combination of a double layer of lipid, particularly cholesterol and glycolipid, and large proteins. These large molecules cause a decrease in the T1 relaxation time of water as myelination progresses. T1-weighted MRI sequences are therefore sensitive at demonstrating the myelination process. Because myelin is hydrophobic, the myelination process is accompanied by a decrease in the water content of the brain. T2-weighted sequences are particularly sensitive to the water content of tissues, and are therefore of value in demonstrating the secondary events as myelination progresses. In summary, T1-weighted sequences are better for the actual myelination process, while T2-weighted sequences are better for the secondary water loss.[152]

A recent study demonstrated that T1 changes were seen earlier than T2 changes using a 1.5T magnet and spin-echo sequences. The T1 sequences were especially helpful in the evaluation of brain development in the first 6 to 8 months of life, while the T2-weighted sequences were better after 6 months of age.[152] T1-enhancing sequences such as inversion recovery may be even more sensitive to the early myelination process. A recent report suggests that a double-echo STIR sequence (TR/TI/TE = 3,000/148/2383 ms) is very sensitive for assessing brain maturation and enabling early diagnosis of delayed myelination.[158]

The patterns of myelination can be grossly characterized as follows: the neonatal T1-weighted spin-echo image looks like the adult T2-weighted image, and the neonatal T2-weighted sequence looks like the adult T1 sequence.[152] Using a 1.5T magnet, the time of myelination appearance for various structures is given in Table 24–5. In general, myelination proceeds from inferior to superior, from posterior to anterior, and from central to peripheral. The more archaic structures are myelinated before the more advanced structures.[159]

A study of both normal and abnormal infants and children on magnets of 0.3 to 0.35T field strength suggests division of normal myelination into the infantile, the isointense, and the adult forms as myelination progresses.[159] This work relies primarily on

TABLE 24–5.

Ages When Changes of Myelination Appeared*

Anatomic Region	T1-Weighted Images†	T2-Weighted Images‡
Middle cerebellar peduncle	Birth	Birth to 2 mo
Cerebellar white matter	Birth to 4 mo	3–5 mo
Posterior limb internal capsule		
Anterior portion	Birth	4–7 mo
Posterior portion	Birth	Birth to 2 mo
Anterior limb internal capsule	2–3 mo	7–11 mo
Genu corpus callosum	4–6 mo	5–8 mo
Splenium corpus callosum	3–4 mo	4–6 mo
Occipital white matter		
Central	3–5 mo	9–14 mo
Peripheral	4–7 mo	11–15 mo
Frontal white matter		
Central	3–6 mo	11–16 mo
Peripheral	7–11 mo	14–18 mo
Centrum semiovale	2–4 mo	7–11 mo

* From Barkovich AJ, Kjos BO, Jackson DE, et al: *Radiology* 1988; 166:173–180. Used by permission.
† T1-weighted sequence was spin-echo TR 600, TE 20.
‡ T2-weighted sequence was TR 2,500, TE 70.

T2-weighted sequences. The infantile pattern extends from birth through 6 months, the isointense from 8 to 12 months, and the early adult pattern thereafter. Total myelination does not occur until early adolescence.[5, 157, 159]

An understanding of these patterns of myelination may help in the evaluation of patients presenting with developmental delay, and in the diagnosis of dysmyelinating and demyelinating diseases. A further discussion of these diseases is provided in Chapter 13.

CONGENITAL TUMORS

The teratomatous tumors, intracranial hamartomas, and lipomas are discussed extensively in Chapter 18. The hamartomatous lesions of the

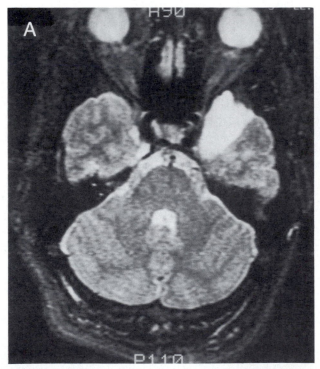

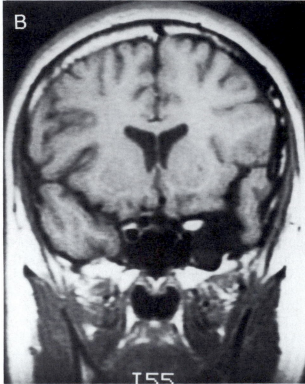

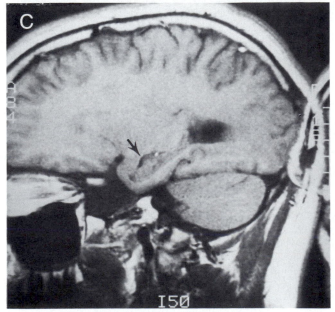

FIG 24–72.
Arachnoid cyst with left temporal lobe hypoplasia. **A,** the long TR/TE MR scan (TR 2,500, TE 80) demonstrates the arachnoid cyst in the anterior portion of the left temporal fossa. The cyst has an intensity equal to CSF. The T1-weighted (TR 700, TE 20) coronal **(B)** and sagittal **(C)** images nicely show the hypoplasia of the anterior portion of the left temporal lobe. The left temporal horn **(C,** *arrow*) is not deformed. Rather, the temporal lobe appears to have normal formation of gray and white matter but appears short.

phakomatoses, including neurofibromatosis, the Sturge-Weber syndrome, and tuberous sclerosis, are also presented in Chapter 18. Craniopharyngioma is discussed in Chapter 23.

Various neuroectodermal tumors occur during early infancy and are considered to be on a congenital basis. These tumors, including astrocytomas, ependymomas, and the various forms of the primitive neuroectodermal tumor (PNET), are discussed extensively in Chapter 16.

CYSTS

Rathke's Pouch Cyst and Neuroepithelial Cyst

Rathke's pouch cyst is a congenital cystic lesion found within the pituitary gland and is discussed in Chapter 23. Neuroepithelial cysts, including colloid cyst, are epithelial-lined cysts found in cerebral parenchyma and are discussed in Chapter 16.

Arachnoid Cyst

Arachnoid cysts have been discussed extensively in Chapter 17. Briefly, most arachnoid cysts are congenital in origin, although they may occasionally occur following trauma or infection.[160]

Arachnoid cysts are sharply marginated lesions, as opposed to low-density nonenhancing neoplasms. Some neoplasms, such as oligodendroglioma and astrocytoma, have CT attenuation coefficients as low CSF, and therefore may mimic an arachnoid cyst.[161] Irregularity of margins is usually present with a neoplasm as opposed to the sharp margination of an arachnoid cyst. MRI is excellent in making this differentiation, based on the intensity of the lesion. An arachnoid cyst has an intensity pattern like that of CSF on the multiple imaging sequences. If the lesion differs in its intensity pattern from intraventricular CSF, suspicion must be raised as to the presence of a neoplastic lesion.[162]

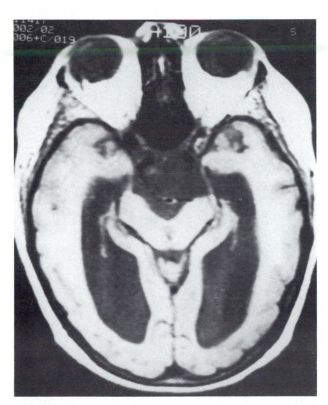

FIG 24–73.
Suprasellar arachnoid cyst. The suprasellar arachnoid cyst as demonstrated on this axial MR image (TR 600, TE 20) has an intensity equal to CSF within the dilated lateral ventricles. The cyst exerts mass effect on the mesencephalon, with an increased size of the interpeduncular fossa and splaying of the cerebral peduncles. The patient was asymptomatic for this suprasellar mass.

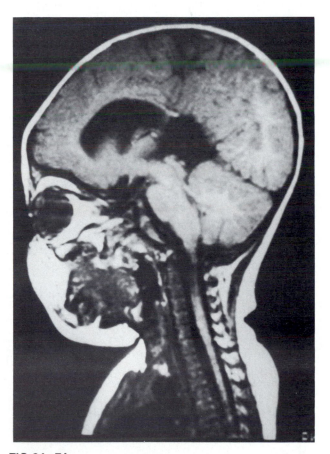

FIG 24–74.
Quadrigeminal plate cistern arachnoid cyst. A sagittal MR scan (TR 700, TE 20) demonstrates a large cystic lesion in the cistern of the quadrigeminal plate. The lesion exerts mass effect, with anterior displacement and dilatation of the lateral ventricles.

Hypoplasia is present with many arachnoid cysts, owing to the congenital nature of the lesion and secondary maldevelopment of the underlying parenchyma (Fig 24–72). However, an arachnoid cyst may slowly expand and produce local mass effect (Figs 24–73 and 24–74).

ABNORMAL VASCULATURE

Arteriovenous malformations and aneurysms are discussed in Chapter 11. The Sturge-Weber syndrome is presented in Chapter 18.

REFERENCES

1. Ludwin SK, Malamud N: Pathology of congenital anomalies of the brain, in Newton TH, Potts DG (eds): *Radiology of the Skull and Brain,* vol 3. St Louis, CV Mosby Co, 1977, pp 2979–3015.
2. DeMyer W: Classification of cerebral malformations. *Birth Defects* 1971; 7:78–93.
3. Hans JS, Benson JE, Kaufman B, et al: MR imaging of pediatric cerebral anomalies. *J Comput Assist Tomogr* 1985; 9:103–114.
4. Pennock JM, Bydder GM, Dubowitz LMS, et al: Magnetic resonance imaging of the brain in children. *Magn Reson Imaging* 1986; 4:1–9.
5. Lee BCP, Lipper E, Nass R, et al: MRI of the central nervous system in neonates and young children. *AJNR* 1986; 7:605–616.
6. Hadley DM, Teasdale GM: Magnetic resonance imaging of the brain and spine. *J Neurol* 1988; 235:193–206.
7. Kemp SS, Zimmerman RA, Bilaniuk LT, et al: Magnetic resonance imaging of the cerebral aqueduct. *Neuroradiology* 1987; 29:430–436.
8. Wolpert SM, Anderson M, Scott RM, et al: Chiari II malformation: MR imaging evaluation. *AJR* 1987; 149:1033–1042.
9. Barkovich AJ, Chuang SH, Norman D: MR of neuronal migration anomalies. *AJNR* 1987; 8:1009–1017.
10. Krawinkel M, Steen HJ, Terwey B: Magnetic resonance imaging in lissencephaly. *Eur J Pediatr* 1987; 146:205–208.
11. Lee BCP, Engle M: MR of lissencephaly. *AJNR* 1988; 9:804.
12. Dunn V, Mock T, Bell WE, et al: Detection of heterotopic gray matter in children by magnetic resonance imaging. *Magn Reson Imaging* 1986; 4:33–39.
13. Smith AS, Weinstein MA, Quencer RM, et al: Association of heterotopic gray matter with seizures: MR imaging. *Radiology* 1988; 168:195–198.
14. Hayden SA, Davis KA, Stears JC, et al: MR imaging of heterotopic gray matter. *J Comput Assist Tomogr* 1987; 11:878–879.
15. Deeb ZL, Rothfus WE, Maroon JC: MR imaging of heterotopic gray matter. *J Comput Assist Tomogr* 1985; 9:1140–1141.
16. Weiner SN, Pearlstein AE, Eiber A: MR imaging of intracranial arachnoid cysts. *J Comput Assist Tomogr* 1987; 11:236–241.
17. Harsh GR, Edwards MSB, Wilson CB: Intracranial arachnoid cysts in children. *J Neurosurg* 1986; 64:835–842.
18. Crawford SC, Boyer RS, Harnsberger R, et al: Disorders of histogenesis: The neurocutaneous syndromes. *Semin US CT MR* 1988; 9:247–267.
19. Oot RF, New PFJ, Pile-Spellman J, et al: The detection of intracranial calcification by MR. *AJNR* 1986; 7:801–809.
20. El-Gammal T, Mark EK, Brooks BS: MR imaging of Chiari II malformation. *AJR* 1988; 150:163–170.
21. Curnes JT, Oakes WJ, Boyko OB: MR imaging of hindbrain deformity in Chiari II patients with and without symptoms of brainstem compression. *AJNR* 1989; 10:293–302.
22. Nakano S, Hojo H, Kataoka K, et al: Age related incidence of cavum septi pellucidi and cavum vergae on CT scans of pediatric patients. *J Comput Assist Tomogr* 1981; 5:348–349.
23. Cowley RA, Moody DM, Alexander E Jr, et al: Distinctive CT appearance of cyst of the cavum septi pellucidi. *AJR* 1979; 133:548–550.
24. Ludwiczak R, Dietemann JL, Wackenheim A: CT and pneumographic studies of membranous occlusion of the aqueduct of Sylvius. A case report. *Neuroradiology* 1979; 18:53–55.
25. Sherman JL, Citrin CM, Barkovich AJ, et al: MR imaging of the mesencephalic tectum: Normal and pathologic variations. *AJNR* 1987; 8:59–64.
26. El-Gammal T, Allen MB Jr, Brooks BS, et al: MR evaluation of hydrocephalus. *AJNR* 1987; 8:591–597.
27. Logue V: Fourteenth Crookshank lecture. Syringomyelia: A radiodiagnostic and radiotherapeutic saga. *Clin Radiol* 1971; 22:2–16.
28. Logue V, Edwards MR: Syringomyelia and its surgical treatment—An analysis of 75 patients. *J Neurol Neurosurg Psychiatry* 1981; 44:273–284.
29. Aboulezz AO, Sartor K, Geyer CA, et al: Position of cerebellar tonsils in the normal population and in patients with Chiari malformation: A quantitative approach with MR imaging. *J Comput Assist Tomogr* 1985; 9:1033–1036.
30. Spinos E, Laster DW, Moody DW, et al: MR evaluation of Chiari I malformations at 0.15T. *AJNR* 1985; 6:203–208.
31. Carmel PW, Markesbery WB: Early descriptions of the Arnold-Chiari malformation. The contribution of John Cleland. *J Neurosurg* 1972; 37:543–547.
32. Paul KS, Lye RH, Strang AF, et al: Arnold-Chiari

malformation: Review of 71 cases. *J Neurosurg* 1983; 58:183–187.

33. Barkovich AJ, Wippold FJ, Sherman JL, et al: Significance of cerebellar tonsillar position on MR. *AJNR* 1986; 7:795–799.

34. Naidich TP, McClone DG, Fulling KH: The Chiari II malformation: Part IV. The hindbrain deformity. *Neuroradiology* 1983; 25:179–197.

35. Gilbert JN, Jones KL, Rorke LB, et al: Central nervous system anomalies associated with meningomyelocele, hydrocephalus and the Arnold-Chiari malformation: Reappraisal of theories regarding the pathogenesis of posterior neural tube closure defects. *Neurosurgery* 1986; 18:559–564.

36. Bell WD, Charney EB, Bruce DA, et al: Symptomatic Arnold-Chiari malformation: Review of experience with 22 cases. *J Neurosurg* 1987; 66:812–816.

37. Venes JL, Black KL, Latack JT: Preoperative evaluation and surgical management of the Arnold-Chiari II malformation. *J Neurosurg* 1986; 64:363–370.

38. Variend S, Emery JL: The weight of the cerebellum in children with myelomeningocele. *Dev Med Child Neurol [Suppl]* 1973; 15(29):77–83.

39. Emery JL: Deformity of the aqueduct of Sylvius in children with hydrocephalus and myelomeningocele. *Dev Med Child Neurol [Suppl]* 1974; 16(32):40–48.

40. Yuh WTC, Segall HD, Senac MD, et al: MR imaging of Chiari II malformation associated with dysgenesis of cerebellum and encephaloceles defined through the use of three-dimensional reconstruction of computed tomography. *Pediatr Neurosci* 1985; 86:18–22.

41. Yamada H, Nakamura S, Tanaka Y, et al: Ventriculography and cisternography with water-soluble contrast media in infants with meningomyelocele. *Radiology* 1982; 143:75–83.

42. Naidich TP, Pudlowski RM, Naidich JB: Computed tomographic signs of the Chiari II malformation. III. Ventricles and cisterns. *Radiology* 1980; 134:657–663.

43. Naidich TP, Pudlowski RM, Naidich JB, et al: Computed tomographic signs of the Chiari II malformation. Part I: Skull and dural partitions. *Radiology* 1980; 134:65–71.

44. Britton J, Marsh H, Kendall B, et al: MRI and hydrocephalus in childhood. *Neuroradiology* 1988; 30:310–314.

45. Lemire RJ, Loeser JD, Leech RW, et al: *Normal and Abnormal Development of the Human Nervous System.* Hagerstown, Md, Harper & Row, 1975.

46. Epstein LG, Berman CZ, Sharer LR, et al: Unilateral calcification and contrast enhancement of the basal ganglia in a child with AIDS encephalopathy. *AJNR* 1987; 8:163–165.

47. Dunn D, Weisberg LA: Serial changes in a patient with congenital CNS toxoplasmosis as observed with CT. *Comput Radiol* 1984; 8:133–139.

48. Diebler C, Dusser A, Dulac O: Congenital toxoplasmosis: Clinical and neuroradiological evaluation of the cerebral lesions. *Neuroradiology* 1985; 27:125–130.

49. Egger J, Kendall BE: CT in mitochondrial cytopathy. *Neuroradiology* 1981; 22:73–78.

50. Seigel RS, Seeger JF, Gabrielsen TO, et al: Computed tomography in oculocraniosomatic disease (Kearns-Sayre syndrome). *Radiology* 1979; 130:159–164.

51. Moossy J: The neuropathology of Cockayne's syndrome. *J Neuropathol Exp Neurol* 1967; 26:654–660.

52. Kendall B, Cavanagh N: Intracranial calcification in paediatric computed tomography. *Neuroradiology* 1986; 28:324–330.

53. Marksbery WR: Lactic acidemia, mitochondrial myopathy and basal ganglia calcification. *Neurology* 1979; 29:1057–1061.

54. Burke JW, Williamson BRJ, Hurst RW: "Idiopathic" cerebellar calcifications: Association with hypothyroidism? *Radiology* 1988; 167:533–536.

55. Camp JD: Symmetrical calcification of the cerebral basal ganglia: Its roentenologic significance in the diagnosis of parathyroid insufficiency. *Radiology* 1947; 49:568–577.

56. Babbitt DP, Tang T, Dobbs J, et al: Idiopathic familial cerebrovascular ferrocalcinosis (Fahr's disease) and review of differential diagnosis of intracranial calcification in children. *AJR* 1969; 105:352–358.

57. Olson W, Engel WK, Walsh GO, et al: Oculocraniosomatic neuromuscular disease with "ragged-red" fibers. *Arch Neurol* 1972; 26:193–211.

58. Kuriyama M, Umezaki H, Fukuda Y, et al: Mitochondrial encephalomyopathy with lactate-pyruvate elevation and brain infarctions. *Neurology (NY)* 1984; 34:72–77.

59. Yamamoto T, Beppu H, Tsubaki T: Mitochondrial encephalomyopathy: Fluctuating symptoms and CT. *Neurology (NY)* 1984; 34:1456–1460.

60. Hasuo K, Tamura S, Yasumori K, et al: Computed tomography and angiography in MELAS (mitochondrial myopathy, encephalopathy, lactic acidosis and stroke-like episodes): Report of 3 cases. *Neuroradiology* 1987; 29:393.

61. Savolaine ER, Gerber AM: Computerized tomography studies of congenital and acquired intraventricular membranes: Report of two cases. *J Neurosurg* 1981; 54:388–391.

62. Harwood-Nash D, Fitz CR: *Neuroradiology in Infants and Children.* St Louis, CV Mosby Co, 1976.

63. Gonsette R, Potvliege R, Andre-Balisaux G, et al: La méga grande citerne: étude clinique, radi-

ologique at anatomopathologique. *Acta Neurol Belg* 1968; 68:559.

64. Blake JA: The roof and lateral recesses of the fourth ventricle considered morphologically and embryologically. *J Comp Neurol* 1900; 10:79.

65. Raybaud C: Cystic malformations of the posterior fossa. *J Neuroradiol* 1982; 9:103–133.

66. Barkovich AJ, Kjos BO, Norman D, et al: Revised classification of posterior fossa cysts and cystlike malformations based on the results of multiplanar MR imaging. *AJNR* 1989; 10:977–988.

67. Raimondi AJ, Samuelson G, Yarzagaray L, et al: Atresia of the foramina of Luschka and Magendie: The Dandy-Walker cyst. *J Neurosurg* 1969; 31:202–216.

68. Hanigan WC, Wright R, Wright S: Magnetic resonance imaging of the Dandy-Walker malformation. *Pediatr Neurosci* 1985–1986; 12:151–156.

69. Banna M: Syringomyelia in association with posterior fossa cysts. *AJNR* 1988; 9:867–873.

70. Hart NM, Malamud N, Ellis WG: The Dandy-Walker syndrome. A clinicopathological study based on 28 cases. *Neurology* 1972; 22:771–780.

71. Sawaya R, McLaurin RL: Dandy-Walker syndrome clinical analysis of 23 cases. *J Neurosurg* 1981; 55:89–98.

72. Yamamoto Y, Waga S: Asymptomatic Dandy-Walker variant in congenital cerebellar hypoplasia. *Clin Genet* 1985; 27:373–382.

73. Masdeu JC, Dobben GD, Azar-Kia B: Dandy-Walker syndrome studied by computed tomography and pneumoencephalography. *Radiology* 1983; 147:109–114.

74. Carmel PW, Antemes JL, Hilal SK, et al: Dandy-Walker syndrome: Clinicopathological features and reevaluation of modes of treatment. *Surg Neurol* 1977; 8:132–138.

75. D'Agostino AN, Kernohan JW, Brown JR: The Dandy-Walker syndrome. *J Neuropathol Exp Neurol* 1963; 22:450–470.

76. Golden JA, Rorke LB, Bruce DA: Dandy-Walker syndrome and associated anomalies. *Pediatr Neurosci* 1987; 13:38–44.

77. Sautreaux JL, Giroud M, Dauvergne M, et al: Dandy-Walker malformation associated with occipital meningocele and cardiac anomalies: A rare complex embryologic defect. *J Child Neurol* 1986; 1:64–66.

78. Hirsch JF, Pierre-Kahn A, Renier D, et al: The Dandy-Walker malformation. *J Neurosurg* 1984; 61:515–522.

79. Strother CM, Harwood-Nash DC: Congenital malformations, in Newton TH, Potts DG (eds): *Radiology of the Skull and Brain.* St Louis, CV Mosby Co, 1978, pp 3712–3748.

80. Gutierrez Y, Friede RL, Kaliney WJ: Agenesis of arachnoid granulations and its relationship to com-

municating hydrocephalus. *J Neurosurg* 1975; 43:553–558.

81. DeMyer W: Holoprosencephaly (cyclopia-arhinencephaly), in Vinken PJ, Bruyn GW (eds): *Handbook of Neurology,* vol 30. Amsterdam, North Holland Publishing Co, 1977, pp 431–478.

82. Manelfe C, Sevely A: Neuroradiological study of holoprosencephalies. *J Neuroradiol* 1982; 9:15–45.

83. Byrd SE, Harwood-Nash DC, Fitz CR, et al: Computed tomography evaluation of holoprosencephaly in infants and children. *J Comput Assist Tomogr* 1977; 1:456–463.

84. Hayashi T, Yoshida M, Kuramoto S, et al: Radiological features of holoprosencephaly. *Surg Neurol* 1979; 12:261–265.

85. Derakhshan I, Sabouri-Deylami M, Lofti J: Holoprosencephaly: Computerized tomographic and pneumographic findings with anatomic correlation. *Arch Neurol* 1980; 37:55–57.

86. Osaka K, Matsumoto S: Holoprosencephaly in neurosurgical practice. *J Neurosurg* 1978; 48:787–803.

87. Warkany J, Lemire RJ, Cohen MM: *Mental Retardation and Congenital Malformations of the Central Nervous System,* Chicago, Year Book Medical Publishers, Inc, 1981.

88. DeMyer W, Zeman W: Alobar holoprosencephaly (arhinencephaly) with median cleft lip and palate: Clinical, electroencephalographic, and nosologic considerations. *Confinia Neurologica* 1963; 23:1–36.

89. Fitz CR: Holoprosencephaly and related entities. *Neuroradiology* 1983; 25:225–238.

90. DeMyer W, Zeman W, Palmer C: The face predicts the brain: Diagnostic significance of median facial anomalies for holoprosencephaly (arhinencephaly). *Pediatrics* 1964; 34:256–263.

91. Berry SA, Pierpont ME, Gorlin RJ: Single central incisor in familial holoprosencephaly. *J Pediatr* 1984; 104:877–880.

92. Leech RW, Shuman RW: Holoprosencephaly and related midline cerebral anomalies: A review. *J Child Neurol* 1986; 1:3–18.

93. Shanks DE, Wilson WG: Lobar holoprosencephaly presenting as spastic diplegia. *Dev Med Child Neurol* 1988; 30:380–386.

94. Hayashi T, Takagi S, Kuramoto S: A case of holoprosencephaly with possible association of Dandy-Walker cyst. *Brain Dev* 1981; 3:97–101.

95. Arslanian SA, Rothfus WE, Foley TP Jr, et al: Hormonal, metabolic and neuroradiologic abnormalities associated with septo-optic dysplasia. *Acta Endocrinol* 1984; 107:282–288.

96. Byrd SE, Naidich TP: Common congenital brain anomalies. *Radiol Clin North Am* 1988; 26:755–772.

97. Wilson DM, Enzmann DR, Hintz RL, et al: Computed tomographic findings in septo-optic dyspla-

sia: Discordance between clinical and radiological findings. *Neuroradiology* 1984; 26:279–283.

98. Acers TE: Optic nerve hypoplasia: Septo-optic pituitary dysplasia syndrome. *Trans Am Ophthalmol Soc* 1981; 79:425–457.

99. Barkovich AJ, Norman D: Absence of the septum pellucidum: A useful sign in the diagnosis of congenital brain malformation. *AJNR* 1988; 9:1107–1114.

100. Loeser JD, Alvord EC Jr: Agenesis of the corpus callosum. *Brain* 1968; 91:553–570.

101. Barkovich AJ, Norman D: Anomalies of the corpus callosum: Correlation with further anomalies of the brain. *AJNR* 1988; 9:493–501.

102. Parrish ML, Roessman U, Levinsohn MW: Agenesis of the corpus callosum: A study of frequency of associated malformation. *Ann Neurol* 1979; 6:349–354.

103. Jeret JS, Serur D, Wisniewski KE, et al: Clinicopathological findings associated with agenesis of the corpus callosum. *Brain Dev* 1987; 9:255–264.

104. Kendall BE: Dysgenesis of the corpus callosum. *Neuroradiology* 1983; 25:239–256.

105. Igidbashian V, Mahboubi S, Zimmerman RA: CT and MR findings in Aicardi syndrome. *J Comput Assist Tomogr* 1987; 11:357–367.

106. Atlas SW, Zimmerman RA, Bilaniuk LT, et al: Corpus callosum and limbic system: Neuroanatomic MR evaluation of developmental anomalies. *Radiology* 1986; 160:355–362.

107. Fujii T, Takao T, Ito M, et al: Lipoma of the corpus callosum: A case report with a review. *Comput Radiol* 1982; 6:301–304.

108. Yock DH: Choroid plexus lipomas associated with lipoma of the corpus callosum. *J Comput Assist Tomogr* 1980; 4:678–682.

109. Reinarz SJ, Coffman CE, Smoker WRK, et al: MR imaging of the corpus callosum: Normal and pathologic findings and correlation with CT. *AJNR* 1988; 9:649–656.

110. Curnes JT, Laster DW, Koubek TD, et al: MRI of corpus callosal syndromes. *AJNR* 1986; 7:617–622.

111. Jeret JS, Serur D, Wisniewski K, et al: Frequency of agenesis of the corpus callosum in the developmentally disabled population as determined by computed tomography. *Pediatr Neurosci* 1985; 86:101–103.

112. Brun A, Probst F: The influence of associated cerebral lesions on the morphology of the acallosal brain. A pathological and encephalographic study. *Neuroradiology* 1973; 6:121–131.

113. Heschl R: Gehirndefekt und Hydrocephalus. *Prag Vierteljahresschr Prakt Heilkd* 1859; 61:59–74.

114. Yakovlev PI, Wadsworth RC: Schizencephalies. A study of the congenital clefts in the cerebral mantle. I—Clefts with fused lips. *J Neuropathol Exp Neurol* 1946; 5:116–130.

115. Yakovlev PI, Wadsworth RC: Schizencephalies. A study of the congenital clefts in the cerebral mantle. II—Clefts with hydrocephalus and lips separated. *J Neuropathol Exp Neurol* 1946; 5:169–206.

116. Raybaud C: Destructive lesions of the brain. *Neuroradiology* 1983; 25:265–291.

117. Friede RL: *Developmental Neuropathology.* New York, Springer-Verlag, 1975.

118. Sidman RL, Rakic P: Neuronal migration with special reference to developing human brain: A review. *Brain Res* 1973; 62:1–35.

119. Osborn RE, Byrd SE, Naidich TP, et al: MR imaging of neuronal migrational disorders. *AJNR* 1988; 9:1101–1106.

120. Barkovich AJ, Norman D: MR imaging of schizencephaly. *AJNR* 1988; 9:297–302.

121. Barkovich AJ: Abnormal vascular drainage in anomalies of neuronal migration. *AJNR* 1988; 9:939–942.

122. Jung JH, Graham JM, Schultz N, et al: Congenital hydranencephaly/porencephaly due to vascular disruption in monozygotic twins. *Pediatrics* 1984; 73:467–469.

123. Bird CR, Gilles FH: Type I schizencephaly: CT and neuropathologic findings. *AJNR* 1987; 8:451–454.

124. Reference deleted in proof.

125. Zimmerman RA, Bilaniuk LT, Grossman RI: Computed tomography in migratory disorders of human brain development. *Neuroradiology* 1983; 25:257–263.

126. Dobyns WB, McCluggage CW: Computed tomographic appearance of lissencephaly syndromes. *AJNR* 1985; 6:545–550.

127. Byrd SE, Bohan TP, Osborn RE, et al: The CT and MR evaluation of lissencephaly. *AJNR* 1988; 9:923–927.

128. Larroche J-C: Malformations of the nervous system, in Adams JH, Corsellis JAN, Duchen LW (eds.): *Greenfield's Neuropathology.* New York, Wiley Medical Publishers, 1984, pp 390–391.

129. Joubert M, Eisenring JJ, Robb JP, et al: Familial agenesis of the cerebellar vermis: A syndrome of episodic hyperpnea, abnormal eye movements, ataxia, and retardation. *Neurology* 1969; 19:813–825.

130. Curatolo P, Mercuri S, Cotroneo E: Joubert syndrome: A case confirmed by computerized tomography. *Dev Med Child Neurol* 1980; 22:362–366.

131. King MD, Dudgeon J, Stephenson JBP: Joubert's syndrome with retinal dysplasia: Neonatal tachypnoea as a clue to a genetic brain-eye malformation. *Arch Dis Child* 1984; 59:709–718.

132. Caesar P, Vles JSH, Deulieger H, et al: Variability of outcome in Joubert syndrome. *Neuropediatrics* 1984; 16:43–45.

133. Nova HR: Familial communicating hydrocephalus, posterior cerebellar agenesis, mega cisterna magna, and port-wine nevi: Report of five members in one family. *J Neurosurg* 1979; 51:862–865.

134. Yoshida M, Nakamura M: Complete absence of the cerebellum with arthrogryposis multiplex congenita diagnosed by CT scan. *Surg Neurol* 1982; 17:62–65.

135. Diebler C, Dulac O: Cephaloceles: Clinical and neuroradiological appearance. *Neuroradiology* 1983; 25:199–216.

136. Ingraham FD, Swan H: Spina bifida and cranium bifidum: A survey of 546 cases. *N Engl J Med* 1943; 228:559–563.

137. Simpson DA, David DJ, White J: Cephaloceles: Treatment, outcome and antenatal diagnosis: *Neurosurgery* 1984; 15:14–21.

138. Charoonsmith T, Suwanwela C: Frontoethmoidal encephalomeningocele with special reference to plastic reconstruction. *Clin Plast Surg* 1984; 1:271–284.

139. Hemmy DC, David DJ: Skeletal morphology of anterior encephaloceles defined through the use of three-dimensional reconstruction of computed tomography. *Pediatr Neurosci* 1985; 86:18–22.

140. Younus M, Coode PE: Nasal glioma and encephalocele: Two separate entities. *J Neurosurg* 1986; 64:516–519.

141. Yokota A, Matsukado Y, Fuwa I, et al: Anterior basal enaphalocele of the neonatal and infantile period. *Neurosurgery* 1986; 19:468–478.

142. Manelfe C, Starling-Jardim D, Touibi S, et al: Transsphenoidal encephalocele associated with agenesis of corpus callosum: Value of metrizamide computed cisternography. *J Comput Assist Tomogr* 1978; 2:356–361.

143. Cohen MM, Lemire RJ: Syndromes with cephaloceles. *Teratology* 1982; 25:161–172.

144. Brambilla GL, Pizzotta S, Rognone F: CT scan and craniostenosis. *J Neurosurg Sci* 1981; 25:13–16.

145. DeMyer W: Megalencephaly: Types, clinical syndromes, and management. *Pediatr Neurol* 1986; 2:321–328.

146. DeMyer W: Megalencephaly in children. *Neurology (NY)* 1972; 22:634–643.

147. Fitz CR, Harwood-Nash DC, Boldt DW: The radiologic features of unilateral megalencephaly. *Neuroradiology* 1978; 15:145–148.

148. DeMyer W: Megalencephaly in children: Clinical syndromes, genetic patterns, and differential diagnosis from other causes of megalencephaly. *Neurology* 1972; 22:634–643.

149. Patronas NK, Zeldowitz M, Levin K: Ventricular dilatations in neurofibromatosis. *J Comput Assist Tomogr* 1982; 6:598–600.

150. Mueller SM, Bell W, Cornell S, et al: Achondroplasia and hydrocephalus: A computerized tomographic, roentgenographic, and psychometric study. *Neurology (NY)* 1977; 27:430–434.

151. Mueller SM: Enlarged central ventricular system in infant achondroplastic dwarf. *Neurology (NY)* 1980; 30:767–769.

152. Barkovich AJ, Kjos BO, Jackson DE, et al: Normal maturation of the neonatal and infant brain: MR imaging at 1.5T. *Radiology* 1988; 166:173–180.

153. Mintz MC, Grossman RI, Isaacson G, et al: MR imaging of fetal brain. *J Comput Assist Tomogr* 1987; 11:120–123.

154. Brody BA, Kinney HC, Kloman AS, et al: Sequence of central nervous system myelination in human infancy. I. An autopsy study of myelination. *J Neuropathol Exp Neurol* 1987; 46:283–301.

155. Kinney HC, Brody BA, Kloman AS, et al: Sequence of central nervous system myelination in human infancy. I. Patterns of myelination in autopsied infants. *J Neuropathol Exp Neurol* 1988; 47:217–234.

156. Martin E, Kikins R, Zuerrer M, et al: Developmental stages of human brain: An MR study. *J Comput Assist Tomogr* 1988; 12:917–922.

157. Holland BA, Haas DK, Norman D, et al: MRI of normal brain maturation. *AJNR* 1986; 7:201–208.

158. Finn JP, Connelly A, Hall-Craggs MA, et al: Brain maturation: An alternative approach to the assessment of myelination using high-field MRI. Presented at the 28th Annual Meeting of the American Society of Neuroradiology, Los Angeles, March 1990.

159. Dietrich R, Bradley WG, Zaragoza EG, et al: MR evaluation of early myelination patterns in normal and developmentally delayed infants. *AJNR* 1988; 9:69–76.

160. Latchaw RE, Nadell J: Intra- and extracellular arachnoid cyst. *AJR* 1976; 126:629–633.

161. Latchaw RE, Gold LHA, Moore JS, et al: The nonspecificity of absorption coefficients in the differentiation of solid tumors and cystic lesions. *Radiology* 1977; 125:141–144.

162. Kjos BO, Brandt-Zawadzki M, Kucharczyk W, et al: Cystic intracranial lesions: Magnetic resonance imaging. *Radiology* 1985; 155:363–369.

PART X

The Orbit

Introduction

William E. Rothfus, M.D.

Magnetic resonance imaging (MRI) and computed tomography (CT) have unquestionably changed the diagnostic approach to pathology of the orbit by obviating more invasive or less informative tests such as conventional tomography, venography, and arteriography. Their ability to differentiate soft tissues within the orbit, to image small objects, and to obtain and display information in multiple projections have made them applicable to a wide variety of clinical settings. Both modalities have superb ability to define the anatomy of the orbit. Orbital pathology can be localized, and information about the extent of involvement is easily elucidated. Whereas CT is particularly useful in orbital trauma where it can detect penetrating metallic foreign bodies and clearly depict bone fractures, MRI is not as useful. However, MRI is applicable in a variety of other disease processes because of its ability to easily obtain multiplanar images, better visualize the orbital apex, and visualize the intracanalicular portion of the optic nerve. Thus, each modality has particular advantages in fulfilling the anatomic role of orbital scanning.

The other major role of orbital scanning is to attempt to characterize pathologic processes. Neoplasm, noninfectious masses, and vascular abnormalities can be characterized by more than anatomic description. CT is used in defining texture, density, and contrast enhancement as well as method of spread and shape, factors that give insight into the specific nature of a pathologic process. MRI often gives additional information due to its ability to scan with multiple parameters and thus be able to do things like detect abnormal flow and characterize hemorrhage. Disease of the globe is particularly well elucidated by MRI.

The purpose of this section is twofold. First, it is to emphasize the utility of high-resolution orbital scanning in a variety of clinical contexts, all of which require precise anatomic information. Second, it is to provide some structure for the analysis of this anatomic information. Thus, this section is divided into chapters representing problems that are commonly present on scans of the orbit. Solving some of these problems, e.g., infection or trauma, simply requires an orderly anatomic approach. Other problems, e.g., tumors or an enlarged optic nerve sheath, are more difficult. They have a variety of differential diagnostic possibilities that must be considered. The more frequent differentials are discussed in the appropriate chapters.

It is emphasized that an exact histologic diagnosis is often not possible on the basis of scanning alone. As in any radiologic approach to differential diagnosis, different diseases may present similarly. Being in the right "ballpark," however, is frequently as important as getting the exact diagnosis because it affects the course of further diagnostic studies and therapeutic measures.

25

Normal Orbital Anatomy and Scanning Techniques

William E. Rothfus, M.D.

NORMAL ANATOMY

The bony orbit forms a cavity that is shaped like a four-sided pyramid, the apex of which is the optic foramen. Its roof, which slopes inferiorly from anterior to posterior, is made up mostly of the orbital portion of the frontal bone, with a posterior component from the lesser wing of the sphenoid. The medial wall, which is oriented in the sagittal plane, is composed of the nasal process of the maxilla, lacrimal bone, lamina papyracea of the ethmoid, and part of the greater wing of the sphenoid. The floor, which slants upward, is formed by the zygomatic bone and orbital processes of the maxilla and palatine bones. The lateral wall is angled about 45 degrees from the sagittal plane and does not extend anteriorly as far as the medial wall. It is formed by the zygomatic bone anteriorly and greater sphenoidal wing posteriorly. The bones are covered by a layer of periosteum called the periorbita. This periorbita is loosely attached, except at the suture lines and foramina. Periosteal reflections (orbital septa) extend from the orbital margins and insert at the tarsal plates.[1] Thus, the orbital contents are enveloped by a protective "sock" of periosteum.

The orbital boundaries are very thin along the floor and medial wall. These areas of thinning are important sites of potential weakness in trauma, infection, and neoplasm. Actual dehiscences occur in the lamina papyracea and form a direct (although small) connection between the ethmoids and the orbit.

When the bony walls are scanned by computed tomography (CT) or magnetic resonance imaging (MRI), account must be taken of their varying degrees of angulation from the true axial, coronal, and sagittal planes. The medial wall, oriented in the sagittal plane, is most easily evaluated in the usual axial (−10 degrees from the orbitomeatal baseline) and coronal sections. The other walls diverge from these planes and are therefore scanned obliquely. Complete evaluation of the walls, e.g., in a complex fracture of the orbits, must take this into account. The use of reconstruction techniques or off-axis sagittal and coronal planes is often needed to gain adequate three-dimensional information about the walls.

CT is generally considered better than MRI at defining the bony walls of the orbit (Figs 25–1 to 25–6). While the orbits stand out on CT as obvious hyperdensities against less dense orbit fat and/or sinus air, the hypointense cortical bones seen on MRI is more difficult to discern against hypointense sinus air. Short TR/TE sequences make it easier to see the bony wall because of its juxtaposition against hyperintense fat (Fig 25–3) than do long TR/TE sequences in which fat is less dense. The bony wall is more easily defined in regions where it is thick and contains fatty marrow (e.g., the lateral wall).

The bony margins of the orbit have variable thickness. Natural areas of thinning, mentioned previously, may be so thin that the bone cannot be resolved. Instead, the air of the sinus appears to abut directly against extraconal fat. Besides the floor and medial wall, the roof and lateral walls may have such areas of thinning. Knowledge of

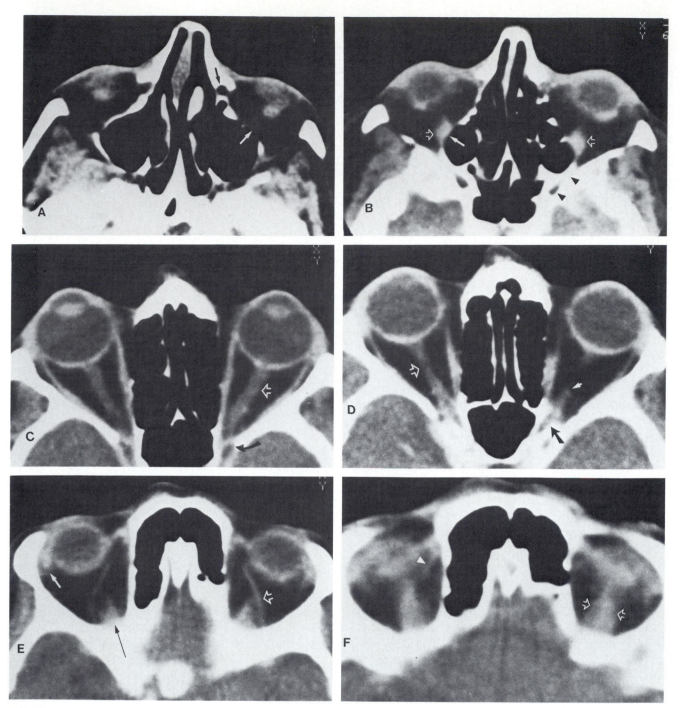

FIG 25-1.

Normal axial CT anatomy. **A,** normal orbit, inferior level, axial section. The lateral maxillary wall *(white arrow)* is quite thin, looking as though it is nonexistent. The nasolacrimal duct *(black arrow)* is a well-defined foramen running coronally from the anteromedial orbit to the nasal cavity. **B,** normal orbit, inferior level, axial section. The lateral wall of the ethmoid sinus *(closed arrow)* is so thin that it appears to be absent. The inferior orbital fissure *(arrowheads)* is seen posteriorly behind the inferior rectus muscle *(open arrows).* **C,** normal orbit, midlevel, axial section. The superior orbital fissure *(curved arrow)* provides communication between the orbit and cavernous sinus. Its walls are well defined. The globe is divided into anterior and posterior chambers by the lens. The medial and lateral recti are thin fusiform structures inserting into the posterior globe. The left optic nerve sheath *(open arrow)* is uniform in caliber, having been sectioned directly down its axis. **D,** normal orbit, midlevel, axial section. The posterior portion of the intraorbital optic nerve is seen entering the anterior aspect of the optic canal *(black arrow).* The optic nerve sheath is sectioned above its "knee." Partial volume averaging causes apparent caliber and density change *(open arrow).* Portions of the ophthalmic artery *(white arrow)* are seen coursing over the optic nerve. **E,** normal orbit, superior level, axial section. The lacrimal gland *(white arrow)* is a small soft-tissue structure just lateral and superior to the globe. Posteriorly, it is outlined by fat. Only the posterior aspect of the superior rectus/superior levator palpebrae muscle complex *(long arrow)* is seen because of the scan angle. The midportion of the superior ophthalmic vein is easily identified *(open arrow).* **F,** normal orbit, superior level, axial section. The superior rectus/superior levator palpebrae muscle complex *(open arrows)* is seen as a rectangular density extending toward the posterosuperior globe. The most anterior part of the superior ophthalmic vein *(arrowhead)* lies just medial to the superior globe. Just anterior to this is a portion of the superior oblique muscle that is draped over the globe.

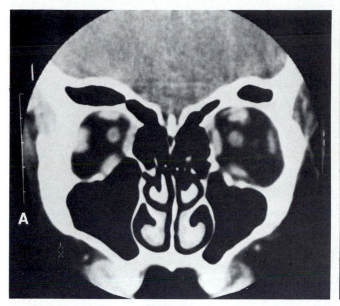 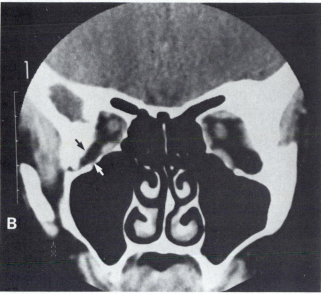

FIG 25–2.
A, normal orbit, direct coronal CT sections. Midorbital sections behind the globe project the optic nerves in the medial half of the orbit. The rectus muscles are clearly seen. The superior oblique can be distinguished just above the medial rectus, and the levator palpebrae superioris can be identified just above the superior rec-

tus in the orbit to the reader's right. **B,** normal orbit, direct coronal CT section. This section is taken just posterior to photo **A.** The orbits CT have changed shape from round to triangular. Because the patient's head is slightly oblique, a portion of the inferior orbital fissure is seen on the left *(arrows)* but not on the right.

these areas is essential to avoid misdiagnosing wall destruction by inflammatory or neoplastic disease.

Normal foramina present as bony defects with smooth, corticated margins. Familiarization with the major foramina is important because they serve as important neurovascular conduits for the orbital extension of extraorbital disease. The superior orbital fissure is a triangular-shaped orifice extending between the superior and lateral walls and running from the cranial cavity to the orbit.[1] Best delineated in an axial section, it is shown on sequential scans just anterior to the cavernous sinus (Figs 25–1 and 25–3). The inferior orbital fissure is between the lateral and inferior walls anterior to the superior orbital fissure. It connects the inferior orbit with the pterygopalatine fossa posteriorly and the infratemporal fossa anteriorly.[1] It is best appreciated in axial or coronal sections (Figs 25–1 and 25–2). The optic canal projects anteriorly, laterally, and inferiorly from the cranial cavity to the orbital apex. Just superior to the superior orbital fissure, it is evaluated well in axial scans, particularly if performed in a plane −40 degrees to the orbitomeatal baseline.[2] With less severe angulation, portions of the canal are seen sequentially (Fig 25–1). The nasolacrimal canal runs coronally from the anteromedial portion of the orbital floor to the nasal cavity and can be seen on axial or coronal scans (Figs 25–1 and 25–3).

The Globe and Lacrimal Gland

The globe dominates the structures of the anterior orbit. Roughly spherical in shape, it lies slightly closer to the lateral wall than the medial wall and closer to the roof than the floor.[3] It is made up of two chambers separated by the lens and iris. The anterior chamber is volumetrically much smaller than the posterior. It is covered by cornea, while the posterior chamber is covered by retina, vascular choroid, fibrous sclera, and Tenon's capsule. These walls and their enclosed chambers are well defined by CT. The walls are uniform in width and density, except for a slight protuberance and change in density at the insertion of the optic nerve posteriorly (papilla). The various layers of the walls cannot be distinguished by CT. The aqueous and vitreous chambers have a uniformly low density, while the lens stands out as a higher-density structure in the anterior portion of the globe (see Fig 25–1).

MRI has been shown to be able to define the anatomy of the globe more intricately than CT, at least when using a high–field strength magnet with ex vivo specimens.[4] The studies of Gomori et al. proved that MRI could distinguish the iris and the ciliary body lateral to the lens, lens nucleus, and cortex of the lens and inner retina and choroid from the outer portion of the sclera. In practice,

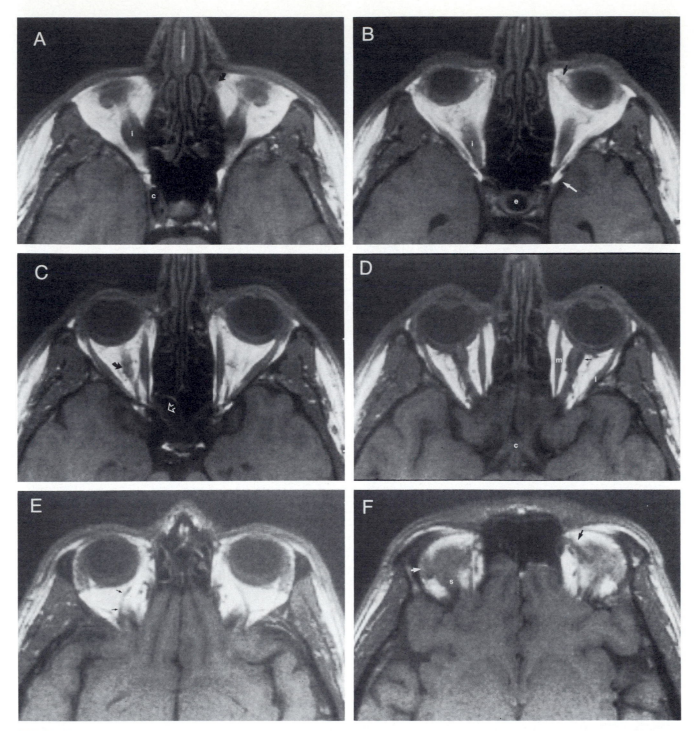

FIG 25-3.

Normal orbit. Axial, short TR/TE MR sections depict similar anatomy to axial CT sections in Figure 25-1. **A,** inferior level. The isointense inferior rectus *(i)* is seen through most of its length due to more angulation than in Figure 25-1. Although seen, the nasolacrimal duct *(curved arrow)* is not as clearly delineated. Signal void from air defines the ethomoid and sphenoid sinuses. Void is also seen in the intracavernous carotid *(c)*. **B,** inferior level. A small amount of high-signal fat is seen in the anterior cavernous sinuses *(white arrow)*. Fibers of the inferior oblique *(black arrow)* spread medially to the inferior globe. Incidental note is made of an empty sella *(e)*. **C,** midlevel. The inferiorly dipping midportion of the optic nerve is barely seen on the right *(curved arrow)*. The intracanalicu-lar portion of the nerve *(arrow)* can be seen surrounded by hypointense cortical bone and aerated sinus. **D,** midlevel. Medial *(m)* and lateral *(l)* rectus muscles are clearly seen. Isointense optic nerve is surrounded by hypointense cerebrospinal fluid (CSF) within the nerve sheath *(arrow)*. The optic chiasm *(c)* is well seen. Chemical shift and motion artifact combine to give the posterior globe wall a bilayer appearance. **E,** superior level. The superior ophthalmic vein midportion *(arrows)* is well seen due to flow void. **F,** superior level. The superior levator/superior rectus *(s)* extends posteriorly to the globe, while (anterior) superior oblique fibers spread over the medial globe *(black arrow)*. The lacrimal gland is isointense *(white arrow)*.

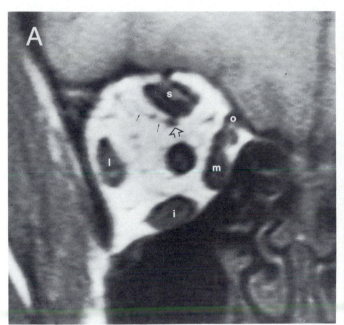

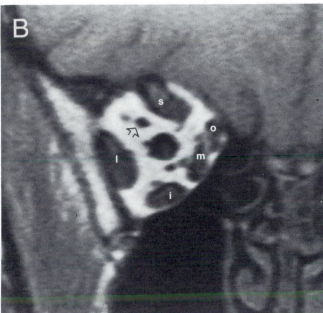

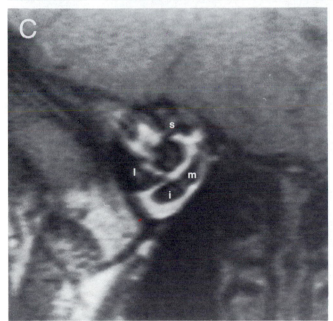

FIG 25–4.
Normal orbit, coronal MR sections. **A–C,** short TR/TE surface coil images extend posteriorly from the globe. The rectus muscles (medial rectus, *m;* lateral rectus, *l;* superior rectus–superior levator, *s;* inferior rectus, *i;* superior oblique, *o*) surround the optic nerve sheath complex. Hypointense CSF forms a ring around the isointense nerve. Note the exquisite detail with which the annulus of Zinn is depicted in **C.** Also note the ability to discern some of the fine septations within the orbital fat, including the "hammock" under the superior rectus (**A,** *small black arrows*) that is associated with the superior ophthalmic artery (**A,** *open arrow*).

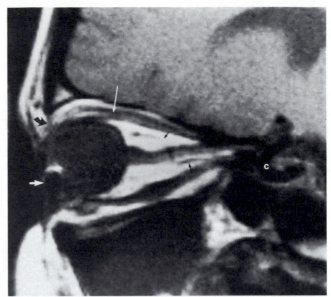

FIG 25–5.
Normal orbit, oblique sagittal short TR/TE MR section. This midorbital section shows a longitudinal view of the optic nerve. The ophthalmic artery is seen swinging from below the nerve posteriorly to above it more anteriorly *(small black arrows)*. The orbital septum is a thin density extending into the tarsus from the superior orbital rim *(curved black arrow)*. A dense black artifact results from metal in eye makeup *(short white arrow)*. The superior rectus and superior levator palpebrae can be seen diverging from their common sheath *(thin white arrow)*. The cavernous carotid artery *(c)* is easily seen due to signal void.

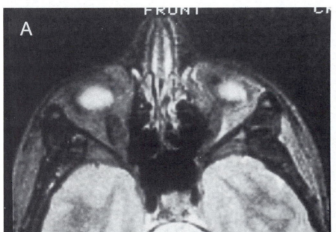

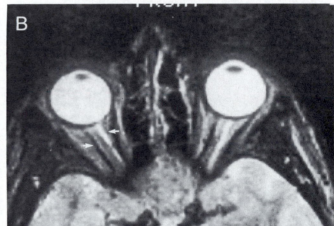

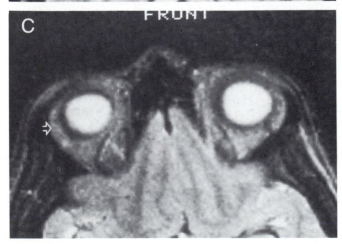

FIG 25–6.
Normal orbit, axial long TR/TE MR sections. **A,** inferior level; **B,** midlevel; **C,** superior level. The extraocular muscles are somewhat less intense than in Figure 25–3, while orbital fat has decreased markedly. A chemical shift misregistration artifact creates bands of high and low signal perpendicular to the frequency-encoding gradient along the interface of orbital fat and the optic nerve *(B, arrows)*. The lacrimal glands remain isointense *(C, arrow)*.

eye movement during scanning and chemical shift artifact diminish the inherent advantages of MRI in defining precise eye anatomy. In a cooperative patient, however, the lens, iris, ciliary body, globe wall, optic nerve head, and aqueous and vitreous chambers are usually distinguishable (see Fig 25–3).[5, 6]

Various methods to evaluate globe proptosis have evolved. One easy method is to project a line from one zygomatic process to the other on a well-positioned midorbital axial scan. Normally, about one third of the globe should project behind this line. Less than one third suggests significant exophthalmos.[7]

The lacrimal gland resides in the superolateral aspect of the anterior orbit just medial to the zygomatic process of the frontal bone. It is most accurately defined on coronal and axial scans. A well-defined oval or bean-shaped structure, it has homogenous CT density roughly equal to that of muscle; so too on MRI, lacrimal gland intensity is similar to that of muscle. Its posterior aspect is the most easily distinguished by virtue of being outlined by extraconal fat (see Figs 25–1 and 25–3).

The Extraocular Muscles

The recti muscles arise from a common tendinous ring at the orbital apex. This ring, the annulus of Zinn, surrounds the medial portion of the superior orbital fissure and the optic foramen.[8] It therefore has a critical relationship to important nervous and vascular structures. From the annulus, the muscles extend anteriorly, gradually diverging as they parallel the orbital walls, thus forming the well-known muscle cone. At their most anterior portions, the muscles have fairly dense tendinous sheaths that insert into different quadrants of Tenon's capsule. This capsule surrounds the posterior portion of the globe, attaches to the sclera and optic nerve, and forms the base of the cone. Two major surgical spaces are defined by the muscle cone—the intraconal space and the extraconal space. Although an intermuscular fascial membrane has been described that further separates the intraconal and extraconal spaces,[9] recent anatomic work suggests that the structure is more defined anteriorly than posteriorly.[10]

The superior oblique muscle also originates at the apex. It courses close to the superomedial wall of the orbit to reach the trochlea, where it bends laterally to insert into the capsule. The shorter inferior oblique muscle originates in the anterior and medial sections of the orbit and runs laterally just inferior to the inferior rectus. The levator palpebrae superioris parallels the superior rectus along much of its course. Lying just above the rectus, it has several fascial attachments to it but inserts into the skin of the upper lid.[8]

The recti are easily defined by CT and MRI. However, the extent to which each muscle is evaluated depends on the plane of sectioning. For example, in the usual axial scanning angle (−10 degrees), the medial and lateral recti are best visualized because the scan slice runs longitudinally down the course of each muscle. The inferior and superior recti, on the other hand, run obliquely through this scanning plane. As a result, only serial portions of these muscles are seen on scans (Figs 25–1 and 25–3). Oblique sagittal images are better to visualize these in a longitudinal fashion (Fig 25–5). Coronal scans, because they cut across all of the muscles except the inferior oblique, are very useful in precisely determining muscle topography (Figs 25–2 and 25–4). Some caution must be used when interpreting direct coronal scans. Because the muscles diverge from the direct coronal plane, different parts of each muscle are imaged, e.g., the midportion of the medial rectus is imaged at the same time as the anterior portion of the lateral rectus. Therefore, it is often difficult to compare muscle size and contour within one orbit unless off-axis coronal images can be obtained.

Generally, the recti have either rectangular or fusiform shapes. They are homogenously isodense on CT and isointense on MRI and enhance uniformly. The superior rectus and levator palpebrae superioris usually cannot be distinguished separately in the posterior portion of the orbit but can be separated anteriorly. The inferior oblique is best identified on coronal scans just under the midportion of the globe. At the orbital apex, the muscles, optic nerves, and vascular structures are quite compact and often inseparable. MRI is generally better than CT in defining the anatomy at the apex (see Fig 25–4).[11]

Orbital Fat

Orbital "fat" is really a collection of fibroareolar tissue that invests well-defined areas of the orbit. By convention, the orbit is separated into intraconal and extraconal compartments. The intraconal compartment is the larger and is formed by the recti and posterior portion of the globe. The extraconal fat lies between the recti and periorbita and abuts the orbital septum anteriorly. In old age, the orbital septum weakens, and fat may protrude through it. On CT scan, the fat is homogenous except where vessels and nerves pass through it. There is clear delineation of the muscle-fat interface. The orbital septum is variably outlined, depending on the amount and turgor of the extraconal fat pressing against its posterior aspect. Short TR/TE MRI sequences are particularly useful in examining orbital fat. Hyperintense fat contrasts easily against less intense muscles and the globe. With appropriate windowing, some of the complex septal structure of the fat, as delineated in anatomic studies by Koorneef,[10] becomes apparent (see Fig 25–4).

The Optic Nerve

Because of its sinuous course within the orbit, the optic nerve may have a nonuniform, distorted appearance on thin axial and sagittal scan sections. The midportion of the nerve is the most common part to show caliber or density variation because it is here that the nerve makes simultaneous vertical and horizontal bends. These bends can become accentuated or effaced by changes in eye position away from primary gaze. Age, too, affects the tortuosity of the optic nerve, which is greater in elderly patients with less retro-orbital fat.[12]

Exiting from the supermedial aspect of the globe, the optic nerve courses slightly laterally and inferiorly. Further posteriorly, the nerve makes a rather marked bend to form a knee directed outward and downward.[13] It then courses upward and medially to enter the optic canal. The intracanalicular nerve continues in a superomedial direction, approximately 40 degrees from the orbitomeatal line.[14]

The appearance of the nerve will vary, depending on the angle of scanning and the thickness of the scan slice.[13] Axial scan sections made at −10 degrees from the orbitomeatal baseline are most apt to display the entirety of the nerve from papilla to optic canal. If a thin section cuts directly down the nerve, it will make the nerve appear uniform in density (intensity) and thickness (see Fig 25–1). However, if the section includes the portion of the nerve that bends, partial volume averaging of fat occurs, and that portion of the nerve is imaged as less dense and less wide (see Fig 25–3). Similar distortions may be present in sagittal views, even when made obliquely along the course of the nerve.

Clearly, evaluation of the exact size, density, and contour of the optic nerve should take into account scan angle, slice thickness, patient eye position, and patient age. Comparison with the contralateral nerve and scrutiny of suspect areas with other planes are necessary to overcome the inherent problems of thin-section techniques.

The Optic Nerve Sheath Complex

While the preceding section has described the features of the normal "optic nerve," this term is actually a misnomer. What the scan images is the optic nerve sheath complex, that is, the nerve and its surrounding pial, arachnoidal, and dural coverings, not simply the optic nerve itself. All three of these membranes are continuous with comparable intracranial membranes that extend along the entire course of the intraorbital nerve. Thus, intracranial and intraorbital subarachnoid spaces are contiguous.

On CT, even with thin sections, it is often difficult to distinguish the various components of the nerve sheath complex. When contrast has been administered, the dura increases in density, which allows it to be separated from the other water-density structures of the complex. Near the back of the globe there is often dilatation of the CSF spaces around the optic nerve, so the nerve can be seen separately from the dura. MRI more frequently depicts the optic nerve as a separate structure.[5] The nerve has the same intensity as white matter. CSF surrounding the intraorbital portion of nerve produces a surrounding ring (coronal) or line (sagittal or axial) along the nerve, with characteristic hypointensity on short TR/TE or hyperintensity on long TR/TE sequences (Figs 25–3 and 25–7). It must be distinguished from chemical shift artifact, which is associated with linear black and white lines (see Fig 25–6).[15] The intracanalicular portion of the nerve is particularly well demonstrated on MRI.[15] The nerve is easily delineated against hypointense bone or sinus (see Fig 25–3).

Vascular and Nervous Structures

High-resolution scanners are able to resolve a number of different veins, arteries, and nerves within the orbit.[5, 6, 16] Obviously, the structures most easily recognized are those that are surrounded by appreciable amounts of fat, those that enhance to the greatest degree, or those that are largest. The superior and inferior ophthalmic

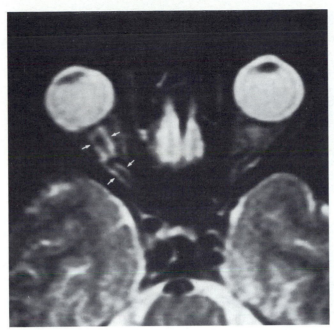

FIG 25–7.
Normal orbit, axial midlevel long TR/TE MR section. Hyperintense CSF *(arrows)* surround the optic nerve. Some patulousness of the perineural space allows the CSF to be seen over much of its intraorbital course.

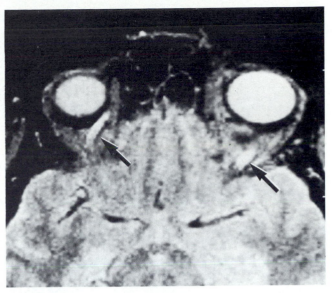

FIG 25–8.
Normal orbit, axial superior-level long TR/TE MR section. The midportion *(right)* and posterior portion *(left)* of the superior ophthalmic veins *(arrows)* are hyperintense due to diastolic pseudogating or flow-related enhancement, normal phenomena.

veins, ophthalmic artery, and isolated branches of cranial nerves III and V meet these criteria.

The superior ophthalmic vein can be identified on all axial scans. The vein originates anteriorly in the medial orbit and then courses posteriorly and laterally below the superior rectus–levator palpebrae muscle complex to cross over the optic nerve. At the orbital apex, it swings medially and dives through the annulus of Zinn to enter the superior orbital fissure. It is the midportion of the vein that is most commonly seen on axial scans (Figs 25–1, 25–3, and 25–8). The diameter of the vein is 2.0 to 3.5 mm.[17] On MRI, the intensity of the superior ophthalmic vein is usually quite hypointense due to flow void. Occasionally, however, the vein is hyperintense due to a flow-related phenomenon (Fig 25–8). This appearance can simulate thrombosis and may require flow-sensitive gradient echo sequences to confirm patency.

The inferior ophthalmic vein is identified less easily than the superior ophthalmic vein.[16] Its course, which is between the inferior rectus and optic nerve, roughly parallels that of the superior ophthalmic vein; it also enters the superior orbital fissure. The mid and anterior portions are the easiest to recognize.

The ophthalmic artery passes through the optic canal below the optic nerve to enter the orbital apex. It then swings laterally over the optic nerve. Finally, it follows a sinuous course toward the superomedial orbit and terminates in nasal, frontal, and palpebral branches. On a scan, the most apparent portions of the ophthalmic artery are where it courses through medial orbital fat and where it passes over the optic nerve (Figs 25–5 and 25–9). The major branches of the artery are variably seen on axial sections.

In general, nerves can be differentiated from vascular structures by virtue of their straighter course. The nervous structures most commonly identified by high-resolution scanning are the frontal branch of the ophthalmic division of the fifth cranial nerve and the inferior division of the third cranial nerve.[16] The former is seen on superior scans to run above the levator palpebrae; the latter is seen on inferior scans to run lateral and inferior to the optic nerve.

ROUTINE CT SCANNING TECHNIQUE

Patients are most effectively evaluated by axial 2.0- to 3.0-mm scans initially. These are usually sufficient to survey the small structures of the orbit. They are routinely performed at −10 degrees to the oribitomeatal baseline, the best angle for imaging the intraorbital optic nerve[13] and displaying the orbital contents well. Coronal scans usually

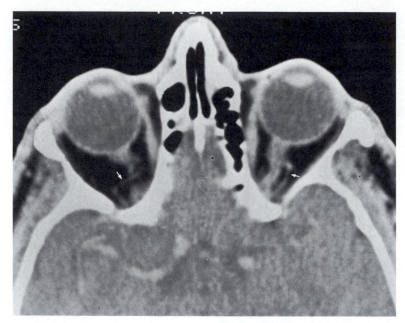

FIG 25–9.
Normal orbit, axial midlevel CT section. The ophthalmic arteries *(arrows)* are seen to swing laterally to medially over the optic nerves.

supplement the axial views. These are performed in either prone or head-hanging positions so that the head is extended about 70 degrees. They can be limited by the patient's ability to extend his neck. Even with larger gantries and improved gantry tilt, metallic artifacts from dental fillings often compromise the quality of coronal scans. Reformatted images require small sections of 1.5 to 2.0 mm to approach the resolution of direct images. Unfortunately, this takes longer to perform but gives some flexibility in that various projections may be obtained at one sitting. Three-dimensional reconstructions are not performed routinely but are quite useful when evaluating trauma or congenital malformations.

Because of inherently large density differences in the orbit, normal structures and pathologic masses are relatively well outlined without the use of contrast enhancement. Intravenous (IV) contrast does cause change in attenuation values of structures within the orbit. Most notable are the rectus muscles, which show the largest amount of enhancement, followed by the sclera and optic nerve. However, the change in density is small when compared with the density differences that already exist within the orbit.[18] It would seem, then, that the routine use of contrast in all patients is unwarranted.

When should contrast be used? Although most pathology of the orbit can be recognized on CT without contrast, some lesions require the use of contrast for further characterization. There are certain contexts in which the use of contrast would seem to be appropriate. A few of these are as follows:

1. Vascular lesions.—Although vascular structures, particularly if enlarged, are delineated without contrast, their nature and extent is better evaluated after contrast. For example, an arteriovenous malformation (AVM) will be highlighted after contrast. A varix can be more easily delineated before or after provocative (Valsalva) maneuvers that follow contrast enhancement.

2. Neoplastic or inflammatory lesions with suspected intracranial involvement.—Contrast enhancement is crucial in defining intracranial extension.

3. Optic nerve thickening.—Enhancement of the optic nerve sheath would indicate a meningioma or an inflammatory condition separate from the optic nerve itself.

4. Certain retrobulbar masses.—Contrast enhancement may help in distinguishing one type of well-circumscribed mass from another (e.g., hemangioma from neurilemmoma).

ROUTINE MRI TECHNIQUE

Prescriptions for effective orbital MRI vary, but at present revolve around spin-echo techniques. A complex set of factors including magnet strength, signal-to-noise ratio, field of view, pixel size, slice thickness, and pulse sequence contribute to the information obtained and image quality. Readers are referred to the article by Wehrli and Kanal for a concise description of the interaction of these parameters on spin-echo sequences.[19]

Most orbital scanning is initiated with short TR/TE (TR = 600 to 800 ms; TE = 20 to 80 ms) images. A 3-mm slice thickness, allowing for interslice gap, is needed to examine small structures of the orbit. The use of (monocular or binocular) surface coils maintains a high signal-to-noise ratio, so the number of exitations may be minimized. Unfortunately, there is signal drop-off with distance from the surface coil. Therefore, pathology at the orbital apex usually has to be imaged with a head coil.

Short TR/TE images provide considerable anatomic detail, but long TR/TE images (TR = 2 to 3 sec; TE = 20 to 100 ms) are usually required in at least one plane to further characterize an abnormality. Since these sequences take longer to obtain, there is usually degradation of image quality. Head coil images may thus be preferable to surface coil images for these sequences.[6]

MAGNETIC RESONANCE ARTIFACTS

One of the most vexing problems in orbital imaging with spin-echo sequences is the chemical shift artifact.[6, 15, 21] This artifact is caused by a slight variance in resonance of water and lipid protons. A misregistration pixel shift occurs along the frequency-encoding direction at interfaces between orbital fat and other "water" structures like the optic nerve, extraocular muscle margins, and scleral margin. This misregistration effect causes low-intensity or high-intensity bands to occur at interfaces, with a subsequent loss of information about the orbital structures forming the interfaces (see Fig 25–6). A number of methods have been described to attenuate the chemical shift artifact, including (1) positioning the patient so that the object of interest (e.g., the optic nerve) is parallel to the frequency-encoding gradient[15]; (2) short inversion time inversion recovery sequence (STIR) to suppress the signal from orbital fat while maintain-

ing somewhat nonspecific sensitivity to pathologic T1 and T2 prolongation[20] (Fig 25–10); (3) chopper fat suppression when using the Dixon method in which there is some reduction in the signal-to-noise ratio[22]; and (4) phase-dependent contrast proton spectroscopic imaging when using the Dixon technique, which cancels fat signal and allows for edge enhancement of orbital structures and better characterization of pathology than does STIR imaging.[6, 23] The practicality of these techniques needs to be tested so that definitive protocols can be applied to specific clinical contexts.

The other major artifact comes from eye movement during scanning. Motion artifact occurs in the phase-encoding direction and is particularly troublesome in evaluating the optic nerve. Relatively long scan times require intense "coaching" of the patient to keep his eyes immobile. Placing the phase-encoding gradient across the scan keeps eye motion from degrading images of the rest of the orbital contents.

The use of IV contrast, such as gadolinium-DTPA, has not been fully explored in the orbit. This is partly because short TR/TE sequences are used. In these sequences, most pathology is seen as hypointense areas juxtaposed against hyperintense fat. In enhancing the pathology with gadolinium, the contrast between pathology and fat actually decreases, thus making it harder to see. In addition, vascular lesions like AVMs and varices can be identified by virtue of their own flow char-

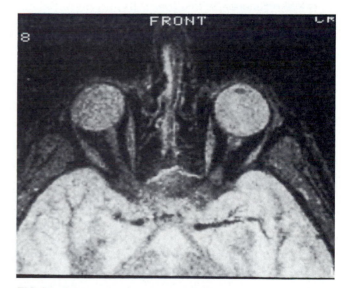

FIG 25–10.
Normal orbit, axial midlevel MR section, STIR sequence. The isointense extraocular muscles and optic nerve stand out against the hypointense "suppressed" orbital fat.

acteristics; no contrast is needed to bring them out more clearly. Therefore, the use of gadolinium would seem to be limited unless fat suppression techniques are used. Cases in which pathology relates to the bony walls (e.g., sphenoid wing meningioma, metastasis) or extends intracranially (e.g., optic nerve glioma) (see Chapter 27) would seem to most benefit from the use of gadolinium.

Which projections are obtained depends on the nature of the suspected orbital pathology. Complex orbital trauma often requires coronal and sagittal images to learn the extent and relationship of the fracture fragments. Orbital infection usually requires axial and coronal sections to determine the location of involvement and to evaluate any associated sinus disease. Retrobulbar masses need at least axial and coronal views, while sagittal views usually help to determine the relationship of the mass to the optic nerve and apex. Optic nerve lesions require axial and coronal projections, with other intracranial views if intracranial spread is questioned. Sphenoid wing pathology usually requires axial and coronal projections. Pathology of the superior or inferior orbit benefits by sagittal imaging.[6]

REFERENCES

1. McCotter RE, Fralick FB: *A Comprehensive Description of the Orbit, Orbital Content and Associated Structures With Clinical Applications.* Omaha, Douglas Printing Co, 1943, pp 3–13.
2. Hammerschlag SB, O'Reilly GVA, Naheedy M: Computed tomography of the optic canals. *AJNR* 1981; 2:593–594.
3. Jacobs L, Weisberg LA, Kinkel WR: *Computed Tomography of the Orbit and Sella Turcica.* New York, Raven Press, 1980, pp 38–44.
4. Gomori JM, Grossman RI, Shields JA, et al: Ocular MR imaging and spectroscopy: An ex vivo study. *Radiology* 1986; 160:201–205.
5. Langer BG, Mafee MF, Pollock S, et al: MRI of the normal orbit and optic pathway. *Radiol Clin North Am* 1987; 25:429–446.
6. Atlas SW: Magnetic resonance imaging of the orbit: Current status. *Magn Reson Q* 1989; 5:39–96.
7. Hilal SK, Trokel SL: Computerized tomography of the orbit using thin sections. *Semin Roentgenol* 1977; 12:137–147.
8. Wolff E, Last RJ: *Anatomy of the Eye and Orbit*, ed
6. Philadelphia, WB Saunders Co, 1968, pp 256–271.
9. Poirier P, Charpy A: Les Organes du sens, in *Traite d'Anatomie Humanie*, vol 5. Paris, Masson, 1911, pp 558–559.
10. Koorneef L: Details of the orbital connective system in the adult. *Acta Morphol Neerl Scand* 1977; 15:1–34.
11. Daniels DL, Yu S, Pech P, et al: Computed tomography and magnetic resonance imaging of the orbital apex. *Radiol Clin North Am* 1987; 25:803–817.
12. Salvolini U, Cabanis EA, Rodallec A, et al: Computed tomography of the optic nerve: I. Normal results. *J Comput Assist Tomogr* 1978; 2:141–149.
13. Unsold R, DeGroot J, Newton TH: Images of the optic nerve: Anatomical-CT correlation. *AJNR* 1980; 1:317–325.
14. Potter GD, Trokel SL: Optic canal, in Newton TH, Potts DG (eds): *Radiology of the Skull and Brain: The Skull*, vol 2. St Louis, CV Mosby Co, 1971, pp 487–489.
15. Daniels DL, Kneeland JB, Shimakawa A, et al: MR imaging of the optic nerve and sheath: Correcting the chemical shift misregistration effect. *AJNR* 1986; 7:249–253.
16. Weinstein MA, Modic MT, Risius B, et al: Visualization of the arteries, veins, and nerves of the orbit by sector computed tomography. *Radiology* 1981; 138:83–87.
17. Bacon KT, Duchesneau PM, Weinstein MA: Demonstration of the superior ophthalmic vein by high resolution computed tomography. *Radiology* 1977; 124:129–131.
18. Watanabe TJ, LeMasters D, Turski PA, et al: Contrast enhancement of the normal orbit, in Felix R, Kazner E, Wegener OH (eds): *Contrast Media in Computed Tomography.* Amsterdam, Excerpta Medica, 1981, pp 130–136.
19. Wehrli FW, Kanal E: Orbital imaging: Factors determining magnetic resonance imaging appearance. *Radiol Clin North Am* 1987; 25:419–427.
20. Johnson G, Miller DH, Tofts PS, et al: STIR sequences in NMR imaging of the optic nerve. *Neuroradiology* 1987; 29:238–245.
21. Atlas SW, Grossman RI, Hackney DB, et al: STIR MR imaging of orbital lesions. *AJNR* 1988; 9:969–974.
22. Simon J, Szumanowski J, Totterman S, et al: Fat suppression MR imaging of the orbit. *AJNR* 1988; 9:961–968.
23. Atlas SW, Grossman RI, Axel L, et al: Orbital lesions: Proton spectroscopic phase dependent contrast MR imaging. *Radiology* 1987; 64:510–514.

26

Orbital Trauma and Infection

William E. Rothfus, M.D.

ORBITAL TRAUMA

Computed tomography (CT) is now a well-established method of evaluating the orbit in direct and indirect trauma.[1-3] In fact, with high-resolution and image reformation capabilities, it has become the evaluative standard, making conventional radiography and complex motion tomography relatively obsolete.[4] This is especially true in the context of complex maxillofacial fractures, which require multiplanar imaging to evaluate the extent and localization of all fractures. By making it possible to determine damage to the soft tissue (globe, optic nerve, extraocular muscles, and retrobulbar fat), CT has a marked advantage over other radiographic techniques. Detection and localization of intraorbital foreign bodies have been greatly facilitated by CT scanning. The role of magnetic resonance imaging (MRI) in the evaluation of orbital trauma is evolving. The ease with which multiplanar and off-axis sections can be completed makes it ideal for evaluating the orbital walls and contents after fracture.[5, 6] Potential aggravation of injury, however, makes MRI contraindicated in the context of a metallic foreign body.

Mechanical injuries to the eye and orbit can be categorized under two main headings: (1) perforating missile and nonmissile injuries and (2) concussions by blunt objects. The role of the radiologist in evaluating either of these is to determine the anatomic extent of soft-tissue and bone injury, characterize the type of injury (e.g., hematoma, avulsion), and identify possible sources of posttraumatic complication (e.g., retained foreign body as a source of infection).

Penetrating Missile and Nonmissile Injury

Up to half of traumatic eye injuries are caused by penetrating objects.[7] Some of the objects remain within the globe or orbits as retained foreign bodies. These usually are metal, but organic materials such as wood may also be retained. Identification and localization of the object are crucial for therapeutic planning. Prior to CT, localization was imprecise and cumbersome, often requiring multiple radiographs and contact lens techniques.[8] Because of its ease, accuracy, and definition of anatomic detail,[9] CT has become the mainstay of localization. The ability of CT to detect a foreign body depends upon the object size and composition. Experimental work performed by Tate and Cupples[10] proves that steel and copper bodies as small as 0.06 mm^3 can be detected by high-resolution scanning. Aluminum and glass bodies need to be larger to be detected, 1.5 to 1.8 mm^3. Wooden bodies are often difficult to localize; their CT densities may vary in the same range as fat and other orbital soft tissues.[11]

Foreign bodies may be extraocular, intraocular, or retro-ocular (Figs 26–1 and 26–2). Extraocular bodies are easily detected on physical examination, but CT may be done to rule out deeper penetration. Intraocular bodies are usually from flying particles entering the eye through the cornea, iris, pupil, or sclera. Because most of the flying objects are metal and carry significant momentum, they usually penetrate to the posterior portion of the globe and lodge in the retina, cornea, or sclera.[8] Particles with less momentum (i.e., less velocity or less mass like plastic or wood) travel a shorter distance into the globe and remain in the anterior

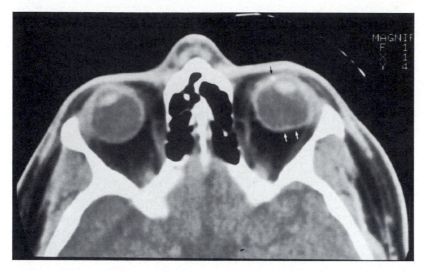

FIG 26–1.
Missile trauma. A small metallic radiodensity is lodged in the cornea *(black arrow)*. Another fragment (not shown) has passed through the globe and caused a rupture of the vitreous. There is resultant loss of turgor of the globe wall, as evidenced by wall flattening *(white arrows)*.

chamber or lens. Particles may course through or around the globe to come to rest behind it or in or near the optic nerve, extraocular muscle, or bony wall.

Missile or nonmissile penetrating trauma is frequently associated with a local hemorrhage. As expected, hematoma appears as a high-density mass. Generally, the larger the hematoma, the more heterogeneous it looks. The hematoma may be local, confined to the globe wall, vitreous cavity, or optic nerve sheath, or more diffuse, spreading over the retrobulbar space. Orbital emphysema may be present, usually as small collections of air along the tract of penetration (Fig 26–3). Structures in the path of the offending object are seen to be disrupted on CT scanning. For example, the lens may be displaced or the optic nerve severed. When the globe has become perforated by a foreign body, its

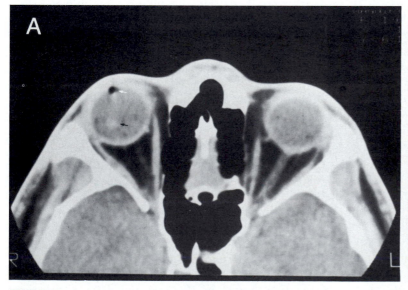
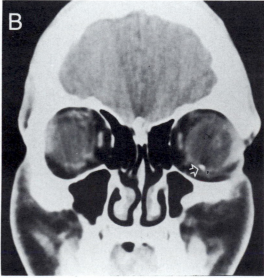

FIG 26–2.
Missile trauma. Axial **(A)** and coronal **(B)** scans show the path of a small metal foreign body *(open arrow)* that entered anterosuperiorly and embedded in the inferior globe wall. A small collection of air is seen at the site of penetration *(white arrow)*; vitreous hemorrhage is present in the midglobe *(black arrow)*.

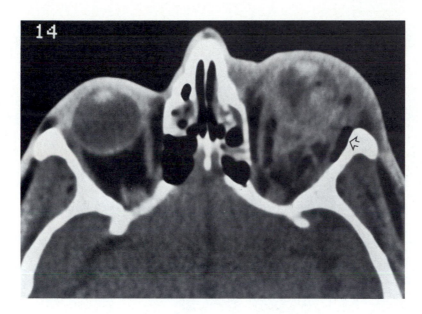

FIG 26–3.
Missile trauma. A large metallic foreign body has passed through the globe into the retrobulbar space. Exuberant hematoma is identified within the vitreous cavity and the posterior globe wall. The optic nerve sheath is also involved by hematoma. A small collection of air is seen along the lateral orbit *(arrow)*. Perforation of the globe has decompressed it, leaving the sclera thickened and flattened.

contents may rupture. The globe becomes shrunken, with the sclera being less rounded in contour and thickened in width (Figs 26–1 and 26–3).[12] Commonly there is blood or air within the globe or orbit (Fig 26–2).

Concussion Injury

Concussions of the orbit result from the impact of a blunt force, as from a large object or fall.[13] The force may be directed at the globe itself or at its bony surroundings; thus, orbital soft-tissue injury may be from direct or indirect forces.

When the striking force lands directly on the globe, the globe is pushed backward, and intraorbital pressure increases. If the pressure is high enough, it will fracture the thinnest portions of the body wall[14] and "blow them out" away from the orbit. Usually, the orbital floor is the site of such a fracture because of its delicate bony structure. Bone fragments and orbital soft tissues are pushed inferiorly into the maxillary sinus, often with resultant hemorrhage. Varying amounts of orbital contents may protrude through the defect in the wall, with varying degrees of enophthalmos resulting. Orbital fat and the inferior rectus and/or inferior oblique muscles are displaced through the floor defect. They may be kinked or entrapped in the herniation and cause impairment of globe mo-

tility and diplopia. Motility abnormalities may also stem from entrapment or fibrosis of orbital connective tissue within the fracture.[15]

The use of CT is ideal for evaluation of these inferior wall blowout fractures. Coronal and oblique sagittal images are particularly well suited to delineating the bone fragments and prolapsed muscle or fat (Fig. 26–4).[15–18] Determining the location and amount of muscle herniation and kinking is of great importance. Assessment of the relationship of muscle to bony wall will help indicate whether the muscle is truly entrapped and thus requires surgical intervention. The nature of the fracture itself is also important to assess because it may have prognostic significance to the clinician. It has been stated that focal or markedly displaced fractures will have a high likelihood of entrapping and incarcerating orbital contents because of their sharp margins and acute angles.[19] Fractures with bowed margins and obtuse angles would not be so prone to entrapment but would be associated with enophthalmos, which also requires surgery but may not be manifested in the acute phase.

Medial wall blowout fractures are less common than floor fractures, but frequently accompany them.[19, 20] These fractures occur through the thin lamina papyracea and displace bony fragments, fat, or muscle into the ethmoid sinuses. To evaluate these fractures, axial and coronal sections are most

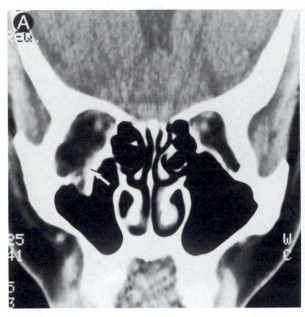
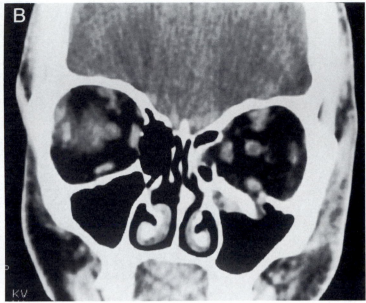

FIG 26–4.
Blunt trauma. Both of these patients had upward gaze motility disorders. **A,** the posterior portion of the inferior rectus *(arrow)* is pulled down into the maxillary sinus with the fracture fragment. **B,** the swollen inferior rectus is not entrapped, but surrounding fascia is displaced into the acutely angled fracture.

helpful (Figs 26–5 and 26–6). As the medial wall fractures, muscle entrapment can occur, and scans in these projections can best evaluate the true position of the medial rectus and superior oblique muscles in relation to bone. The other major clinical problem with medial wall fracture is enophthalmos. In fact, the degree of medial wall blowout seems to be a major determinant of clinically significant enophthalmos.[21] Again, scans provide the essential information in establishing the need and planning for cosmetic surgery.

Orbital roof blowout fractures can occur due to the inherent thinness of the orbital floor of the anterior cranial fossa.[22] These are best evaluated with coronal or sagittal sections.

MRI has strong capabilities in evaluation of blowout fractures in the nonemergent patient.[5, 6] Short repetition time/echo time (TR/TE) sequences can be used because of the high tissue contrast between orbital fat, muscle, and sinus wall (and air). Distortions of the muscle and fat through orbital defects can be easily examined in multiple planes as necessitated by the location of the pathology (i.e., coronal and oblique sagittal planes for floor or roof fractures, axial and coronal planes for medial wall fracture) (see Fig 26–6). Although entrapment or kinking of the muscles and protrusion of fat can be defined, the presence and location of

bony fragments are not as well depicted as with CT.

Orbital walls can be fractured in combination with extensive maxillofacial injury. Le Fort types II and III fractures most notably involve the orbits because they traverse lines of weakness in the midfacial skeleton.[14, 23] The Le Fort type II frac-

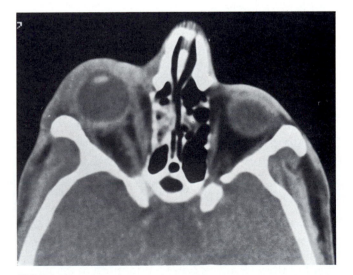

FIG 26–5.
Blunt trauma. A smooth right orbit medial wall fracture is associated with opacification of ethmoid air cells and enlargement of the medial rectus from hemorrhage. The muscle is not entrapped.

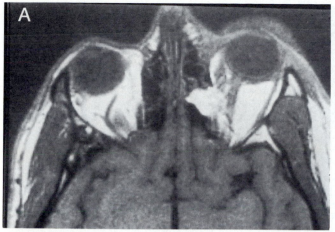

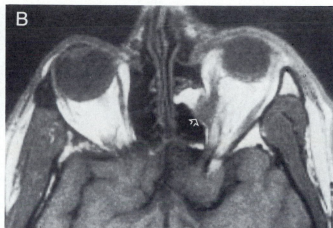

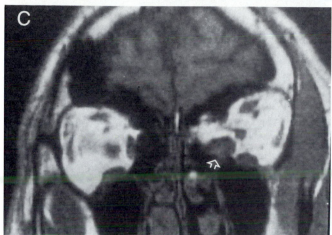

FIG 26–6.
Blunt trauma, medial wall blowout fracture. Axial **(A** and **B)**
and coronal **(C)** short TR/TE sections show an acutely
angled fracture with prolapse of high-intensity fat into it.
Although the medial rectus *(arrows)* was pulled into the
fracture, no ocular motility disorder was present.

ture extends bilaterally from the nasal bones across
the frontal processes of the maxillae, along the medial wall and the floor of the orbits, through the infraorbital rims, through the anterior and lateral
maxillary sinus walls, and finally to the posterior
maxillary sinus walls and pterygoids. Le Fort type
III fractures also involve the nasal bones and frontal process of the maxillae, but extend more posteriorly through the medial wall of the orbit to involve the infraorbital fissures and lateral orbital
walls, then the zygomaticofrontal sutures and zygomatic arches. These Le Fort fractures need not be
pure, and combinations of the fractures may exist
in the same patient (Fig 26–7).

Another major facial fracture affecting the orbit
is the zygomatic complex, or malar tripod, fracture.
The zygoma is separated downward, inward, and
posteriorly, with resultant fractures through the inferior orbital rim, zygomaticofrontal suture, and zygomatic arch. Severe fractures of these types cause
comminuted fracture of the orbital floor and herniation of orbital structures into the maxillary si-

nus.[14] Fractures of the zygoma and maxilla are particularly amenable to three-dimensional image reconstruction techniques (Fig 26–8). These techniques are quite useful in planning surgery.

Other fractures may involve the orbit in crucial
areas. Orbital roof, basal skull, and sphenoid wing
fractures are especially important in that they may
involve the optic canal. Confined by its bony surroundings and held rigidly by its dural attachment,
the optic nerve is most susceptible to injury at this
location. Fractures may damage the optic nerve directly, with bony fragments from the orbital roof,
optic canal, or anterior clinoid process impinging
or transecting the nerve (Fig 26–9).[24, 25] Indirect
injury occurs from nerve shearing or contusion at
the cranial opening of the canal where the nerve is
tethered. Vascular insufficiency and hemorrhage
can contribute to injury as well.[25]

Clearly, the complexity of canal fractures
makes evaluation and surgical planning difficult. A
critical role is played by CT in defining both bony
and soft-tissue abnormalities. Imaging in conven-

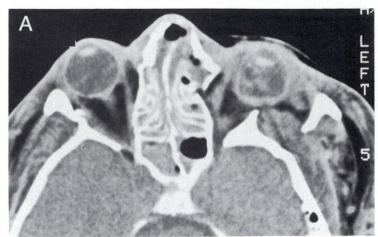

FIG 26–7.
Blunt trauma, complex zygomaxillary fracture. Axial **(A)** and coronal **(B** and **C)** CT scans show the walls of the left orbit to be markedly disrupted. There is fracture of the medial wall as well as displaced fractures through the zygomaticofrontal suture, orbital floor, and maxilla. The globe is hemorrhagic and ruptured.

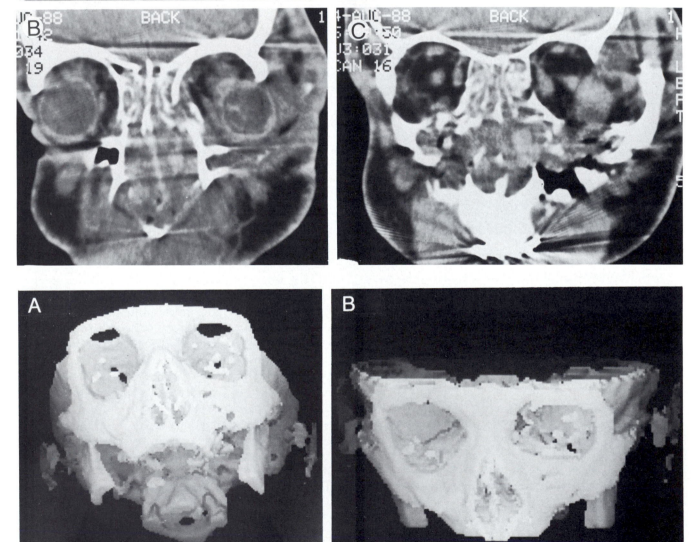

FIG 26–8.
Blunt trauma. A depressed fracture of the right maxilla and orbital floor is evident in various angles **(A** and **B)** of this three-dimensional reconstruction, which was completed with contiguous 2-mm scan sections.

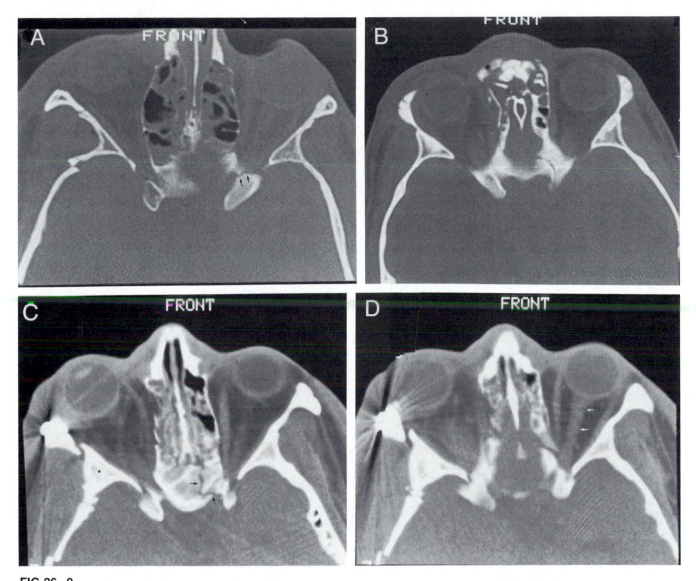

FIG 26–9.
Blunt injury, spectrum of optic canal fractures causing (left) blindness. **A,** nondisplaced fracture of the lateral and inferior canal walls *(arrows).* **B,** nondisplaced transverse fracture of the canal roof. **C** and **D,** contiguous sections through a displaced canal fracture *(black arrows).* Note the tubular enlargement of the left optic nerve sheath complex due to hemorrhage and edema *(white arrows),* as well as a contralateral sphenoid buttress fracture *(star)* and a medial wall fracture.

tional axial and coronal projections can be supplemented by direct or reformatted (including three-dimensional) images in other planes to adequately assess the extent of injury.[23] The role of MRI in these injuries has not been defined; it would seem to be an ideal agent, however, for evaluation of the intracanalicular portion of the nerve as well as the retrobulbar and prechiasmatic portions.

As in penetrating trauma, concussion injury results in a variety of soft-tissue abnormalities. These are easily detected by CT scanning. Orbital emphysema is a frequent concomitant of blowout fractures but may be seen in malar and Le Fort fractures because of sinus involvement.[14] The air is readily distinguished from air trapped behind the eyelid, a distinction sometimes difficult with radiographs alone. Orbital emphysema should be expected to resolve fairly rapidly and have no mass effect. These features distinguish it from the more serious complication of intraorbital aerocele, an encapsulated collection of air under pressure.[26]

Severe blunt trauma is accompanied by shearing forces that lead to tears of the globe walls, rupture of the globe, subluxation of the lens, or avulsion of the optic nerve. Hemorrhages are common and occur focally in the aqueous or vitreous chambers, globe wall, optic nerve sheath, or extraocular muscles (Figs 26–5, 26–7, 26–10, and 26–11). Diffuse hemorrhage may also occur. As in penetrating trauma, CT is excellent in defining these abnormalities and their degree of severity.

ORBITAL AND PERIORBITAL INFECTION

Acute orbital or periorbital infection is rarely subtle clinically. Eyelid swelling is manifested early in infection, whether it be from reactive edema, cellulitis, or abscess. However, swelling may become so tense that physical examination of the globe and vision is hindered. Thus, it may be impossible to determine clinically the extent of disease and take appropriate therapeutic measures.[27, 28] The use of CT or MRI is integral in evaluating the orbit in this circumstance. Not only can the presence or absence of deeper involvement be assessed, but associated bony and intracranial disease can be evaluated.[28–33] A large percentage of cases of periorbital and orbital cellulitis are secondary to sinusitis or trauma. The use of scanning again becomes essential in determining the location and presence of sinus disease or an intraorbital foreign body serving as the nidus of infection. It is repeated that MRI may be contraindicated if a metallic foreign body is suspected.

Clinically and radiologically, infectious disease can be separated into two basic anatomic groups— preseptal or postseptal—based on the location of the infection in relation to the orbital septum, the tough fascial projection extending from the periosteum of the orbital margin toward the tarsal plates.[34] The septum is a well-recognized barrier to the spread of various orbital pathologic processes including infection.

Preseptal Inflammation

By definition, preseptal or "periorbital" inflammation does not affect the orbital contents. It may arise from a local infection such as cellulitis or abscess. Alternatively, it may stem from sinusitis, usually ethmoid sinusitis.[31, 35] The mechanism of the latter is believed to be reactive edema, caused by elevated pressure in valveless veins that connect the sinuses with the soft tissues of the face and lids.[36] Preseptal infection is commonly a disease of children less than 1 year old, as opposed to postseptal infection, which occurs in older children.[32] The CT manifestation of preseptal inflammation is swelling of the soft tissues of the lid and face. The orbital septum forms a clear line of demarcation between the expanded soft tissue of the lid and the normal extraconal fat (Fig 26–12). The appearance of the swelling is identical in cellulitis, abscess, or reactive edema—fairly homogeneous increased density. Location of swelling and presence of sinus opacity are therefore important features in assessing the CT scan. Soft-tissue edema is usually most prominent near the affected sinus. In ethmoid sinusitis, maximal swelling is commonly over the frontal process of the maxilla; in frontal sinusitis, it is in the upper lid. Progressively severe sinus infection causes extensive swelling, which spreads over the nose, cheek, and brow.

In general, preseptal inflammatory disease runs a much more benign course than postseptal disease does.[31, 32]

Postseptal Inflammation

Postseptal inflammation, commonly referred to as "orbital cellulitis," actually constitutes a spec-

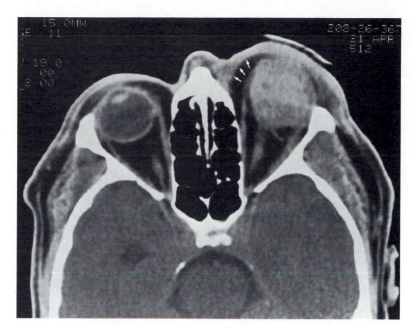

FIG 26–10.
Blunt trauma. Hemorrhage into the left globe has obscured normal anatomy and expanded the eye. There is considerable preseptal soft-tissue hemorrhage, defined nicely along its posterior margin by the septum *(arrows)*.

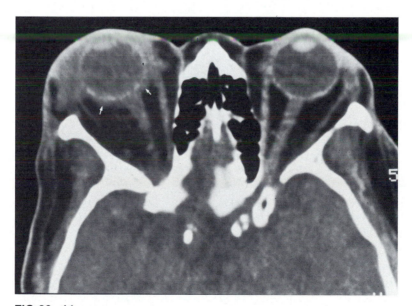

FIG 26–11.
Blunt trauma. A peribulbar hemorrhage dissects around the globe wall and infiltrates into Tenon's capsule *(arrows)*.

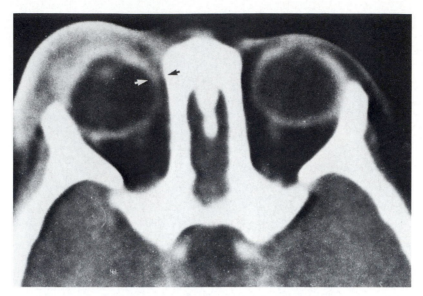

FIG 26–12.
Preseptal inflammation. The soft tissues anterior to the globe are markedly swollen. The orbital septum *(arrows)* is displaced poste-riorly but forms a line of separation between the extraconal fat and swollen tissues.

trum of infection located in various anatomic compartments. Diagnostically and therapeutically, it is helpful to separate this group into anatomically distinct categories based on the major location of disease. Thus, the major subgroupings are (1) sub-periorbital, (2) retrobulbar, and (3) bulbar.

Subperiorbital (subperiosteal) cellulitis or abscess usually propagates from contiguous sinus inflammation, either by direct spread through the sinus wall or by progressive thrombophlebitis.[36] Since the usual site of spread is from the ethmoid or frontal sinus, most involvement is of the medial or superior portions of the orbit. Edema fluid and pus accumulate within the subperiosteal space. They form an expanding mass that bows the periorbita away from the orbital wall. Because the periorbita is relatively tethered at the sutures and foramina,[37] the subperiorbital collection usually attains a convex shape. Adjacent structures, e.g., extraconal fat and the rectus muscle, are pushed away from the orbital walls as well.

The CT scan shows the subperiorbital collection as a convex homogeneous or heterogeneous density along the orbital wall (Fig 26–13). The collection has a sharp inner border, which is defined by the periorbita. The periorbita may be visualized because it enhances or because it is thickened by inflammation. When the collection is totally confined by the periorbita and has not spread to the orbit proper, a thin lucent cleavage plane of nor-mal extraconal fat is present between the collection and the displaced rectus muscle. The collection may vary in size and may have an air-fluid level or contain air. MRI depicts the inflammatory subperiorbital collection as hypointense on short TR/TE and hyperintense on long TR/TE sequences (Fig 26–14). Again, multidirectional capabilities make MRI ideal in evaluating the extent of spread.

The periosteum and orbital septa are major deterrents to the spread of inflammatory disease, but can be breached in severe infection (e.g., sinusitis, osteomyelitis, masseteric abscess). Additionally, the primary focus of infection may begin within the periosteum. In either case, retrobulbar inflammation occurs. This is potentially more dangerous and less surgically accessible than subperiorbital infection is, but fortunately it is less frequent.[38] The CT findings of infection in this compartment include obscuration of normal soft-tissue planes, increased density of retrobulbar fat, and swelling and enhancement of involved extraocular muscles (Fig 26–15).[28, 32, 39] When inflammation matures from cellulitis to actual abscess, a definable mass, ring enhancement, or air collection occurs.[30, 40] Proptosis may be marked. MRI descriptions of deep orbital infection are lacking, but it is expected that MRI would reflect diminished muscle-fat contrast in all sequences and show increased muscle and fat intensity on long TR/TE sequences.

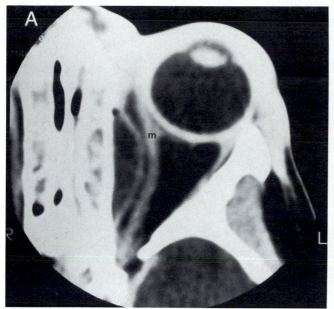

FIG 26–13.

Subperiorbital abscess. Axial **(A)** and coronal **(B)** projections show a large medial subperiorbital collection with a well-demarcated enhancing margin. The medial rectus *(m)* is swollen and displaced laterally but is separated from the collection by a thin strip of extra-conal fat. Note the optic nerve "hydrops" *(arrow)*, as shown by lucent cerebrospinal fluid surrounding the optic nerve in the coronal section.

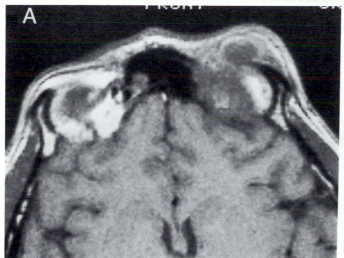

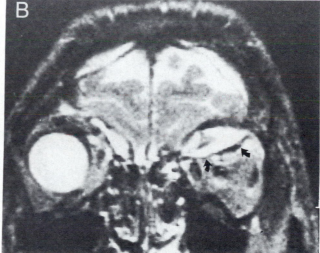

FIG 26–14.

Subperiorbital abscess. Axial short TR/TE **(A)** and coronal long TR/TE **(B)** MRI show the abscess to be well defined by the hypointense periorbita *(arrows)*. As is common with abscesses, the collection is isointense on short TR/TE and hyperintense on long TR/TE sequences. A small hypointensity within the abscess **(B)** represents focal hemorrhage following attempted needle aspiration.

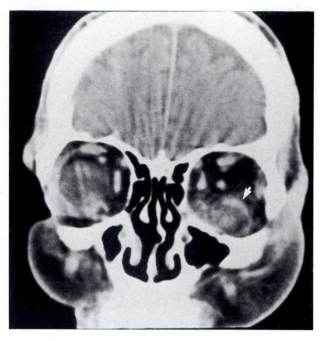

FIG 26–15.
Retrobulbar abscess. The enhancing inferior rectus *(arrow)* is displaced around an intermediate-density abscess beneath it. Note the irregular density around the abscess, which represents adjacent fat inflammation.

It is noteworthy that extensive postseptal infection (especially fungal) can be present with only minimal scan (CT or MRI) findings.[39]

Deep bulbar infection (endophthalmitis) can be present with or without other forms of postseptal disease. The most common CT appearance is ocular wall thickening of a nodular or uniform character with homogeneous enhancement (Fig 26–16).[28] When retrobulbar disease is present, bulbar swelling is marked in the region of the most active cellulitis. The soft-tissue density of the globe wall most likely represents a combination of actual scleral swelling and effusion distending Tenon's capsule.[40]

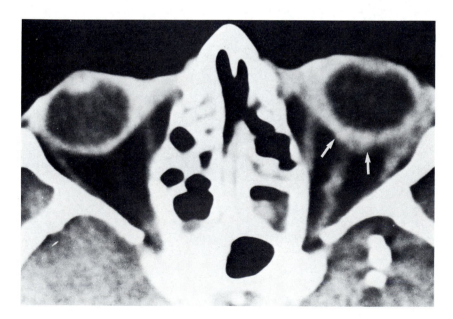

FIG 26–16.
Bacterial endophthalmitis. The posterior globe wall is thickened and enhances homogeneously *(arrows)*. There appears to be involvement of the insertion of the lateral rectus by adjacent inflammation.

REFERENCES

1. Grove AS: Orbital trauma evaluation by computed tomography. *Comput Tomogr* 1979; 3:267–278.
2. Grove AS, Tadmor R, New FFJ, et al: Orbital fracture evaluation by coronal computed tomography. *Am J Ophthalmol* 1978; 85:679–685.
3. Rowe LD, Miller E, Brant-Zawadzki M: Computerized tomography in maxillofacial trauma. *Laryngoscope* 1981; 91:745–757.
4. Brant-Zawadzki MN, Minagi H, Federle MP, et al: High resolution CT with image reformation in maxillofacial pathology. *AJNR* 1982; 3:31–37.
5. McArdle CB, Amparo EG, Mirfakhraee M: MR imaging of orbital blow-out fractures. *J Comput Assist Tomogr* 1986; 10:116–119.
6. Tonami H, Nakagawa T, Ohguchi M, et al: Surface coil MR imaging of orbital blowout fractures: A comparison with reformatted CT. *AJNR* 1987; 8:445–449.
7. Nirnanen M: Perforating eye injuries—a comparative epidemiological prognostic and socioeconomic study of patients treated 1930–1939 and 1950–1959. *Acta Ophthalmol Suppl (Copenh)* 1978; 135:1–87.
8. Lloyd GAS: *Radiology of the Orbit.* Philadelphia, WB Saunders Co, 1975, pp 197–210.
9. Kadir S, Aronow S, Davis KR: The use of computerized tomography in the detection of intraorbital foreign bodies. *Comput Tomogr* 1977; 1:151–156.
10. Tate E, Cupples H: Detection of orbital foreign bodies with computed tomography: Current limits. *AJNR* 1981; 2:363–365.
11. Hansen JE, Gudeman SK, Holgate RC, et al: Penetrating intracranial wood wounds: Clinical limitations of computerized tomography. *J Neurosurg* 1988; 68:752–756.
12. Seuel D, Krausz H, Ponder T, et al: Value of computed tomography for the diagnosis of a ruptured eye. *J Comput Assist Tomogr* 1983; 7:870–875.
13. Duke-Elder S, MacFaul PA: *System of Ophthalmology,* vol 14. *Injuries,* pt 1. London, Henry Kimpton, 1972, pp 63–291.
14. Lloyd GAS: *Radiology of the Orbit.* Philadelphia, WB Saunders Co, 1975, pp 180–188.
15. Koornneef L, Zonneveld FW: The role of direct multiplanar high resolution in the assessment and management of orbital trauma. *Radiol Clin North Am* 1987; 25:753–766.
16. Hammerschlag SB, Hughes S, O'Reilly GV, et al: Blow-out fractures of the orbit: A comparison of computed tomography and conventional radiography with anatomical correlation. *Radiology* 1982; 143:487–492.
17. Ball JB: Direct oblique sagittal CT of orbital wall fractures. *AJNR* 1987; 8:147–154.
18. Zonneveld FW, Koornneef L: Patient positioning for direct sagittal CT of the orbit parallel to the optic nerve. *Radiology* 1986; 158:547–549.
19. Zilkha A: Computed tomography of blow-out fracture of the medial orbital wall. *AJNR* 1981; 2:427–429.
20. Dodick JM, Galin MA, Littleton JT, et al: Concomitant medial wall fracture and blow-out fracture of the orbit. *Arch Ophthalmol* 1971; 85:273–276.
21. Hammerschlag SB, Hughes S, O'Reilly GV, et al: Another look at blow-out fractures of the orbit. *AJNR* 1982; 3:331–335.
22. Curtin HD, Wolfe P, Schramm V: Orbital roof blow-out fracture. *AJR* 1982; 139:969–972.
23. Gerlock AJ, Sinn DP, McBride KL: *Clinical and Radiographic Interpretation of Facial Fractures.* Boston, Little, Brown & Co, Inc, 1981, pp 137–144.
24. Guyon JJ, Brant-Zawadzki MB, Seiff SR: CT demonstration of optic canal fractures. *AJNR* 1984; 5:575–578.
25. Kline LB, Morawetz RB, Swaid SN: Indirect injury of the optic nerve. *Neurosurgery* 1984; 14:756–763.
26. Holler ML, Brockup AH, Shiffman F: Intraorbital aerocele. *Arch Ophthalmol* 1980; 98:1612–1613.
27. Goldberg F, Berne AS, Oski FA: Differentiation of orbital cellulitis from preseptal cellulitis by computed tomography. *Pediatrics* 1978; 62:1000–1005.
28. Zimmerman RA, Bilaniuk LT: CT of orbital infection—its cerebral complications. *AJR* 1980; 134:45–50.
29. Leo JS, Halpern J, Sackler JRL: Computed tomography in the evaluation of orbital infections. *Comput Tomogr* 1980; 4:133–138.
30. Fernback SK, Naidich TP: CT diagnosis of orbital inflammation in children. *Neuroradiology* 1981; 22:7–13.
31. Gellady AM, Shulman ST, Ayoub EM: Periorbital and orbital cellulitis in children. *Pediatrics* 1978; 61:272–276.
32. Spires JR, Smith RJH: Bacterial infections of the orbital and periorbital soft tissues in children. *Laryngoscope* 1986; 96:763–767.
33. Towbin R, Han B, Kaufman RA, et al: Postseptal cellulitis: CT in diagnosis and management. *Radiology* 1986; 158:735–737.
34. Putterman AM, Urist MJ: Surgical anatomy of the orbital septum. *Ann Opthalmol* 1974; 6:290–294.
35. Smith TF, O'Day D, Wright PF: Clinical implications of preseptal (periorbital) cellulitis in childhood. *Pediatrics* 1978; 62:1006–1009.
36. Chandler JR, Langenbrunner DJ, Stevens ER: The pathogenesis of orbital complications in acute sinusitis. *Laryngoscope* 1970; 80:1414–1428.
37. Whitnall WE: *Anatomy of the Human Orbit and Accessory Organs of Vision* (facsimile of 1921 edi-

tion). New York, Robert E. Krieger Publishing Co, Inc, 1979, pp 85–86.

38. Morgan PR, Morrison WV: Complications of frontal and ethmoid sinusitis. *Laryngoscope* 1980; 90:661–666.

39. Greenberg MR, Lippman SM, Grinnell VS, et al: Computed tomographic findings in orbital mucor. *West J Med* 1985; 143:102–103.

40. Harr DL, Quencer RM, Abrams GW: Computed tomography and ultrasound in the evaluation of orbital infection and pseudotumor. *Radiology* 1982; 142:395–401.

27

Orbital Masses

William E. Rothfus, M.D.

In this chapter we wish to emphasize a framework on which a differential diagnosis of orbital masses can be developed. Several authors point out difficulties in making histologic diagnoses of orbital masses on the sole basis of scan appearance.[1-6] Indeed, it is not surprising that computed tomography (CT) and magnetic resonance imaging (MRI) fall short in differentiating processes in which histology, method of spread, and anatomic preference are similar, as is the case in many orbital tumors and pseudotumors. However, some groups of orbital masses do have similarities on scans that seem to separate them from other groups of masses.

Thus we have endeavored to combine pathologic entities with somewhat similar CT or MRI appearances into four differential categories: (1) the well-circumscribed mass has distinct margins separate from the surrounding orbital structures. This type is usually round or oval in shape; histologically, it usually has a capsule. (2) The infiltrative, or less well-marginated mass has less definite margins than the well-circumscribed mass does. It characteristically involves multiple orbital structures and is not encapsulated. Although a portion of the mass may be fairly distinct, other portions blend into the surrounding structures. (3) The serpiginous mass has a knobby exterior but well-defined margins. (4) The thickened optic nerve sheath complex has tubular, fusiform, or excrescent enlargement of the optic nerve or its sheath.

WELL-CIRCUMSCRIBED MASSES

Cavernous Hemangioma

Cavernous hemangioma is a common tumor, being among the five most common orbital neoplasms.[7] It is encapsulated and has smooth or mildly lobulated exteriors. Slow growing, it usually remains isolated from other orbital structures; invasion of the optic nerve or extraocular muscles is uncommon. This tumor is made up of multiple vascular channels; thus they contain a large blood pool.

As predicted by its histology, the hemangioma is a well-delineated round or oval mass on CT scan.[8-10] Because of its highly vascular composition, its inherent density is high, and it enhances following contrast administration. This enhancement is homogeneous or heterogeneous[8] depending on the size of the vascular channels within the tumor (Fig 27-1). When dynamic contrast injection methods are used, enhancement tends to be rather delayed, which differs from other tumors (e.g., capillary hemangiomas) with more rapid circulation.[11] Calcified phleboliths may be present. Although the characteristic location is intraconal and superolateral, hemangiomas may occur anywhere, intraconally or extraconally (Fig 27-2). The optic nerve may be displaced, but rarely invaded. The tumor may cause adjacent orbital wall remodeling.

Cavernous hemangioma is easily detected on MRI scans by virtue of its well-defined margins

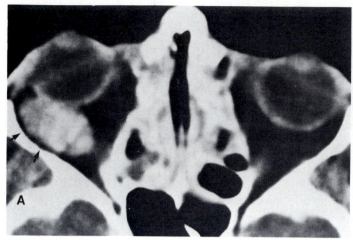
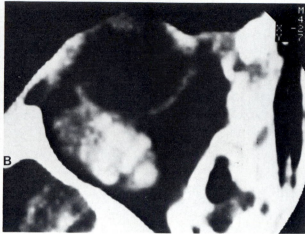

FIG 27–1.
Cavernous hemangioma. **A,** a well-defined oval mass sits in the superolateral retrobulbar space. Diffuse, although inhomogeneous enhancement is noted. Notice the slight remodeling of the lateral orbital wall *(arrows).* **B,** a magnified view at a wider window setting brings out tumor heterogeneity caused by vascular (thus contrast) pools.

and contrast with orbital fat. It is isointense to hypointense on short repetition time/echo time (TR/TE) images and hyperintense on long TR/TE images (Fig 27–3).[11, 12] Focal areas of hyperintensity or hypointensity can be scattered through the tumor, presumably reflecting areas of blood flow (either slow or fast) within the more solid portions of tumor.

Hemangiopericytoma

Pathologically, hemangiopericytoma has vascular channels, is well circumscribed, and has a fibrous coat.[13] It is easy to see, then, why this tumor has a CT/MRI appearance that is similar to hemangioma.[2] Enhancement may be heterogeneous or homogeneous, but is usually prominent. This tumor grows slowly, so it too may cause expansion of bony walls. The natural history of this tumor is different from hemangioma in that local invasion of muscles and bone is more common and recurrences (local and metastatic) more frequent.[13]

Neurofibroma, Schwannoma

Schwannoma and the isolated form of neurofibroma (i.e., nonplexiform) are benign, encapsulated tumors that are well defined when presenting in the orbit. They may not be associated with other features of neurofibromatosis. In general, they become apparent in the adult years. They tend not to be vascular and are made up of a fairly uniform population of cells.[14] On CT, they are oval-shaped

or fusiform easily delineated masses with fairly uniform texture and enhancement. Round or swirl-like areas of lucency may occur due to cystic necrosis, xanthomatous change, or local hypocellularity (Fig 27–4).[15] Enhancement is usually less pronounced than in hemangioma or hemangiopericytoma. On MRI schwannomas and neurofibromas are hypointense to isointense on short TR/TE images and hyperintense on long TR/TE images (Fig 27–5). The capsule may be represented by a con-

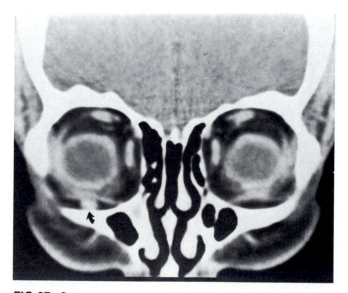

FIG 27–2.
Cavernous hemangioma. A small, homogeneously enhancing cavernous hemangioma *(arrow)* sits beneath the globe. Although no significant mass effect is present, it was palpable through the lower lid.

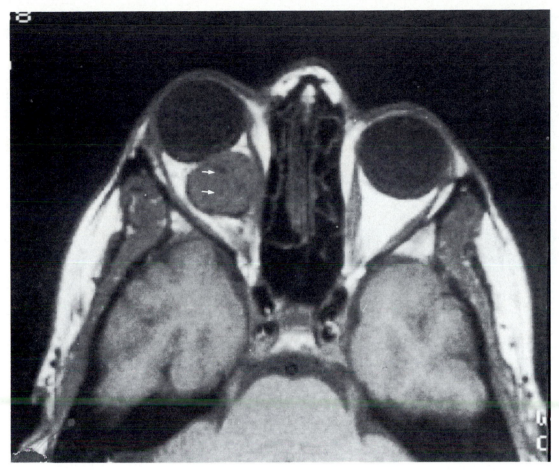

FIG 27–3.
Cavernous hemangioma. A short TR/TE axial MR scan shows the well-defined tumor causing distortion of the medial rectus and pos-terior globe wall. Small vascular channels are present as foci of hy-pointensity within the tumor *(arrows)*.

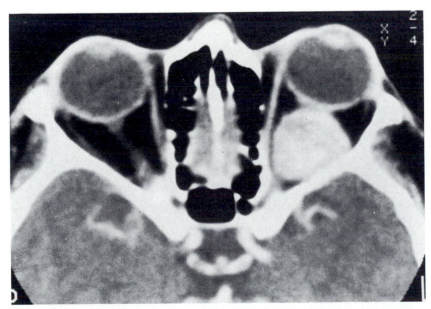

FIG 27–4.
Neurofibroma. This well-defined mass shows slight inhomogeneity, with scattered lucent swirls and dots.

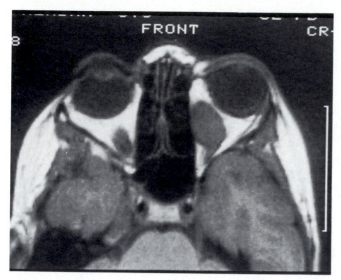

FIG 27–5.
Neurofibroma. Short TR/TE MR axial study with a homogeneous encapsulated tumor of the medial portion of the orbit.

tinuous peripheral rim of decreased intensity that is distinguishable from the partial artifactual rim of chemical shift.

This appearance is decidedly different from the plexiform type of neurofibroma, the other major form of neurofibroma. Grossly cordlike, the plexiform type is nodular on scans. It is more vascular and diffuse than the isolated form[14] and can be seen to entangle itself around normal orbital structures. Plexiform neurofibroma is discussed with serpiginous masses.

Dermoid

Of the well-defined masses, the dermoid cyst may be the easiest to differentiate. The pathogno-

monic appearance includes a smooth, uniformly thin wall surrounding a central cyst that has low attenuation (at or near fat density) on CT (Fig 27–6) or has fatty characteristics (high signal on short TR/TE, low signal on long TR/TE) on MRI.[16–18] Contiguous bony scalloping, sinus tract, remodeling, or sclerosis is also common.[18] Not all dermoids show typical features, however. Debris within a cyst or associated inflammation may alter the appearance of the cyst or the wall. The more keratin and the less cholesterin the dermoid cyst contains, the less typical is its appearance on MRI (Fig 27–7).

Other Masses

Fibromas, extradural meningiomas, angioleiomyoma, and fibrous histiocytomas are also types of well-defined orbital masses.[11, 19] They are homogeneous, high-density lesions that enhance with contrast. Occasionally an orbital varix will have a round contour that simulates a neoplasm.[20] Contrast enhancement is pronounced and homogeneous. As discussed later (under serpiginous masses) provocative maneuvers may significantly alter the shape of a varix, thus helping to distinguish it from other vascular masses. The MRI appearance of a varix may vary with the type of flow within it. Hypointensity results from rapid flow, while the more usual hyperintensity results from flow-related enhancement or even-echo rephasing (Fig 27–8).

Subacute hematomas may appear as well-defined masses. As with extraorbital hematomas, density and intensity changes vary with time because the CT density of a subacute hemangioma may be quite variable, and differential diagnosis is diffi-

FIG 27–6.
Dermoid. This thin-walled mass *(arrow)* has on CT a low-absorption interior measuring in the fat range. Some higher-density material (debris) is seen within the cyst. Remodeling of the lamina papyracea is present.

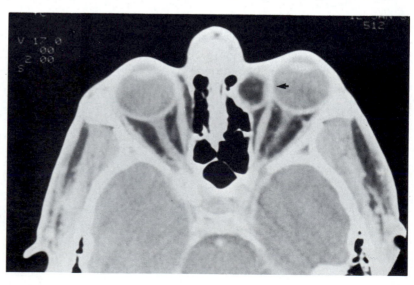

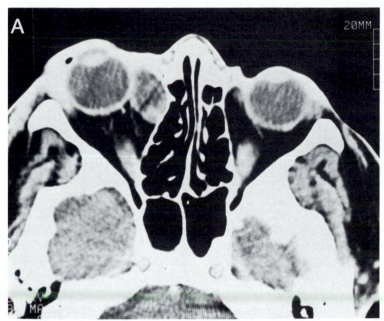

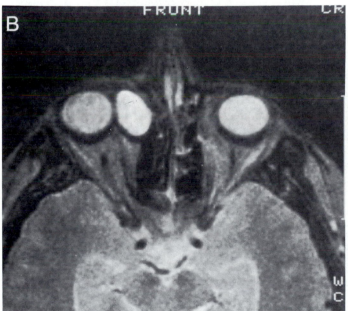

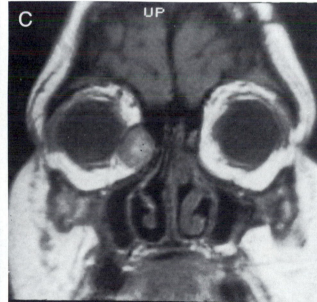

FIG 27–7.
Dermoid with atypical MRI characteristics. **A,** a lucent encapsulated mass has caused remodeling of the medial portion of the right orbit similar to Figure 27–6. **B,** a long TR/TE axial MR section shows marked hyperintensity. **C,** a short TR/TE coronal sequence shows relative isointensity. The cyst was highly keratinized.

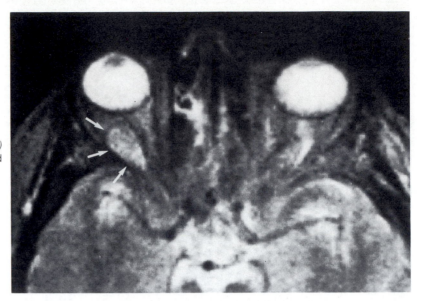

FIG 27–8.
Varix. This surgically confirmed varix *(arrows)* is well defined and hyperintense on MR and simulates a neoplasm.

cult. However, MRI is usually more distinctive. Hyperintensity predominates due to the presence of methemoglobin on both short and long TR/TE images (Fig 27–9).

INFILTRATIVE MASSES

Pseudotumor

An orbital pseudotumor is a reactive inflammatory lesion that in many ways simulates a neoplasm. The etiology of the reactive process is unknown, and its clinical course is unpredictable. Pseudotumors are common, being the fourth most frequent orbital mass in a large Mayo Clinic series.[21] Its clinical presentation, especially in the acute phase, suggests the inflammatory nature of the disease with proptosis, chemosis, limitation of eye motion, pain, and lid swelling. Proptosis, however, may dominate the more-inflammatory–type symptoms, and thus, the clinical presentation is more like a tumor. Pseudotumor usually is unilateral. Corticosteroid therapy and low-dose radiotherapy have been effective in most cases in alleviating or curing symptoms.

Pathologically, pseudotumor may be diffuse and affect many orbital structures or be local and mainly affect muscle (myositis), the lacrimal gland (dacryoadenitis), the posterior portion of the globe (periscleritis), the optic nerve (perineuritis), or orbital fat (diffuse pseudotumor). Histologically, lymphocytic infiltration predominates, often being so extensive that the underlying tissue is replaced. The maturity of the lymphocytes and presence of other cell types, e.g., polymorphonuclear leukocytes and plasma cells, emphasize some features of acute inflammation.[21, 22] More chronic forms of pseudotumor have a fibrous stroma intermingled with the pleomorphic inflammatory cells.

Various authors have described CT findings in orbital pseudotumor.[23–28] Being a disease with multiple expressions, pseudotumor can manifest a host of different scan appearances. However, some classification is possible when based on the regional nature of disease involvement.[27] That is, pseudotumor largely limited to the muscle can be separated from pseudotumor of the lacrimal gland, which can be separated from pseudotumor of the retrobulbar and extraconal fat.

The dominant CT characteristics of a pseudotumor mass, wherever it is located, is its tendency toward homogeneous texture. This correlates well with the pathologic process, which is a relatively uniform inflammation that obliterates normal structures. The periphery of the mass spreads irregularly through orbit fat when it originates behind or around the globe. Thus, on CT, the mass usually has irregular, sometimes quite indistinct margins (Fig 27–10). Because the retrobulbar inflammatory process invariably involves contiguous muscle, fat, and connective tissue, the CT scan shows obscuration of soft-tissue planes by the mass. Thus, the mass seems to combine the affected structures into an enhancing conglomerate (Fig 27–11). Occasionally, the pseudotumor mass is relatively confined to the extraconal or intraconal space. As such, the muscles and their associated fascial structures limit the mass and give it a more defined appearance

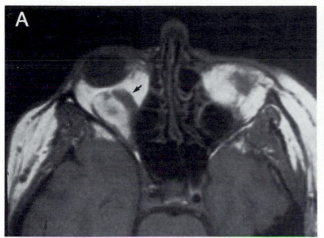

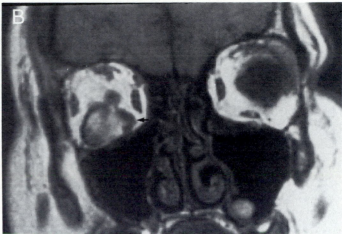

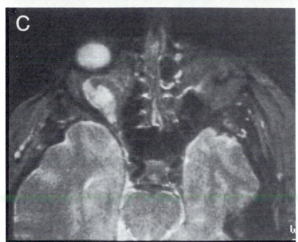

FIG 27–9.
Subacute hematoma. Both axial **(A)** and coronal **(B)** short TR/TE and axial **(C)** long TR/TE MR sequences demonstrate hyperintensity within this spontaneous hematoma. The hypointense lateral rim is probably a combination of hemosiderin and chemical shift. The inferior rectus *(arrows)* has been displaced medially.

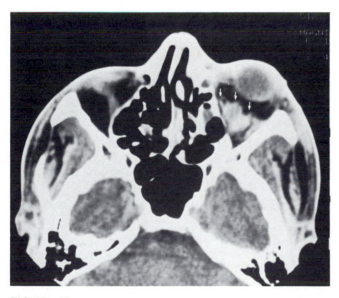

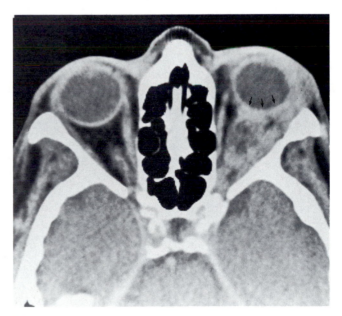

FIG 27–10.
Pseudotumor. An enhancing pseudotumor of the posterior portion of the orbit shows irregular fingers of inflammation *(arrows)* extending into the orbital fat.

FIG 27–11.
Pseudotumor. Extensive orbital involvement is seen, with pseudotumor infiltrating multiple structures and obscuring normal soft-tissue planes. Notice some scleral thickening and enhancement *(arrows)*.

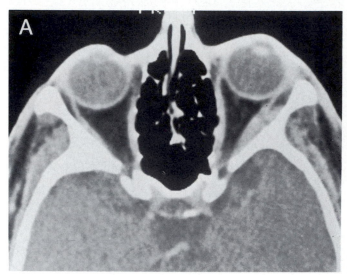
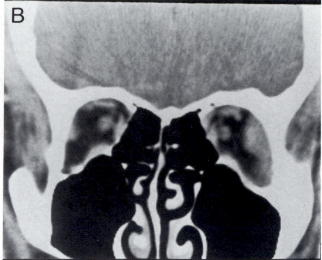

FIG 27–12.
Pseudotumor. Axial **(A)** and coronal **(B)** CT views show a homogeneous extraconal mass contiguous to the lateral rectus that is being confined by fascia related to the muscle.

(Fig 27–12). In these cases, some part of the mass may be marginated while another part may be a more typical ill-defined margin.

Nugent and colleagues[27] have noted the tendency for acute retrobulbar pseudotumors to be located either anteriorly, posteriorly, or diffusely in the orbital cone. The anterior masses relate closely to the back of the globe and are associated with swelling and enhancement of the scleral margin (see Fig 27–11). Such scleral involvement is believed to be highly characteristic but not pathognomomic of pseudotumor.[26] The posterior type originates at the apex and obliterates the tissue planes near the annulus of Zinn. Diffuse-type involvement obscures all structures from the back of the globe to the apex. Because localized disease has been observed to progress to the diffuse type, it is likely that the latter represents the severest stage of disease progression. Bilateral retrobulbar pseudotumor can exist but may be a concomitant of a systemic disorder such as Wegener's granulomatosis, polyarteritis nodosa, sarcoidosis, multifocal fibrosclerosis, or thyroiditis.[21] Bony wall erosion or intracranial extension are uncommonly seen.[29, 30]

Pseudotumor has a fairly distinctive appearance on spin-echo sequences.[31, 32] It is usually hypointense to fat and isointense to muscle on short TR/TE and hypointense to isointense to fat and muscle on long TR/TE sequences (Fig 27–13). Thus, pseudotumor may be distinguished from metastatic tumors (hyperintense on long TR/TE) and hematoma (hyperintense on both long and short TR/TE). However, other inflammatory lesions like sarcoid and other infiltrative neoplasms like leukemia have shown a similar appearance to pseudotumor.[11, 31, 32]

Lymphoma and Lymphoid Hyperplasia

Orbital lymphoma is a common cause of proptosis, in one series following only inflammatory conditions and hemangiomas in frequency.[33] It occurs principally in and after middle age and usually presents clinically as a mass with swelling and proptosis. Occasionally, symptoms and signs may be more inflammatory, thus making distinction from pseudotumor difficult. As well, it may be difficult histologically and radiologically to distinguish lymphomas from pseudotumor. Microscopically, the conditions look alike, having a predominance of lymphocytes. Special immunopathologic techniques may be necessary to help separate the two. Similarly, the microscopic appearance of lymphoid hyperplasia mimics a well-differentiated lymphoma. Often the only way to distinguish these is by searching for other evidence of systemic lymphoma.[22]

Because of pathologic similarity, lymphoma and lymphoid hyperplasia have many of the same CT features as pseudotumors. In particular, the lymphomatous mass has a homogeneous texture both before and after contrast administration. It may be intraconal or extraconal. The mass also obscures nearby muscle because of the contiguity of

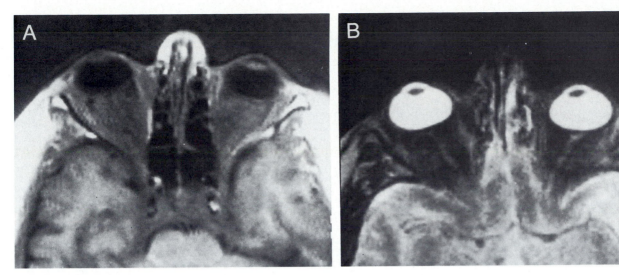

FIG 27–13.
Diffuse pseudotumor-vasculitis. Axial scans demonstrate isointensity of the diffusely infiltrative process on short TR/TE **(A)** and hypointensity on long TR/TE **(B)** MR sequences.

similar CT densities and, in some cases, frank invasion of muscle. Lymphomas may be primarily irregular, with poorly delineated margins on CT corresponding with the gross appearance of a lumpy, ill-defined tumor (Fig 27–14). On the other hand, the gross and CT characteristics are commonly more defined, especially in the superior and anterior portions of the orbit. In such a case, the tumor mass conforms more to the orbital space and forms a cast within the orbit fat (Fig 27–15). Lymphoma may show a tendency to "coat" the globe; the homogeneous mass of tumor seems to extend in a blanketlike manner around the periphery of the globe (Fig 27–16). Diffuse spread of tumor throughout the orbit, contiguous extraorbital spread, and bony destruction, although uncommon, are indicative of highly malignant forms of lymphoma.

The MRI appearance of lymphoma mimics CT in terms of location and contour. Lymphomas are generally hypointense or isointense on short TR/TE sequences. Intensity is more variable on long

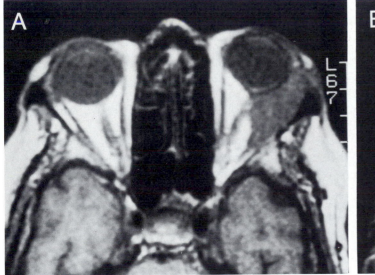

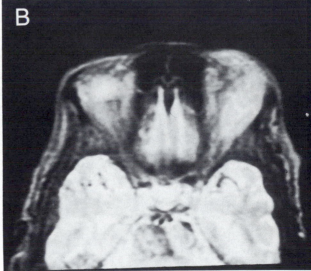

FIG 27–14.
Lymphoma. The tumor mass, which on MR is isointense on short TR/TE **(A)** and hyperintense on long TR/TE **(B)**, spreads through the lateral portion of the orbit with a clear sulcus between it and surrounding structures.

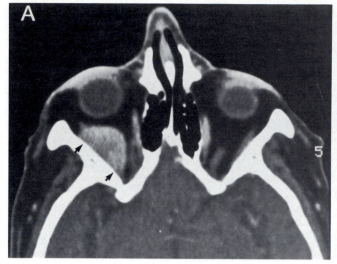

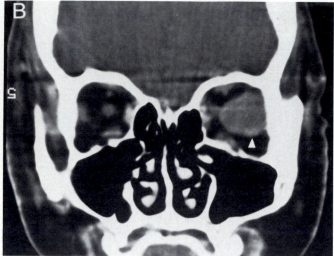

FIG 27–15.
Lymphoma. Axial **(A)** and coronal **(B)** CT scans show a well defined tumor mass protruding into the orbit and displacing the lateral rectus *(B, arrowhead)*. Even though the medial aspect of the tumor is well defined, the mass is not wholly circumscribed and has a broad base with rather obtuse angles *(A, arrows)* to the orbit wall.

TR/TE, with tumor appearing either isointense or hyperintense (see Fig 27–14).[34–37] Therefore, it may be rather difficult to effectively separate lymphomas from other infiltrative masses on the basis of intensity characteristics alone.

Metastatic Tumor

Most metastatic involvement of the orbit is by carcinoma, particularly adenocarcinomas, with the breast and lung being the most frequent primary sites. Incidence is chiefly in the adult age group, with a peak in the seventh decade. Interestingly,

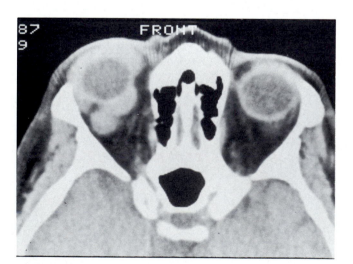

FIG 27–16.
Lymphoma. Lumpy homogeneous masses drape the periphery of the right globe.

in a significant number of cases, the orbit is the first site of presentation, with the primary tumor being found later. Proptosis, diplopia, pain, eyelid swelling, and ophthalmoplegia are all common symptoms.

Metastases occur in the orbital wall, globe, retrobulbar soft tissues, or optic nerve sheath.[38] When involving the soft tissues alone, tumor may be located intraconally or extraconally, focally or diffusely. On CT, the margins of the metastatic tumor mass are usually irregular and reflect their infiltrative nature, although occasionally, more bulbous areas are seen. Enhancement is variable; texture is commonly inhomogeneous. By MRI, most metastases have relatively low intensity on short TR/TE and high intensity on long TR/TE sequences.[31, 32, 38] One exception is scirrhous adenocarcinoma, which is hypointense on long TR/TE sequences due to its high fibrous content (Fig 27–17).

Most retrobulbar metastases have mass effect and cause proptosis of the globe. Uniquely, scirrhous adenocarcinoma, regardless of the primary site of origin, causes a retraction of orbital contents (enophthalmos) as it infiltrates them. Thus, an infiltrative mass associated with enophthalmos is likely to be a scirrhous type of metastatic adenocarcinoma.

Capillary Hemangioma

Capillary hemangioma occurs at an earlier age than does cavernous hemangioma and does not

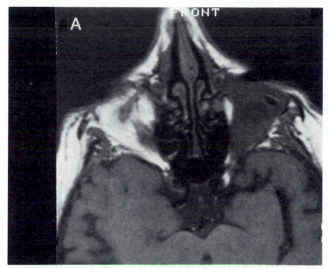

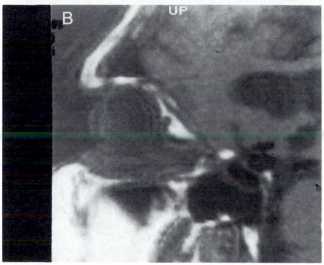

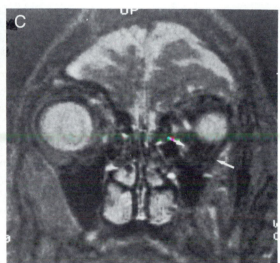

FIG 27–17.
Scirrhous carcinoma. There is an infiltrative mass of the inferior aspect of the left globe. On short TR/TE axial **(A)** and sagittal **(B)** MR images, the mass is isointense to hypointense, while on a coronal long TR/TE image **(C),** it is hypointense *(arrows),* much like the pseudotumor in Figure 27–13. Note enophthalmos in **B,** which suggests the diagnosis.

have a true capsule. It tends to be more aggressive and infiltrate local structures, which makes surgical removal difficult.[7] Some of these tumors involve the face, eyelids, or scalp and extend back into the orbit for a variable distance. The cutaneous lesions are easily seen and may change in size with alteration in intravascular pressure.

The CT/MRI scans delineate the extent of this tumor well. Because capillary hemangioma possesses more stromal tissue and fewer vascular channels than cavernous hemangiomas do, it has a more homogeneous pattern before and after contrast administration. The tumor insinuates through and around the orbital septum and presents as an enhancing mass over the involved portions of the face and scalp (Fig 27–18). This type of tumor has a tendency to involute.[39] As it does, it may develop a capsule and thus appear more circumscribed.

Lymphangioma

Lymphangioma is a benign tumor of young age that clinically may simulate features of hemangioma—proptosis, fluctuation in size, strabismus, orbital enlargement, and cutaneous lesions. Histologically, it is made up of numerous lymph-filled channels surrounded by a stromal framework.[40] The proportion of lymph channels to stroma may vary. Bleeding into the cysts is common and may be enough to compromise vision. Difficult to remove surgically, this infiltrative tumor may extend through large portions of the orbit, intraconally or extraconally, and has a tendency to recur locally.

Because of the variable histologic makeup of the tumor, the CT appearance of lymphangiomas is likewise variable. The spectrum ranges from relatively homogeneous density to high irregular density, depending on the uniformity of vascular spaces and the presence or absence of bleeding

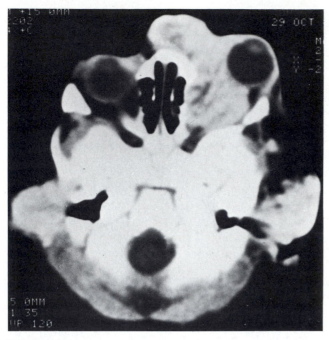

FIG 27–18.
Capillary hemangioma. A large enhancing tumor extends from the nose and face through the orbital septum into the retrobulbar space. It extends irregularly through the retro-ocular fat.

within the tumor cysts. Although one end of the CT spectrum is toward tumor homogeneity, lymphangioma is not usually as uniform in texture as lymphomas or pseudotumor (Fig 27–19). Only half of lymphangiomas show enhancement[8]; when they do, it is usually not prominent.

Most lymphangiomas have indistinct margins because of their invasive character and lack of a capsule. When the tumor is limited by the muscle cone or fascial structure or there is frank hematoma formation, the periphery becomes more delineated.

The MRI appearance of lymphangioma is fairly characteristic. A rather isointense matrix is distinguished among loculated regions of hyperintensity on long TR/TE sequences. These loculations may be hypointense (representing proteinaceous fluid) or hyperintense (representing methemoglobin in chocolate cyst fluid) on short TR/TE sequences. The overall effect is of a bubbly appearance (Fig 27–20). Occasionally chocolate cysts may be quite large and contain levels of differing intensities due to various blood constituents (Fig 27–21).

There is no particular location in which orbital lymphangioma occurs. It may be entirely intraconal (the most common location) or extraconal or bridge between the spaces. It may even extend through large portions of the orbit and may be diffuse. Calcification may occur and is usually focal and dense. Expansion of the orbital walls can sometimes be demonstrated by scan and documents the slow growth of this tumor.

Other Neoplastic or Neoplastic-Like Conditions

Wegener's granulomatosis fairly commonly involves the orbital structures.[41] When presented as a

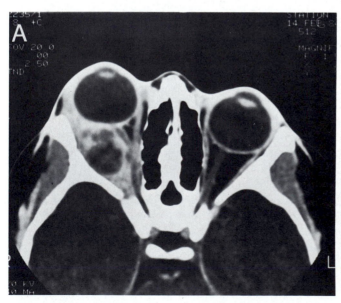
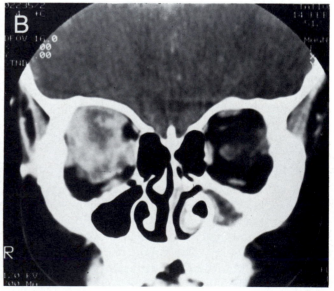

FIG 27–19.
Lymphangioma. Axial **(A)** and coronal **(B)** CT scans show that the inhomogeneously enhancing mass infiltrates through much of the retrobulbar space. The large central lucency represents a hemorrhagic cyst; it contributes to mass effect and displaces the optic nerve medially.

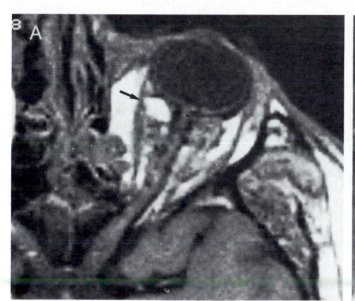

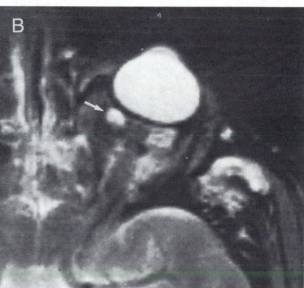

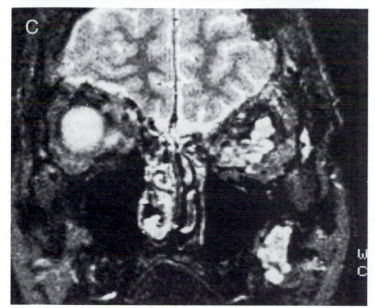

FIG 27–20.
Lymphangioma. **A,** a short TR/TE axial MR image
demonstrates a mixed-intensity tumor surrounding the optic
nerve. The focal area of hyperintensity just behind the globe
(arrow) is a chocolate cyst, as confirmed by similar
hyperintensity *(arrow)* on a comparable long TR/TE section
(B). The coronal section **(C)** brings out the bubbly
appearance of the tumor. Note also the more extensive
lymphangiomatosis involving the infratemporal fossa.

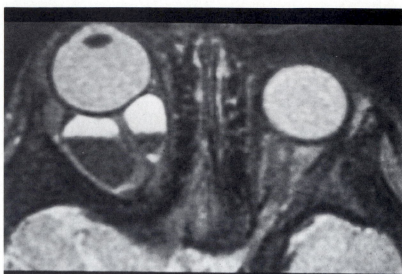

FIG 27–21.
Lymphangioma. An axial long TR/TE MR section shows a large hemorrhagic cyst containing a debris-fluid level caused by posterior sedimentation of blood products containing deoxyhemoglobin.

retrobulbar mass, the CT scan shows a local or diffuse infiltrative mass with homogeneous density and variable enhancement[42] that is indistinguishable from pseudotumor. Involvement may be unilateral or bilateral. One distinguishing characteristic of Wegener's granulomatosis is the presence of a sinus mass or sinus bone destruction, neither of which need to be contiguous with the orbital mass. Other granulomatous and autoimmune diseases such as sarcoidosis, histiocystosis, polyarteritis nodosa, lupus erythematosus, rheumatoid arthritis, and fibrosclerosis may simulate pseudotumor on CT or MRI. One clue to these diagnoses is their tendency to be bilateral.[28]

Infiltrative leukemia, carcinoid, and amyloid can mimic pseudotumor with diffuse orbital involvement and characteristic long TR/TE homogeneous hypointensity.[11, 43] So too, myeloma (primary or secondary) can mimic pseudotumor.[44] It may be localized to the retro-ocular spaces or involve adjacent globe, bone, and facial soft tissue.

To summarize, infiltrative masses have irregular margins, except where they are confined by normal anatomic boundaries (e.g., the orbital septum). They often obscure the soft-tissue planes within the orbit, which makes normal structures "melt" into the density of the mass itself. Simply, they can be thought of as comprising two major groups: childhood and adulthood. Hemangiomas and lymphangiomas predominate in the childhood group. Of these two, hemangiomas tend to be more vascular and enhance vigorously. Lymphangiomas enhance less than hemangiomas do and may be quite variable in texture. MRI of lymphangiomas is usually distinctive. The adult infiltrative masses—

pseudotumor, lymphoma, lymphoid hyperplasia, and metastasis—can appear similar on scans. The lymphoid tumors tend to be globular. Most metastases and lymphomas are hyperintense on long TR/TE sequences, which helps distinguish them from pseudotumor and pseudotumor mimics that are hypointense.

SERPIGINOUS MASSES

Arteriovenous Malformation

Arteriovenous malformation (AVMs) may occur anywhere in the orbit. When in the retrobulbar space, it can present with exophthalmos, chemosis, bruit, ophthalmoplegia, or visual loss. Supplied by branches of the ophthalmic and/or external carotid arteries, it has the typical appearance of enlarged, serpiginous vessels. Usually an AVM wraps around the normal structures but may penetrate them as well.

The CT scan appearance of an intraorbital AVM is fairly characteristic.[45] Tortuous densities are seen that represent dilated arteries and veins. These enhance very prominently, especially when rapid dynamic scanning is done. Portions of the AVM may be composed of tightly entwined vascular channels that cannot be individually distinguished. Rather, they appear as a densely enhancing mass with a multinodular periphery. Calcifications occasionally occur within the AVM. Muscle enlargement may be an accompanying finding, especially if the AVM intimately involves the muscle. Rarely, an AVM may cause bony wall remodeling. On MRI, the AVM is easily distin-

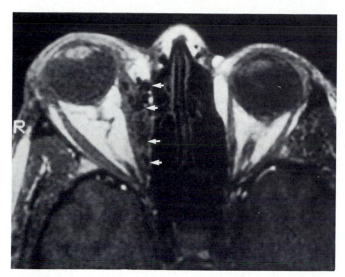

FIG 27–22.
AVM. Multiple round hypointensities (flow voids) are present along the medial portion of the orbit and within the medial rectus *(arrows)*. Chronic pulsatile pressure has remodeled the medial wall.

guished by tubular, serpiginous, or round conglomerates of hypointensity caused by a flow void (Fig 27–22).

Some of the above findings (enlarged, prominently enhancing vascular structures and muscle enlargement) can be seen with another arteriovenous communication, carotid-cavernous sinus fistula. Usually, a distinction between the two can be made. Carotid-cavernous sinus fistula enlarges only venous structures, especially the superior ophthalmic vein.[46] It has no definable vascular "mass"; muscle enlargement affects multiple muscles rather than one.

Venous Varix

Venous malformation, specifically the varix characteristically causes intermittent exophthalmos. Exophthalmos can be provoked by such maneuvers as jugular compression, the Valsalva maneuver, straining, or dropping the head. The malformation may be developmental or associated with an AVM.[47]

On CT in the resting patient, the varix may be inapparent or only a small lobulated linear or round density. Even contrast administration can fail to make it stand out sufficiently. Provocative maneuvers done at the time of scanning with contrast enhancement can accentuate the volume of the varix, sometimes strikingly (Fig 27–23).[48] MRI can be somewhat deceiving, especially if the varix is large. Due to slow, turbulent flow or diastolic pseudogating, it can appear hyperintense like a tumor (see Fig 27–8). Maneuvers may alter the size of the varix, but obviously, clinical suspicion must be high to anticipate the need for such maneuvers. Varices, like AVMs, may have phlebolithic calcification and can cause deformity of the orbit wall (Fig 27–24).

Plexiform Neurofibroma

Plexiform neurofibroma is invariably associated with neurofibromatosis. As previously stated, it is a knobby, ropelike tumor that can be quite diffuse. It envelopes normal structures like the optic nerve, extraocular muscles, and lacrimal gland; contiguous involvement of the eyelids and face is

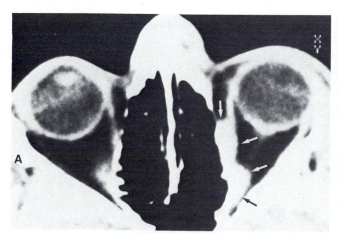
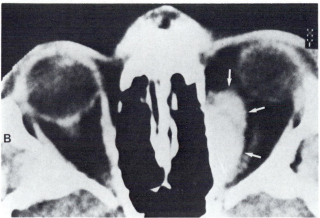

FIG 27–23.
Varix. **A,** in normal head position, the varix is seen as a thin, slightly tortuous enhancing density along the medial aspect of the orbit *(arrows)*. **B,** a scan in the head-hanging position illustrates marked dilatation of the varix *(arrows)*. Note the associated flattening of the orbital wall, probably a result of chronic pulsatile pressure.

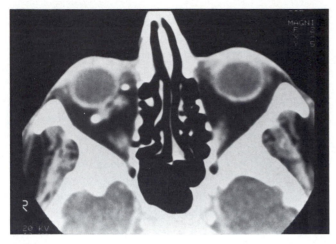

FIG 27–24.
Varix. A knobby varix just behind the right globe contains two calcified phleboliths.

common.[49, 50] On the CT scan, nodular thickening occurs longitudinally along the object affected by the tumor (Fig 27–25). Because the tumor is relatively vascular, enhancement occurs, but not nearly to the same degree as in an AVM. Nodular thickening along the periphery of the optic nerve sheath and increased density of the orbital fat can result from involvement of small orbital nerves.[50] Associated bony dysplasia of the sphenoid wing, another common finding in neurofibromatosis, may be seen with these tumors. On MRI most plexiform neurofibromas are hypointense on short TR/TE and hyperintense on long TR/TE sequences (Fig 27–26).

THE ENLARGED OPTIC NERVE SHEATH COMPLEX

Enlargement of the optic nerve sheath complex presents a differential diagnosis encompassing a wide variety of disease processes. The most dramatic are primary optic nerve glioma and meningioma, but nonneoplastic conditions like papilledema or Graves' disease can similarly expand the sheath. Thin-section CT is usually not sufficient to distinguish the optic nerve from its surrounding sheath; so too, MR is frequently complicated by patient motion and chemical shift artifact. Thus, differentiating primary optic nerve pathology from pathology of the nerve sheath or the enclosed cerebrospinal fluid (CSF) spaces becomes difficult. Most often, differential diagnosis is accomplished by evaluating size, shape, growth patterns, and patient age.

Optic Nerve Sheath Meningioma

Modern imaging techniques have led to the awareness that optic nerve sheath meningioma is not as rare as once thought. Clinically, it presents with early visual loss, optic atrophy, and late proptosis in a middle-aged patient. Understanding the scan appearance comes from consideration of the site of origin and nature of growth.[51, 52]

Intraorbital meningioma arises from the arachnoid attached to the dura of the sheath. Early growth is usually confined to the area between the optic nerve and sheath, so the tumor spreads in a sheetlike manner along the CSF space surround-

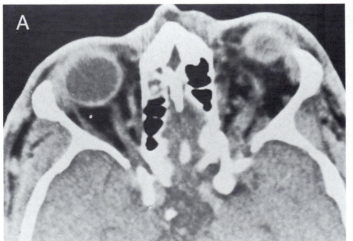
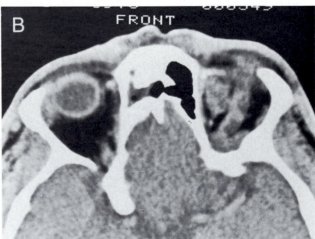

FIG 27–25.
Plexiform neurofibroma. **A** and **B,** knobby and beadlike masses are dispersed through the left orbit with associated proptosis.

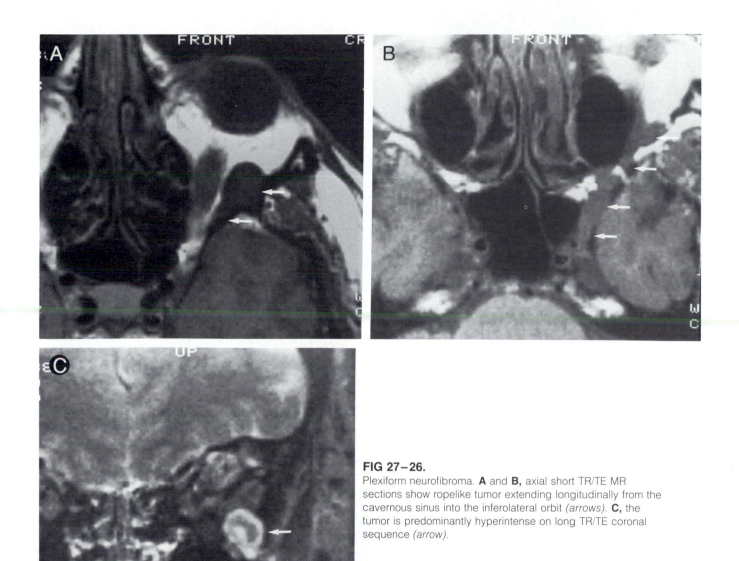

FIG 27–26.
Plexiform neurofibroma. **A** and **B,** axial short TR/TE MR
sections show ropelike tumor extending longitudinally from the
cavernous sinus into the inferolateral orbit *(arrows).* **C,** the
tumor is predominantly hyperintense on long TR/TE coronal
sequence *(arrow).*

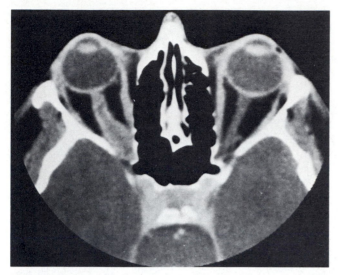

FIG 27–27.
Optic meningioma. The posterior aspect of the intraorbital optic nerve is surrounded by enhancing tumor, which forms a fusiform enlargement of the nerve sheath complex.

ing the nerve. With progressive growth, there is compression of the optic nerve. Finally, the enlarging tumor may break through the dura and produce an exophytic intraconal tumor mass.

The CT appearance of intraorbital meningioma tends to fall into two patterns, one corresponding to the "subdural" mode of growth and the other to the "exophytic" mode. Subdural growth, which is limited by the dura, produces tubular enlargement of the nerve sheath complex. This enlargement may affect the entire intraorbital length of the nerve (Fig 27–27) or be more segmental, depending on the extent of tumor extension through the

perineural space. Longitudinal growth usually stops at the optic canal, although extension into the optic canal can be associated with canal widening and hyperostosis. Occasionally, this meningioma calcifies to produce a smooth, sleevelike focal calcification surrounding the nerve (Fig 27–28).

The exophytic meningioma shows wide-based tumor extending from the optic nerve sheath complex and projecting into the surrounding orbit. Although sometimes lobulated, the mass is well defined. As with other meningiomas, enhancement is prominent and homogeneous. With thin sections, the enhancing tumorous optic nerve sheath can usually be distinguished from the lucent optic nerve (Fig 27–29).[52, 53] Occasionally, the meningioma may become so large as to encompass the nerve completely and give an image of the optic nerve "ghost." The tumor may become eccentric enough to displace the nerve, but keeps a broad attachment to it.

MRI is extremely useful in depicting optic nerve sheath meningioma. Tumor is generally less intense than the nerve, which makes the nerve stand out in relief (Fig 27–30). The ability to evaluate multiple projections, especially parasagittally along the axis of the nerve, gives MRI a distinctive advantage over CT in evaluating these tumors; however, calcification is poorly detected by MRI, so a plaquelike calcified tumor can potentially be missed. In cases in which the sheath is enlarged but the optic nerve cannot be clearly distinguished, gadolinium enhancement can be used to increase contrast between tumor and nerve (Fig 27–31).

FIG 27–28.
Optic meningioma. This noncontrast CT scan shows a large plaquelike calcification along the lateral aspect of the more lucent optic nerve (arrow).

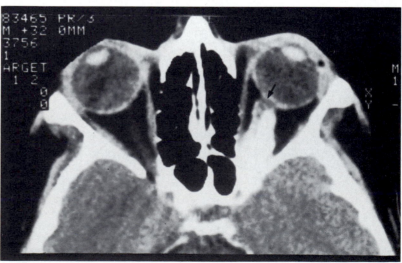

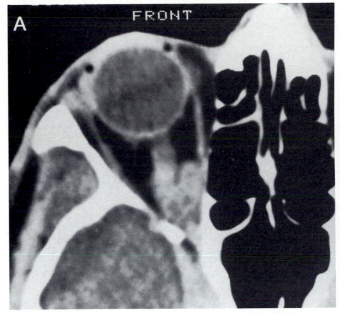
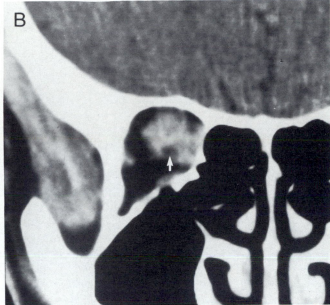

FIG 27–29.
Optic meningioma. This tumor as seen on axial **(A)** and coronal **(B)** CT scans differs from the more tubular and fusiform types described above because it demonstrates more exophytic growth away from the nerve sheath. The optic nerve *(arrow)* is still clearly distinguishable from the tumor.

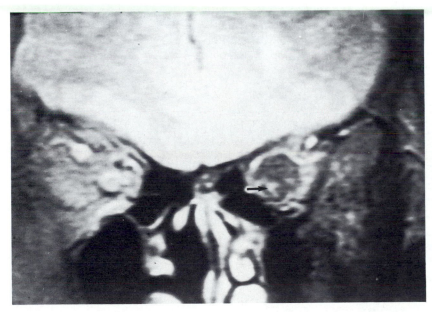

FIG 27–30.
Optic meningioma. A coronal long TR/TE MR sequence shows a fairly hypointense tumor surrounding the isointense optic nerve *(arrow)*.

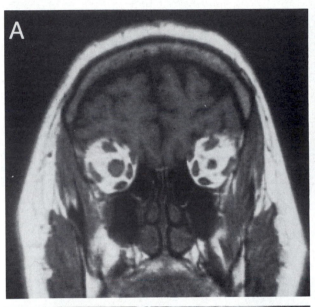

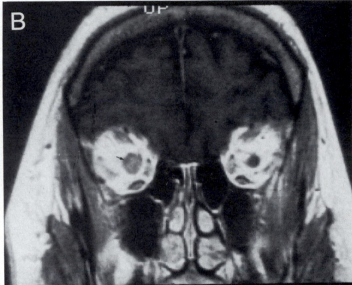

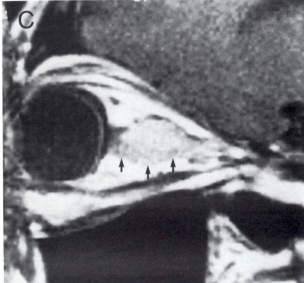

FIG 27–31.
Optic meningioma. **A,** although the enlargement of the right optic nerve sheath complex is present, the nerve cannot be distinguished from tumor because both are isointense. **B,** following gadolinium administration, intensity of the tumor increases sufficiently to be able to distinguish tumor from the less intense nerve *(arrow)*. **C,** a sagittal enhanced short TR/TE study from another patient helps distinguish isointense nerve *(arrows)* from the more intense tumor above it.

Optic Nerve Glioma

Primary optic nerve glioma usually presents in a younger age group than does meningioma and is one of the most prevalent orbital tumors in children. Diminished visual acuity and some proptosis are common clinical findings. Often seen in the context of von Recklinghausen's disease, gliomas may be bilateral.

One typical CT appearance is of smooth, fusiform widening of the optic nerve,[52, 54] which is related to a pattern of circumferential growth of tumor and/or circumferential proliferation of adjacent arachnoid.[55] The widening may be focal in early stages but slowly progresses to diffuse bulging in later stages (Fig 27–32). Occasionally, the tumor may lose its characteristic spindle shape and develop bulbous, rounded excrescences where it has stretched or penetrated the dura. Even so, the tumor remains well defined and usually uniform in density. If tumor growth is primarily longitudinal, that is, along the nerve axis, the CT image becomes one of a uniformly thickened nerve.[52] When this happens, the nerve often becomes tortuous or kinked (Fig 27–33 and 27–34).

Optic nerve glioma is usually easy to differentiate from meningiomas. In general, it has lower precontrast density than does meningioma and enhances to a lesser degree. It does not exhibit a central lucency within the tumor mass, as does meningioma, and thus is fairly homogeneous in enhancement.[52] Calcification, although more frequent in meningiomas, rarely occurs in optic gliomas and is usually conglomerate.

MRI shows the optic nerve tumor as hypointense or isointense in short TR/TE sequences and

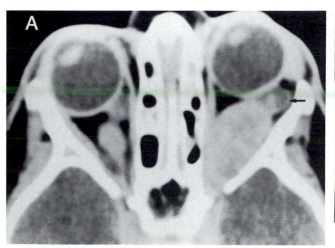

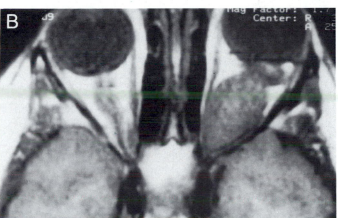

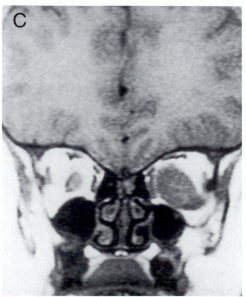

FIG 27–32.
Optic nerve glioma. **A,** axial enhanced CT shows a fusiform homogeneously enhancing tumor that fails to disclose any optic nerve-tumor density difference. The anterior aspect of the optic nerve sheath complex is kinked forward, with some distension of the perineural space *(arrow).* **B** and **C,** axial and coronal short TR/TE MRI confirms the lack of nerve-tumor discriminability due to infiltration of tumor through the nerve.

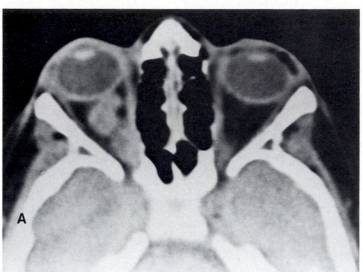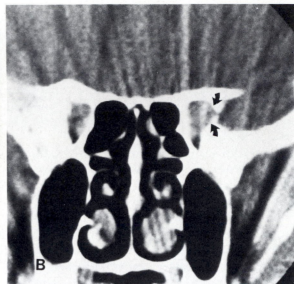

FIG 27–33.
Optic nerve glioma. There is tubular enlargement of the right optic nerve along with tortuosity and kinking. Note the absence of nerve lucency.

only slightly hyperintense in long TR/TE sequences. Again, tumor texture is usually homogeneous and not easily detected as separate from the nerve itself (see Fig 27–32).[56] Because intraorbital glioma is often associated with spread in other portions of the visual pathways, the intracanalicular and intracranial portions of the nerves, optic chiasm, and optic tracts must be evaluated with thin

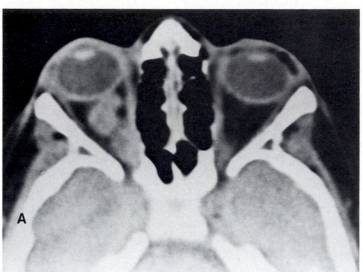

FIG 27–34.
Optic nerve glioma. An axial postgadolinium short TR/TE MR section shows a vaguely enhancing optic nerve tumor growing longitudinally down the left nerve. The nerve sheath complex is tortuous; some distinction of the perineural CSF space is present.

head-coil sections.[57, 58] Although conventional spin-echo sequences can usually survey these areas, the use of gadolinium enhancement can streamline the examination (Fig 27–35).

Other Neoplasms

Metastatic involvement of the optic nerve or nerve sheath is uncommon. It represents about 1% of all orbital and ocular metastases.[59] Breast, stomach, and lung account for most cases. Deposits occur more frequently in the nerve sheath than the nerve parenchyma.[60] For this reason, it would be more common to see a metastasis encircling the lucent nerve than expanding the nerve on scan, thus mimicking meningioma.[52]

Leukemias and lymphomas are pathologically different from metastasis in that they infiltrate the leptomeninges and the nerve together. The scan appearance then has tubular expansion of the nerve sheath complex, with homogeneous involvement of both nerve and sheath and no demonstration of separate optic nerve lucency.[52]

Schwannoma, hemangioblastoma, and choristoma can arise in the optic nerve and simulate fusiform optic glioma.[61, 62]

Papilledema

The CT appearance of the optic nerve in papilledema is one of uniformly increased nerve sheath caliber. Raised intracranial pressure pro-

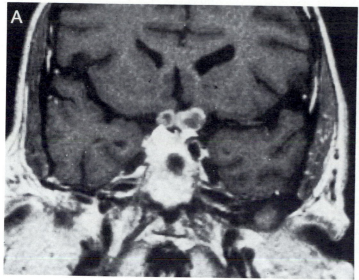
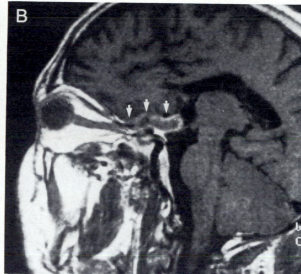

FIG 27–35.
Optic nerve glioma. The optic chiasm and intracranial optic nerves enhance with gadolinium *(arrows),* which delineates the extent of malignant glioma spread in coronal **(A)** and sagittal **(B)** MR projections.

duces optic nerve fiber swelling and vascular engorgement, which thicken the nerve itself; heightened subarachnoid space pressure distends the perineural CSF spaces as well.[63, 64] Scans cannot usually distinguish the swollen nerve from the surrounding CSF[52, 65]; however, small sections can usually define protrusion of the optic nerve head into the posterior vitreous.[64] Jinkins has shown diminished profusion within the nerve head when using dynamic contrast CT techniques, which un-derscores hemodynamic changes occurring within the nerve.[64] The normal tortuous intraorbital curve of the optic nerve becomes accentuated in papilledema.[65] Nerve sheath enlargement usually occurs bilaterally, but may be asymmetrical (Fig 27–36).

Optic Neuritis and Perineuritis

The acute inflammation of optic neuritis leads to nerve edema, cellular infiltrate, and perineural fluid collection. Together these can cause swelling

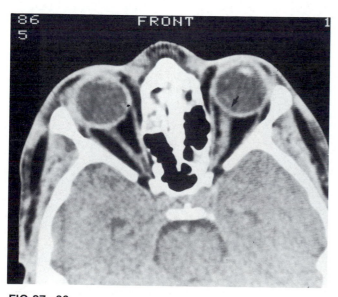

FIG 27–36.
Unilateral papilledema. The left optic nerve sheath complex is swollen without discernible nerve lucency. The papilla protrudes slightly *(arrow).*

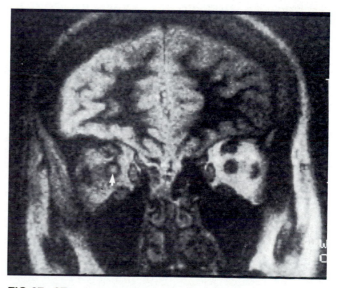

FIG 27–37.
Optic neuritis. A STIR coronal sequence shows diffuse hyperintensity of the swollen right optic nerve *(arrow).*

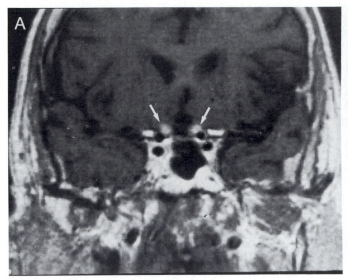

FIG 27–38.
Optic neuritis. Postgadolinium short TR/TE coronal **(A)** and sagittal **(B)** MR views show enhancement *(arrows)* of the optic nerves. No-

of the optic nerve sheath complex enough to be detected on CT scan.[66] Swelling is uniform and usually without detectable nerve vs. sheath differentiation.[52]

MRI has particular utility in patients with presumed optic neuritis. First, it can be used to survey the nerve in multiple projections. Second, because of its unique sensitivity to pathologic water, it can define changes within the nerve sheath complex with a high degree of accuracy. To effectively evaluate the intraorbital nerve, techniques that attenuate chemical shift are usually necessary. Short inversion time inversion recovery sequence (STIR) imaging has been shown to be successful in detecting optic neuritis, the pathologic nerve complex being hyperintense[67] (Fig 27–37). Because inflamed nerves enhance with intravenous (IV) contrast, gadolinium may be used to show active disease (Fig 27–38). Third, since a significant portion of patients with optic neuritis have or will develop more diffuse multiple sclerosis,[68] MRI can be used to evaluate the rest of the visual pathways and brain for involvement.[69]

Perineuritis involves inflammation of the sheath more prominently than the nerve, usually of granulomatous (sarcoid) or idiopathic (pseudotumor) cause. On CT, the expanded optic nerve sheath complex has a shaggy outline due to enhancing sheath and/or reactive changes in the contiguous orbital fat.[28, 70, 71] The optic nerve can usually be seen separate from the inflamed sheath (Fig 27–39).[52]

tice that enlargement of the nerve is only mild, as compared with more severe swelling seen with glioma (see Fig 27–34).

The Patulous Subarachnoid Space

The perioptic subarachnoid space, which communicates with the intracranial subarachnoid space, can vary in size, depending on age, CSF pressure, and the extent of communication between the two spaces.[72] Several authors have documented the passage of intrathecal contrast around the optic nerve during cisternography,[72–74] thus confirming the presence of the patulous, freely

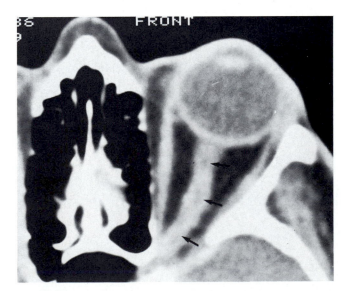

FIG 27–39.
Perineuritis. The optic nerve sheath is expanded by irregular enhancement. Vaguely seen optic nerve lucency *(arrows)* proves that the process is perineural. A slight prominence of retrobulbar fat density suggests inflammation spreading into the fat.

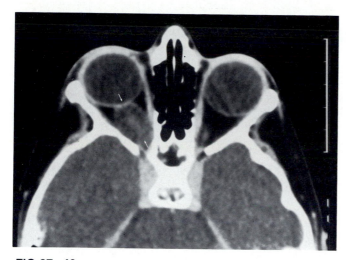

FIG 27–40.
Patulous subarachnoid space. The dura is expanded, with lucent CSF separating it from the right optic nerve *(arrows)* in a patient with neurofibromatosis.

communicating perioptic subarachnoid space in some patients. Such a communication may occur normally or as the result of optic nerve atrophy.

A dilated perioptic space can be seen in patients with neurofibromatosis without glioma (Fig 27–40). This is presumably a reflection of a dural ectasia. A variety of other lesions that compress the optic nerve also result in optic "hydrops."[75] Tumors near the apex or apical muscle enlargement from Graves' orbitopathy can block CSF flow by nerve sheath compression.[76, 77] Contiguous inflammation may cause nerve compression or "sympathetic" effusion, thus dilating the sheath.

Trauma

Direct or indirect mechanical trauma of the optic nerve can produce nerve swelling or hematoma within the nerve sheath. Both of these then produce widening of the nerve sheath complex on CT scan. Occasionally, acute blood within the sheath can be identified as a hyperdensity outlining the lucent optic nerve.[52]

REFERENCES

1. Gyldensted C, Lester J, Fledelius H: Computed tomography of orbital lesions—a radiological study of 144 cases. *Neuroradiology* 1977; 13:141–150.
2. Forbes GS, Sheedy PF, Waller RR: Orbital tumors evaluated by computed tomography. *Radiology* 1980; 136:101–111.
3. Knochel J, Osborne AG, Wing DS: Differential diagnosis of lateral orbital masses. *J Comput Tomogr* 1981; 5:11–15.
4. Hawkes RC, Holland GN, Moore WS, et al: NMR imaging in the evaluation of orbital tumors. *AJNR* 1983; 4:254–256.
5. Han JS, Benson JE, Bonstelle CT, et al: Magnetic resonance imaging of the orbit: A preliminary experience. *Radiology* 1984; 150:755–759.
6. Li KC, Poon PY, Hinton P, et al: MR imaging of orbital tumors with CT and ultrasound correlations. *J Comput Assist Tomogr* 1984; 8:1039–1047.
7. Henderson JW: *Orbital Tumors.* New York, Brian C Decker, 1980, pp 128–133.
8. Davis KR, Hesselink JR, Dallow RL, et al: CT and ultrasound in the diagnosis of cavernous hemangioma and lymphangioma of the orbit. *J Comput Tomogr* 1980; 4:98–104.
9. Forbes GS, Earnest F, Waller RR: Computed tomography of orbital tumors, including late-generation scanning techniques. *Radiology* 1982; 142:387–394.
10. Lloyd GAS: CT scanning in the diagnosis of orbital disease. *Comput Tomogr* 1979; 3:227–239.
11. Mafee MF, Putterman A, Valvassori GE, et al: Orbital space-occupying lesions. Role of computed tomography and magnetic resonance imaging. An analysis of 145 cases: *Radiol Clin North Am* 1987; 25:529–559.
12. Fries PD, Char DH, Norman D: MR imaging of orbital cavernous hemangioma. *J Comput Assist Tomogr* 1987; 11:418–421.
13. Henderson JW: *Orbital Tumors.* New York, Brian C Decker, 1980, pp 136–143.
14. Henderson JW: *Orbital Tumors.* New York, Brian C Decker, 1980, pp 261–279.
15. Cohen LM, Schwartz AM, Rockoff SD: Benign schwannomas: Pathologic basis for CT inhomogeneities. *AJR* 1986; 147:141–143.
16. Blei L, Chambers J, Liotta L, et al: Orbital dermoid diagnosed by computed tomographic scanning. *Am J Ophthalmol* 1978; 85:58–61.
17. Hesselink JR, Davis KR, Dallow RL, et al: Computed tomography of masses in the lacrimal gland region. *Radiology* 1979; 131:143–147.
18. Nugent RA, Lapointe JS, Rootman J, et al: Orbital dermoids: Features on CT. *Radiology* 1987; 165:475–478.
19. Jacobs L, Weisberg L, Kinkel W: *Computerized Tomography of the Orbit and Sella Turcica.* New York, Raven Press, 1980, p 105.
20. Lloyd GAS: Vascular anomalies in the orbit: CT and angiographic diagnosis. *Orbit* 1982; 1:45–54.
21. Henderson JW: *Orbital Tumors.* New York, Brian C Decker, 1980, pp 512–526.
22. Jakobiec FA, Font RL. Orbit, in Spencer WH (ed): *Ophthalmic Pathology.* Philadelphia, WB Saunders Co, 1986, pp 2663–2812.
23. Harr DL, Quencer RM, Abrams CW: Computed to-

mography and ultrasound in the evaluation of orbital infection and pseudotumor. *Radiology* 1982; 142:395–401.
24. Wilner HI, Gupta KL, Kelly JK: Orbital pseudotumor: Association of orbital vein deformities and myositis. *AJNR* 1980; 1:305–309.
25. Enzmann DR, Donaldson SS, Marshall WH, et al: Computed tomography in orbital pseudotumor (idiopathic orbital inflammation). *Radiology* 1976; 120:597–601.
26. Bernardino ME, Zimmerman RD, Citrin CM, et al: Scleral thickening: A CT sign of orbital pseudotumor. *AJR* 1977; 129:703–706.
27. Nugent RA, Rootman J, Robertson WD, et al: Acute orbital pseudotumors: Classification and CT features. *AJNR* 1981; 2:431–436.
28. Curtin HD: Pseudotumor. *Radiol Clin North Am* 1987; 25:583–599.
29. Noble SC, Chandler WF, Lloyd RV: Intracranial extension of orbital pseudotumor: A case report. *Neurosurgery* 1986; 18:798–801.
30. Kaye AH, Hahn JF, Craciun A, et al: Intracranial extension of inflammatory pseudotumor of the orbit. Case Report. *J Neurosurg* 1984; 60:625–629.
31. Atlas SW, Grossman RI, Savino PJ, et al: Surface-coil MR of orbital pseudotumor. *AJNR* 1987; 8:141–146.
32. Bilaniuk LT, Atlas SW, Zimmerman RA: Magnetic resonance imaging of the orbit. *Radiol Clin North Am* 1987; 25:509–528.
33. Jakobiec FA, Jones IS: Lymphomatous, plasmacytic, histiocytic, and hematopoietic tumors, in Jones IS, Jakobiec FA (eds): *Diseases of the Orbit.* Hagerstown, Md, Harper & Row Publishers, Inc, 1979, pp 309–315.
34. Char DH, Sobel D, Kelly WM, et al: Magnetic resonance scanning in orbital tumor diagnosis. *Ophthalmology* 1985; 92:1305–1310.
35. Edwards JH, Hyman RA, Vicirca SJ, et al: O.G.T. magnetic resonance imaging of the orbit. *AJNR* 1985; 6:253–258.
36. Sullivan JA, Harms SE: Surface-coil MR imaging of orbital neoplasms. *AJNR* 1986; 7:29–34.
37. Flanders AE, Espinsoa GA, Markiewicz DA, et al: Orbital lymphoma. Role of CT and MRI. *Radiol Clin North Am* 1987; 25:601–613.
38. Peyster RG, Shapiro MD, Haik BG: Orbital metastasis: Role of magnetic resonance imaging and computed tomography. *Radiol Clin North Am* 1987; 25:647–662.
39. Jakobiec FA, Jones IS: Vascular tumors, malformations, and degenerations, in Duane TD (ed): *Clinical Opthalmology,* vol 2. Philadelphia, Harper & Row Publishers, Inc, 1981, pp 1–6.
40. Henderson JW: *Orbital Tumors.* New York, Brian C Decker, 1980, pp 147–152.
41. Haynes BF, Fishman ML, Fauci AS, et al: The ocular manifestations of Wegener's granulomatosis: Fif-

teen years' experience and review of the literature. *Am J Med* 1977; 63:131–141.
42. Vermess M, Haynes BF, Fauci AS, et al: Computer assisted tomography of orbital lesions in Wegener's granulomatosis. *J Comput Assist Tomogr* 1978; 2:45–48.
43. Braffman BH, Bilaniuk LT, Eagle RC, et al: MR imaging of a carcinoid tumor metastatic to the orbit. *J Comput Assist Tomogr* 1987; 11:891–894.
44. Price HI, Danzinger A, Wainwright HC, et al: CT of orbital multiple myeloma. *AJNR* 1980; 1:573–575.
45. Ambrose JAE, Lloyd GAS, Wright JE: A preliminary evaluation of fine matrix computerized axial tomography (EMI scan) in the diagnosis of orbital space-occupying lesions. *Br J Radiol* 1974; 47:747–751.
46. Merrick R, Latchaw RE, Gold LHA: Computerized tomography of the orbit in carotid-cavernous sinus fistula. *Comput Tomogr* 1979; 4:127–132.
47. Jakobiec FA, Jones IS: Vascular tumor, malformations and degenerations, in Duane TD (ed): *Clinical Ophthalmology,* vol 2. Philadelphia, Harper & Row Publishers, Inc, 1981, pp 15–18.
48. Winter J, Centeno RS, Bentson JR: Maneuver to aid diagnosis of orbital varix by computed tomography. *AJNR* 1982; 3:39–40.
49. Zimmerman RA, Bilaniuk LT, Metzger RA, et al: Computed tomography of orbital facial neurofibromatosis. *Radiology* 1983; 146:113–116.
50. Reed D, Robertson WD, Rootman J, et al: Plexiform neurofibromatosis of the orbit: CT evaluation. *AJNR* 1986; 7:259–263.
51. Wright JE: Primary optic nerve meningioma: Clinical presentation and management. *Trans Am Acad Ophthalmol Otolaryngol* 1977; 83:617–625.
52. Rothfus WE, Curtin HD, Slamovits TL, et al: Optic nerve/sheath enlargement. A differential approach based on high-resolution CT morphology. *Radiology* 1984; 150:409–415.
53. Daniels DL, Williams AL, Syvertsen A, et al: CT recognition of optic nerve sheath meningioma: Abnormal sheath visualization. *AJNR* 1982; 3:181–183.
54. Byrd SE, Harwood-Nash DC, Fitz CR, et al: Computed tomography of intraorbital optic nerve gliomas in children. *Radiology* 1978; 129:73–78.
55. Hogan MJ, Zimmerman LE: *Ophthalmic Pathology: An Atlas and Textbook,* ed 2. Philadelphia, WB Saunders Co, 1962, pp 617–619.
56. Haik BG, Saint Louis L, Bierly J, et al: Magnetic resonance imaging in the evaluation of optic nerve gliomas. *Ophthalmology* 1987; 94:709–717.
57. Pomeranz SJ, Shelton JJ, Tobias J, et al: MR of visual pathways in patients with neurofibromatosis. *AJNR* 1987; 8:831–836.
58. Brown EW, Riccardi VM, Mawad M, et al: MR imaging of optic pathways in patients with neurofibromatosis. *AJNR* 1987; 8:1031–1036.

59. Ferry AP, Font RL: Carcinoma metastatic to the eye and orbit: I. A clinicopathologic study of 227 cases. *Arch Ophthalmol* 1974; 92:276–286.

60. Eggers H, Jakobiec FA, Jones IS: Optic nerve gliomas, in Duane TD (ed): *Clinical Ophthalmology,* vol 2. Philadelphia, Harper & Row Publishers, Inc, 1981, pp 1–14.

61. Azar-Kia B, Naheedy MH, Elias DA, et al: Optic nerve tumors: Role of magnetic resonance imaging and computed tomography. *Radiol Clin North Am* 1987; 25:561–581.

62. Lauten GJ, Eatherly JB, Ramirez A: Hemangioblastoma of the optic nerve: Radiologic and pathologic features. *AJNR* 1981; 2:96–99.

63. Hayreh SS: Pathogenesis of edema of the optic disc. *Doc Ophthalmol* 1968; 24:298–411.

64. Jinkins JR: "Papilledema": Neuroradiologic evaluation of optic disk protrusion with dynamic orbital CT. *AJNR* 1987; 8:681–690.

65. Cabanis EA, Salvolini U, Rodallec A, et al: Computed tomography of the optic nerve: II. Size and shape modifications in papilledema. *J Comput Assist Tomogr* 1978; 2:150–155.

66. Howard CW, Osher RH, Tomsok RL: Computed tomographic features in optic neuritis. *Am J Opthalmol* 1980; 89:699–702.

67. Miller DH, Newton MR, van der Poel JC, et al: Magnetic resonance imaging of the optic nerve in optic neuritis. *Neurology* 1988; 38:175–179.

68. Rizzo JF, Lessell S: Risk of developing multiple sclerosis after uncomplicated optic neuritis: A long term prospective study. *Neurology* 1988; 38:185–190.

69. Rosenblatt MA, Behrens MM, Zweifach PH, et al: Magnetic resonance imaging of optic tract involvement in multiple sclerosis. *Am J Ophthalmol* 1987; 104:74–79.

70. Som PN, Sacher M, Weitzner I, et al: Sarcoidosis of the optic nerve. *J Comput Assist Tomogr* 1982; 6:614–616.

71. Krochel GB, Charles H, Smith RS: Granulomatous optic neuropathy. *Arch Ophthalmol* 1981; 99:1053–1055.

72. Chambers EF, Manelfe C, Cellerier P: Metrizamide CT cisternography and perioptic subarachnoid space imaging. *J Comput Assist Tomogr* 1981; 5:875–880.

73. Fox AJ: Intrathecal metrizamide enhancement of the optic nerve sheath. *J Comput Assist Tomogr* 1979; 3:653–656.

74. Manelfe C, Pasquini U, Bank WO: Metrizamide demonstration of the subarachnoid space surrounding the optic nerves. *J Comput Assist Tomogr* 1978; 2:545–547.

75. Jinkins JR: Optic hydrops: Isolated nerve sheath dilatation demonstrated by CT. *AJNR* 1987; 8:867–870.

76. Healy JR, Rosenkrantz H: Enlargement of the optic nerve sheath complex in thyroid ophthalmopathy. *J Comput Tomogr* 1981; 5:8–10.

77. Kennerdell JS, Rosenbaum AE, El-Hoshy MH: Apical optic nerve compression of dysthyroid optic neuropathy on computed tomography. *Arch Ophthalmol* 1981; 99:807–809.

28

Differential Problems in Orbital Diagnosis

William E. Rothfus, M.D.

EXTRAOCULAR MUSCLE ENLARGEMENT

Although it is now possible to make volumetric computed tomographic (CT) measurements of the extraocular muscles to determine whether they are larger than normal limits,[1] it is often more practical to determine enlargement empirically. Close scrutiny of the muscles in more than one projection is necessary, as is comparison with the opposite side. Muscle shape, size, and pattern of muscle involvement are critical clues in narrowing the differential diagnosis of extraocular muscle enlargement; so too are changes in orbital fat, the bony walls, the globe, or the superior ophthalmic vein.[2, 3]

Graves' Disease

Muscular involvement in Graves' disease (thyrotoxic or euthyroid) can be unilateral or bilateral, symmetrical or asymmetrical, singular or multiple, subtle or marked. However bilateral, symmetrical thickening of multiple muscles is most frequent.[4] Single muscle involvement is relatively unusual.[3] The inferior and medial rectus muscles are most commonly involved.[5, 6]

Pathologically, the muscles are infiltrated with mucopolysaccharides, edema, fluid, and round cells from a diffuse inflammatory reaction.[7] As expected, enhancement of the affected muscle is commonly seen on CT scanning.[8] Characteristically, the enhancement is uniform. The muscle attains a fusiform shape as the muscle belly enlarges; the tendon sheaths are usually spared[2, 9] (Fig 28–1). The midportion of the muscle belly usually enlarges most, but in some instances, there is preferential enlargement of the posterior muscle. The latter type is often associated with apical compressive syndromes. In general, there is a correlation between the clinical severity of disease and the extent of muscle involvement.[10]

Graves' disease is a diffuse disease of the orbital contents. As such, muscle swelling is usually accompanied by alterations in other structures of the orbit. Orbital fat, for instance, may increase in volume and cause proptosis of the globe and prolapse of the orbital fat anteriorly (Figs 28–1 and 28–2).[2, 3, 5, 9, 11] In addition, the character of the fat may change and show a finely reticulated, "dirty-fat" appearance, presumably reflecting venous congestion and/or thickened soft-tissue septations (Fig 28–3). Interestingly, these findings can occur in the absence of muscle thickening. The globe, besides being displaced forward, may rarely show episcleral enhancement at the point of attachment of an inflamed muscle tendon. When multiple muscles are enlarged, especially at the orbital apex, the optic nerve can become swollen, either from associated inflammatory change or compression.[12, 13] Optic neuropathy, which occurs in about 5% of Graves' disease patients is usually caused by compression at the apex. However, optic nerve enlargement is not an invariable accompaniment.[14]

The lacrimal glands and eyelids can also become swollen and displaced in severe disease (see Fig 28–2). Orbital wall remodeling results from chronic direct pressure and hyperemia.[15] Superior ophthalmic vein engorgement from vascular compression at the orbital apex may be apparent on scanning (Fig 28–4). The combination of muscle thickening and superior ophthalmic vein enlargement may therefore mimic a carotid-cavernous sinus fistula.[2]

Despite the presence of inflammatory cells and mucopolysaccharides, the muscles in chronic

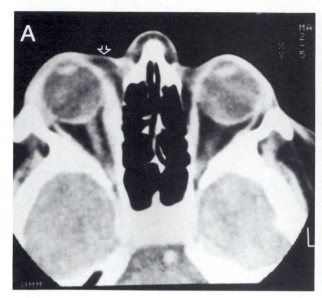 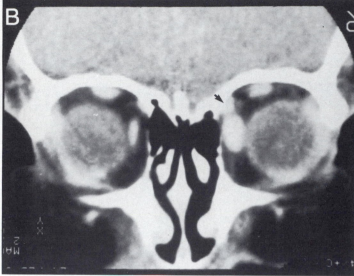

FIG 28–1.
Graves' disease. Axial **(A)** and coronal **(B)** contrast CT examination shows fusiform enlargement of the uniformly enhancing right medial rectus. The anterior muscle tapers to a fairly normal sheath. The orbital septum is prolapsed near the involved muscle *(open arrow)*. Note the enlargement of the contiguous superior oblique in **(B)** *(black arrow)*.

Graves' disease may not show marked intensity changes on magnetic resonance imaging (MRI). The muscles tend to take on a fairly hypointensive appearance that may relate to chronic fibrotic changes (Fig 28–5). However, active muscle inflammation can be identified in selected cases by hyperintensity on long repetition time/echo time (TR/TE) spin-echo sequences (Fig 28–6). In long-standing disease, focal fatty infiltration of the muscle may occur[16]; thus, muscle intensity on short TR/TE sequences would be expected to increase focally. Because MRI can effectively depict septations within orbital fat, these can be seen to be thickened in Graves' orbitopathy. Secondary changes in the fat volume, lacrimal glands, etc., can also be depicted.

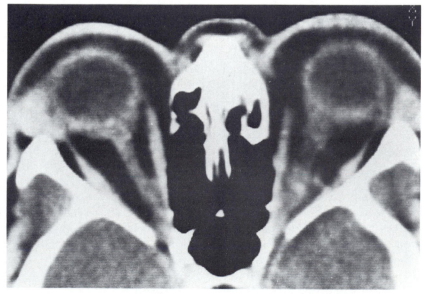

FIG 28–2.
Graves' disease. Marked exophthalmos is accompanied by eyelid swelling and pronounced enhancement of the lacrimal glands.

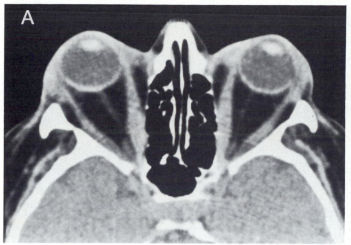

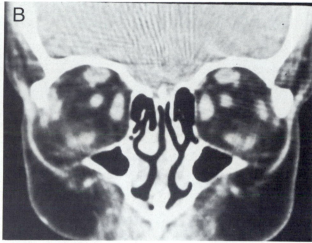

FIG 28–3.
Graves' disease. Bilateral symmetrical multiple muscle enlargement is associated with marked proptosis and orbital septal pro-

lapse **(A).** Thickened fine septations are faintly visible as a reticulated density within the orbital fat **(B).**

Myositic Pseudotumor

In many ways, the CT appearance of the pseudotumor myositis mimics that in Graves' orbitopathy. In fact, clinically and radiographically it may be difficult to distinguish them. Because it too originates from reactive inflammation, muscle swelling and myositis is fusiform[17] and accompanied by uniform enhancement. The inflammatory response usually also involves the contiguous muscle tendon and sclera (Fig 28–7).[2, 9, 18] Although

myositis has been reported to have an irregular muscle contour,[3] this has not been a reliable indicator. There may be increased density in the orbital fat contiguous to the involved muscle due "spillover" of the inflammatory process[5] (Fig 28–8). This gives the muscle contour a less distinct edge, as opposed to Graves' orbitopathy, which has a very sharp edge. The pattern of muscle swelling varies in the two diseases. While solitary muscle swelling is uncommon in thyroid disease (except for inferior rectus involvement), it is

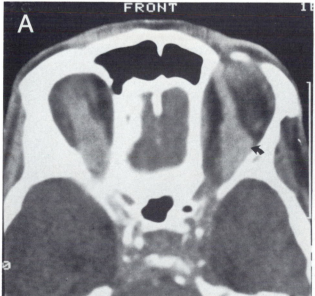

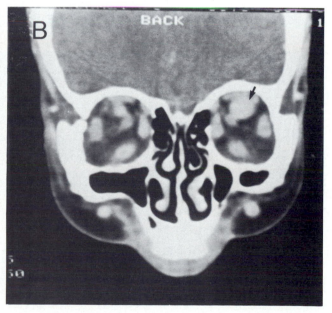

FIG 28–4.
Graves' disease. Axial **(A)** and coronal **(B)** unenhanced CT study shows multiple bilateral muscle enlargement is present, more

marked on the left. The superior ophthalmic vein is distended and forms a large varicosity *(arrows).*

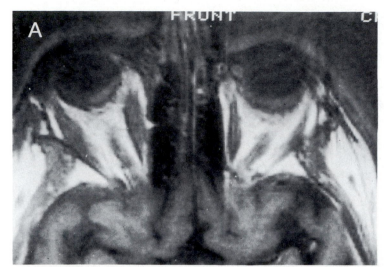

FIG 28—5.
Graves' disease. Axial **(A)** and coronal **(B)** short
TR/TE and axial long TR/TE sequences **(C).** Although
there is more significant muscle enlargement on the
right, a reticular increase in fat intensity is noticeable
bilaterally. The muscles are isointense to
hypointense throughout.

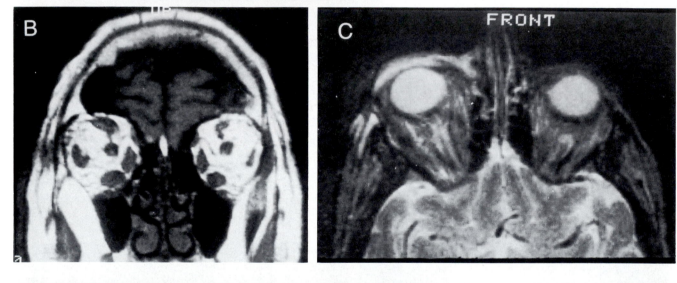

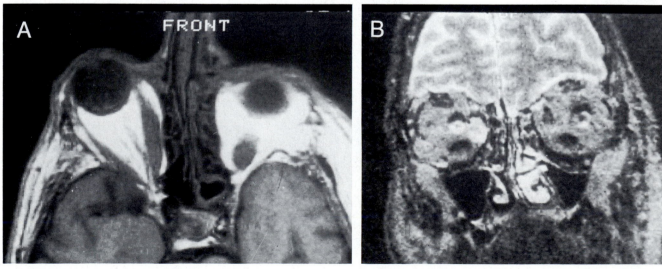

FIG 28—6.
Graves' disease. Axial short TR/TE **(A)** and coronal long TR/TE **(B)**
sequences show marked enlargement of the right medial rectus.

The muscle is hyperintense on long TR/TE sequences; this reflects
acute inflammation, which correlated with dysmotility.

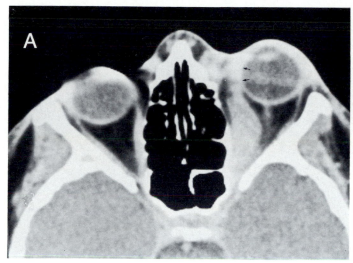
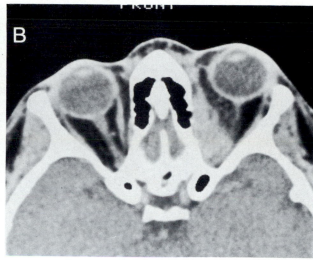

FIG 28–7.

A and **B,** myositic pseudotumor. The left medial rectus is markedly enlarged and enhances homogeneously. There is involvement of the muscle tendon and subjacent globe wall *(arrows)*. Note the reticulated density of inflammation in the contiguous orbital fat.

said to be the rule in pseudotumor myositis.[3] Isolated lateral rectus involvement is rare in Graves' disease[5] and much more common in myositis. Pseudotumor is not usually associated with fat bulging the orbital septum or with an increase in orbital fat volume.[2, 3] Unfortunately, exceptions do exist, and pseudotumor may present with multiple muscle enlargement and proptosis (Fig 28–8). In these cases, clinical information and response to steroids may provide the key to differential diagnosis.[19, 20]

Most MRI descriptions of myositic pseudotumor illustrate the pseudotumor to be hypointense to fat and isointense to muscle on short TR/TE sequences and isointense to muscle and fat on long TR/TE sequences.[21, 22] This appearance probably reflects a fibrotic response present in subacute or chronic cases.[5] Identical findings are seen in infectious myositis, sarcoid, and metastatic (fibroblastic) carcinoid.[21, 23] Less commonly, there is hyperintensity on long TR/TE sequences,[21] probably from a more acute inflammatory response.

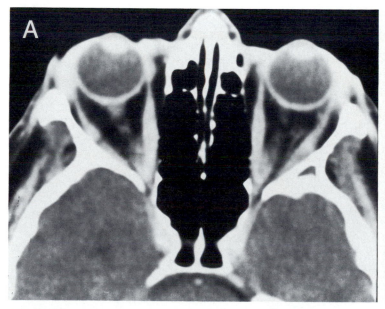
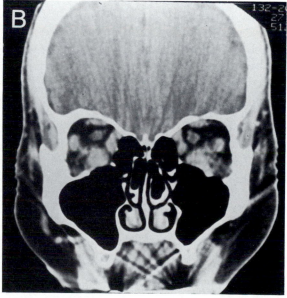

FIG 28–8.

A and **B,** myositic pseudotumor. Multiple bilateral muscle enlargement. The inferior recti are most markedly enlarged. The fat surrounding these muscles has reticulated density from spreading inflammation **(B).**

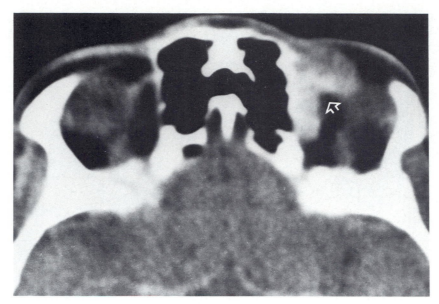

FIG 28–9.
Rhabdomyosarcoma. The superior oblique muscle is diffusely enlarged by homogeneously enhancing tumor. Note the bend in the tumor at the site of the trochlea *(arrow).*

Acromegaly

Diffuse extraocular muscle enlargement can occur in acromegaly.[24, 25] The findings mimic those of Graves' disease, but proptosis is not a prominent feature. The degree of muscle enlargement is usually moderate and shows no direct correlation with growth hormone levels.[2, 26]

Primary and Secondary Neoplasm

The enlargement of a rectus muscle that results from tumor can be from direct extension of neoplasm within or around the muscle or from venous outflow compression.[2, 3] Primary muscle tumors, i.e., rhabdomyosarcoma, which occur most commonly in children,[27] directly infiltrate the muscle and form a local or diffuse, usually enhancing mass (Fig 28–9).[28, 29] With further growth, the aggressive nature of the tumor is demonstrated by contiguous bone destruction and progressive orbital extension.

Orbital lymphoma may affect one or more muscles and be indistinguishable from Graves' disease or pseudotumor. Involvement of the superior rectus-levator complex is characteristic (Fig 28–10).[30] Secondary neoplasms can deposit and grow within an extraocular muscle,[2, 9, 31] thus causing the muscle to segmentally enlarge. Usually the focus of growth has a local irregular margin. Contiguous involvement of a muscle by tumor from an orbital wall, paranasal sinus, or orbital foramen is more common. Tumor at the orbital apex or cavernous sinus may obstruct venous outflow and cause passive congestion of the muscles with concomitant mild ipsilateral enlargement. Whatever the cause of secondary involvement, tumor is usually evident as a area of homogeneous or heterogeneous enhancement on CT. Characteristically on MRI, metastasis is isointense or hypointense on short TR/

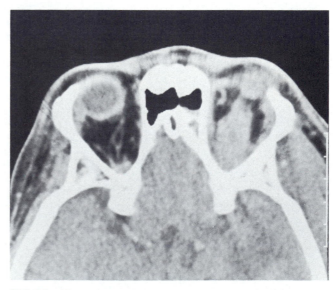

FIG 28–10.
Lymphoma. The superior rectus-levator complex is enlarged and has a slightly lobulated periphery.

TE and hyperintense on long TR/TE sequences.[31] Thus metastasis may be distinguished from the usual presentation of thyroid orbitopathy or pseudotumor.

Arteriovenous Malformations and Fistulas

Arteriovenous malformations (AVMs) and fistulas involving the cavernous sinus produce fairly uniform enlargement of the rectus muscle or muscles. The muscle swelling seems to be the result of increased venous pressure, supported by the commonly associated finding of a dilated superior ophthalmic vein (Fig 28–11).[2, 3, 32] In fact, this latter finding is important in distinguishing the AVM-fistula category of muscle swelling from thyroid and pseudotumor swelling, which also cause uniform diffuse muscle thickening and proptosis, but less commonly cause superior ophthalmic vein enlargement. Superior ophthalmic vein dilatation is not pathognomonic of arteriovenous shunting, but may occur in any disease (Graves' orbitopathy, apical tumor) in which apical compression is significant. Shunt-based muscle enlargement does not characteristically have the fat prolapse so frequently seen in Graves' orbitopathy.[2, 3] Rarely, an AVM growing within the orbit may insinuate itself within an extraocular muscle. In this case, the serpiginous AVM can be distinguished by serpiginous enhancement on contrast CT or by flow void on MRI (see Fig 27–22).

Other Orbital Inflammations

Although not emphasized in the literature, swelling of an extraocular muscle may occur from contiguous orbital or sinus infection. Ordinarily muscle thickening is just one of a constellation of scan findings related to an orbital abscess or cellulitis (see Chapter 26). In this context, moderate uniform swelling and enhancement arise from cellular infiltrate, edema, and hyperemia (see Fig 26–13).

THE ENLARGED SUPERIOR OPHTHALMIC VEIN

As previously discussed, the normal superior opthalmic vein is frequently seen on all good-quality CT scans of the orbit.[33] The vein has a tortuous course and increases in width from anterior to posterior. Measurements of the normal vein have been made with CT and give a diameter of 2.0 mm anteriorly and 3.5 mm posteriorly.[34] The superior ophthalmic vein can be enlarged in a number of pathologic processes. Basically, however, there are two main etiologic categories for the dilatation—increased flow through the vein or congestion of venous outflow.

Those lesions with increased flow include carotid-cavernous sinus fistulas, AVMs, and highly vascular tumors.[34, 35] A carotid-cavernous sinus fistula is suggested on scans by associated findings of proptosis, extraocular muscle enlargement, and di-

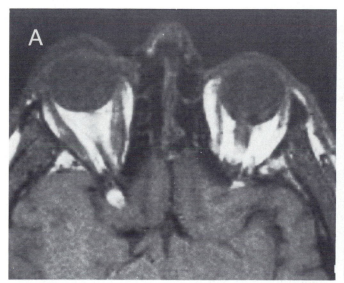 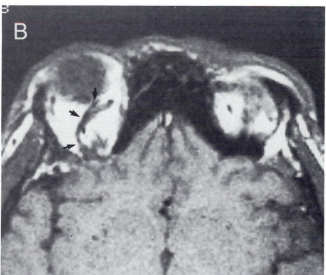

FIG 28–11.
Carotid-cavernous sinus fistula. **A,** there is fairly uniform enlargement of the right extraocular muscles. Proptosis is mild. **B,** the superior ophthalmic vein is distended *(arrows)* due to the high-flow state.

latation of the ipsilateral cavernous sinus.[32] Clinically, chemosis and engorged conjunctival vessels are seen, and a bruit may be heard (see Fig 28–11). While intraorbital AVMs might clinically simulate carotid-cavernous sinus fistulas, the scan appearance of regular serpiginous enhancing or flow void structures would distinguish them. A vascular tumor large enough to cause significant shunting through the superior ophthalmic vein would be readily apparent on a scan, which makes the differential diagnosis simple.

The lesions causing venous congestion may be compressive or destructive. The most common area of venous compression is at the orbital apex where orbital structures are most confined and in closest proximity. Apical tumors and enlarged muscles at the annulus of Zinn, such as are present in Graves' disease, may extrinsically compress the superior ophthalmic vein enough to cause venous congestion (see Fig 28–4); so too, an obstructed or compressed cavernous sinus may rarely result in venous congestion that dilates the vein.[34] High-resolution scans can, in most instances, separate apical tumor from apical muscle thickening. This is especially easy when there is supportive evidence of Graves' orbitopathy or myositic pseudotumor on the scan (see the preceding section extraocular muscle enlargement). Superior ophthalmic vein enlargement can rarely occur in the setting of Graves' disease without apical compression; the etiology is obscure.

Superior ophthalmic vein enlargement from a fistula or compression may result in thrombosis of the vein. By CT, it is difficult to distinguish a thrombosed vein because of its inherently high density. MRI may be able to demonstrate a loss of signal flow void in the vein. Care must be taken in interpreting hyperintensity in the vein, however, to ensure that it is not due to chemical shift artifact or flow-related phenomena like diastolic pseudo-gating. The use of phase-dependent spectroscopic imaging or gradient echo imaging may be necessary to confidently diagnose thrombosis.[36]

LACRIMAL GLAND ENLARGEMENT

Masses of the lacrimal gland are largely confined to the superolateral aspect of the anterior portion of the orbit. The lacrimal gland fossa, bounded by the orbital septum anteriorly, the globe and levator palpebrae medially, the perior-

bital surface of the frontal bone laterally, and extraconal fat posteriorly, provides a significant restrictive barrier to other than the most aggressive disease processes. Easily palpated, these masses displace the globe medially and inferiorly. Lacrimal globe tumors are the most common primary extraconal tumors.

Unilateral Enlargement

Tumors constitute about half of lacrimal gland masses. Benign (pleomorphic or mixed) types tend to remain localized to the fossa, although they may enlarge the bony walls of the fossa.[37] Well defined, these tumors variably enhance.[38] Since they usually originate in the posterior (orbital lobe) portion of the gland, growth is posterior into the extraconal space. The posterior aspect of the tumor is well defined and rounded. Tumors often indent the subjacent globe wall (Fig 28–12). Malignant tumors (primary and metastatic) show no consistent enhancement pattern. When small, they are usually confined, but with growth they may invade the orbital wall or irregularly extend posteriorly, encase the lateral rectus, and displace the optic nerve.[38]

Lymphoid tumors and inflammatory conditions, like acute or chronic dacryoadenitis and pseudotumor, may radiographically mimic the appearance of tumor. These masses affect the entire gland. They have less well defined margins but have a fairly homogeneous appearance on CT or MRI (Figs 28–13 and 28–14). Occasionally more rimlike enhancement can be seen in chronic dacryoadenitis. As opposed to tumors that indent the globe, lymphoid and inflammatory lesions tend to mold around the globe.[5, 39, 40] They do not cause bony erosion.

Dermoid cyst is the only lacrimal gland mass that has an unequivocal CT and MRI appearance—a well-defined oval wall and cystic interior of low absorption on CT and hyperintensity on short TR/TE MRI, and smooth erosion or a sinus tract of the contiguous bony wall (Fig 28–15).[38, 41] A fluid level is sometimes seen in the cyst.[42] Although scalloped erosion of the orbital wall is typical, other slow-growing masses of the gland can cause a similar appearance (Fig 28–16).

Bilateral Enlargement

Bilateral lacrimal gland enlargement may be a manifestation of sarcoidosis, Mikulicz's syndrome,

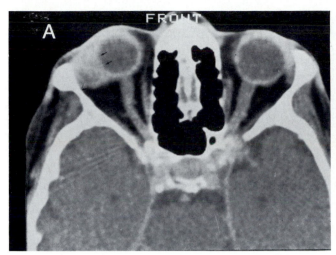

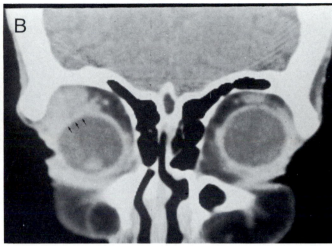

FIG 28–12.
Lacrimal gland, mixed pleomorphic adenoma. **A** and **B**, a slightly heterogeneously enhancing tumor displaces the right globe medially and inferiorly. Note the flattening of the globe wall *(arrows)*.

Sjögren's syndrome, Graves' disease, myxedema, amyloidosis, blood dyscrasias, and occasionally pseudotumor and lymphoid hyperplasia.[40, 43] Because most of these are composed of a round cell infiltrate with accompanying chronic inflammatory changes, the CT appearance of these numerous entities is similar; that is, well-defined, homogeneous enlargement of both glands (Figs 28–17 to 28–19). Mikulicz's syndrome and Sjögren's syndrome may show prominent enhancement.[38]

There is a paucity of MRI description related to the lacrimal gland. Typical dermoids would be expected to be hyperintense on short TR/TE and hypointense on long TR/TE sequences if the cholesterol content is high enough. Epithelial tumors should show some hyperintensity on long TR/TE sequences.[40] Subacute or chronic inflammatory conditions would be expected to be relatively hypointense on short and long TR/TE sequences (Fig 28–19). Until a large series of lacrimal gland masses is evaluated with MRI, it is uncertain whether that modality can further improve the differential diagnosis.

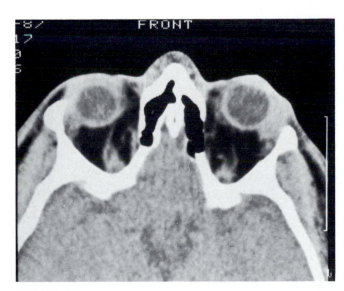

FIG 28–13.
Lacrimal gland, benign lymphoepithelial tumor. The left lacrimal gland is enlarged; irregular spread of tumor causes a spiculated density behind the gland.

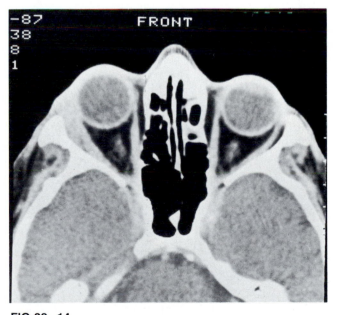

FIG 28–14.
Right lacrimal gland lymphoma. A homogeneous tumor is spreading posteriorly, filling much of the extraconal space.

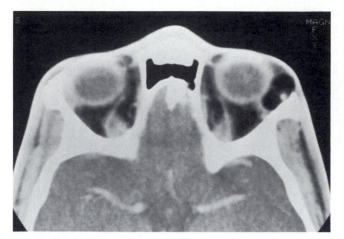

FIG 28–15.
Lacrimal gland dermoid. The left gland is replaced by encapsulated tumor with a typical interior fat-density.

MASSES OF THE POSTERIOR ASPECT OF THE GLOBE

Although CT and MRI are useful in demonstrating a variety of ocular disease processes,[44, 45] funduscopic examination and ultrasound are the initial methods of examination. Even with the current high resolution, scans often cannot reach the level of sensitivity of ultrasound regarding detail of

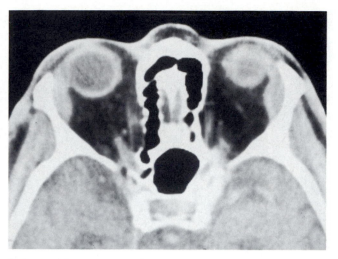

FIG 28–17.
Lacrimal gland lymphoma. Both lacrimal glands are enlarged and enhance homogeneously. Unilateral involvement is more typical of lymphoma.

the chambers, lens, and globe wall or give the same level of tissue characterization of masses in the globe.

One of the primary uses for scanning in ocular diseases is delineating masses of the posterior globe walls, specifically in determining the presence and extent of extraocular spread. Direct evaluation of the globe may be hindered by leukokoria (white ocular light reflex) or by the presence of hemorrhage. Such an evaluation is especially crucial for neoplasms because it largely determines the subsequent course of management. Ultrasound

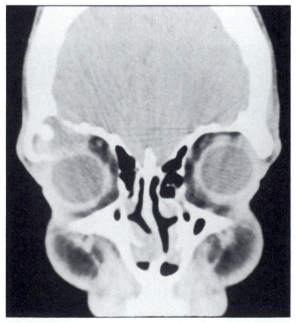

FIG 28–16.
Lacrimal gland epidermoid. The enlarged right lacrimal gland causes a scalloped erosion of the orbital wall that simulates dermoid changes.

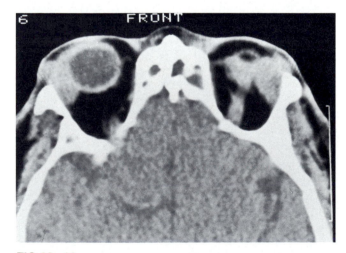

FIG 28–18.
Lacrimal gland Wegener's granulomatosis. The bilateral enlargement is typical of systemic disease; it is indistinguishable from enlargement seen in other conditions like sarcoidosis and Sjögren's syndrome.

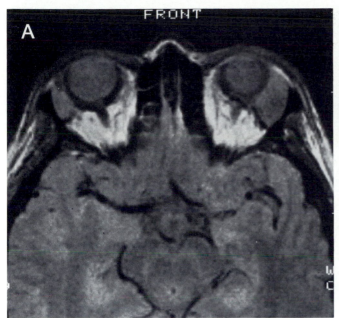 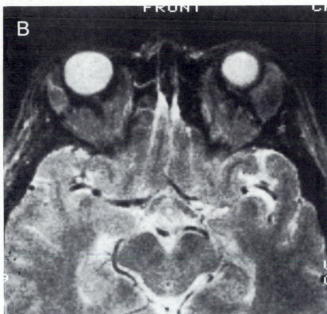

FIG 28–19.
Lacrimal gland pseudotumor. Short TR/TE **(A)** and long TR/TE **(B)** MR axial images show bilateral asymmetrical lacrimal gland en-largement. The glands stay relatively hypointense in both se-quences.

alone may be unsatisfactory, especially if the mass contains calcium or if there is extensive retrobul-bar spread.

Retinoblastoma and Its Mimics

Retinoblastoma is by far the most common in-traocular malignancy of childhood. Usually pre-senting in the first 2 years of life, it is multicentric and occurs bilaterally in about one third of pa-tients. It is highly malignant and spreads by local invasion and hematogenous metastasis. Locally, the tumor extends from the retina through the other layers of the globe wall, along the perivascu-lar and perineural tissue planes, and into the sub-arachnoid space. Determination of the extent of ex-traocular tumor is critical in these patients because its presence forebodes a poor prognosis.[46, 47]

Characteristics of retinoblastoma on CT scan include a well-defined high-density global wall mass, conglomerate areas of calcifications, and slight contrast enhancement (Fig 28–20).[46–50] The mass may protrude a variable distance into the vit-reous and be flat or papillated. It may be difficult to distinguish tumor from associated dense subret-inal effusion unless contrast is used.[50] Calcification is present in almost all tumors; its presence is nearly pathognomonic in children less than 3 years

old.[50] When there is extraocular spread of tumor, a soft-tissue density of slight-to-moderate enhance-ment bulges from the globe, commonly along the optic nerve. Calcification is more common in the intraocular than the extraocular portion of the tu-mor.[46]

On MRI, retinoblastomas are isointense or slightly hyperintense to vitreous with short TR/TE sequences. With longer TR/TE sequences, they are less intense than vitreous.[50, 51] Calcifications are more difficult to discern than on CT. However, gradient echo images can be utilized to depict cal-cification if necessary.[36] Hypointensity results from local magnetic susceptibility effects. The MRI character of retinoblastomas is sufficiently different from its mimickers (discussed below) to be diagnostic in most cases.

The differential diagnosis of retinoblastoma in-cludes Coats' disease, persistent hyperplastic pri-mary vitreous (PHPV), retrolental fibroplasia, scle-rosing endophthalmitis, and phthisis bulbi. Coats' disease, a retinal vascular anomaly, is associated with a subretinal exudate that can be quite exten-sive. The exudate causes increased retrolental den-sity, occasionally in a "V" shape so characteristic of retinal detachment.[50–52] On MRI, the exudate is hyperintense on both short and long TR/TE se-quences.[50, 51] PHPV is a congenital retention of the

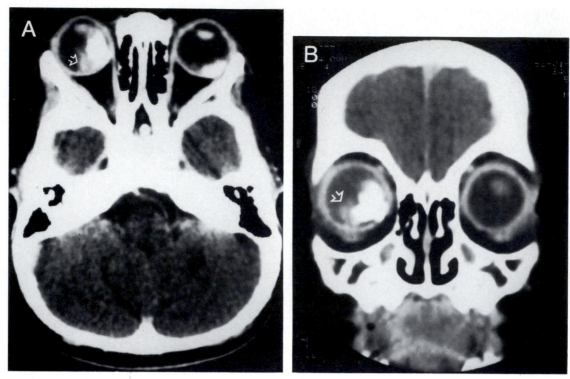

FIG 28–20.
Retinoblastoma. Axial **(A)** and coronal **(B)** CT scans show dense calcifications in both globes. A modestly enhancing portion of tumor is noted on the right *(arrow)*.

embryonic hyaloid vascular system, usually with associated subretinal hemorrhage. The CT appearance is variable but shows increased retrolental density without calcification, microphthalmos, and sometimes posterior layering of blood[49, 50, 53] (Fig 28–21). MRI reflects the hemorrhagic component with hyperintensity on short and long TR/TE spin-echo sequences. The appearance of retrolental fibroplasia may be similar to PHPV with noncalcified retinal detachments.[50] These detachments are usually along the temporal aspect of the globe.[49] Sclerosing endophthalmitis from *Toxocara canis* infestation produces a homogeneous retrolental density without a discrete mass on CT; this proteinaceous subretinal exudate is hyperintense on MRI sequences.[50] Phthisic inflammatory changes are dense on CT and hypointense on MRI unless there is evidence of residual retinal hemorrhage, in which case hyperintensity will be seen.

Malignant Melanoma

Malignant melanoma is the most common primary intraocular tumor of adulthood. Originating in the choroid layer of the wall, it spreads quickly and metastasizes early. The tumor can extend through the wall and form a retrobulbar mass in 15% of cases.[54] By CT, melanoma presents a well-defined nodular or convex eccentric thickening of the global rim.[44, 55] It shows high density on the unenhanced scan and enhances moderately follow-

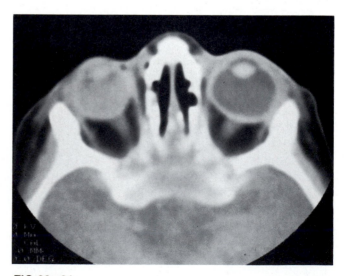

FIG 28–21.
Persistent hyperplastic primary vitreous. The right globe is shrunken, and there is increased retrolental density due to hemorrhage.

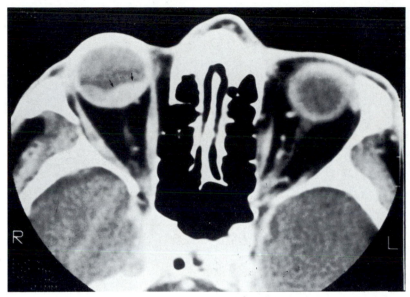

FIG 28–22.
Melanoma. An enhanced axial CT scan demonstrates a density difference between the enhancing tumor *(arrows)* and adjacent subretinal fluid.

ing contrast administration. Calcification is not present. Since subretinal fluid is a common accompaniment of melanoma, contrast may be necessary to separate the densities of the enhancing tumor and nonenhancing fluid (Fig 28–22).

MRI is usually characteristic in the diagnosis of melanoma. The melanin content of the tumor leads to a paramagnetic shortening of T1 and T2[56–61]; the degree of shortening roughly corresponds to the melanin content.[56] Thus melanotic melanomas are usually hyperintense to vitreous on short TR/TE and hypointense on long TR/TE sequences, depending on the melanin content (Figs 28–23 and 28–24). Adjacent subretinal fluid can easily be distinguished from tumor due to its hyperintensity on long TR/TE sequences. Metastatic mucin-secreting adenocarcinoma, metastatic carcinoid, and subacute choroidal hematoma may simulate the MRI features of melanotic melanoma.[31, 58, 62] Amelanotic melanoma is isointense

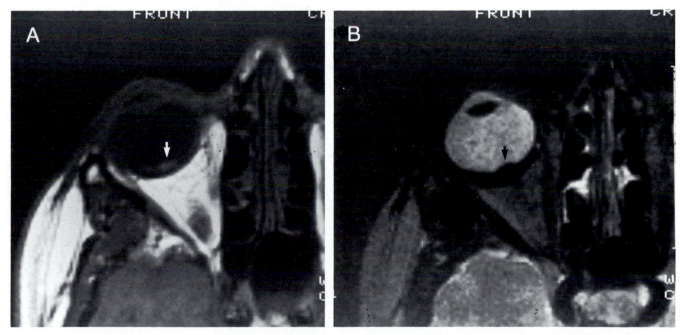

FIG 28–23.
Melanoma (melanotic). Characteristic hyperintensity *(arrow)* is present on short TR/TE **(A)**, while hypointensity *(arrow)* is present on long TR/TE sequences **(B).**

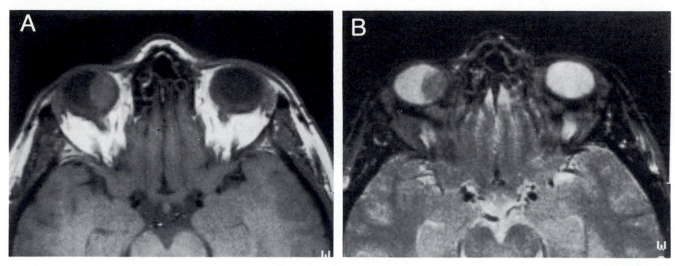

FIG 28–24.
Melanoma (amelanotic). Tumor of right globe is relatively isointense on both short **(A)** and long **(B)** TR/TE sequences due to a lack of paramagnetic melanin.

on short TR/TE and hypointense on TR/TE sequences, an appearance similar to metastasis (Fig 28–24).[61]

Metastatic and Other Tumors

Metastatic disease of the eye is probably more common than primary malignant melanoma is. In adults, the richly vascularized choroid layer is the most common site of implantation. Spread of tumor into the orbit from the globe is seen in a significant number of patients. Breast, lung, and kidney carcinomas have the highest incidence of ocular involvement.[63] The CT scan may show a globular thickening of the wall or a more diffuse, smooth expansion (Fig 28–25). Subretinal fluid frequently adjoins the metastasis, so as with melanoma, distinction between tumor and fluid may be difficult. Enhancement may be variable. MRI can more easily make the distinction of tumor vs. fluid. The MRI appearance of metastasis too may vary, becoming either more or less intense from short to long TR/TE sequences.[31, 58–60] Most metastases are isointense on short TR/TE and hypointense on long TR/TE sequences.[61]

Lymphoid lesions can usually be distinguished from other ocular tumors in that they tend to involve the globe secondarily. That is, they wrap around the globe wall without indenting or invading the globe itself (Fig 28–26). Choroidal hemangioma, sometimes associated with Sturge-Weber-Krabbé syndrome, represents another type of enhancing lesion with associated retinal fluid. It

enhances more briskly than do melanomas on CT[55] and are of higher intensity than are melanomas on MRI.[58, 61]

Inflammation of the sclera, which may accompany systemic illness (e.g., sarcoidosis, rheumatoid arthritis, Wegener's granulomatosis), can usually be distinguished from tumor. The globe wall is more uniformly thickened and enhanced in scleritis than in tumor[64] (Fig 28–27).

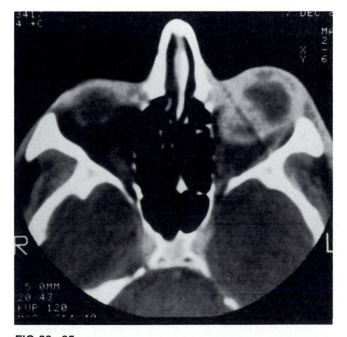

FIG 28–25.
Globe metastasis. A large heterogeneously enhancing choroidal breast metastasis has broken through the globe wall to invade the retrobulbar fat.

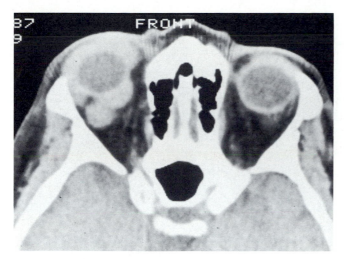

FIG 28–26.
Lymphoma. A globular homogeneous tumor enwraps the right globe.

Retinal and Choroidal Fluid

Retinal and choroidal detachments alone may cause enough density in the globe on CT or intensity variation in the globe on MRI to raise the possibility of tumor. Scrutiny of their configuration gives a clue to their identity. Retinal detachments are commonly V-shaped, with thin edges converging at the optic discs (Fig 28–28); anteriorly, retinal detachments will stop behind the ciliary body (the location of the ora serrota, the terminal part of the retina).[65, 66] Most retinal detachments are hyperintense on MRI. Choroidal effusions are either semilunar or oval shaped with thicker edges. Their edges converge less acutely (Fig 28–29). Density

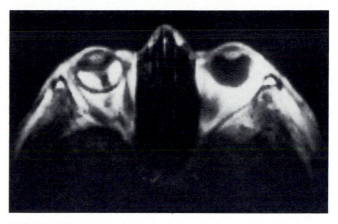

FIG 28–28.
Retinal detachment. A short TR/TE axial MR image with hyperintense V-shaped fluid collections in right globe.

on CT may vary, but intensity is usually high on long and short TR/TE images.[66] Choroidal hematomas (hemorrhagic choroid detachments) are biconvex. CT density and MRI intensity varies with the age of the hematoma. As with other hematomas, CT density decreases with time. MRI intensity is acutely low, but with time, intensity increases, first on short TR/TE sequences and later with long TR/TE.[66]

NONTRAUMATIC DISEASE AFFECTING THE ORBITAL WALLS

The orbital walls may be abnormal as a result of a wide variety of congenital, developmental, or acquired diseases. Because of this variety, some

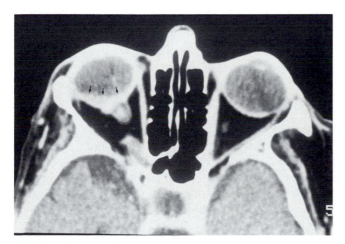

FIG 28–27.
Scleritis. The posterior right globe wall is thickened and enhances exuberantly *(arrows)*.

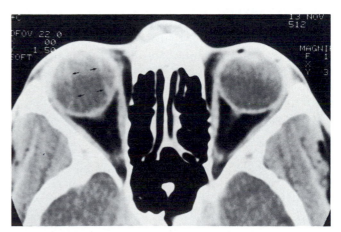

FIG 28–29.
Choroidal effusion. The margins of the effusion are rather thick *(arrows)* and run a more parallel course than a retinal detachment does.

categorization of disease manifestation is useful and helps to limit the differential diagnosis. One approach to orbital wall disease is as follows: (1) the small orbit, (2) the large orbit, (3) lucent abnormalities of the wall, and (4) sclerotic abnormalities of the wall (after S.A. Kieffer, 1971).[67] These categories are based on conventional radiographic findings but may be applied easily to CT. Application to MRI is possible by recognizing alterations in the normal form or intensity patterns of the orbital walls. In general, sclerotic abnormalities cause normal cortical-marrow relationships to be altered by hypointensity on both short and long TR/TE images. Lucent abnormalities are usually more hyperintense, especially on long TR/TE images.

The Small Orbit

The vast majority of small orbits result from congenital and developmental disease. Microphthalmos and anophthalmos, both congenital diseases, have well-formed orbits that are disproportionately small in relation to the rest of the head. On scan, anophthalmos is seen as bilaterally small bony orbits containing soft-tissue structures that represent rudimentary orbital parts. Microphthalmos, which is unilateral or bilateral, has more defined internal structures, often with a perceptible globe and muscles. The optic nerve may be missing or the globe partially calcified (Fig 28–30).[68]

Craniosynostosis and diseases associated with craniosynostosis (e.g., Crouzon's disease) are distinguished by foreshortening of the bony orbits.[69] The scan shows shallow orbits with proptosis of the globes as well as an oddly shaped calvarium. Of the craniosynostoses, oxycephaly and plegiocephaly most often produce orbital abnormalities.[70]

Because growth of the orbital contents stimulates development of the bony orbit, enucleation takes away the stimulus for orbital expansion. Therefore, if an adequate prosthesis is not provided, the orbit becomes proportionally smaller.[71]

A mucocele, by slowly expanding and reforming the walls of a paranasal sinus, can contract the size of the orbit without causing an obvious lytic defect. Easy identification of the mucocele is possible by a CT water-density (or MRI hyperintense) mass. The orbit is otherwise normal.[72]

Fibrous dysplasia, by virtue of the thickening caused by bony involvement, may compromise the

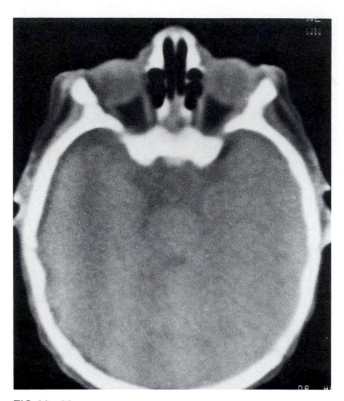

FIG 28–30.
Microphthalmos. Both globes and orbits are small in relation to head size. A hypoplastic optic nerve is barely seen in the right orbit; none is present in the left orbit.

size of the orbit. Especially when involvement is diffuse, the orbital space becomes shrunken and exophthalmos pronounced (Fig 28–31). The diagnostic features of fibrous dysplasia are discussed later with sclerotic lesions.

The Large Orbit

Enlargement of the orbit usually results from an intraorbital mass.[67] It may be diffuse or local, depending on the underlying etiologic process. Diffuse orbital expansion occurs in congenital glaucoma, serous cysts, and neurofibromatosis. In congenital glaucoma, or buphthalmos, heightened intraocular pressure causes enlargement of the globe, which then serves to enlarge the entire orbit. This condition is easily identified by scan (Fig 28–32). Serous cysts occur in the context of anophthalmos or microphthalmos. Orbital wall dysplasia from neurofibromatosis may lead to generalized expansion of the entire orbit.[73] There is a defect of the greater wing of the sphenoid bone of varying size that is illustrated well by scanning. Herniation of a portion of the temporal lobe into the orbit may

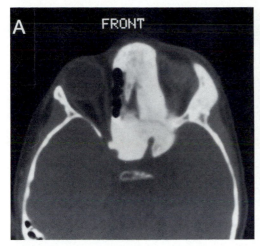
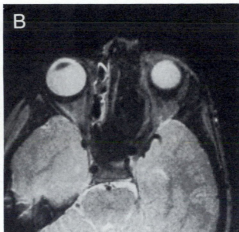
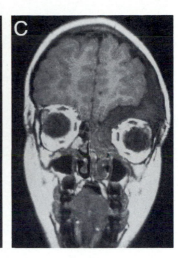

FIG 28–31.
Fibrous dysplasia. An axial CT scan **(A)** shows typical ground-glass sclerosis of the involved lateral orbital wall, ethmoid, and sphenoid that is causing contraction of the orbit. A comparable axial long TR/TE MR image **(B)** reflects fibro-osseous overgrowth with low signal intensity. A coronal short TR/TE sequence depicts areas of involvement as less hypointense. Note additional involvement of the lateral frontal bone **(C).**

also contribute to orbital enlargement. Occasionally, schwannoma may be the cause of the sphenoid wing (superior ophthalmic fissure) defect (Fig 28–33).

Other tumors may cause diffuse or focal expansion. Generally, younger patients and patients with intraconal rather than extraconal masses have a greater tendency to have diffusely enlarged orbits. So too, long-standing slow-growing tumors are more prone to remodel their bony surroundings. Thus, hemangiomas, optic gliomas, and pseudotumors have a propensity to cause enlargement of the entire orbit.[67] Focal remodeling is more likely in adult tumors and in those with an extraconal location. Hemangiomas, hemangiopericytomas, neurofibromas, and lacrimal gland tumors can all focally affect the wall. Venous varix, a tumorlike condition in many ways, can by its chronic pulsations erode the orbital wall.

Maxillary sinus hypoplasia or aplasia results in orbital enlargement because of depression of the orbital floor. This diagnosis can be confirmed by scan findings that include thickening of the antral wall, lateral expansion of the ipsilateral nasal cavity, hypoplasia of the zygomatic recess of the an-

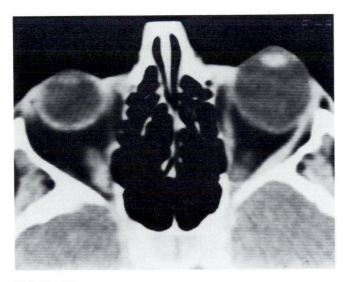

FIG 28–32.
Buphthalmos. The left globe is markedly enlarged, and there is atrophy of the globe wall. The orbital walls are slightly expanded by the enlarged globe. (Courtesy of Reza Raji, M.D., Pittsburgh.)

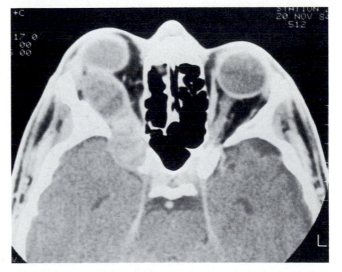

FIG 28–33.
Schwannoma. A huge tumor expands the right superior orbital fissure in its growth from the cavernous sinus into the orbit.

trum, and ipsilateral inferior turbinate hypertrophy.[74]

Lucent Abnormalities of the Wall

Congenital lucencies of an orbital wall are noted in neurofibromatosis and encephalocele. As previously described, neurofibromatosis may be manifested by the absence of a portion of the greater sphenoid wing. A dysplastic change, this bony defect has a smoothly tapered margin and no associated mass and affects the medial aspect of the bone (Fig 28–34). Long-standing temporal fossa masses, e.g., subarachnoid cyst, can produce a similar plain radiographic picture, but scans easily identify these. Encephaloceles have well-defined, circumscribed bony defects, usually near the midline. A mass may protrude into the medial portion of the orbit.[67] CT (or MR) scanning illustrates the defect containing cerebrospinal fluid (CSF) or a brain density (or intensity) and any associated anomaly of the globe or brain. Other well-defined defects of bone may result from slow-growing orbital tumors like dermoids, lacrimal gland adenomas, hemangiomas, or neurofibromas. The accompanying tumor is readily apparent on scans.

Secondary tumors from local or distant neoplasia are the most common source of lucent defects.

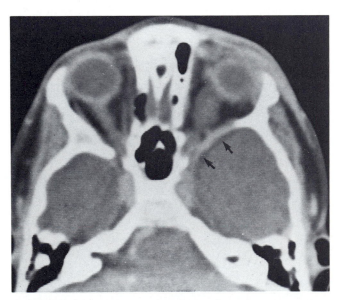

FIG 28–34.
Neurofibromatosis. There is a well-defined defect of the greater wing of the left sphenoid bone *(arrows)*. In this particular case, the temporal lobe does not herniate through the defect; the enhancing dura covers the defect. The posterior optic nerve is involved by glioma. (Courtesy of Reza Raji, M.D., Pittsburgh.)

Sinus, nasal cavity, and nasopharyngeal tumors frequently invade the orbit, usually by direct extension through the orbital walls. Thus, destruction of the bony walls occurs at the medial wall and floor in ethmoid and maxillary sinus, nasal cavity, and nasopharyngeal tumors and at the orbital roof in frontal sinus tumors. Tumors may also extend through orbital foramina to enter the orbit.[75] Orbital involvement by malignant tumor is characterized by irregular, permeative destruction of bone and an invasive soft-tissue mass, while benign tumor has less irregular destruction and a well-defined mass.[76]

Metastatic spread from distant primary sites to the orbital wall accounts for about 12% of all metastatic orbital and ocular disease.[63] Most of these deposits are from breast, lung, and kidney carcinomas in the adult and from neuroblastoma and Ewings' sarcoma in children. These metastases are primarily lytic rather than sclerotic. Destruction of the wall is usually irregular on the CT scan and has an associated enhancing soft-tissue component. Varying amounts of orbital invasion are seen; the tumor mass may be confined by the periorbita or break through it and involve fat and muscle by a fairly defined or irregular mass. Metastatic destruction of the orbital wall may be more obviously seen and more easily characterized on MRI than CT. Tumor mass, which is usually hyperintense on long TR/TE sequences, will stand out from surrounding (less intense) orbital fat, bony wall, or aerated sinus.

Eosinophilic granuloma may be difficult to distinguish from metastatic disease by CT. The bony defect is fairly well delineated with smoothly tapered edges; usually only a small soft-tissue mass is present (Fig 28–35). Although the frontal bone is most often affected, other bones of the orbit can be involved.

Osteomyelitis may result from sinusitis, trauma, or hematogenous spread. Lytic defects are usually irregular with acute disease, but can be sclerotic with chronic disease (Fig 28–36). A soft-tissue mass from adjacent cellulitis or an abscess is likely to accompany the bony changes. When orbital bone destruction accompanies mucosal thickening of several sinuses in the absence of air-fluid levels, fungal disease (i.e., mucormycosis or aspergillosis) should be suspected.[77] Mucoceles cause remodeling of the expanded sinus walls and makes them thin enough to appear destroyed. The soft-tissue mass of the mucocele is generally well defined and may have a thin bony margin. On MRI

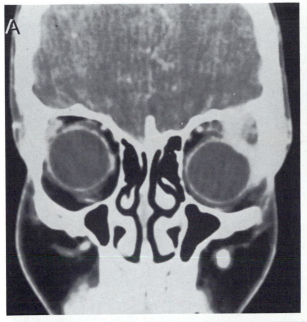
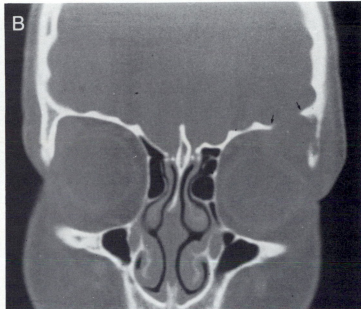
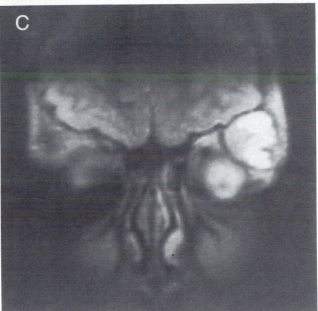

FIG 28–35.
Eosinophic granuloma. An enhancing left superior orbital mass **(A)** is associated with bone destruction **(B)** having typical beveled margins *(arrows)*. A comparable coronal long TR/TE MR sequence **(C)** shows varied intensity most likely related to recent hemorrhage (confirmed at surgery).

a mucocele is usually hyperintense due to its high protein content (Fig 28–37).

Extensive lysis of bone may accompany very aggressive meningiomas that extend directly into the orbit. Generally, the soft-tissue component is large. Such tumors may become so extensive that they obliterate all definable bony and soft-tissue structures (Fig 28–38).

Rarely, intraorbital malignancies such as rhabdomyosarcoma will invade the adjacent bony wall. The resultant bony destruction and mass are easily identified by scan.

Sclerotic Abnormalities of the Wall

Sphenoid wing meningiomas generally cause hyperostosis and thickening. They often have a high-density, soft-tissue component that protrudes into the posterior portion of the orbit and/or middle cranial fossa. On CT, homogeneous enhancement is characteristic. The extraconal tumor, displacement of extraocular muscles, and proptosis are apparent (Fig 28–39). These meningiomas may be extensive and compromise the superior orbital fissure, optic foramen, and associated neurovascu-

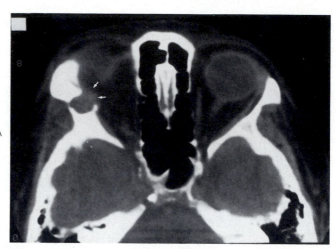

FIG 28–36.
Chronic osteomyelitis. A well-defined defect is seen in the right
lateral orbital wall. The rest of the wall is thickened and sclerotic. A
small soft-tissue mass accompanies the lytic defect *(arrows)*.

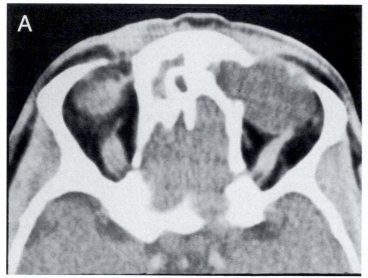

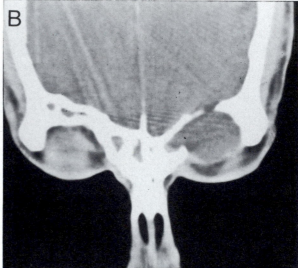

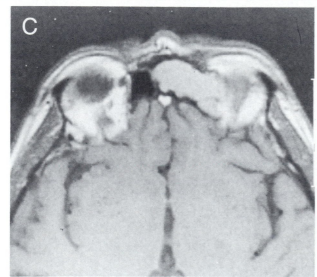

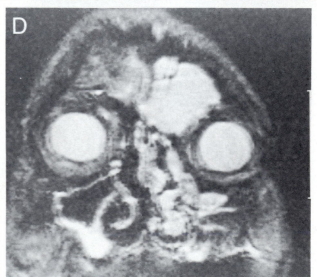

FIG 28–37.
Mucocele. Axial **(A)** and coronal **(B)** CT scans show expansion of
the left frontal sinus with remodeling of the orbital roof and extension of a well-defined mass into the orbit. On short TR/TE **(C)** and
long TR/TE **(D)** sequences the mucocele is hyperintense, thus reflecting the high protein content.

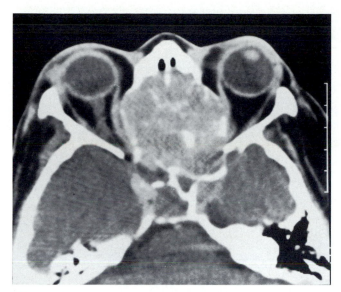

FIG 28–38.
Meningioma. A large subfrontal meningioma is expanding and destroying the ethmoid sinuses and bulging into both orbits.

lar structures (Fig 28–40). Meningiomas of the orbital roof, also sclerotic, are less likely than sphenoid wing meningiomas are to invade the orbit. Those meningiomas that arise in the parasellar region and from the medial sphenoid wing may gain access to the orbit by invading the superior orbital fissure.[75] Most meningiomas are hypointense on MRI spin-echo sequences, thus making them difficult to distinguish from normal bony wall.[78, 79] Where they protrude into the orbit, they are outlined by hyperintense orbital fat (on the short TR/

TE sequence). Enhancement with gadolinium is usually prominent and homogeneous (Fig 28–41).

Fibrous dysplasia can involve any of the bones of the orbit. With its thickened, sclerotic appearance, it may in some instances simulate meningioma. Bone involved with fibrous dysplasia tends to have extremely high density and homogeneous texture on CT. There is no significant soft-tissue component as in meningioma. Fibrous dysplasia also occurs at a younger age group than meningioma does. On MRI, areas of involvement are uniformly hypointense (see Fig 28–31).

Bony dysplasias, like osteopetrosis and Engelmann's disease, cause uniform dense bony thickening that is hypointense on MRI. Foraminal encroachment may be defined by both CT and MRI (Fig 28–42).

Paget's disease unusually affects the orbit and only rarely in a solitary fashion. The involved bone is expanded and shows both lytic and sclerotic areas. On CT, sclerosis is irregular with areas of low density interspersed within the thickened bone. Foraminal openings may be severely compromised. MRI of Paget's disease reveals relatively high signal within the expanded diploic space; the inner and outer tables are irregular.[80]

Metastases to the orbital wall can be sclerotic as well as lytic. Carcinomatous implants from the prostate or breast are the most common blastic metastasis to the orbit (Fig 28–43). As in Paget's disease, sclerosis is irregular. Bony thickening, however, is not as prominent as in Paget's disease, and

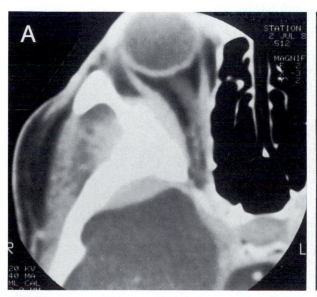
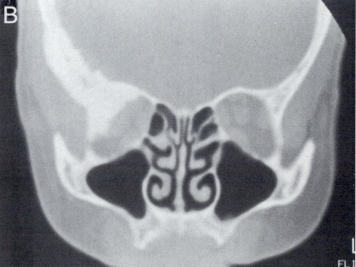

FIG 28–39.
Sphenoid wing meningioma. Axial **(A)** and coronal **(B)** CT scans show sclerosis and expansion of the right sphenoid wing. A soft-tissue tumor extends into the lateral portion of the orbit, middle cranial fossa, and temporalis region.

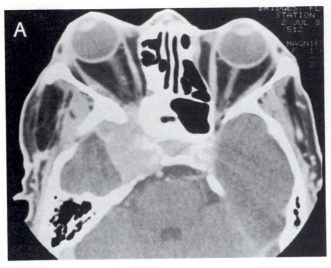 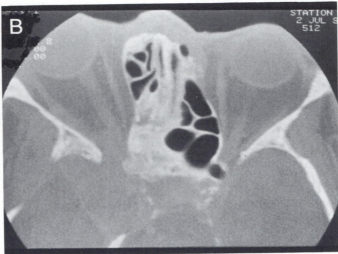

FIG 28–40.
Cavernous sinus meningioma. A large homogeneous meningioma expands the right cavernous sinus and protrudes slightly into the widened superior orbital fissure **(A).** Magnified bone windows **(B)** show sclerosis of the sphenoid on either side of the fissure.

a soft-tissue mass is present. By scan, the most difficult differential possibility to exclude is an aggressive meningioma, which may have sclerotic and lytic areas and a prominent soft-tissue mass.

CT-GUIDED FINE-NEEDLE BIOPSY

Fine-needle aspiration biopsy techniques have proved to be useful and safe in orbital diagnosis.[81–85] Whether done blindly or guided by ultrasound or CT, they have applicability in several clinical contexts, most notably inoperable orbital masses presenting diagnostic (and thus therapeutic) dilemmas.

When done with CT guidance, the biopsy is performed with a 22- or 23-gauge needle usually placed through the lid just below the outer canthus. Once the needle is inserted, its position is checked by contiguous 5-mm (or less) scans (Fig 28–44). If needed, repositioning and rescanning are performed. The biopsy is made by a combina-

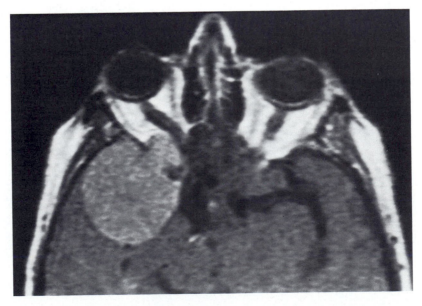

FIG 28–41.
Sphenoid wing meningioma. Axial short TR/TE gadolinium enhanced MRI shows a large homogeneous tumor extending into the right middle cranial fossa. A lip of tumor prolapses into the superior orbital fissure.

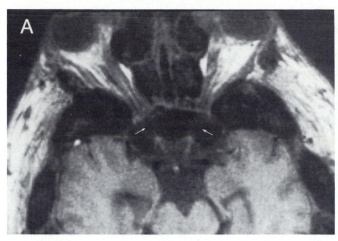
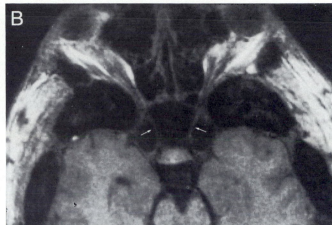

FIG 28–42.
Engelmann's disease. **A** and **B,** short TR/TE MRI. Densely (hypointense) sclerotic, expanded sphenoid bones narrow the optic foramina and leave just enough room for the optic nerves *(arrows).*

tion of suction and agitation of the needle.[81, 83] Cytologic analysis is then made on the specimen. It is emphasized that this is a cytologic test; as such, it is limited by specimen sampling.

As various techniques have been attempted and modified, indications for CT-guided biopsy have developed. Thus, CT guidance has been found to be unnecessary for relatively superficial lesions and extraconal lesions, which can undergo biopsy without CT localization. Large intraconal masses, especially if anteriorly placed, are more amenable to biopsy with ultrasound guidance.[84] Additionally, aspiration biopsy is not indicated in well-circumscribed intraconal or extraconal masses. Some of these masses, e.g., hemangiopericytoma and mixed lacrimal gland tumor, can become locally aggressive if their capsule is violated.[81]

Infiltrative lesions like lymphoma and metastases are usually amenable to CT localization and biopsy techniques. Even deep-seated apical lesions extending from the cavernous sinus may undergo biopsy with care.[85] Although fine-needle aspiration has led to histologic diagnosis of a number of optic nerve lesions (e.g., meningioma, astro-

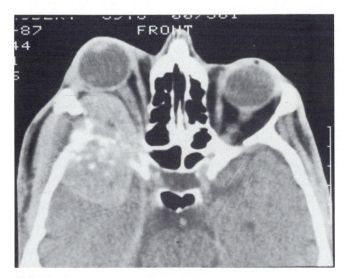

FIG 28–43.
Prostate metastasis. Partially calcified tumor erodes the right sphenoid wing and lateral orbital wall. Tumor extends into the lateral portion of the orbit, middle cranial fossa, and temporalis region and simulates the appearance of meningioma.

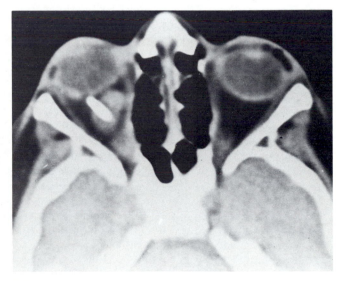

FIG 28–44.
Fine-needle aspiration biopsy. A biopsy needle has been placed into the enlarged optic nerve. The scan confirms the needle position. Biopsy established the diagnosis of optic nerve glioma (same patient as in Figure 27–33).

cytoma, leukemia),[82] it should be used judiciously to avoid further compromising vision.

In summary, however, fine-needle aspiration biopsy is limited by the amount of specimen obtained and the inability to determine the extent of disease; in the appropriate clinical setting diagnostic information may be gained easily and safely and save the patient major surgery.

REFERENCES

1. Forbes G, Gehring DG, Gorman CA, et al: Volume measurements of normal orbital structures by computed tomographic analysis. *AJNR* 1985; 6:419–424.
2. Rothfus WE, Curtin HD: Extraocular muscle enlargement: A CT review *Radiology* 1984; 151:677–681.
3. Trokel SL, Hilal SK: Recognition and differential diagnosis of enlarged extraocular muscles in computed tomography. *Am J Ophthalmol* 1979; 87:503–512.
4. Enzmann DR, Donaldson SS, Kriss JP: Appearance of Graves' disease on orbital computed tomography. *J Comput Assist Tomogr* 1979; 3:815–819.
5. Curtin HD: Pseudotumor: *Radiol Clin North Am* 1987; 25:583–599.
6. Forbes G, Gorman CA, Brennan MD, et al: Ophthalmopathy of Graves' disease: Computerized volume measurements of the orbital fat and muscle. *AJNR* 1986; 7:651–656.
7. Robbins S: *Pathologic Basis of Disease.* Philadelphia, WB Saunders Co, 1974, p 1336.
8. Brismar J, Davis KR, Dallow RL, et al: Unilateral endocrine exophthalmos: Diagnostic problems in association with computed tomography. *Neuroradiology* 1976; 12:21–24.
9. Trokel SL, Jakobiec FA: Correlation of CT scanning and pathologic features of ophthalmic Graves' disease. *Ophthalmology* 1981; 88:553–564.
10. Enzmann DR, Marshall WH, Rosenthal AR, et al: Computed tomography in Graves' ophthalmopathy. *Radiology* 1976; 118:615–620.
11. Peyster RG, Ginsberg F, Silber JH, et al: Exophthalmos caused by excessive fat: CT volumetric analysis and differential diagnosis. *AJNR* 1986; 7:35–40.
12. Healy JF, Rosenkrantz H: Enlargement of the optic nerve sheath complex in thyroid ophthalmopathy. *J Comput Tomogr* 1981; 5:8–10.
13. Kennerdell JS, Rosenbaum AE, El-Hoshy MH: Apical optic nerve compression of dysthyroid optic neuropathy on computed tomography. *Arch Ophthalmol* 1981; 99:807–809.
14. Barrett L, Glatt HJ, Burde RM, et al: Optic nerve dysfunction in thyroid eye disease: CT. *Radiology* 1988; 167:503–507.
15. Healy J, Metcalf JH, Brahme FJ: Thyroid ophthalmopathy: Bony erosion on CT and increased vascularity on angiography. *AJNR* 1981; 2:472–474.
16. Rothfus WE: CT demonstration of lipomatosis of extraocular muscles in dysthyroid orbitopathy. *Orbit* 1983; 4:227–229.
17. Nugent RA, Rootman J, Robertson WD, et al: Acute orbital pseudotumors: Classification and CT features. *AJNR* 1981; 2:431–436.
18. Bernardino ME, Zimmerman RD, Citrin CM, et al: Scleral thickening: A CT sign of orbital pseudotumor. *AJR* 1977; 129:703–706.
19. Jellinek EH: The orbital pseudotumor syndrome and its differentiation from endocrine exophthalmos. *Brain* 1969; 92:35–58.
20. Blodi FC, Gass JDM: Inflammatory pseudotumor of the orbit. *Br J Ophthalmol* 1968; 52:79–93.
21. Atlas SW, Grossman RI, Savino PJ, et al: Surface-coil MR of orbital pseudotumor. *AJNR* 1987; 8:141–146.
22. Sullivan JA, Harms SE: Characterization of orbital lesions by surface coil MR imaging. *Radiographics* 1987; 7:9–28.
23. Braffman BH, Bilaniuk LT, Eagle RG, et al: MR imaging of a carcinoid tumor metastatic to the orbit. *J Comput Assist Tomogr* 1987; 11:891–894.
24. Mastaglia FL, Barwick DD, Hall R: Myopathy in acromegaly. *Lancet* 1970; 2:907–909.
25. Nagulesparen M, Trickey R, Davies MJ, et al: Muscle changes in acromegaly. *Br Med J* 1976; 2:914–915.
26. Dal Pozzo G, Boschi MC: Extraocular muscle enlargement in acromegaly. *J Comput Assist Tomogr* 1982; 6:706–707.
27. Jones IS, Reese AB, Kraut J: Orbital rhabdomyosarcoma: An analysis of 62 cases. *Am J Ophthalmol* 1966; 61:721–736.
28. Knochel JQ, Osborn AG, Wing DS: Differential diagnosis of lateral orbital masses. *J Comput Tomogr* 1980; 5:11–15.
29. Forbes GS, Sheedy PF, Waller RR: Orbital tumors evaluated by computed tomography. *Radiology* 1980; 136:101–111.
30. Hornblass A, Jakobiec FA, Reifler DM, et al: Orbital lymphoid tumors located predominantly within extraocular muscles. *Ophthalmology* 1987; 94:688–697.
31. Peyster RG, Shapiro MO, Haik BG: Orbital metastasis: Role of magnetic resonance imaging and computed tomography. *Radiol Clin North Am* 1987; 25:647–662.
32. Merrick R, Latchaw RE, Gold LHA: Computerized tomography of the orbit in carotid-cavernous sinus fistulae. *Comput Tomogr* 1980; 4:127–132.
33. Weinstein MA, Modic MT, Risius D, et al: Visualization of the arteries, veins, and nerves of the orbit by sector computed tomography. *Radiology* 1981; 138:83–87.

34. Bacon KT, Duchesneau PM, Weinstein MA: Demonstration of the superior ophthalmic vein by high resolution computed tomography. *Radiology* 1977; 124:129–131.
35. Dubois PJ, Kennerdell JS, Rosenbaum AE: Advantages of a fourth generation CT scanner in the management of patients with orbital mass lesions. *Comput Tomogr* 1979; 3:279–290.
36. Atlas S: Magnetic resonance imaging of the orbit: Current status. *Magn Reson Q* 1989; 5:39–96.
37. Lloyd GAS: *Radiology of the Orbit.* Philadelphia, WB Saunders Co, 1975, pp 132–134.
38. Dallow RL: Reliability of orbital diagnostic tests: Ultrasonography, computerized tomography and radiography. *Ophthalmology* 1978; 85:1218–1228.
39. Jakobiec FA, Yeo JH, Trokel SL, et al: Combined clinical and computed tomographic diagnosis of primary lacrimal fossa lesions. *Am J Ophthalmol* 1982; 94:785–807.
40. Mafee MF, Haik BG: Lacrimal gland and fossa lesions: Role of computed tomography. *Radiol Clin North Am* 1987; 25:767–779.
41. Blei L, Chambers J, Liotta L, et al: Orbital dermoid diagnosed by computed tomographic scanning. *Am J Ophthalmol* 1978; 85:58–61.
42. Wright JE, Stewart WB, Krohel GB: Clinical presentation and management of lacrimal gland tumors. *Br J Ophthalmol* 1979; 63:600–606.
43. Duke-Elder S, McFaul PA: Diseases of the lacrimal gland in the ocular adenexa: Part II, in *System of Ophthalmology.* St Louis, CV Mosby Co, 1974, pp 595–674.
44. Bernardino ME, Danzinger J, Young SE, et al: Computed tomography in ocular neoplastic disease. *AJR* 1978; 131:111–113.
45. Brandt-Zawadzki M, Enzmann DR: Orbital computed tomography: Calcific densities of the posterior globe. *J Comput Assist Tomogr* 1979; 3:503–505.
46. Danzinger A, Price HI: CT findings in retinoblastoma. *AJR* 1979; 133:783–785.
47. Price HI, Batnitzky S, Danzinger A, et al: The neuroradiology of retinoblastoma. *Radiographics* 1982; 2:7–24.
48. Goldberg L, Danzinger A: Computed tomographic scanning in the management of retinoblastoma. *Am J Ophthalmol* 1977; 84:380–382.
49. Hopper KD, Kate NNK, Dorwart RH, et al: Childhood leukokoria: Computed tomographic appearance and differential diagnosis with histopathologic correlation. *Radiographics* 1985; 5:377–394.
50. Mafee MF, Goldberg MF, Greenwald MJ, et al: Retinoblastoma and simulating lesions: Role of CT and MR imaging. *Radiol Clin North Am* 1987; 25:667–682.
51. Haik BG, Saint Louis L, Smith ME, et al: Magnetic resonance imaging in the evaluation of leukocoria. *Ophthalmology* 1985; 92:1143–1152.
52. Sherman JL, McLean IW, Braillier DR: Coat's disease: CT-pathologic correlation in two cases. *Radiology* 1983; 146:77–78.
53. Mafee MF, Goldberg MF, Valvassori GE, et al: Computed tomography in the evaluation of patients with persistent hyperplastic primary vitreous (PHPV). *Radiology* 1982; 145:713–715.
54. Grimson BS, Cohen KL, McCartney WH: Concomitant ocular and orbital neoplasms. *J Comput Assist Tomogr* 1982; 6:617–619.
55. Mafee MF, Peyman GA, McKusick MA: Malignant uveal melanoma and similar lesions studied by computed tomography. *Radiology* 1985; 156:403–408.
56. Gomori JM, Grossman RI, Shields JA, et al: Choroidal melanomas: Correlation of NMR spectroscopy and MR imaging. *Radiology* 1986; 158:443–445.
57. Mafee MF, Peyman GA, Grosolano JE, et al: Malignant uveal melanoma and simulating lesions: MR imaging evaluation. *Radiology* 1986; 160:773–780.
58. Mafee MF, Peyman GA, Peace JH, et al: Magnetic resonance imaging in the evaluation and differentiation of uveal melanoma. *Ophthalmology* 1987; 94:341–348.
59. Haik B, Saint Louis L, Smith ME, et al: Magnetic resonance imaging in choroidal tumors. *Ann Ophthalmol* 1987; 19:218–238.
60. Chambers RB, Davidorf FH, McAdoo JF, et al: Magnetic resonance imaging of uveal melanomas. *Arch Ophthalmol* 1987; 105:917–921.
61. Peyster RH, Augsburger JJ, Shields JA, et al: Intraocular tumors: Evaluation with MR imaging. *Radiology* 1988; 168:773–779.
62. Spencer G, Lufkin R, Simons K, et al: MR of melanoma simulating ocular neoplasm. *AJNR* 1987; 8:921–922.
63. Ferry AP, Font RL: Carcinoma metastatic to the eye and orbit: I. A clinicopathologic study of 227 cases. *Arch Ophthalmol* 1974; 92:276–286.
64. Johnson MH, DeFilipp GJ, Zimmerman RA, et al: Scleral inflammatory disease. *AJNR* 1987; 8:861–865.
65. Mafee MF, Peyman GA: Retinal and choroidal detachments: Role of magnetic resonance imaging and computed tomography. *Radiol Clin North Am* 1987; 25:487–507.
66. Mafee MF, Linder B, Peyman GA, et al: Choroidal hematoma and effusion: Evaluation with MR imaging. *Radiology* 1988; 168:781–786.
67. Kieffer SA: Orbit, in Newton TH, Potts DG (eds): *Radiology of the Skull and Brain*, vol 1, book 2. St Louis, CV Mosby Co, 1971, pp 463–485.
68. Jacobs L, Weisberg LA, Kinkel WR: *Computerized Tomography of the Orbit and Sella Turcica.* New York, Raven Press, 1980, pp 275–278.
69. Blodi FC: Pathologic changes of the orbit bones. *Trans Am Acad Ophthalmol Otolaryngol* 1976; 81:26–57.

70. Jacobs L, Weisberg LA, Kinkel WR: *Computerized Tomography of the Orbit and Sella Turcica.* New York, Raven Press, 1980, pp 255–257.

71. Kennedy RE: The effect of early enucleation on the orbit in animals and humans. *Am J Ophthalmol* 1965; 60:277–306.

72. Hesselink JR, Weber AL, New PFJ, et al: Evaluation of mucoceles of the paranasal sinuses with computed tomography. *Radiology* 1979; 131:397–400.

73. Binet EF, Kieffer SA, Martin SH, et al: Orbital dysplasia in neurofibromatosis. Radiology 1969; 93:820–833.

74. Modic MT, Weinstein MA, Berlin AJ, et al: Maxillary sinus hypoplasia visualized with computed tomography. *Radiology* 1980; 135:383–385.

75. Hesselink JR, Weber AL: Pathways of orbital extension of extraorbital neoplasms. *J Comput Assist Tomogr* 1982; 6:593–597.

76. Parsons C, Hodson N: Computed tomography of paranasal sinus tumors. *Radiology* 1979; 132:641–645.

77. Centeno RS, Bentson JR, Mancuso AA: CT scanning in rhinocerebral mucormycosis and aspergillosis. *Radiology* 1981; 140:383–389.

78. Spagnoli MV, Goldberg HI, Grossman RI, et al: Intracranial meningiomas: High-field MR imaging. *Radiology* 1986; 161:369–375.

79. Zimmerman RD, Fleming CA, Saint-Louis LA, et al: Magnetic resonance imaging of meningiomas. *AJNR* 1985; 6:149–157.

80. Tjon-A-Tham RTO, Bloem JL, Folk THM, et al: Magnetic resonance imaging in Paget disease of the skull. *AJNR* 1985; 6:879–881.

81. Kennerdell JS, Dekker A, Johnson BJ, et al: Fine needle aspiration biopsy: Its use in orbital tumors. *Arch Ophthalmol* 1979; 97:1315–1317.

82. Kennerdell JS, Dekker A, Johnson BJ: Orbital fine needle aspiration biopsy: The results of its use in 50 patients. *Neuro-ophthalmology* 1980; 1:117–121.

83. Dubois PJ, Kennerdell JS, Rosenbaum AE, et al: Computed tomographic localization for fine needle aspiration biopsy of orbital tumors. *Radiology* 1977; 131:149–152.

84. Spoor TC, Kennerdell JS, Dekker A, et al: Fine needle aspiration biopsy with B-scan guidance. *Am J Ophthalmol* 1980; 89:274–277.

85. Rowed DW, Kassel EE, Lewis AJ: Transorbital intracavernous needle biopsy in painful ophthalmoplegia. *J Neurosurg* 1985; 62:776–780.

PART XI

MR and CT Imaging
in Otolaryngology

29

The Temporal Bone

Katherine Shaffer, M.D.

Methods of temporal bone imaging have undergone considerable change in the last two decades. Complex-motion tomography replaced conventional films in the late 1960s. It, in turn, was supplanted by high-resolution, thin-section computed tomography (CT) in the 1980s. CT remains the preferred method to study most temporal bone abnormalities because of its exquisite bone detail and improved soft-tissue resolution. Magnetic resonance imaging (MRI), introduced in the 1980s, is becoming the procedure of choice for specific abnormalities, particularly acoustic neuroma.

IMAGING TECHNIQUE

The temporal bone is usually imaged in two planes, most frequently axial and coronal, with both CT and MRI. Sagittal scans are also occasionally used, depending on the particular anatomic area to be studied within the temporal bone.[1] Sagittal reformatted images of 1.5-mm-thick CT scans can also be obtained. Unless otherwise noted, all CT scans were done on a General Electric Medical Systems 9800 scanner and all MRI scans on a General Electric Signa scanner (General Electric Medical Systems, Milwaukee.)

Computed Tomography

Contiguous 1.5-mm-thick scans are usually done in the coronal and axial planes to evaluate temporal bone abnormalities. Sections may be overlapped (1.5-mm-thick sections at 1-mm intervals) to evaluate tiny areas such as the oval window or ossicular prostheses. Axial scans can be angled relative to the orbitomeatal line for optimal visualization of particular structures.[2] Routinely, axial scans are parallel to the infraorbitomeatal line since most temporal bone anatomy can be seen well with this angulation and the eye is not in the scanning beam. Direct coronal scans can be performed with the patient either in the hanging-head position or prone. Extension of the patient's neck combined with maximum gantry angulation helps attain a true coronal plane. Angled scanning planes to duplicate views obtainable with conventional tomography (e.g., Stenvers)[3] have not been popular in the United States. Radiation to the eyes from scanning in two planes is minimal if the x-ray beam does not pass directly through them during the axial scans.[4]

CT technique depends on the type of scanner and detector used. In general, high kilovoltage (kVp) (120 to 140) is necessary to penetrate the temporal bone. The mAs (milliampere-seconds) is adjusted depending on whether areas of high inherent contrast (the bone and air spaces) or low contrast (the internal auditory canal and cerebellopontine angle) are of primary interest. High mAs will improve the signal-to-noise ratio in soft tissues when 1.5-mm slices are used.

The reconstruction algorithm and the window width used for displaying temporal bone scans are important factors to produce an optimal image. Because the temporal bone is the densest bone in the body, a very wide window (3,000 to 4,000 Hounsfield units [HU]) is required for differentiation of inner- and middle-ear structures.[5] Multiple reconstruction algorithms are now available on scanners; a bone detail algorithm, which enhances edges, is best to reconstruct all temporal bone scans except those done for acoustic neuroma. However, artifacts are also introduced with this algorithm, and this makes the same images viewed at a narrow window unsatisfactory to evaluate intracranial soft tissues. Therefore, reconstruction of data with two different algorithms, one for bone and one for soft tissue, is necessary when evaluating a patient for acoustic neuroma. The resulting scans are viewed at wide and narrow windows, respectively. Reconstructing a portion of the scan data (zoom or target reconstruction) will improve spatial resolution in those scanners that collect more data than is displayed with conventional reconstruction. Target reconstruction is preferred over simple image magnification because of the improved resolution.

Magnetic Resonance Imaging

Axial, coronal, and occasionally sagittal T1-weighted spin-echo sequences with a short repetition time (TR) and short echo time (TE) are used to study patients for acoustic neuroma. Three-millimeter-thick contiguous slices are obtained with a multislice acquisition technique. In patients with other pathology, T2-weighted images (long TR and TE) are added. The standard head coil is used so that both ears and adjacent brain can be evaluated simultaneously, or surface coils may be chosen to improve detail.[6–8]

NORMAL ANATOMY

Previous anatomic studies have confirmed that CT scans of the temporal bone correspond well with anatomic sections.[9, 10] Normal temporal bone anatomy is illustrated in axial and coronal CT scans. (Figs 29–1 and 29–2). MRI of the temporal

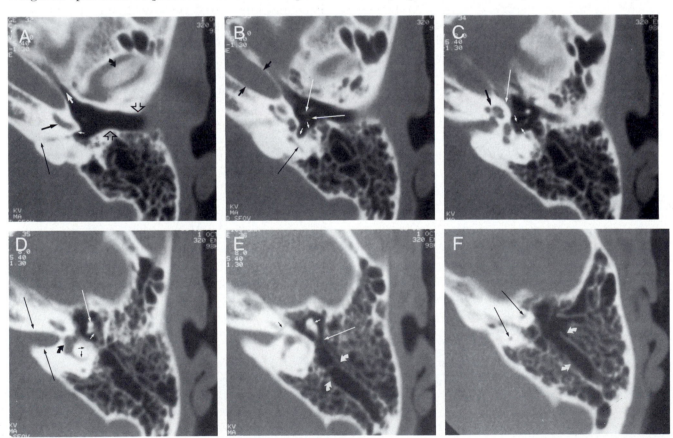

FIG 29–1.

Normal left ear, axial CT scans. **A,** most inferior section: eustachian tube *(white arrow)*, basal turn of the cochlea *(short black arrow)*, mandibular condyle *(curved black arrow)*, round window niche *(small white arrow)*, anterior and posterior walls of the bony external canal *(open arrows)*. **B,** posterior semicircular canal *(long black arrow)*, handle of the malleus (anterior) and long process of the incus *(long white arrows)*, carotid canal *(short black arrows)*, sinus tympani (medial) and pyramidal eminence *(short white arrows)*. **C,** stapes crura *(short white arrows)*, tensor tympani *(long white arrow)*, cochlea *(black arrow)*. **D,** 3 mm superior to **C:** short process of the incus *(short white arrow)*, lateral semicircular canal *(short black arrows)*, internal auditory canal *(long black arrows)*, malleus head *(long white arrow)*, vestibule *(curved arrow)*. **E,** joint between the malleus (anterior) and incus in the attic *(short white arrow)*, aditus ad antrum *(long white arrow)*, mastoid antrum *(curved white arrows)*, labyrinthine portion of the facial nerve canal *(black arrow)*. **F,** limbs of the superior semicircular canal *(black arrows)*, mastoid antrum *(white arrows)*.

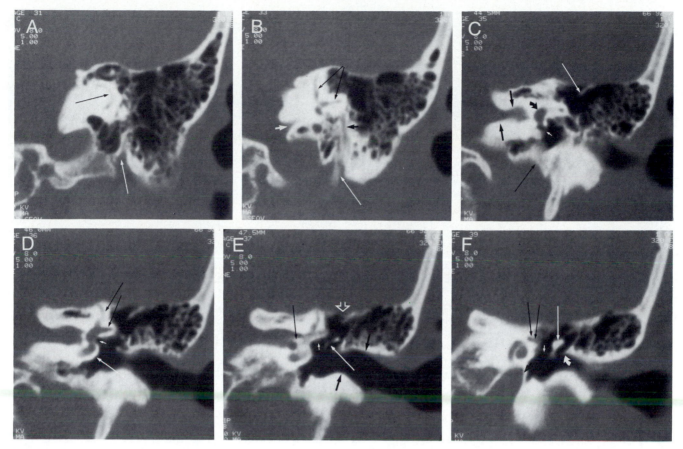

FIG 29–2.

Normal left ear, coronal CT scans. **A,** most posterior section: posterior semicircular canal *(black arrow)*, stylomastoid foramen *(white arrow)*. **B,** 3 mm anterior to **A:** posterior limbs of the superior and lateral semicircular canals *(long black arrows)*, descending facial nerve canal *(short black arrow)*, styloid process *(long white arrow)*, cochlear aqueduct opening *(short white arrow)*. **C,** 3 mm anterior to **B:** Körner's septum in the mastoid antrum *(long white arrow)*. Posterior internal auditory canal *(short black arrows)*, round window *(short white arrow)*, small jugular fossa *(long black arrow)*, vestibule *(curved arrow)*. **D,** oval window *(short white arrow)*, basal turn of the cochlea *(long white arrow)*, anterior limbs of the superior and lateral semicircular canals *(long black arrows)*. **E,** long process of the incus *(long white arrow)*, facial nerve under the lateral semicircular canal *(short white arrow)*, falciform crest in the internal auditory canal *(long black arrow)*, tegmen tympani *(open white arrow)*, superior and inferior walls of the bony external auditory canal *(short black arrows)*. **F,** 3 mm anterior to **E:** malleus *(long white arrow)*, drum spur or scutum *(curved white arrow)*, bone over the carotid artery *(short black arrow)*, canals for the facial nerve above the cochlea *(long black arrows)*, tensor tympani tendon *(small white arrow)*.

bone has also been correlated with cryomicrotome sections (Fig 29–3).[6, 11]

The temporal bone consists of five parts: the petrous portion, mastoid, tympanic bone, squamous portion, and styloid process. The squamous part of the temporal bone forms the skull above the ear and the superior surface of the bony external auditory canal; it also contributes the posterior half of the zygomatic arch. The styloid process, from which muscles and ligaments in the hyoid and glossal regions originate, is generally unimportant when evaluating the temporal bone except in cases of trauma where the facial nerve may be injured.

The petrous portion of the temporal bone is a wedge-shaped bone forming part of the skull base between the occipital and sphenoid bones. All of the inner-ear structures are located within this small area, including the cochlea, semicircular canals, vestibule, internal auditory canal, much of the facial nerve canal, and the cochlear and vestibular aqueducts. The petrous apex, the most anteromedial portion of the bone, is pneumatized in about one third of the population.

The mastoid creates the posterior superior surface of the external auditory canal and contains the mastoid antrum (Figs 29–1,E and 29–2,C) and air cells. Several muscles attach to the mastoid process, including the digastric and sternocleidomastoid. Mastoid pneumatization is quite variable, de-

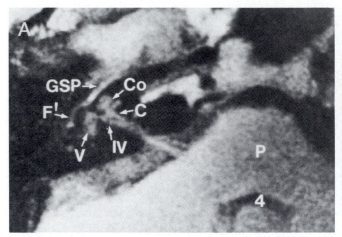 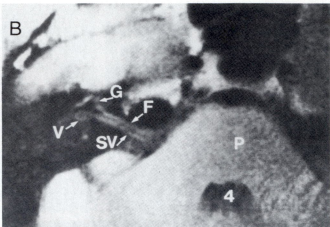

FIG 29–3.
Normal right ear, axial MRI. **A,** T1-weighted partial saturation scan, 350-ms TR, 256 × 256 matrix, four averages, 3 mm thick: cisternal and intracanalicular segments of the inferior vestibular *(IV)* and cochlear *(C)* nerves, vestibule *(V)*, cochlea, *(Co)*, horizontal segmental *(F)* of the facial nerve, and greater superficial petrosal nerve *(GSP)* contrast with the low-intensity signal from the cerebrospinal fluid and petrous bone. The cochlear nerve is anterior to the inferior vestibular nerve. *P* = pons; *4* = fourth ventricle. **B,** T1-weighted partial saturation scan, 350-ms TR, 256 × 256 matrix, two averages, 5 mm thick. The characteristic appearance of the facial nerve *(F)* and its geniculate ganglion *(G)* distinguishes it from the superior vestibular nerve *(SV)* coursing more posteriorly. *V* = vestibule; *4* = fourth ventricle. (From Daniels DL, Schenk JF, Foster T, et al: *AJR* 1985; 145:469–472. Used by permission.)

pending primarily on heredity and the presence of childhood infection, but both ears are usually symmetrical.[12] The aditus ad antrum is a narrow air passage between the attic (epitympanum) anteriorly and the mastoid antrum posteriorly (Fig 29–1,E). The antrum may be quite large; it is often divided superiorly by a thin bony partition, Körner's septum, which is a remnant of the petrosquamosal suture (Fig 29–2,C).[13]

The tympanic bone joins the mastoid to form the anterior and inferior bony external auditory canal and the nonarticulating portion of the mandibular fossa. The bony external canal, about 1.5 cm long, occupies two thirds of the entire canal; the lateral one third is cartilaginous (Figs 29–1,A and 29–2,E). The external canal may be somewhat S shaped and angled, so it is not in the coronal plane. Several sutures adjacent to the bony external canal should not be mistaken for fractures, particularly the tympanosquamosal and more medial petrosquamosal sutures, which are anterior to the canal.[14] The tympanic membrane attaches obliquely to a bony ring at the medial end of the external canal, so the canal is longer anteriorly and inferiorly. The majority of the tympanic membrane (pars tensa) has a middle fibrous layer. The wedge-shaped pars flaccida superiorly in the membrane lacks this middle fibrous layer, so it is more susceptible to retraction into the middle ear. Laterally, the tympanic membrane is covered by the

squamous epithelium of the external auditory canal; medially it is lined by middle-ear mucosa.

The middle ear is a small pyramidal air-containing space divided into the epitympanum above the level of the tympanic membrane, mesotympanum medial to it, and hypotympanum inferiorly. The middle-ear space is bounded by the tympanic membrane laterally, inner ear medially, tegmen superiorly, and floor inferiorly, which includes the bone covering the carotid artery and jugular vein. Anteriorly, the eustachian tube connects the middle ear to the nasopharynx to provide exchange of air and equalize pressure changes in the ear (see Fig 29–1,A). The posterior wall of the middle ear is quite complex and has a somewhat variable appearance. The facial recess, pyramidal eminence, sinus tympani, and round window niche occupy the posterior portion of the middle ear laterally to medially (Fig 29–1,A and B). More detailed discussion of middle-ear anatomy can be found in articles by Virapongse et al.,[13] Swartz,[15] and Mafee et al.[16]

The malleus, incus, and stapes are suspended in the middle ear to conduct sound from the vibrations of the tympanic membrane into the inner ear at the oval window. Main parts of the malleus are the head, a club-shaped structure in the attic, neck, and handle (manubrium), which attaches to the tympanic membrane (Figs 29–1,D and 29–2,F). The tensor tympani muscle originates anteriorly adjacent to the eustachian tube; its tendon turns across the middle ear and inserts on the neck of the malleus (Fig 29–1,C). The incus, shaped like an anvil, is posterior to the malleus. The body of the incus articulates with the malleus head in the attic (Fig 29–1,E), and the short process projects posteriorly into the fossa incudis, a space just below the aditus (Fig 29–1,D). The long process extends inferiorly parallel to the malleus handle (Figs 29–1,B and 29–2,E). The lenticular process, at the end of the long process, articulates with the capitulum of the stapes. The stapes consists of the capitulum, two crura, and the footplate, which is held in the oval window of the vestibule by the annular ligament. The footplate is not normally visible even with CT. However, the two crura can be identified with thin high-resolution scans, particularly in the axial plane (Fig 29–1,C). The stapedius tendon originates from the pyramidal eminence and extends forward to attach to the posterior crus of the stapes. Superior, lateral, and anterior malleal ligaments, which help suspend the ossicles, may be seen with CT.[15, 17] Other normal ligaments and mucosal folds are important in middle-ear inflammatory disease, but they are not seen unless abnormally thickened.[16]

The inner ear contains organs of both hearing and balance in a complex arrangement. Abnormalities of the inner ear are seen only indirectly due to changes in the bony labyrinth, which encases the membranous labyrinth. The membranous labyrinth, filled with endolymph, is composed of the utricle and saccule in the vestibule, semicircular canals, cochlear duct, and the endolymphatic duct and sac. These structures are connected by several small ducts. The sensory portion of the inner ear is in the membranous labyrinth; it is surrounded by perilymph in the bony labyrinth.

The cochlea is responsible for sensorineural hearing by converting vibrations of the endolymph into electrical impulses, which are transmitted to the eighth nerve. The snail-shaped cochlea, consisting of 2½ to 2¾ turns, is in the anterior-inferior portion of the inner ear; it can be seen well in both coronal and axial scans (Figs 29–1,A and C, and 29–2, D and F). The round window opening in the basal turn is covered by a membrane to allow counterpulsation of the vibrations initiated by stapes footplate motion (Fig 29–2,C).

The vestibule is an oval structure behind the cochlea and contains the oval window (Figs 29–1,D and 29–2,C). Sound pulsations first enter the inner ear through stapes vibrations in the oval window (Fig 29–2,D). The semicircular canals are connected at both ends to the vestibule.

Balance is controlled by the posterior, superior, and lateral semicircular canals, which are perpendicular to each other and are oriented to the axis of the petrous pyramid, so they are not in true coronal, axial, or sagittal planes (Figs 29–1,B and D, and F and 29–2,A, B, and D). The canals connect with the vestibule at both ends by five openings since the superior and posterior canals share one opening, the common crus. The arcuate eminence is a bulge on the upper surface of the temporal bone above the superior semicircular canal.

The internal auditory canal transmits the seventh and eighth nerves between the cerebellopontine angle cistern and the inner ear (Figs 29–1,D and 29–2,E). The canals are usually oriented in a nearly coronal plane with parallel walls, but variations occur. They may angle posteriorly, flare medially at the porus acusticus, or bulge in the midportion. Any variability should be symmetrical within 2 mm. The falciform crest, a bony partition that separates the superior and inferior portions of the canal laterally, is often visible on coronal scans (Fig 29–2,E). Four separate nerves occupy the internal canal: the superior and inferior vestibular nerves in the posterior canal, the cochlear nerve in the anterior inferior canal, and the facial nerve in the anterior superior canal (Fig 29–3). The nerves leave the internal canal through multiple openings at or near its lateral end.

The intratemporal facial nerve is divided into labyrinthine, tympanic, and mastoid segments, with two genus or bends dividing them. The nerve exits the internal canal in the first or labyrinthine portion of the facial canal and arcs anteriorly above the cochlea. This portion of the canal is easily seen in axial sections (Fig 29–1,E), and it appears as the medial of two holes above the cochlea in coronal scans (Fig 29–2,F). The opening between the internal canal and the labyrinthine segment is the narrowest part of the facial nerve canal.[18] At the first genu, anterior to and above the cochlea, the geniculate ganglion is formed, and the greater superficial petrosal nerve passes anteriorly. The facial nerve bends back upon itself, going posteriorly first above the cochlea, then along the medial wall of the middle ear under the lateral semicircular canal and above the stapes (Fig 29–2,E). A thin bony covering over the nerve in the middle ear may be normally dehiscent, sometimes allowing the nerve to protrude into the middle ear.[19] At the second genu, behind the middle ear, the nerve bends inferiorly down through the mastoid in its vertical segment. The facial nerve passes out of the temporal bone at the stylomastoid foramen, after which it soon enters the parotid (Fig 29–2,A and B).

The cochlear aqueduct lies below the internal auditory canal (Fig 29–2,B). The medial portion of the aqueduct may be quite large and funnel shaped, thus causing confusion with the medial internal canal on axial scans. They can be easily differentiated in the coronal plane. The lateral end of the aqueduct near the cochlea is not normally visible. The cochlear aqueduct allows theoretical communication between CSF and perilymph in the cochlea. The vestibular aqueduct is a narrow bony canal that contains the endolymphatic duct. The duct connects the endolymphatic sac on the posterior surface of the temporal bone to the vestibule. The course of the vestibular aqueduct is best identified in the sagittal plane as it travels superiorly and anteriorly. The diagnosis of a small vestibular aqueduct cannot be made with CT, but in some inner-ear anomalies, the aqueduct may be enlarged and easily seen (see Fig 29–8).

The carotid artery loops beneath the cochlea as it enters the skull base. The thin bone separating the artery from the hypotympanum is visible in the coronal plane (Fig 29–2,F). An absence of this bone implies a congenital anomaly of the artery. A spur of bone seen on low axial or sagittal scans separates the carotid artery from the jugular vein posteriorly.

The jugular vein is visible under the vestibule in coronal scans (Fig 29–2,C). Right and left veins often vary in size, with the right being larger in about three fourths of patients,[20] but a bony covering should separate even a large jugular vein from the middle ear. The jugular foramen is just posterior and inferior to the temporal bone. The jugular vein is in the larger pars venosa along with the vagus nerve and spinal accessory nerve. Anteromedially, the inferior petrosal sinus and glossopharyngeal nerve occupy the pars nervosa. Like the jugular veins, the jugular foramina are often asymmetrical, with the right usually being larger.[21]

MRI, particularly with surface coils, can evaluate nerves in the internal auditory canal and jugular foramen better than CT can (Fig 29–3).[6, 22] The course of the facial nerve can also be studied with MRI,[8] but MRI is poor for directly visualizing bony structures such as ossicular erosions in inflammatory disease. MRI does have some use for studying the normal fluid-filled inner-ear structures.[23]

CONGENITAL ANOMALIES

Congenital anomalies of the temporal bone are quite variable, both anatomically and in the type and severity of resulting hearing loss. Abnormalities causing conductive hearing loss are amenable to detection by CT, but patients with sensorineural hearing loss may appear radiographically normal. Sensorineural hearing loss may be congenital or acquired, of genetic or nongenetic etiology. Half of sensorineural deafness is estimated to be congenital in origin.[24]

Congenital malformations usually affect either the middle and external ear or the inner ear because of their varying embryology. The external auditory canal originates when the first branchial groove invaginates to form the cartilaginous canal at 6 weeks of fetal age. The medial external canal and the outer surface of the tympanic membrane develop by canalization of an epithelial core of cells. Connective tissue around the core ossifies at about 12 weeks and creates the tympanic bone. The auricle develops around the first branchial groove from six hillocks of tissue on the first and second branchial arches; these fuse by the third fetal month. The ossicular chain is formed from the first and second branchial arches, forerunners of the ossicles being produced at weeks 5 to 11 and more mature ossicles developing between weeks 11 to 26.[25] The first branchial arch (Meckel's cartilage) forms the malleus head, tensor tympani muscle and tendon, and the body and short process of the incus. The stapedius muscle and tendon, remainder of the ossicles except the stapes footplate, the mandibular condyle, facial canal, and styloid process develop from the second branchial arch (Reichert's cartilage). The first pharyngeal pouch becomes the pneumatized portion of the temporal bone at 22 to 30 weeks.

The inner ear originates earlier than the middle ear as the otic placode invaginates at 3 weeks to become the otic vesicle. The membranous labyrinth begins to develop at 5 weeks, reaching nearly adult size at 25 weeks. The osseous labyrinth forms from 14 ossification centers from cartilage between 16 to 23 weeks, and it also reaches adult dimensions by midpregnancy. The medial stapes footplate and annular ligament also originate with the inner ear.[25]

Because of their similar embryology, malformations of the external ear, external auditory canal, and middle ear usually occur concomitantly. Often, the malformations are obvious on clinical examina-

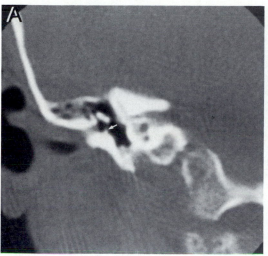
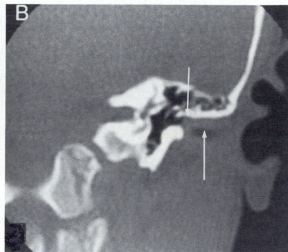

FIG 29–4.
Small external auditory canals (CT scan). **A,** right coronal scan, co-chlear level. The small external canal is filled with soft tissue. The malleus handle is fused to the bony prominence *(arrow).* There is no complete bony atresia plate. **B,** left coronal scan, vestibular level. The small external canal is filled with soft tissue *(arrows).*

tion, and they may be unilateral or bilateral. Soft-tissue atresia of the external auditory canal is less common than tympanic bone hypoplasia is, which produces a small or absent bony canal (Fig 29–4). With tympanic bone hypoplasia, the medial end of the external canal is frequently occupied by a bony atresia plate of varying thickness in the position of the tympanic membrane (Fig 29–5,B), and the gle-noid fossa is correspondingly large posteriorly. Mastoid pneumatization tends to be inversely re-lated to the severity of the congenital malforma-tion, so well-developed mastoids may be seen with minor anomalies. Mastoid size also is a prognostic

factor for success of surgical reconstruction. The middle-ear space is often attenuated in these mal-formations, particularly posteriorly, and this leads to an abnormal course of the facial nerve in its sec-ond and third portions (Fig 29–5,A). The course of the nerve must be identified if reconstructive sur-gery is planned so that the nerve is not inadvert-ently injured. External auditory canal deformities have been classified as slight, moderate, or severe, depending upon the size of the mastoid and mid-dle-ear space, presence of ossicular anomalies, atresia plate thickness, and extent of tympanic bone hypoplasia.[26] Less obvious ossicular deformi-

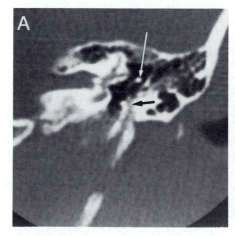
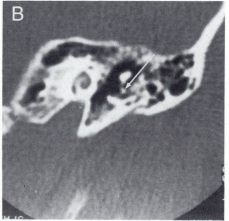

FIG 29–5.
Congenital anomaly of the external auditory canal, pinna, and mid-dle ear. **A,** coronal scan through the internal canal. The mastoid is well developed, and the incus appears normal *(white arrow).* The vertical portion of the facial nerve canal is anterior to the normal position *(black arrow).* **B,** the malleus handle is fused to the bony atresia plate *(arrow).* No external canal is present in either scan.

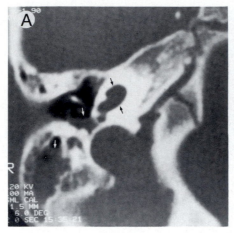 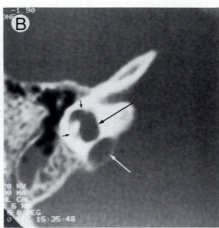

FIG 29–6.
Mondini malformation in a child with recent pneumococcal meningitis and ear infections. **A,** abnormal cochlea with a decreased number of turns *(black arrows),* fluid in the middle ear and mastoid *(white arrows).* **B,** a higher scan shows a large vestibule *(long black arrow)* and a short lateral semicircular canal with a dilated anterior limb *(short black arrows).* The jugular diverticulum protrudes behind the vestibule *(white arrow).*

ties can cause conductive hearing loss in patients who have normal-appearing ears; these dysplasias most commonly affect the distal incus and stapes.[25]

Inner ear malformations are usually isolated, although 11% to 30% are reported to occur together with middle- and external-ear anomalies.[26] Patients with congenital sensorineural hearing loss may be divided into those who have recognizable syndromes, those without any syndrome, and those with microtia.[24] The following syndromes may be associated with sensorineural hearing loss: Apert, Crouzon, Usher, Klippel-Feil, Waardenburg, Hurler, and cervico-oculo-acoustic dysplasia (Wildervanck syndrome). Other craniofacial dysplasias, chromosomal abnormalities, and maternal thalidomide ingestion may produce combined abnormalities of the external middle and inner ear.

There are four named inner-ear anomalies that produce sensorineural hearing loss. The Scheibe malformation, which affects only a portion of the membranous labyrinth, is considered the most common cause of hereditary hearing loss.[24] The Alexander malformation, aplasia of the cochlear duct, likewise has a normal bony labyrinth. The Michel anomaly, lack of development of the inner ear, is rare. The Mondini malformation in its pure form is a decrease in the number of cochlear turns. It may also be associated with other inner-ear abnormalities (Fig 29–6). If nerves to the inner ear do not develop normally, the internal auditory canal may be abnormally small (Fig 29–7). Unnamed malformations include a short broad lateral semicircular canal (which may not produce hearing

loss) and large vestibular or cochlear aqueducts (Fig 29–8). Patients with congenital inner-ear anomalies, particularly Mondini malformation, are at risk for developing meningitis due to potential abnormal communication between the CSF and middle ear.[27–29]

Congenital cholesteatomas, arising in the middle ear and elsewhere in the temporal bone from

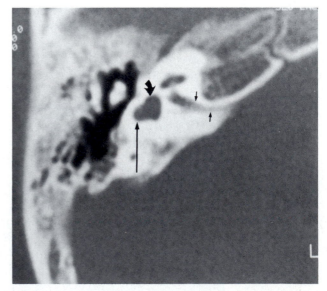

FIG 29–7.
Congenital inner-ear anomaly in a child with congenital right facial paralysis and sensorineural hearing loss. An abnormally small internal canal *(small arrows)* and a short broad lateral semicircular canal *(long arrow)* appear as the diverticulum of the vestibule *(curved arrow).* The cochlea, other semicircular canals, and the middle ear were normal.

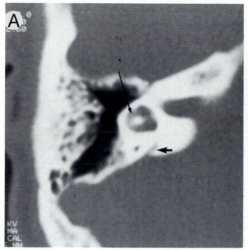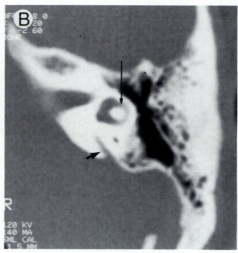

FIG 29–8.
Congenital inner-ear anomalies in a child studied for possible left cholesteatoma. Both lateral semicircular canals *(long arrows)* are short and broad, more so on the right **(A).** Vestibular aqueducts *(short arrows)* are also prominently larger on the left **(B).**

congenital epithelial inclusions, will be discussed under cholesteatomas.

Vascular malformations in the middle ear are important to detect before any surgery is performed. These anomalies may or may not be symptomatic. A high jugular bulb rising above the tympanic annulus occurs in 6% of patients.[30] Dehiscent bone over the dome of a large jugular bulb allows the vein to protrude into the middle ear (Fig 29–9). When this occurs, patients often have pulsatile tinnitus or conductive hearing loss. The bluish mass must not be mistaken for tumor such as glomus jugulare and operated upon. Other types of pathology causing the same appearance on physical examination are hemotympanum, cholesterol granuloma, and other vascular anomalies. The jugular bulb may have a diverticulum superomedially to the level of the internal auditory canal (see Fig 29–6,B), which rarely causes sensorineural hearing loss.[31]

Anomalies of the carotid artery also create pulsatile tinnitus and have severe sequelae if oper-

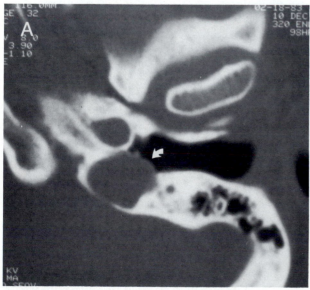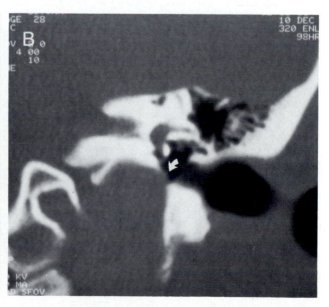

FIG 29–9.
Dehiscent jugular bulb in a woman with left pulsatile tinnitus. **A,** an axial scan through the left hypotympanum shows a large jugular bulb with dehiscent bone *(arrow).* **B,** a coronal scan also demonstrates absent bone *(arrow).*

ated upon unknowingly. These include aberrant carotid artery, persistent stapedial artery, and aneurysm.[32] Normally the vertical portion of the carotid artery, visible in coronal scans below the cochlea, is always covered by bone (Figs 29–2,F and 29–10,D). An absence of this normal appearance indicates an anomalous vessel. The ectopic internal carotid artery is considered the anastomosis of enlarged inferior tympanic and caroticotympanic arteries (Fig 29–10,A and C).[33] The artery enters the middle ear through a large inferior tympanic canaliculus, travels through the middle ear adja-

cent to the cochlea, and exits anteriorly to enter the horizontal portion of the carotid canal. A persistent stapedial artery may be associated with this malformation and is even more rare. The presence of this anomaly is indicated by enlargement of the lateral canal for the facial nerve above the cochlea (Fig 29–10,C) and absence of the foramen spinosum since the persistent stapedial artery forms the middle meningeal artery after leaving the middle ear.[34] Congenital or acquired aneurysms of the internal carotid artery may also occur in the middle ear.[35]

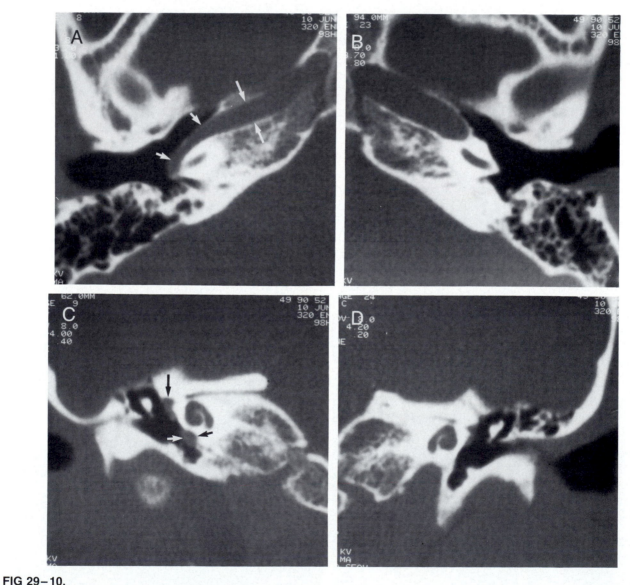

FIG 29–10.
Aberrant right carotid artery with a persistent stapedial artery. **A,** a low right axial scan shows an abnormal vessel in the middle ear *(short arrows)* continuous with the carotid canal *(long arrows).* **B,** normal left ear. **C,** an aberrant vessel erodes the bone of the co-chlea slightly on this coronal scan *(short arrows).* The enlarged facial nerve canal contains a persistent stapedial artery *(long arrow).* **D,** normal left ear.

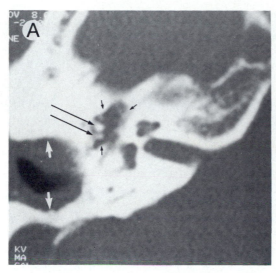 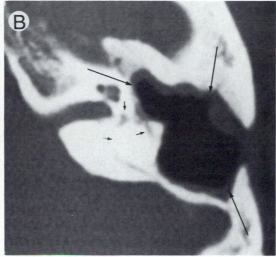

FIG 29–11.
Bilateral mastoidectomies and left labyrinthitis ossificans. **A,** a right mastoidectomy defect contains soft tissue *(white arrows).* The middle ear is opacified *(short black arrows).* The malleus and incus are still visible *(long black arrows).* **B,** a radical left mastoidectomy defect is lined with a small amount of soft tissue *(long arrows).* The vestibule and semicircular canals are obliterated by labyrinthitis ossificans *(short arrows).* The patient had a dead left ear.

INFLAMMATORY DISEASE

Otitis media is common, particularly in children. It may be serous, which is due to eustachian tube dysfunction, bacterial, or viral. Simple otitis media does not need radiologic evaluation, but complications should be studied. Acute otomastoiditis can lead to coalescent mastoiditis with bone destruction and allow infection to rupture through the mastoid tip (Bezold's abscess) or produce an extradural abscess. Other complications of otomastoiditis include meningitis, brain abscess, lateral sinus thrombosis, petrous apicitis, suppurative labyrinthitis, and facial nerve paralysis.[36] Lateral sinus thrombosis can lead to obstructed venous drainage from the brain and otitic hydrocephalus.[36, 37]

While most episodes of acute otitis media clear on treatment, more chronic sequellae also occur. Granulation tissue may form in the middle ear and produce a nonmobile soft-tissue density (Fig 29–11,A). Repeated hemorrhage in granulation tissue can lead to cholesterol granuloma formation.[38] The pathogenesis of cholesterol granuloma is debatable, but cholesterol crystals, old hemorrhage, and giant cells are present. The tympanic membrane frequently appears bluish due to the old hemorrhage.[16]

The tympanic membrane may be perforated, thickened, or retracted in patients with middle-ear inflammatory disease. The normal tympanic membrane is difficult to see on CT, so good visualization implies that it is thickened. Perforations and retraction pockets are not reliably seen on scans. Tympanosclerosis is another complication of repeated middle-ear infections. This may be of fibrous, calcified, and new bone types.[38] Tympanosclerosis most commonly involves the tympanic membrane, where small calcific deposits are visible (Fig 29–12,B). When tympanosclerosis affects the stapes, it is indistinguishable from otosclerosis. New bone formation usually occurs in the epitympanum.[39]

Chronic otitis media and tympanosclerosis can produce conductive hearing loss by ossicular fixation[39] or erosions, even in the absence of infection (dry ear).[40] Chronic ear disease has been divided into the tubotympanic and atticoantral types, which may coexist.[16] These areas are separated by the anterior and posterior tympanic isthmi.[16, 41] Mucosal folds in the middle ear, normally not visible with CT, separate the middle ear into compartments.[16] Obstruction of ventilation at the level of the tympanic isthmus may cause persistent fluid or mucosal disease in the mastoid even though eustachian tube function is normal.

CT is the method of choice to evaluate patients with middle-ear disease and its complications. Contrast is used if intracranial pathology is suspected. Fluid can be differentiated from nonmobile areas of opacification in the middle ear and mastoid by air-fluid levels and a change in the po-

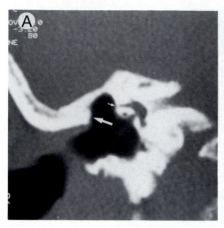
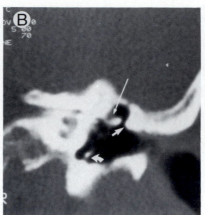
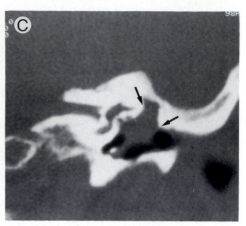

FIG 29–12.
Cholesteatoma with automastoidectomy in a middle-aged woman with a long history of bilateral draining ears. **A,** right automastoidectomy secondary to cholesteatoma. No ossicles are visible, and the lateral attic wall is eroded *(large arrow)*. The bone is thinned over the lateral semicircular canal *(small arrow)*. No fistula was present at surgery. **B,** the left ear has a small soft-tissue mass medial to the malleus *(long arrow)* and an eroded drum spur *(short arrow)*, both suggestive of cholesteatoma. There is a calcified tympanosclerotic focus in the tympanic membrane *(curved arrow)*. **C,** left ear 2½ years later. No surgery had been performed. A large cholesteatoma now fills much of middle ear and attic and has destroyed the ossicles *(arrows)*.

sition of fluid between axial and coronal scans. CT numbers are not useful to distinguish fluid since it may be serous or proteinaceous.[16] Granulation tissue cannot be reliably separated from cholesteatoma; they may be present simultaneously. A soft-tissue mass with ossicular erosion and a bulging tympanic membrane does correlate with cholesteatoma.[16, 42] Minor areas of bone erosion can be seen with chronic inflammatory disease without cholesteatoma, however.[16, 40] MRI is not satisfactory for middle-ear inflammatory disease because subtle bony abnormalities will not be shown.

Petrositis is infection of petrous apex air cells. It is an uncommon complication of middle-ear and mastoid infection, particularly with widespread use of antibiotics. Infection usually extends to the petrous apex via air cell tracts, although petrositis has been seen in very young children.[43] Gradenigo's syndrome, consisting of sixth-nerve paralysis, fifth-nerve pain, and suppurative otitis media, is a less common finding today in patients with petrositis.[44]

Labyrinthitis ossificans, obliteration of labyrinthine spaces by bone, is secondary to an insult to the inner ear, usually suppurative labyrinthitis. Spread of infection from the meninges, middle ear, or blood stream may cause suppurative labyrinthitis. Other causes of labyrinthitis ossificans include tumors, trauma, inner-ear hemorrhage, advanced otosclerosis, and surgery (Figs 29–11,B and 29–13).[45] Patients usually present with severe vertigo and hearing loss. During the acute infection,

the labyrinth will appear normal, but ossification develops over months or years to obliterate the bony cavities.[46] CT and possibly MRI are important to evaluate patients with labyrinthitis ossificans who are being considered for cochlear implants since the findings may determine the type of implant used or the probable surgical success (Fig 29–13).[23]

Malignant external otitis is an uncommon infection usually caused by *Pseudomonas aeruginosa* that occurs in immunocompromised or diabetic patients. It begins as infection with granulation tissue formation in the external auditory canal, at the junction of the bony and cartilaginous portions. Malignant external otitis is divided into early and late stages radiographically by the absence or presence of bone destruction.[47] Late disease with bone destruction is common when patients are radiographically evaluated (Fig 29–14,A). The infection may spread out of the temporal bone into the jugular foramen, temporomandibular joint, skull base, infratemporal fossa, and nasopharynx by extension along fascial planes and through foramina. An inflammatory nasopharyngeal mass due to this infection is indistinguishable from tumor except by history and histology (Fig 29–14,B). Facial nerve paralysis is usually caused by involvement of the horizontal rather than the vertical portion of the nerve,[47] or the nerve may be affected at or below the stylomastoid foramen.[48] Facial nerve paralysis is a grave prognostic sign; in a large series, half of patients who had facial nerve paralysis died.[49] CT

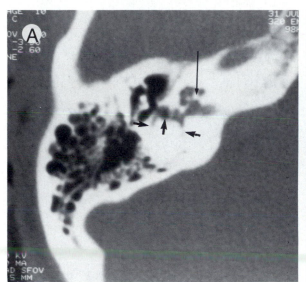

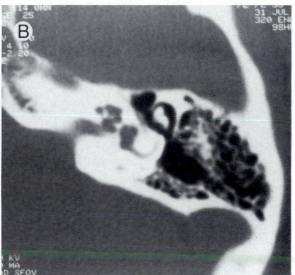

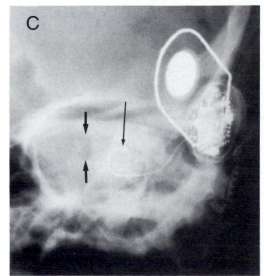

FIG 29–13.
Labyrinthitis ossificans with a cochlear implant in a woman with severe sensorineural hearing loss thought secondary to aminoglycoside therapy for liver and brain abscesses, but more likely due to central nervous system (CNS) infection itself. **A,** axial CT scan, right ear. The focus of calcification is in the cochlea *(long arrow),* and there is partial obliteration of the vestibule and semicircular canals *(short arrows).* **B,** the left ear shows less severe abnormalities. **C,** a 22-channel cochlear implant is seen to be coiled in the left cochlea *(long arrow)* on this postoperative anteroposterior (AP) film. The internal auditory canal is visible *(short arrows).*

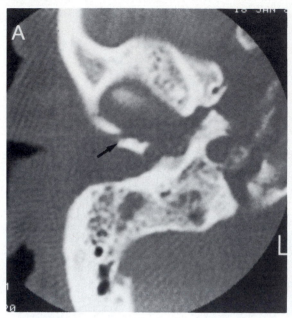 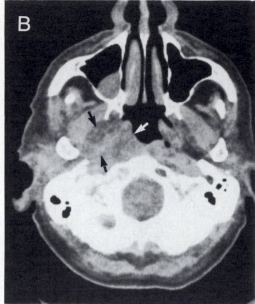

FIG 29-14.
Malignant external otitis (CT scan) in an elderly diabetic with a several-month history of right *Pseudomonas* external otitis. **A,** soft tissue fills the low external auditory canal and has destroyed the posterior bony wall of the temporomandibular joint *(arrow)*. **B,** a lower axial scan (no contrast) shows a mass and obliteration of fat planes in the nasopharynx *(arrows)*. Aggressive infection may be indistinguishable from tumor.

findings of malignant external otitis are not specific; the diagnosis is made by a combination of the radiographic and clinical findings. Nuclear scanning is important for diagnosis and follow-up of these patients. Technetium 99m bone scanning will detect osteomyelitis in the temporal bone and skull base earlier than CT will, but bone scan results remain positive even after infection has cleared. Gallium 67 citrate scans assess the activity of previously treated malignant external otitis.[50, 51]

CHOLESTEATOMA

CT has proved superior to complex-motion tomography to study patients with cholesteatoma. Soft-tissue information is better with CT and axial scans, is useful to evaluate the posterior middle-ear spaces and lateral semicircular canal, and is easily obtained.[52, 53]

Cholesteatoma is a sac lined by squamous epithelium and filled with keratinized debris. When this debris can no longer leave the sac, a mass forms. Cholesteatomas are either congenital (2%) or acquired (98%). Acquired cholesteatomas are further divided into those arising from perforation or retraction of the pars flaccida portion of the tympanic membrane (more common) or the pars tensa

portion. The latter patients have a history of previous middle-ear infection, while the former group may not.[41] The presence of squamous epithelium in the middle ear is usually attributed to epithelial migration from the external canal through a defect in the tympanic membrane.[54] Other etiologies including squamous metaplasia have also been proposed.[41] Negative middle-ear pressure due to eustachian tube dysfunction can produce an attic retraction pocket from the pars flaccida portion of the tympanic membrane. Adults with cholesteatoma usually have poorly developed mastoids, while children often have extensive mastoid pneumatization; this pneumatization may lead to more aggressive mastoid spread of cholesteatomas in children.[41] Bone destruction is present in the majority of patients with acquired cholesteatomas. The mechanical pressure theory of bone destruction has given way to theories of collagenase production, an osteoclast stimulator, and associated inflammation.[41, 54]

Pars flaccida cholesteatomas begin in Prussak's space, between the head of the malleus and body of the incus medially and the upper tympanic membrane and lower lateral attic wall laterally. With CT, a soft-tissue density of only several millimeters can be recognized in this region. Pars flaccida cholesteatomas typically displace the ossicles

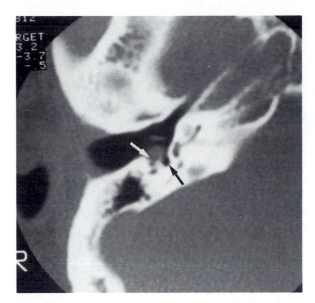

FIG 29–15.
Cholesteatoma (CT scan). A small cholesteatoma is present in the right posterior middle ear in a man who previously had left radical mastoidectomy for cholesteatoma. The mass spares the sinus tympani *(black arrow)* but fills the facial recess *(white arrow)*. The long process of the incus is eroded.

medially. Bone destruction is common with these cholesteatomas, usually involving the drum spur (scutum) and long process of the incus. The stapes superstructure, incus body, and malleus head may also be eroded.[41, 55]

Pars tensa cholesteatomas arise from central perforations or posterior superior retraction pockets. The central cholesteatomas usually displace the ossicles laterally, while the posterior lesions often extend into the posterior recesses of the middle ear. The sinus tympani, medial to the pyramidal eminence, is of particular importance to the surgeon because it is not readily visualized during middle-ear exploration (Fig 29–15). Pars tensa cholesteatomas also frequently erode the ossicles and cause conductive hearing loss (see Fig 29–12,C).

Two significant complications of middle-ear cholesteatomas are exposure of the horizontal portion of the facial nerve and erosion into the lateral semicircular canal to create a fistula (Fig 29–16). The facial nerve is difficult or impossible to differentiate in the middle ear unless it has air adjacent to it or a well-defined bony covering, so the diagnosis of bone erosion over the facial canal is frequently inaccurate even with CT.[56] Cortical destruction of the lateral semicircular canal is seen best with an axial scan plane +30 degrees to the infraorbitomeatal line.[2, 56] Coronal scans also demonstrate erosion, but a false-positive diagnosis can be made if the scan is through the anterior limb of the canal rather than its midportion. Other complications of cholesteatoma include extension into the inner ear (Fig 29–17) and automastoidectomy when sufficient bone erosion has occurred to allow the squamous debris to exit the ear (Figs 29–12,A and 29–18). This may appear as postsurgical change in a patient with no surgical history.[56] Cholesteatomas may become infected and produce the same complications described with acute otomastoiditis (Fig 29–19).

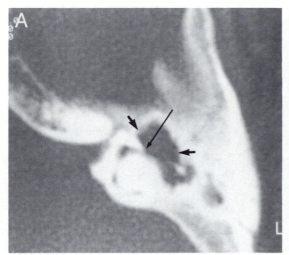
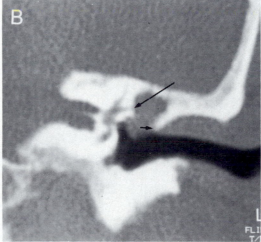

FIG 29–16.
Cholesteatoma with a lateral semicircular canal fistula. The patient became dizzy with left-ear manipulation. **A,** an axial CT scan shows erosion of the anterior limb of the lateral semicircular canal *(long arrow)*. Abnormal soft tissue fills an enlarged attic and aditus *(short arrows)*. **B,** erosion is also seen in this coronal scan *(long arrow)*. The drum spur is eroded *(short arrow)*, and no ossicles are present.

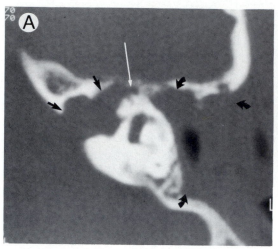

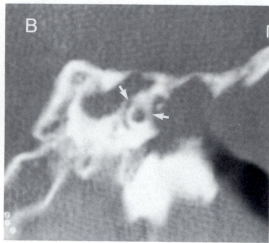

FIG 29–17.
Extensive cholesteatoma in a young man who had previous surgeries for left cholesteatoma, a dead ear, and facial nerve paralysis. **A,** abnormal soft tissue fills the mastoidectomy defect *(curved black arrows).* Cholesteatoma erodes anteriorly through the region of the geniculate ganglion *(white arrow)* medially into the petrous apex and internal auditory canal *(straight black arrows).* **B,** encroachment of cholesteatoma on the cochlea *(arrows)* is seen in this coronal scan.

It is important to understand the postoperative mastoid since many patients will be studied for recurrent disease or cholesteatoma in the opposite ear. Mastoidectomy may be of the closed or open cavity types. Closed cavity types include the simple mastoidectomy (rarely used now) and the intact canal wall operation. Tympanoplasty and middle-ear exploration can be performed without taking down the external auditory canal wall and creating a mastoid cavity, but surgical exposure is decreased, and there is a higher recurrence rate of cholesteatoma with this procedure. In the open cavity mastoidectomy, a mastoid bowl is formed, and the posterior bony external canal wall is removed. During radical mastoidectomy, the tympanic membrane and all ossicles except the stapes are removed. Modified radical mastoidectomy combines tympanoplasty and ossicular preservation or reconstruction. There are five basic types of tympanoplasty, which are classified by the amount

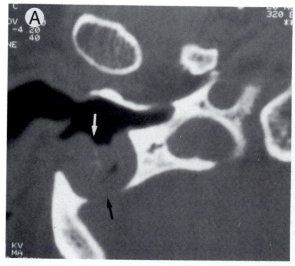

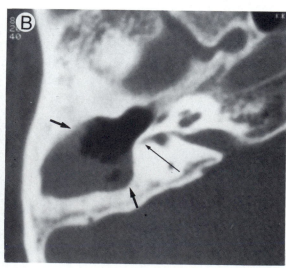

FIG 29–18.
Cholesteatoma in an elderly woman with no prior ear surgery and a chronic draining ear. **A,** a low right axial CT scan shows erosion into the sigmoid sinus *(black arrow)* and posterior inferior external auditory canal *(white arrow).* **B,** a large cavity with abnormal soft tissue seen on a higher scan *(short arrows).* There is no erosion of the lateral semicircular canal *(long arrow).* The entire canal is not seen because of the scan angle.

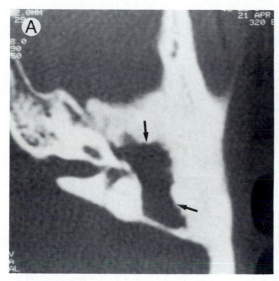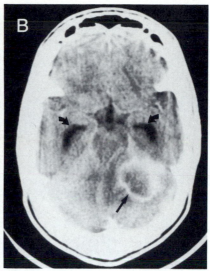

FIG 29–19.
Cholesteatoma with brain abscess. A young man with known cho-lesteatoma who had previously refused surgery was admitted with posterior fossa signs. **A,** extensive mastoid erosion from cho-lesteatoma *(arrows).* **B,** a left cerebellar abscess *(straight arrow)* produces hydrocephalus with dilated temporal horns *(curved arrows).*

of ossicular bypass.[57] Baseline axial CT scans should be performed in patients who are at high risk for recurrent cholesteatoma (particularly those who have had an intact canal wall procedure) about 3 months after surgery.[57, 58] It is usually impossible to distinguish recurrent cholesteatoma from granulation tissue or fibrosis in the operated ear when there is diffuse soft tissue (Figs 29–11,A

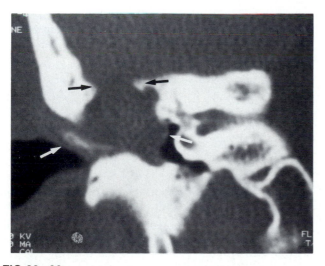

FIG 29–20.
Recurrent cholesteatoma and brain herniation in a 29-year-old man with a history of three previous ear operations, the last 10 years earlier, and a stenotic external auditory canal. The external canal, mastoid, and attic are filled with abnormal soft tissue *(white arrows)* that consisted of fibrotic tissue, recurrent cholesteatoma, and temporal lobe (indistinguishable). A large tegmen defect *(black arrows)* allowed the brain to herniate into the mastoid.

and 29–20). A localized mass is usually recurrent cholesteatoma, however.

Synthetic ossicular replacements are also used in middle-ear surgery, including stapes prostheses (often wire) and partial or total ossicular replacement prostheses (PORP, TORP). These can usually be discerned in the pneumatized ear, but if granulation tissue or cholesteatoma is present, they may be invisible.[59, 60] Tympanostomy tubes may or may not be identifiable, depending on the type of tube and the pneumatization of the middle ear. The easiest tube to see is a metallic bobbin.[57]

External auditory canal cholesteatomas are unrelated to middle-ear cholesteatomas, although they also may be congenital or acquired. Most external canal cholesteatomas are secondary to trapping of epithelium during otologic surgery (Figs 29–21 and 29–22). They can also be complications of temporal bone fracture.[61, 62] *Keratosis obturans* is a term that has been used synonymously with external canal cholesteatoma,[63] but recent otologic literature distinguishes the two. Keratosis obturans is a lamellar plug of keratin in the external canal, while cholesteatoma invades bone and is filled with randomly arranged keratin debris.[64]

Congenital cholesteatoma is thought to occur from ectopic ectodermal rests, although other theories have been proposed.[65] It is found at multiple sites in the temporal bone, including the middle ear, external auditory canal, mastoid, and petrous apex. These epidermoid cysts also arise intracranially, particularly in the cerebellopontine angle.[41] A

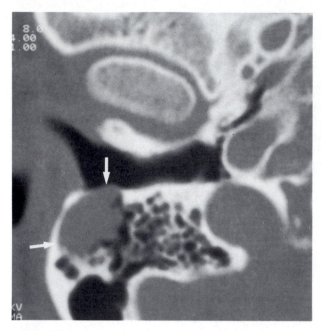

FIG 29–21.
Mastoid cholesteatoma, axial CT scan, right ear. This patient had a previous tympanoplasty, so the cholesteatoma is probably acquired (iatrogenic). A soft-tissue mass in the mastoid erodes into the posterolateral bony external auditory canal *(arrows)*.

middle-ear cholesteatoma is considered congenital if a pearly tumor is seen behind an intact tympanic membrane in a patient with no history of middle-ear disease (Fig 29–23).[66] Most cases present in childhood, and bone destruction can occur as with

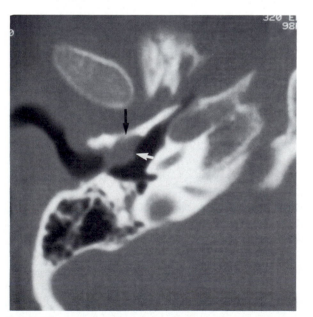

FIG 29–22.
External canal cholesteatoma. This patient had a previous tympanoplasty, so the cholesteatoma is almost certainly iatrogenic. A mass abuts the tympanic membrane *(white arrow)* and erodes the anterior bony canal *(black arrow)*.

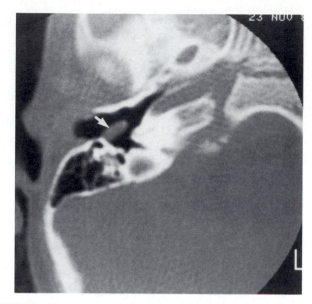

FIG 29–23.
Congenital cholesteatoma (CT scan) in a child with a pearly mass behind an intact right tympanic membrane *(arrow)* without a history of ear infection.

acquired lesions. Sometimes it is impossible to distinguish congenital from acquired cholesteatoma. Cranial nerve palsies, particularly facial palsy, are caused by petrous apex cholesteatomas. The typical CT appearance of a petrous apex cholesteatoma (epidermoid) is a nonenhancing mass that is slightly less dense than brain and smoothly erodes bone (Fig 29–24).

Another petrous apex lesion, cholesterol granuloma, may appear similar to congenital cholesteatoma and produce identical clinical findings, but its origin and treatment are different (Fig 29–25). The cholesterol granuloma (also called a giant cholesterol cyst)[67] forms as it does in the middle ear, secondary to obstructed ventilation, inflammation, hemorrhage, and foreign-body reaction. It probably arises in a pneumatized petrous apex since in one series the opposite petrous apex frequently contained air cells.[68] The cholesterol granuloma contains brownish fluid, while a cholesteatoma is filled with white keratin. Both lesions produce smooth cystic erosion of bone. The cholesterol granuloma is typically isodense in a normal brain on CT, while cholesteatoma is usually hypodense. A cholesteatoma must be surgically removed, but a cholesterol granuloma can be drained into an adjacent air space. MRI can distinguish epidermoid from cholesterol granuloma; epidermoid has a low signal on T1-weighted images and a high signal on T2-weighted images, while cholesterol granuloma is bright on both pulse sequences.[69, 70] The bright signal of the cholesterol

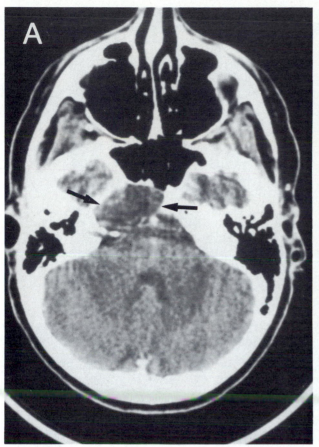

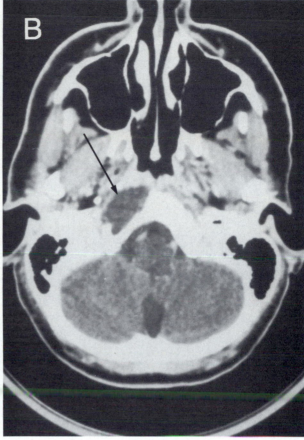

FIG 29–24.
Congenital cholesteatoma (epidermoid), petrous apex, in a 34-year-old woman with right sixth-nerve paresis. **A,** a large smooth-walled mass erodes the right petrous apex and adjacent clivus *(ar-* *rows)*. The CT density is slightly less than adjacent brain. **B,** a scan 2 cm lower demonstrates a mass extending through the skull base *(arrow)*.

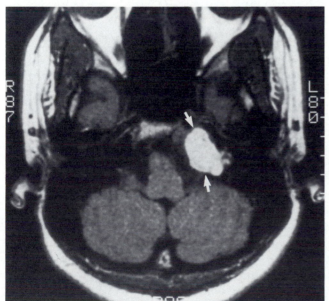

FIG 29–25.
Cholesterol granuloma in a young woman with progressive left hearing loss and tinnitus for 6 months. T1-weighted MRI (TR 600, TE 25, 256 × 256 matrix, 3-mm slice, 2 NEX [number of excitations]) shows a bright expansile mass in the left petrous apex *(arrows)*.

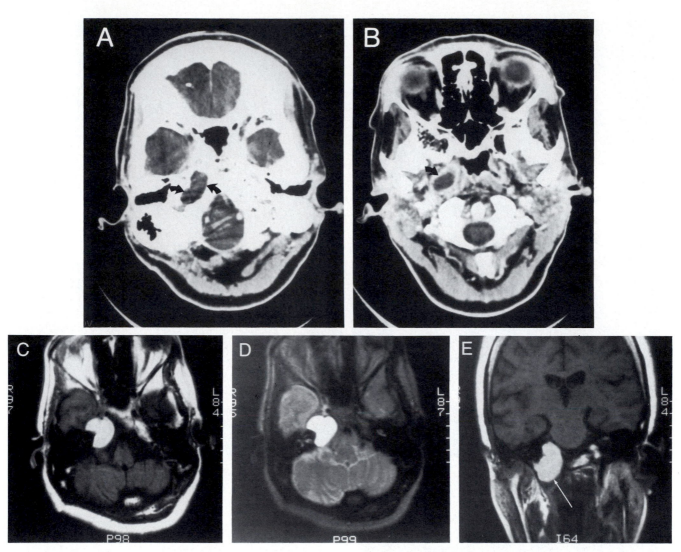

FIG 29–26.
Petrous apex mucous cyst in a middle-aged woman with a history of headache, progressive facial weakness, right sixth-nerve paresis, and posterior fossa surgery 20 years earlier for a temporal bone cystic lesion. **A,** axial CT scan through the skull base. A low-attenuation smooth-walled expansile lesion is present *(arrows).* **B,** a scan 2.5 cm lower shows a cyst extending down to the parapha-ryngeal space *(arrow).* **C,** T1-weighted axial MRI (TR 600, TE 20, 256 × 256 matrix, 5-mm slice, 2 NEX). The mass is very bright. **D,** T2-weighted MRI, same level (TR 2,500, TE 80). The mass remains bright. **E,** a coronal T1-weighted scan better demonstrates the inferior extent of the cyst *(arrow).* At surgery the cyst contained hemorrhage and mucin; it was lined with ciliated columnar epithelium.

granuloma is likely due to old hemorrhage. Other more rare petrous apex lesions include mucocele (Fig 29–26),[71, 72] dermoid,[73] aneurysm, cartilaginous or osseous neoplasms, and secondary bone destruction from contiguous masses or blood-borne lesions.[74]

OTODYSTROPHIES

Otosclerosis

Otosclerosis is a condition of unknown etiology found only in humans and affects the endochon-dral (middle) layer of the otic capsule. The name otospongiosis has been favored by many authors for this condition because the normal dense otic capsule bone is replaced by more vascular bone similar to haversian bone. Otosclerosis is often bilateral, and women are affected more often than men, whites more than nonwhites. The age range of those with otosclerosis is wide, although symptoms often develop in the second decade; two thirds present with tinnitus.[75] Otosclerosis is divided into fenestral and retrofenestral types. The oval and round windows are affected in the fenestral type, while retrofenestral otosclerosis involves

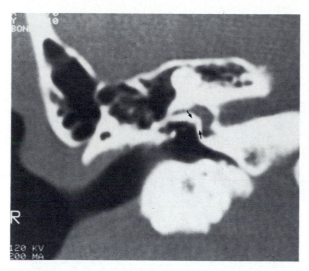

FIG 29–27.
Stapedial otosclerosis with marked bony overgrowth of the stapes footplate *(arrows)* on coronal CT of the right ear.

the remainder of the bony labyrinth.[75] In addition to tinnitus, symptoms include conductive hearing loss, sensorineural hearing loss, or mixed loss. Conductive hearing loss is commonly seen with stapes fixation in the oval window. The etiology of the sensorineural component of hearing loss is more debatable; theories include hyalinization of the spiral ligament of the cochlea,[75] cochlear nerve degeneration,[76] ototoxic factors, and hypoxemia due to venous congestion.[77] Some authors believe

that cochlear otosclerosis with pure sensorineural hearing loss never occurs.[77]

The most common site of an otosclerotic focus, occurring in 80% to 90% of patients, is the fissula ante fenestrum anterior to the oval window.[76] Early lesions of otosclerosis appear lytic, so the oval window may appear indistinct or enlarged. Eventually this vascular bone mineralizes and may lead to obliterative otosclerosis (filling in the oval window with bone) in a small percentage of patients (Fig 29–27).[75]

Cochlear otosclerosis is manifested by lytic foci in the otic capsule, most often around the cochlea, in patients with sensorineural or mixed hearing loss (Fig 29–28,B). CT densitometry has been proposed as a method to identify subtle areas of demineralization before they become visible.[78] Densitometry has also been used to study more advanced cases of cochlear demineralization.[79] Lesions in the cochlea have been shown to correlate with hearing loss documented on audiograms.[80] The areas of demineralization may be subtle or may form an obvious halo around the cochlea (Fig 29–29).[77, 79] When otospongiotic foci mature and remineralize, they are difficult to detect. The bone density is the same as that of the normal otic capsule, but occasionally slight thickening or irregularity is visible.[77, 80]

Patients suspected of having both stapedial and cochlear otosclerosis should be evaluated with

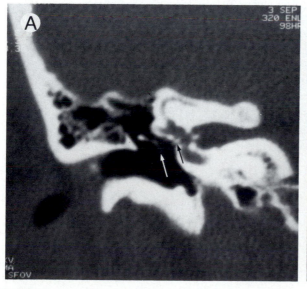 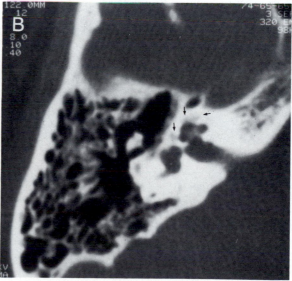

FIG 29–28.
Otosclerosis in a young woman with mixed hearing loss, status poststapedectomy. **A,** coronal scan, right ear. A wire prosthesis is attached to the long process of the incus *(white arrow)* and in the oval window *(black arrow)*. **B,** an axial scan shows small areas of cochlear capsule demineralization *(arrows)*.

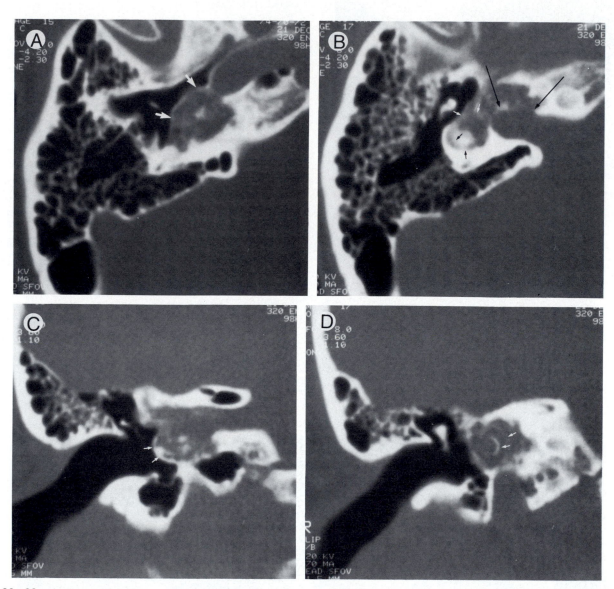

FIG 29–29.
Probable otosclerosis in a young woman with severe sensorineural hearing loss bilaterally and no other evidence of osteogenesis imperfecta or syphilis. Temporal bone abnormalities were bilaterally symmetrical. **A,** axial CT scan, cochlear level, right ear. Severe lytic changes make the cochlea unrecognizable *(arrows)*. **B,** a higher scan shows similar lysis of bone around the internal auditory canal *(long black arrows),* vestibule *(white arrows),* and lateral semicircular canal *(short black arrows).* **C,** coronal scan at the oval window level. The vestibule, superior semicircular canal, and lateral internal canal are difficult to discern. The basal turn of the cochlea is thin but present *(arrows).* **D,** a coronal scan through the cochlea shows a ghost of cochlear coils *(arrows)* surrounded by lytic bone.

CT since the diagnosis can usually be made in both types of otosclerosis and other pathology can be distinguished. The differential diagnosis of stapedial otosclerosis (conductive hearing loss in a normal-appearing ear) includes congenital stapes fixation, ossicular anomalies, traumatic ossicular disruption, tympanosclerosis, and congenital attic cholesteatoma.[75] Lytic changes in the otic capsule similar to those of cochlear otosclerosis can be produced by Paget's disease, syphilitic osteitis, and osteogenesis imperfecta. The latter two conditions are indistinguishable from otosclerosis radiographically.

Patients with a poor result following surgery for stapedial otosclerosis should be studied with CT. Various types of prostheses are in use for stapes replacement, including 35-gauge wire, stainless steel, and synthetic materials. The stainless steel piston prosthesis is not often used now, but it is the easiest to see on CT scans (Fig 29–30). Visualization of all components of the thin-wire or synthetic prostheses is difficult. (see Fig 29–28, A).[81] Complications of stapes surgery include incus necrosis where the prosthesis is crimped onto the long process, granuloma formation, regrowth of otosclerosis across the oval window, prosthesis subluxation (usually posterior and inferior), vertigo, perilymph fistula, and protrusion of a long prosthesis into the vestibule.[81] Some physicians have considered a stapes prosthesis to be a contraindication for MRI, but one study evaluated seven types of metallic prostheses in a 1.5-tesla magnet and found no movement of any kind.[82]

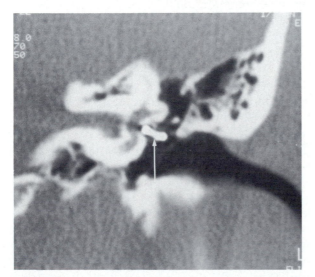

FIG 29–30.
Stapedectomy wire piston prosthesis: an unusually large metallic prosthesis following stapedectomy for otosclerosis *(arrow).*

Paget's Disease

Paget's disease (osteitis deformans) is a progressive condition of unknown etiology that affects primarily the axial skeleton of older adults. Recent experimental evidence suggests that viral infection in osteoclasts produces Paget's disease.[83] There are both lytic and proliferative phases, and the skull is involved in 28% to 70% of patients.[84] The initial lytic phase is followed by disorderly bone formation, the appearance of which varies between individuals. Temporal bone involvement is less frequent than calvarial disease and usually occurs with it. Paget's disease can produce conductive hearing loss by stapes thickening or fixation, sensorineural loss, or mixed hearing loss. The lytic phase predominates in the temporal bone, affects the petrous portion first, and progresses laterally (Fig 29–31).[85] The otic capsule is most resistant to lytic changes. A basilar impression, with upward angulation of the temporal bones, may result from skull base Paget's disease. During the reparative phase, thickened new bone can narrow normal lumina. CT accurately demonstrates the lytic and sclerotic phases of Paget's disease. It may occasionally be difficult to distinguish Paget's disease from otosclerosis, luetic osteitis, labyrinthitis ossificans, or metastatic disease on the basis of temporal bone findings alone, but examination of the remainder of the skull and the patient's history should clarify the situation.

Fibrous Dysplasia

Normal cancellous bone is replaced by abnormal tissue containing variable amounts of fibrous and osseous elements in patients with fibrous dysplasia. This condition, of unknown etiology, may be monostotic, polyostotic, or manifested as the McCune-Albright syndrome, in which polyostotic fibrous dysplasia is associated with skin hyperpigmentation and endocrine disturbances.[86] Lesions of fibrous dysplasia usually develop in childhood or adolescence, and they often stabilize in adulthood.[87] Malignancy has rarely been reported in fibrous dysplasia lesions, but irradiation leads to increased malignant degeneration.[88] In the skull, fibrous dysplasia often affects adjacent bones of the skull base, particularly the frontal fossa. The bone is abnormally thick, and it frequently has a "ground-glass" appearance, but cystic areas of fibrous tissue also occur. The temporal bone is affected in about 18% of patients who have fibrous

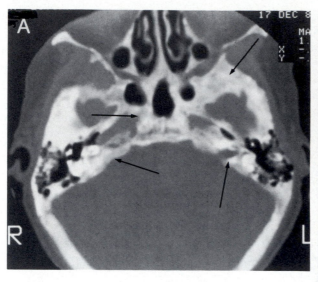
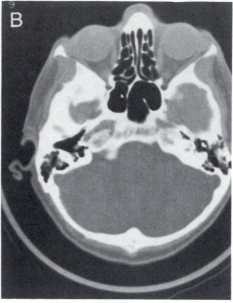

FIG 29–31.
Paget's disease. **A,** axial CT scan shows extensive skull base and temporal bone demineralization *(arrows)* in a 65-year-old woman with bilateral mixed hearing loss. **B,** remineralization after several years of treatment with diphosphonate.

dysplasia involving the skull.[89] Patients with fibrous dysplasia in the temporal bone often present with painless swelling over the mastoid; they may also have conductive hearing loss due to external canal or middle-ear stenosis (Fig 29–32). Differential diagnosis of the sclerotic temporal bone includes meningioma, metastasis, osteopetrosis, osteosarcoma, and ossifying fibroma as well as chronic mastoiditis.[90, 91] CT is the preferred radiologic method to evaluate the sclerotic temporal bone.

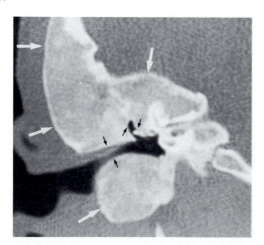

FIG 29–32.
Fibrous dysplasia in a teenager with a long history of conductive hearing loss and temporal swelling. There is markedly expanded bone of the mastoid, tympanic bone, and upper petrous pyramid with a "ground-glass" appearance *(white arrows).* The middle ear and external canal *(black arrows)* are narrow.

TRAUMA

Most temporal bone injuries are caused by moderately severe head trauma, often in motor vehicle accidents, but middle-ear injuries can also occur with blasts, barotrauma, iatrogenic causes, and patient-induced injury such as with cotton swabs. CT should be used to evaluate patients with post-traumatic hearing loss, whether acute or chronic. Thin high-resolution scans must be done because conventional 10-mm-thick sections do not reliably detect fractures.[92] High-resolution thin-section scans should be performed on patients who show mastoid and middle-ear blood on conventional scans since clinically occult fractures can be detected.[93] Most fractures will be visible on axial scans, but coronal or sagittal scans are also important. These can be obtained by reformatting multiple axial slices, particularly if the original scans are overlapped when the patient cannot cooperate for direct coronal scans.[94]

Temporal bone fractures have generally been classified as longitudinal or transverse, determined by whether the direction of the fracture line is parallel or perpendicular to the long axis of the temporal bone.[95] Complex fractures include elements of both types; atypical fractures fit into none of the categories.[93] An oblique classification is added by some authors.[96] Fractures have also been divided into labyrinthine, tympanolabyrinthine, and extralabyrinthine classifications.[97]

Longitudinal fractures, usually caused by temporoparietal blows, are much more common than transverse fractures are, and they are usually less severe. These fractures begin in the squamous portion of the temporal bone, extend anteromedially through the external canal, mastoid, and middle ear, and terminate in the region of the foramen lacerum (Fig 29–33).[92] Patients present with conductive hearing loss due to a torn tympanic membrane, hemotympanum, and/or ossicular injury. Mixed hearing loss indicates concomitant inner-ear trauma, either a fracture or concussive injury. The facial nerve is injured in 10% to 20% of patients with longitudinal fractures,[98] although one series had a significantly higher incidence of facial nerve deficit.[96] Facial weakness may be immediate, due to transection of the nerve or impingement of a bone fragment on it, but more commonly facial paralysis is delayed secondary to nerve compression by hematoma. The most common site of facial nerve injury is near the geniculate ganglion,[92, 93] but the entire course of the nerve must be studied closely, particularly if surgical decompression is planned. CSF otorrhea is a serious complication of longitudinal fractures and is usually associated with dural laceration at the tegmen tympani.[93]

Transverse fractures account for 10% to 20% of temporal bone fractures, often due to occipital or frontal trauma. These fractures cross the inner ear perpendicular to the petrous pyramid, either through the internal auditory canal (medial) or the bony labyrinth (lateral) (Fig 29–34).[93] If a lateral transverse fracture communicates with the middle ear, blood will be seen behind an intact tympanic membrane. Symptoms of transverse fracture include sensorineural deafness, vertigo, and facial paralysis (seen in 40% to 50% of patients).[92] Labyrinthine concussion without detectable fracture can also cause sensorineural hearing loss and vertigo. A dural tear in patients with transverse fractures may lead to CSF rhinorrhea (because the tympanic membrane is intact) or pneumocephalus (Fig 29–35).

Ossicular injuries are common with longitudinal fractures, but they are seen less often in patients who have transverse fractures. Ossicular fracture or dislocation can also occur without temporal bone fracture. Ossicular injury should be suspected when conductive hearing loss greater than 30 decibels (dB) persists after middle-ear blood and fluid have cleared, generally within 2 months.[99] The malleus is stabilized by its attachment to the tympanic membrane, the tensor tympani tendon, and the anterior and lateral mallear ligaments. The stapes footplate is firmly held in the oval window by the annular ligament and the stapedius tendon attached to the posterior crus. The incus, however, does not have similar structures to anchor it; it is suspended between the malleus and stapes at the incudomalleal and incudostapedial joints.[99] Incudostapedial joint subluxation is the most common ossicular injury, with or without fracture of the stapes crura. Separation of the incudomalleal joint is readily seen with axial CT (see Fig 29–33,A).

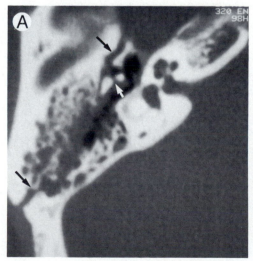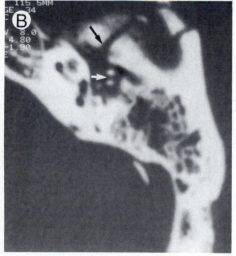

FIG 29–33.
Longitudinal temporal bone fractures. This patient had bilateral conductive hearing loss but no facial paralysis after a motor vehicle accident. **A,** an axial CT scan, right ear, shows a fracture line through the mastoid and attic *(black arrows)* with ossicular dislocation *(white arrow).* **B,** an axial scan, left ear, shows less severe anterior fractures *(black arrow)* and a malleus and incus in the normal position *(white arrow).*

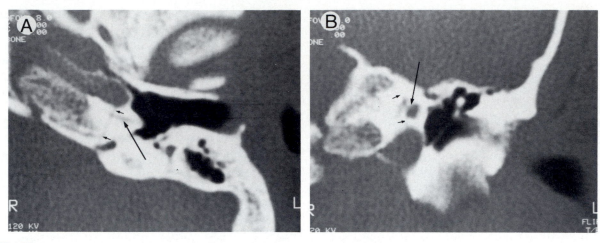

FIG 29–34.
Transverse petrous fracture. This man had a dead left ear following head trauma. A subtle fracture line *(short arrows)* extends through the cochlea *(long arrow)* on axial **(A)** and coronal **(B)** scans.

Stapediovestibular joint injury cannot be seen with CT[99] unless a pneumolabyrinth has developed (Fig 29–36).[100, 101] The resulting perilymph fistula from stapes footplate injury appears as nonspecific middle-ear fluid.

Fractures that do not fit the above general classification include fracture of the anterior wall of the external canal, linear mastoid fracture, and styloid process fracture (which may cause facial nerve paralysis). Foreign bodies such as bullets, shrap-

nel, and cotton swabs produce unpredictable ear injuries.

In addition to common complications of temporal bone trauma such as facial nerve paralysis and CSF leak due to a dural tear, less frequent complications also occur. Paralysis of the sixth or fifth cranial nerves, sigmoid sinus thrombosis, pneumocephalus, meningitis, persistent vertigo, and cholesteatoma may develop in these patients.

MRI has been used to study a small series of patients with temporal bone fractures. MRI could distinguish blood from CSF in the middle ear, and MRI detected more intracranial areas of hemorrhage than CT did. However, MRI did not show

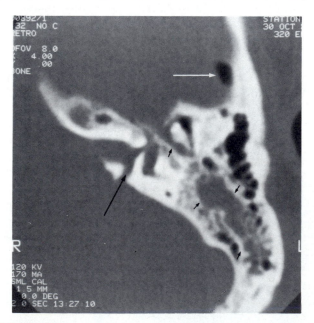

FIG 29–35.
Transverse petrous fracture. Following an assault, this patient had a dead left ear and facial paralysis. There was a fracture through the posterior wall internal auditory canal *(long black arrow)*, partial mastoid and middle-ear opacification *(short black arrows)*, and intracranial gas secondary to a dural tear *(white arrow)*.

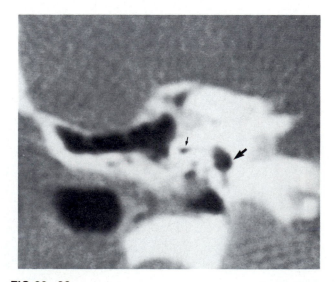

FIG 29–36.
Pneumolabyrinth. This patient had sudden hearing loss 1 week following ossicular replacement surgery. There is air in the vestibule and lateral semicircular canals *(arrows)*.

the fracture lines and ossicular injuries as well as CT did. A partially pneumatized middle ear led to false diagnoses of ossicular dislocation, so CT remains the method of choice to evaluate temporal bone trauma.[102]

BENIGN TUMORS

Acoustic Neuroma

Acoustic neuromas, which account for 80% to 90% of masses in the cerebellopontine angle, are benign tumors originating from cells of the eighth nerve sheath. The term *acoustic neuroma*, while in wide use, is misleading since the tumors are more properly called schwannomas. Most acoustic neuromas originate from the vestibular division of the eighth nerve. In the past, the superior vestibular nerve was thought to be the site of 90% of these tumors, but more recent studies suggest that only half arise from the superior vestibular nerve.[103] The insensitivity of tests for inferior vestibular nerve function accounts for the discrepancy. Most acoustic neuromas arise in the internal auditory canal and expand into the cerebellopontine angle, but a small percentage remain intracanalicular or arise on the nerve outside the canal.

Patients with acoustic neuroma typically present with asymmetrical sensorineural hearing loss and decreased discrimination. Tinnitus, dizziness, and vertigo are also frequent symptoms. Less often, patients suffer sudden hearing loss secondary to vascular compromise by the tumor.[104] Larger tumors expanding into the posterior fossa cause decreased fifth-nerve function (diminished corneal reflex or facial numbness), cerebellar signs, and hydrocephalus. Facial nerve weakness is an uncommon finding, even with large tumors, because the facial nerve is relatively resistant to compression.

Acoustic neuromas are more common in middle-aged patients, but they may occur in a wide age range. Patients with the central form of neurofibromatosis often have bilateral tumors and present earlier than do patients without neurofibromatosis (Fig 29–37). Central neurofibromatosis, an autosomal dominant inherited disorder, may have few or no peripheral manifestations.[105] Wide internal auditory canals secondary to dural ectasia may be seen in neurofibromatosis without acoustic neuroma.[106] In some young adults with acoustic neuromas, the tumors grow quite rapidly. The duration of symptoms and their severity does not al-

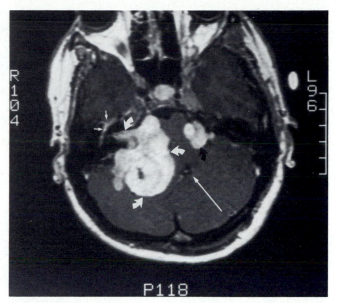

FIG 29–37.
Multiple acoustic neuromas in a young woman with neurofibromatosis who had right progressive hearing loss and facial weakness. A gadolinium-DTPA–enhanced, T1-weighted MR scan (TR 500, TE 20, 256 × 128 matrix, 3-mm slice, 2 NEX) shows a huge right acoustic neuroma filling the internal auditory canal, protruding into the cerebellum *(curved white arrows)*, and displacing the fourth ventricle *(long white arrow)*, smaller left acoustic neuroma *(black arrow)*, and abnormal enhancement of the right facial nerve *(short white arrows)*.

ways correlate with tumor size.[107] Growth rates of acoustic neuromas that have been followed varied from slow (long doubling time or no change) to moderate (doubling time between 205 and 545 days) (Fig 29–38).[108] A mean growth rate of 0.1 cm/yr (with a wide range of variation) was seen in a series of elderly patients whose acoustic neuromas were followed.[109] Unilateral acoustic neuroma not associated with neurofibromatosis has been reported under the age of 15 years in 15 patients, only 5 of whom were under age 10 years of age.[110] Multiple audiologic and radiologic tests have been used to identify individuals who have acoustic neuromas. After obtaining the audiogram, the most sensitive audiologic screening test is the auditory brain stem response (ABR), which is abnormal in 96% to 98% of patients with tumors.[111] There is a high false-positive rate for the test, however. Conventional x-rays and tomograms have no place in screening for acoustic neuroma. Contrast-enhanced CT has been the procedure of choice in the 1980s for detecting both the tumor and an enlarged internal auditory canal. With the approval of gadolinium-diethylenetriamine pentaacetic acid (DTPA) for clinical use, enhanced MRI has replaced CT as

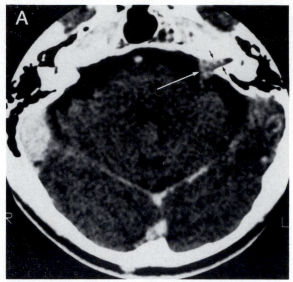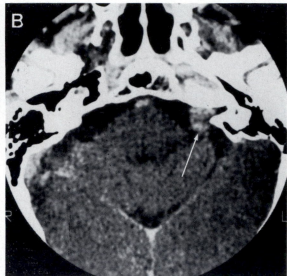

FIG 29–38.
Acoustic neuroma on CT scan. **A,** a 77-year-old man with an enhancing left acoustic neuroma in the internal canal *(black arrows)* and cerebellopontine angle cistern *(white arrow).* **B,** enlargement of the tumor *(arrow)* 1 year later.

the procedure of choice; its use will increase as scanners become more widely available.

On CT scans, an acoustic neuroma typically appears as an enhancing mass projecting into the cerebellopontine angle cistern from the internal auditory canal (Fig 29–38). Scans without contrast seldom add information because the tumors are isodense with brain and calcification is rare. Enhancement is sometimes inhomogenous, particularly in larger tumors. The differential diagnosis of cerebellopontine angle masses will be covered elsewhere. Thin sections (1.5 to 2 mm) through the internal canals are necessary to detect intracanalicular enhancement in a normal-sized canal. These scans must be reconstructed with a soft-tissue algorithm and viewed at a moderately narrow window to see the tumor well. Additional reconstructions with a bone algorithm can be done from the same scan data to see other inner-ear structures. The accuracy of CT in detecting small tumors has increased as the importance of high-resolution thin scans is recognized. A small percentage of acoustic neuromas will still be missed by CT, particularly those that remain intracanalicular and have not significantly enlarged the internal auditory canal.

The gold standard for excluding small acoustic neuromas has been gas CT cisternography, a technique first described in 1979.[112] This replaced posterior fossa myelography with iophendylate (Pantopaque). Water-soluble positive-contrast cisternography has not gained acceptance for identi-

fying acoustic neuromas because it is difficult to determine whether contrast enters the internal canal and because of occasional intracranial complications of the contrast. The technique of gas CT cisternography has been described by many authors. It involves injection of a small amount of gas into the lumbar subarachnoid space and positioning the gas into the affected cerebellopontine angle cistern. The major complication of the procedure is headache, which can be lessened by using a small needle for the lumbar puncture and keeping the patient flat for several hours after the scan. The anatomy of the cerebellopontine angle on gas CT cisternography has been well described.[113] Individual nerves or a nerve bundle is visible, as is a vascular loop frequently (Fig 29–39,A). Identification of individual nerves in the internal canal depends somewhat on the size of the canal; nerves are difficult to distinguish in small canals. A mass indenting the gas in the cerebellopontine angle cistern almost certainly represents tumor (Fig 29–39,B). However, a number of causes of false-positive cisternograms (nonfilling of the internal canal with gas) have been reported. In these instances, the edge adjacent to the gas is seldom convex. A meniscus effect at the interface between the gas and CSF in the internal canal is probably the most common cause of nonfilling of the canal.[114] This problem can be reduced by tapping on the patient's head to dislodge fluid in the canal or repositioning the head. Other causes of false-positive

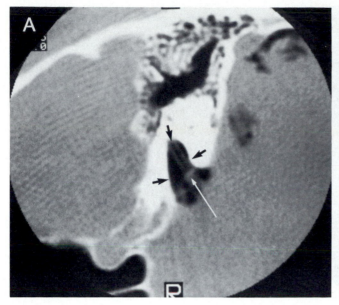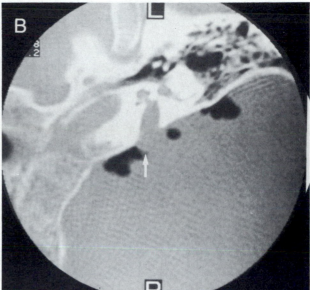

FIG 29–39.
CT/air cisternogram of acoustic tumor. **A,** normal left air cisterno-gram of a patient in the decubitus position. Air surrounds nerves in the internal auditory canal extending to the fundus of the canal *(black arrows).* A vascular loop is visible *(white arrow).* **B,** positive air study. Gas caps tumor protruding into cerebellopontine angle cistern *(arrow).*

gas CT cisternography results include any cerebel-lopontine angle mass, arachnoid adhesions, neuri-tis, a small internal canal, developmental lack of extension of the meninges into the internal ca-nal,[114] and subdural gas injection.[115] A small bub-ble of gas in the lateral internal canal may be a clue to a false-positive cisternogram.[116] False-neg-ative gas CT cisternograms are rare, but small in-tracanalicular filling defects or partial filling of the internal canal with gas should be viewed with suspicion and the study repeated 6 to 12 months later.[116]

MRI has become the radiographic study of choice to screen patients for acoustic neuroma as MRI scanners have become more widespread and the experience of radiologists and clinicians in-creases with MRI. In one series, MRI had a sensi-tivity and accuracy of 100% in detecting small acoustic neuromas, while enhanced CT had a 58% sensitivity rate and detected 19 of 33 tumors.[117] MRI identified all acoustic neuromas in another series in which CT revealed 65% of the tumors.[118] The ideal pulse sequences to detect acoustic neu-roma have been the subject of some controversy. Resolving power, which takes into consideration signal-to-noise ratio, contrast, and spatial resolu-tion, was evaluated for a series of echo and recov-ery times in a spin-echo sequence.[119] For a 1.5-tesla magnet, using a 256 × 256 matrix and 3-mm-

thick sections with a TR of 800 ms produced the highest resolving power with a TE of 25 ms and one average.[117] With this technique, 1-mm-thick nerves can be seen in the internal auditory canal and cerebellopontine angle cistern. Many authors use both T1-weighted sequences (short TR and TE) and T2-weighted sequences (long TR and TE) to evaluate patients for acoustic neuroma, while oth-ers routinely use only T1-weighted sequences.[120] On the T1-weighted images, there is greater con-trast between the seventh and eighth nerves and surrounding CSF (Figs 29–40 and 29–41,A). A T2-weighted pulse sequence can detect the cystic component in an acoustic neuroma.[117] On T1-weighted images, acoustic neuromas are somewhat variable in appearance, usually having signal in-tensity near or slightly less than that of the brain stem.[118, 120] A central band having no anatomic correlate is sometimes seen in intracanalicular tumors[120]; this probably represents truncation arti-fact. High signal and mixed signal have also been seen.[118] On T2-weighted images, acoustic neuro-mas have high signal; small tumors become more difficult to differentiate from CSF, however, be-cause of its increased signal.

Injection of intravenous contrast for MRI scans further increases the sensitivity of MRI for detect-ing small acoustic neuromas. Of several extra-axial intracranial tumors studied before and after injec-

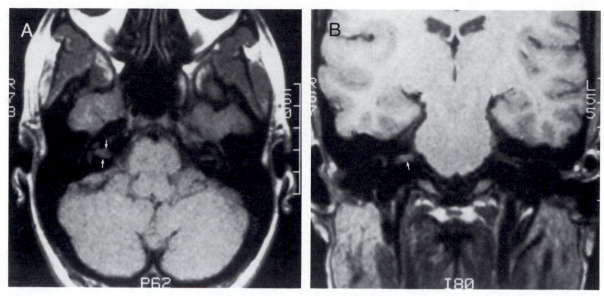

FIG 29–40.
Intracanalicular right acoustic neuroma. T1-weighted axial **(A)** and coronal **(B)** MRI scans (TR 600, TE 20, 256 × 256 matrix, 3-mm slice, 2 NEX) show increased signal of tumor within the right internal auditory canal *(arrows)*.

tion of gadolinium-DTPA, acoustic neuromas showed the greatest enhancement, an average of 300% (Figs 29–37 and 29–41,B).[121] Enhancement is greatest just after intravenous injection and is shown best on T1-weighted scans, with inversion recovery sequences demonstrating the greatest enhancement, followed by spin-echo scans with short TR and TE times.[121, 122] The T1 relaxation time is shortened to a greater extent than is the T2 relaxation time with gadolinium enhancement. The dose of gadolinium used has not been shown to produce any adverse effects.[122] Differential enhancement of extra-axial tumors cannot be reliably used to distinguish types of tumors because of variable enhancement, partial volume artifact, and overlapping data.[121] MRI, particularly if intravenous paramagnetic contrast is given, has replaced CT and gas CT cisternography for the detection of acoustic neuromas, particularly the small intracanilicular ones.

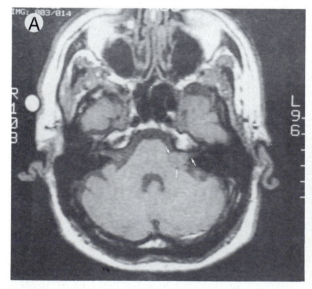
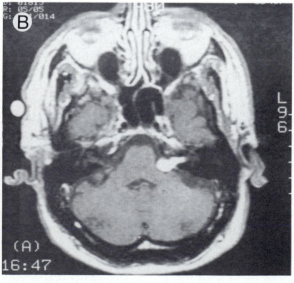

FIG 29–41.
Acoustic neuroma. **A,** a T1-weighted axial MR scan (TR 500, TE 25, 256 × 128 matrix, 3-mm slice, 2 NEX) shows tumor in the left internal canal and cerebellopontine angle cistern *(arrows)*. **B,** marked tumor enhancement after gadolinium-DTPA injection.

Glomus Tumors

Glomus tumors, also called paragangliomas or chemodectomas, are the most common primary tumor arising in the temporal bone (acoustic neuroma is the most common tumor affecting the temporal bone). Glomus tumors are slowly growing vascular masses that originate in chemoreceptor cells. These tumors are usually of nonchromaffin (nonsecretory) cells, although they may rarely be secretory, similar to pheochromocytomas.[123] These lesions of ectodermal origin occur at four major sites in the head and neck: the carotid body, along the vagus nerve, the dome of the jugular bulb, and in the middle ear. They are seen most often in middle-aged females. The temporal bone tumors originate from the jugular bulb, cochlear promontory, and the nerves of Jacobson and Arnold (at the inferior tympanic canaliculus and mastoid canaliculus, respectively).[123] The term *jugulotympanic paraganglioma* has been used for all temporal bone glomus tumors, but most authors still refer to the glomus jugulare and tympanicum classifications for those tumors arising in the jugular bulb and middle ear. Glomus tumors are rarely malignant, with the potential for distant metastases to regional lymph nodes and lung.[124, 125] Up to 10% of tumors are multiple[126]; with evidence of familial tumors, multiplicity may be much higher.[127] The carotid body tumor is the most common familial tumor.[127] Screening for multiple tumors can be performed by digital subtraction venous angiography, radionuclide angioscintigraphy,[127, 128] enhanced CT through the temporal bone and neck, or MRI.[129]

Patients with glomus tumors involving the temporal bone present with otologic or neurologic symptoms. Otologic symptoms are usually the earliest, including pulsatile tinnitus, bruit, and conductive hearing loss. Sensorineural hearing loss is a late symptom of inner-ear invasion.[130] Cranial nerve impairment, most commonly nerves IX, X, and XI in the jugular foramen, is the most frequent neurologic symptom of a glomus tumor. However, large tumors may involve cranial nerves V through XII and invade the posterior fossa.[130]

Radiologic diagnosis of a glomus tumor affecting the temporal bone has depended upon CT and angiography in recent years. The tumor enhances because of its vascularity, but enhancement may fade rapidly during a scan. Dynamic high-resolution CT has been proposed to identify the very vascular glomus tumors more accurately.[131] Moth-eaten destruction of the jugular foramen is typical of glomus jugular tumors (Fig 29–42).[132] Smooth enlargement of the fossa is less common and may also occur with neural tumors arising in the jugular foramen. The glomus tympanicum tumor typically presents as a soft-tissue mass on the cochlear promontory; no bone erosion was reported in a se-

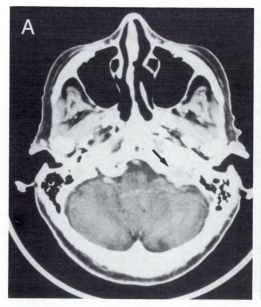
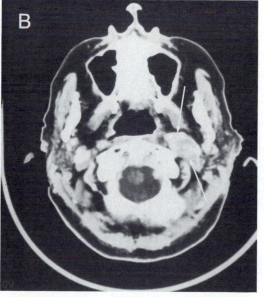

FIG 29–42.
Glomus jugulare tumor. **A,** a contrast-enhanced CT scan shows an enhancing mass with bone destruction in the jugular fossa *(arrow).*   **B,** the mass fills and enlarges the upper cervical jugular vein *(arrows).*

ries of 46 patients, although some tumors filled the middle ear and engulfed the ossicles (Fig 29–43).[133] In large lesions, the site of origin may be difficult to detect. Both types of glomus tumors tend to spread by pathways of least resistance, such as foramina, air cell tracts, and vascular channels,[126] and they can fill the middle ear and mastoid. It is impossible to distinguish glomus jugulare from tympanicum on otoscopic findings alone unless all margins of a small glomus tympanicum on the cochlear promontory are visible.[130] Two main clinical classifications of temporal bone glomus tumors are in use, the Glasscock-Jackson and Fisch classifications. Both relate the anatomic extent of tumor to the type of surgical resection necessary for treatment.[130] Treatment of glomus tumors is usually surgical, but radiation therapy and/ or embolization may be added for larger tumors.[130] Angiography is still often necessary preoperatively to identify feeding vessels.

MRI of glomus tumors is excellent for differentiating these lesions from others found in the same locations because of signal void areas of high-velocity blood flow producing a characteristic "salt-and-pepper" appearance (Fig 29–44). Small areas of increased signal in the second echo of T2-weighted images is due to even-echo rephasing, which indicates slow blood flow. T1-weighted images have better spatial resolution, while the tumor is more conspicuous on T2-weighted images. In the series of patients studied, however, CT provided better demonstration of subtle bone erosion.[129]

The differential diagnosis of glomus tumors of the temporal bone includes a dehiscent jugular bulb, aberrant carotid artery, aneurysm, persistent stapedial artery, cholesterol granuloma, cholesteatoma, neural tumor in the jugular fossa, metastases, and other more rare lesions affecting the temporal bone. CT is the method of choice to distinguish glomus tympanicum from jugulare tumors because bone erosion is seen best. MRI is better for differentiating glomus tumors from other types of lesions.

Facial Nerve Neuroma

Facial nerve neuroma (a term encompassing neurilemoma and neurofibroma) usually arises from Schwann cells of the nerve sheath.[134] These benign tumors may arise anywhere along the course of the nerve, from the cerebellopontine angle to the extratemporal nerve. Neoplastic involvement of the facial nerve usually causes progressive facial weakness, while Bell's palsy is of sudden onset. Hemifacial spasm, not seen in Bell's palsy, may be another differentiating symptom.[135] Facial nerve neuromas cause fewer than 5% of cases of facial nerve weakness while Bell's palsy accounts for about 80% of the cases.[136] The probable site of nerve involvement can be determined by testing lacrimation, the stapedial reflex, taste on the anterior two thirds of the tongue, and facial motor function; this is useful to tailor the CT examination.[137] If a lesion is not found in the intracranial or intratemporal portions of the nerve, evaluation of the extratemporal nerve should be performed. The short segment of nerve between the stylomastoid

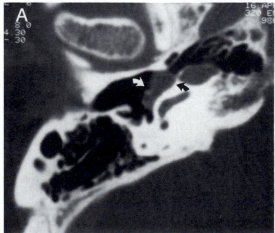
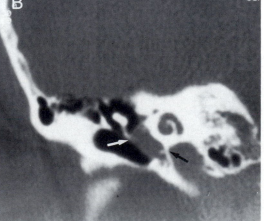

FIG 29–43.
Glomus tympanicum tumor in a 59-year-old woman with right pulsatile tinnitus and a vascular mass behind the tympanic membrane. **A,** an axial CT scan shows a soft-tissue mass low in the middle ear *(arrows).* **B,** the mass is separated from the carotid by bone *(black arrow)* on this coronal scan. The mass fills the anterior middle ear and reaches the malleus *(white arrow).*

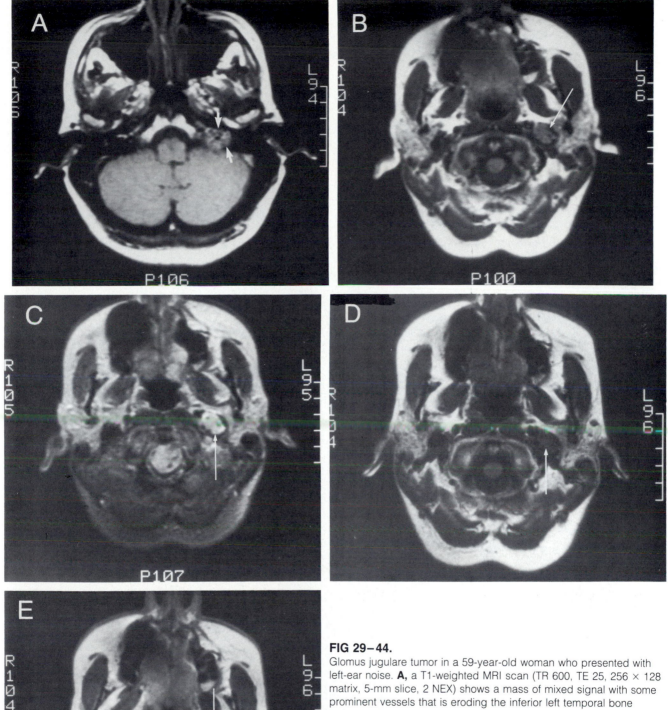

FIG 29–44.
Glomus jugulare tumor in a 59-year-old woman who presented with
left-ear noise. **A,** a T1-weighted MRI scan (TR 600, TE 25, 256 × 128
matrix, 5-mm slice, 2 NEX) shows a mass of mixed signal with some
prominent vessels that is eroding the inferior left temporal bone
(arrows). **B,** a lower scan (same factors) demonstrates tumor in the
jugular vein *(arrow).* **C,** the tumor is brighter on a more T2 weighted
scan *(arrow)* (TR 2500, TE 50, 256 × 128 matrix, 5-mm slice, 2 NEX).
D, a T1-weighted scan 7 months later prior to gadolinium-DTPA
injection (TR 500, TE 20, 256 × 256 matrix, 5-mm slice 2 NEX). The
tumor was embolized but did not change on subsequent
angiography. The tumor has relatively low signal *(arrow).* **E,** mild
enhancement occurs immediately after intravenous injection of
gadolinium-DTPA *(arrow).*

foramen and parotid can be seen in axial CT as a small soft-tissue "dot" surrounded by fat.[138]

Facial nerve neuromas are most common in the region of the geniculate ganglion.[136] The tumors may become quite large before producing symptoms, particularly in the cerebellopontine angle cistern, geniculate ganglion, and horizontal portion of the nerve (Fig 29–45). A geniculate ganglion mass can expand into the middle cranial fossa,[139] and tumor in the horizontal facial nerve can fill the middle ear and cause conductive hearing loss (Fig 29–46). Sensorineural hearing loss is due to compression of the eighth nerve by an internal auditory canal mass. This may occur sooner than facial nerve symptoms because motor nerves are more resistant to compression than sensory nerves are.[136]

The differential diagnosis of facial neuromas can be divided by which portion of the nerve is affected. Intracranial and cerebellopontine angle masses that can cause facial nerve symptoms include benign and malignant tumors, infarcts, and inflammatory conditions. Intratemporal facial paralysis may be secondary to other tumors (particularly hemangioma and carcinoma), congenital or acquired cholesteatoma, other inflammatory disease, malignant external otitis, trauma, or other rare lesions. The extratemporal facial nerve is often involved by adjacent malignant tumors, including those in the parotid, pharynx, and skin. Infections and trauma can also injure this portion of the nerve.[137]

All segments of the facial nerve can be identified on MRI done to study the temporal bone, par-

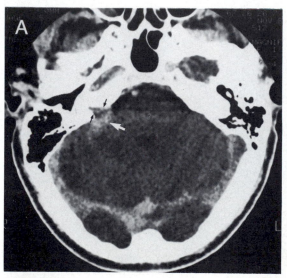

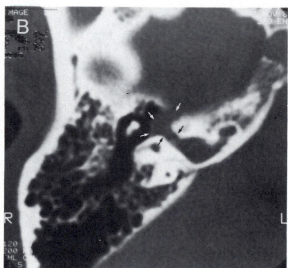

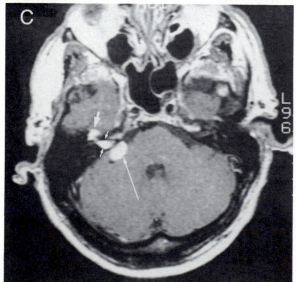

FIG 29–45.
Facial nerve neuroma in a middle-aged man with right sensorineural hearing loss but no facial paralysis. **A,** a contrast-enhanced CT scan shows a wide internal auditory canal *(black arrows)* with an enhancing mass *(white arrow)*. **B,** wide labyrinthine portion of the facial nerve canal *(black arrows)* and a mass in the middle ear and geniculate ganglion *(white arrows)* seen on the CT bone window. **C,** T1-weighted MR scan after gadolinium-DTPA intravenous injection. (TR 500, TE 25, 256 × 128 matrix, 3-mm slice, 2 NEX) Tumor is in cerebellopontine angle cistern *(long arrow),* internal auditory canal *(short arrows),* and middle fossa *(broad arrow).*

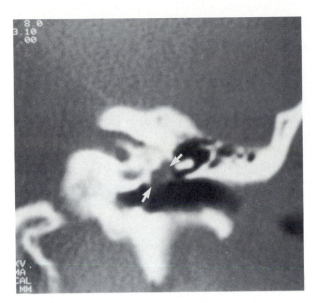

FIG 29—46.
Facial nerve neuroma in a middle-aged man with hearing loss and no facial paralysis. The mass in medial portion of the ear *(arrows)* cannot be differentiated from cholesteatoma.

ticularly if a surface coil is used.[6, 8] The normal facial nerve usually does not enhance after intravenous gadolinium injection, but facial nerve neuroma does. MRI with enhancement may be particularly useful in patients with neurofibromatosis who may have facial neuromas as well as acoustic neuromas (see Fig 29—37).[140]

Other Benign Tumors

Benign intratemporal vascular tumors, including capillary and cavernous hemangiomas and vascular malformations, have recently been recognized as being an increasingly common cause of facial nerve paralysis. In recent reports, these lesions have been as common or more common than facial nerve neuromas.[141, 142] These neoplasms occur at sites of vascular anastomoses in the temporal bone, including the internal auditory canal, geniculate ganglion, and distal turn of the facial canal.[142] The vascular lesions are usually less than 10 mm in size, often producing symptoms that are more severe than facial or acoustic neuromas of the same size.[141] Two distinguishing features of benign vascular tumors in the temporal bone are irregular bone erosion, or "honeycombing,"[141] and production of intratumoral bone (ossifying hemangioma).[142]

Masses primarily affecting the petrous apex, including epidermoid, cholesterol granuloma, and many other rare lesions from which epidermoid and cholesterol granuloma must be distinguished, have been discussed previously.

Meningiomas are common intracranial and cerebellopontine angle neoplasms, but they seldom occur in the temporal bone. Meningiomas arise from arachnoid cells, which have been reported in the temporal bone at the following sites: internal auditory canal, jugular foramen, geniculate ganglion, and along the grooves for the greater and lesser superficial petrosal nerves.[143] A review of 79 cases of meningioma involving the temporal bone determined that only 20 of these appeared confined to the temporal bone.[144] However, in only 3 patients was CT done to determine intracranial involvement, and only 5 patients had long-term follow-up. A temporal bone meningioma may produce hyperostosis, but less bone is produced than by ossifying fibroma.[142]

Osteomas are rare benign tumors of the temporal bone, usually the mastoid (Fig 29—47). Fifty-one of 61 cases reviewed involved the mastoid or squamous portion of the temporal bone.[145] These lesions are usually obvious on physical examination, but osteomas also occur in clinically inaccessible sites.[146] A rare cause of sensorineural hearing loss is osteoma of the internal auditory canal. Osteomas should be distinguished from exostoses, which are not true neoplasms; they are believed to be a reaction to irritation such as swimming in cold water.[145]

Osteoblastoma is a benign expansile vascular

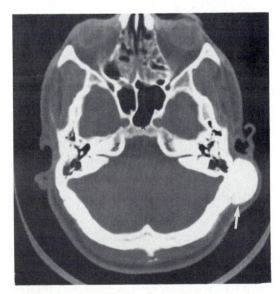

FIG 29—47.
Osteoma in a 39-year-old man with a long history of hard swelling behind his left ear *(arrow)*.

tumor that is rarely found in the temporal bone. It is closely related to osteoid osteoma, and some authors distinguish them only by size.[147] An osteoblastoma may have variable density, although most are described as osteolytic, and angiographic findings are also inconsistent.[147, 148]

Other rare mesenchymal tumors that have been reported in the temporal bone include ossifying fibroma,[91] chondroblastoma,[149] and chondroma.[150] Fibrous dysplasia has been previously discussed.

Schwannomas occur at multiple sites in the temporal bone, with the most common being on the vestibular nerve (acoustic neuroma) and facial nerve and in the jugular fossa. Jugular fossa schwannomas are less common than glomus jugulare tumors are and must be distinguished from them.[151] Both CT and MRI are useful for this differentiation (see glomus tumors). Intralabyrinthine schwannomas are very rare and are usually found incidentally in patients undergoing surgery for Meniere's disease.[152] Radiologic studies are normal in these patients.[152]

Gland cell tumors arising in the external auditory canal, including both benign and malignant lesions, are rare. Benign adenomas of ceruminous glands are less common than is adenoid cystic carcinoma.[153] These adenomas, often called ceruminomas, do not destroy bone but may recur if not completely excised (Fig 29–48).[154] It may be difficult to distinguish a low-grade malignant tumor from a benign one histologically.

MALIGNANT TUMORS

Primary Tumors

Squamous carcinomas constitute over half of the primary malignant tumors of the ear. These lesions may arise on the pinna, where they are easily identified, or in the external auditory canal, where they are more difficult to diagnose and carry a worse prognosis. (Fig 29–49).[155] Patients with squamous carcinoma originating in the external canal often have a history of chronic ear infections and/or external otitis.[156, 157] They usually present with pain and drainage from the ear; facial nerve paralysis or dizziness are later signs.[158] Contrast-enhanced CT is currently the radiologic method of choice to study patients suspected of having tumors because patterns of spread and bone destruction are demonstrated well. (Fig 29–50).[158–160] No MRI series of temporal bone malignancies has been reported, probably because of the rarity of these lesions. MRI may be useful to distinguish a fluid-filled mastoid from extension of tumor or thin extradural plaques of tumor, both of which have caused false-negative CT interpretations of tumor extent.[158] Squamous carcinomas spread locally, often along naturally occurring planes, but they seldom destroy the otic capsule.[160] When the tumor enters the middle ear, determining site of origin

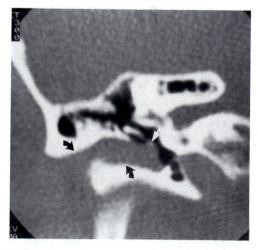

FIG 29–48.
Ceruminoma in an elderly man with a soft-tissue mass filling the external auditory canal and a history of a mass removed elsewhere 5 years earlier. The mass fills bony the external canal *(black arrows)* and protrudes into middle ear *(white arrow).* No bone destruction is seen.

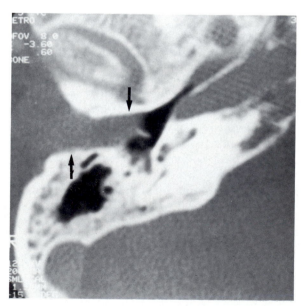

FIG 29–49.
Squamous carcinoma in the external auditory canal of an elderly woman with a long history of a draining ear and a new mass in the external canal *(arrows).* No definite bone destruction is seen, unusual for this lesion. This cannot be distinguished from more benign masses (see Fig 29–48).

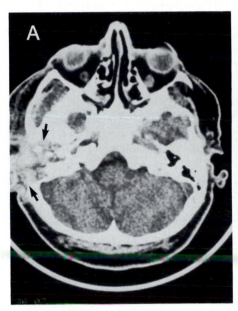

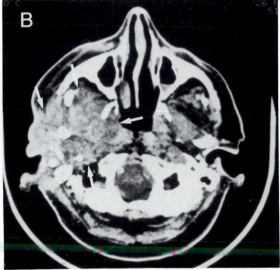

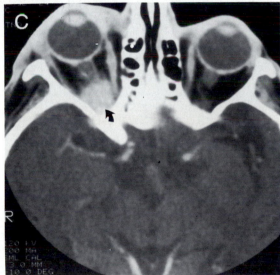

FIG 29–50.
Squamous carcinoma in an elderly woman with a long history of a draining ear and previous operations. **A,** a noncontrast axial scan shows tissue of moderately high attenuation filling the mastoid cavity and eroding into the temporomandibular joint *(arrows).* **B,** in a scan 1.5 cm lower, the infratemporal fossa is filled with abnormal tissue that obliterates fat planes *(arrows).* The tissue was felt to be a cholesteatoma at surgery, but the pathologic diagnosis was well-differentiated squamous carcinoma because of its invasive behavior. **C,** metastatic tumor to the orbit *(arrow)* 6 months after extensive surgical resection.

may be difficult. Metastatic spread is first to preauricular nodes, less frequently to cervical nodes.[159] Distant metastatic disease is rare. Treatment is by surgical removal and irradiation, if the lesion is resectable.

Adenoid cystic carcinoma arises from salivary gland tissue. Minor salivary gland tissue occurs at multiple sites in the upper aerodigestive tract, including the external and middle ear.[161] Adenoid cystic carcinoma is an uncommon tumor, but one that has a poor prognosis because of its tendency to spread by perineural invasion, so tumor cells may be found at some distance from the margins of the primary mass.

Primary adenocarcinoma of the middle ear is also rare and must be distinguished from metastatic disease.[162] There is some controversy over differentiating middle-ear adenomas from low-grade adenocarcinomas.[163, 164] A rare papillary adenocarcinoma that resembled thyroid carcinoma has been reported (Fig 29–51).[165] Ceruminous tumors of the external canal may also be malignant, and the histology is not always a good predictor of tumor behavior.[164]

Melanomas are common on the pinna and may invade the external canal from this location. They are much less common deep in the external auditory canal and middle ear. Only a few primary mid-

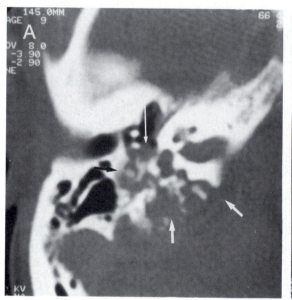

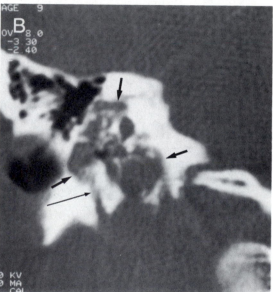

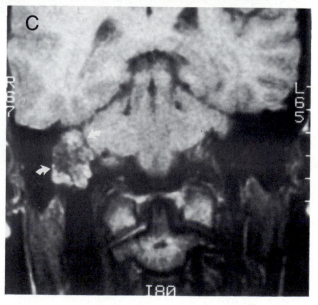

FIG 29–51.
Papillary adenocarcinoma in a teenage boy with dense right facial paralysis. **A,** an axial CT scan shows expansile destruction of the posterior temporal bone *(short white arrows),* with mass extending through the region of the facial nerve *(black arrow)* into the middle ear *(long white arrow).* **B,** a coronal scan behind the internal canal shows a large area of bone destruction *(short arrows)* that involves the descending portion of the facial nerve *(long arrow).* **C,** coronal MRI (TR 600, TE 25, 256 × 256 matrix, 5-mm slice, 2 NEX). The tumor has a mixed signal *(arrows).*

dle-ear melanomas have been reported.[166] CT is essential to exclude intracranial invasion.[167]

Histiocytosis X is a general term that includes three clinical entities characterized by a proliferation of histiocytes: eosinophilic granuloma, Hand-Schüller-Christian syndrome, and Letterer-Siwe disease.[168] Some authors consider these three conditions a continuum,[169] while others point out confusion and disagreement in the classification systems.[170] Hand-Schüller-Christian syndrome was described as a triad of bone lesions, exophthalmos, and diabetes insipidus, but this occurs in only a small percentage of patients.[168] Eosinophilic granuloma is a generally benign lytic bony lesion that may be single or multiple. It is usually a condition of children, although lesions of eosinophilic granuloma do occur in older adults.[171] Fifteen percent of all patients with histiocytosis X in one series had ear involvement.[168] Temporal bone histiocytosis X may present as a mastoid mass, discharge, or polyps and mimic inflammation (Fig 29–52).[172] The middle ear and tympanic membrane are usually normal, a differentiating feature from otitis accompanied by mastoiditis.[169] Therapy for localized lesions includes conservative surgery and low-dose irradiation, with chemotherapy reserved for nonbony disease.[172]

Rhabdomyosarcoma is the most common soft-tissue sarcoma in children. Approximately 50% of these lesions occur in the head and neck, with the

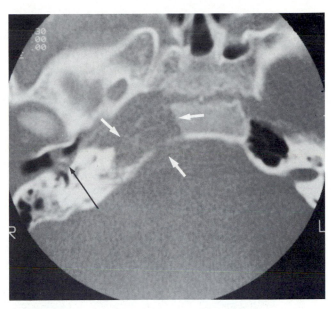

FIG 29–53.
Rhabdomyosarcoma in a 12-year-old boy with progressive right hearing loss over several weeks. There is destruction of the petrous apex and part of the clivus *(white arrows)* and a mass in the middle ear around the ossicles *(black arrow)*.

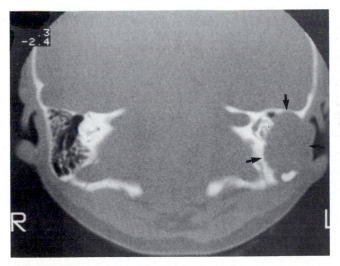

FIG 29–52.
Eosinophilic granuloma on coronal CT scan in a child with known bone lesions, diabetes insipidus, and left deafness. The left mastoid is destroyed and filled with soft tissue *(arrows)*. Some mastoid reconstitution occurred after surgery and irradiation. (Courtesy of Robert Starshak, M.D., Children's Hospital of Wisconsin.)

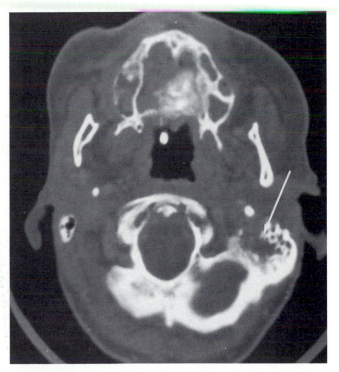

FIG 29–54.
Direct metastasis to the temporal bone in a 54-year-old woman who had large oropharyngeal squamous carcinoma treated with irradiation and radical neck dissection. The tumor recurred and invaded the left mastoid *(arrow)* 6 months later.

temporal bone being the third most frequent site after the orbit and nasopharynx.[173, 174] The tumor often mimics otitis media, granulation tissue, or polyps, which delays diagnosis (Fig 29–53).[175] While rhabdomyosarcoma was once uniformly fatal, now long-term survivals are being reported following irradiation and chemotherapy.[175, 176]

Other sarcomas are rare in the temporal bone. One case of Ewing's sarcoma originating in the ear has been reported.[177]

Metastatic Tumors

Metastatic disease to the temporal bone is seldom reported but probably occurs more frequently in patients with advanced malignancies. Tumors may spread to the temporal bone via hematogenous routes or direct extension. Hematogenous spread is seen most often in tumors that metastasize to bone, including carcinoma of the lung, breast, kidney, and prostate.[85, 178, 179] The marrow spaces of the temporal bone are usually affected

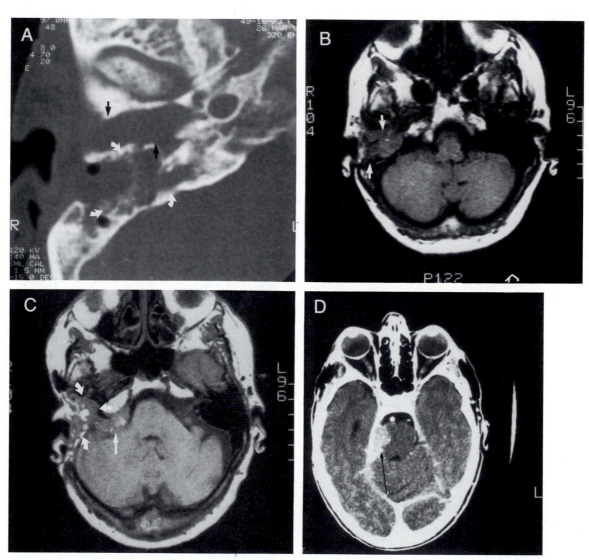

FIG 29–55.
Adenocarcinoma in an elderly woman who had recurrence of a malignant right parotid tumor that invaded the temporal bone 6 years after treatment. **A,** axial CT shows abnormal soft tissue in the external auditory canal *(black arrows)* and mastoid with destruction *(white arrows).* **B,** T1-weighted MRI (TR 600, TE 20, 256 × 128 matrix, 5-mm slice, 2 NEX) has abnormal signal in the same area *(arrows).* **C,** T1 weighted MRI (TR 600, TE 20, 256 × 256 matrix, 3-mm slice, 2 NEX) 8 months after **B,** The patient had temporal bone resection with placement of fat in the defect *(curved arrows).* There was recurrent tumor in the right cerebellopontine angle cistern *(straight arrow).* **D,** CT 5 months after resection of the right cerebellopontine angle mass. The tumor recurred adjacent to the pons *(arrow).*

first by hematogenous metastatic lesions, with relative sparing of the pneumatized mastoid and otic capsule.

Tumors that extend directly along fascial planes, nerves, and foramina to invade the temporal bone include those arising in skin, the parotid, adjacent lymph nodes, the nasopharynx, and meninges (Figs 29–54 and 29–55). Systemic malignancies such as myeloma, leukemia, and lymphoma may rarely affect the ear.

CT is the current method of choice to detect metastatic lesions of the temporal bone, although MRI may play an increasing role. Nonspecific soft-tissue mass and bone destruction are seen with metastatic as well as primary tumors; rare aggressive inflammatory conditions must also be distinguished. A history of a primary malignancy is of major importance to make the diagnosis of temporal bone metastatic disease.

Acknowledgments

Thanks to Victor Haughton, M.D., for reviewing the MRI portions of the manuscript; to David Daniels, M.D., who identified patients with temporal bone pathology on MRI scans; and to Barb Mendenhall for typing the manuscript.

REFERENCES

1. Manzione JV, Rumbaugh CL, Katzberg R: Direct sagittal computed tomography of the temporal bone. *J Comput Assist Tomogr* 1985; 9:417–419.
2. Chakeres DW, Spiegel PK: A systematic technique for comprehensive evaluation of the temporal bone by computed tomography. *Radiology* 1983; 146:97–106.
3. Zonneveld FW, Van Waes PFGM, Damsma H, et al: Direct multiplanar computed tomography of the petrous bone. *Radiographics* 1983; 3:400–449.
4. Shaffer KA, Haughton VM, Wilson CR: High resolution computed tomography of the temporal bone. *Radiology* 1980; 134:409–414.
5. Shaffer KA, Volz DJ, Haughton VM: Manipulation of CT data for temporal-bone imaging. *Radiology* 1980; 137:825–829.
6. Daniels DL, Schenck JF, Foster T, et al: Surface-coil magnetic resonance imaging of the internal auditory canal. *AJR* 1985; 145:469–472.
7. Koenig H, Lenz M, Sauter R: Temporal bone region: High-resolution MR imaging using surface coils. *Radiology* 1986; 159:191–194.
8. Teresi L, Lufkin R, Wortham D, et al: MR imaging of the intratemporal facial nerve by using surface coils. *AJR* 1987; 148:589–597.
9. Beatty CW, Harris LD, Suh KW, et al: Comparative study using computed tomographic thin-section zoom reconstructions and anatomic macrosections of the temporal bone. *Ann Otol Rhinol Laryngol* 1981; 90:643–649.
10. Littleton JT, Shaffer KA, Callahan WP, et al: Temporal bone: Comparison of pluridirectional tomography and high resolution computed tomography. *AJR* 1981; 137:835–845.
11. Daniels DL, Haughton VM: *Cranial and Spinal Magnetic Resonance Imaging, an Atlas and Guide*, New York, Raven Press, 1987.
12. Virapongse C, Sarwar M, Bhimani S, et al: Computed tomography of temporal bone pneumatization: 1. Normal pattern and morphology. *AJR* 1985; 145:473–481.
13. Virapongse C, Rothman SLG, Kier EL, et al: Computed tomographic anatomy of the temporal bone. *AJR* 1982; 139:739–749.
14. Virapongse C, Sarwar M, Sasaki C, et al: High resolution computed tomography of the osseous external auditory canal: 1. Normal anatomy. *J Comput Assist Tomogr* 1983; 7:486–492.
15. Swartz J: High-resolution computed tomography of the middle ear and mastoid. Part I: Normal radioanatomy including normal variations. *Radiology* 1983; 148:449–454.
16. Mafee MF, Aimi K, Kahen HL, et al: Chronic otomastoiditis: A conceptual understanding of CT findings. *Radiology* 1986; 160:193–200.
17. Chakeres DW, Weider DJ: Computed tomography of the ossicles. *Neuroradiology* 1985; 27:99–107.
18. Valavanis A, Kubik S, Oguz M: Exploration of the facial nerve canal by high-resolution computed tomography: Anatomy and pathology. *Neuroradiology* 1983; 24:139–147.
19. Swartz JD: The facial nerve canal: CT analysis of the protruding tympanic segment. *Radiology* 1984; 153:443–447.
20. Moretti JA: Highly placed jugular bulb and conductive deafness. *Arch Otolaryngol* 1976; 102:430–431.
21. Daniels DL, Williams AL, Haughton VM: Jugular foramen: Anatomic and computed tomographic study. *AJR* 1984; 142:153–158.
22. Daniels DL, Schenck JF, Foster T, et al: Magnetic resonance imaging of the jugular foramen. *AJNR* 1985; 6:699–703.
23. Harnsberger HR, Dart DJ, Parkin JL, et al: Cochlear implant candidates: Assessment with CT and MR imaging. *Radiology* 1987; 164:53–57.
24. Mafee MF, Selis JE, Yannias DA, et al: Congenital sensorineural hearing loss. *Radiology* 1984; 150:427–434.
25. Swartz JD, Glazer AU, Faerber EN, et al: Congen-

ital middle-ear deafness: CT study. *Radiology* 1986; 159:187–190.

26. Swartz JD, Faerber EN: Congenital malformations of the external and middle ear: High-resolution CT findings of surgical import. *AJR* 1985; 144:501–506.

27. Kaseff LG, Nieberding PH, Shorago GW, et al: Fistula between the middle ear and subarachnoid space as a cause of recurrent meningitis: Detection by means of thin-section, complex-motion tomography. *Radiology* 1980; 135:105–108.

28. Herther C, Schindler RA: Mondini's dysplasia with recurrent meningitis. *Laryngoscope* 1985; 95:655–658.

29. Curtin HD, Vignaud J, Bar D: Anomaly of the facial canal in a Mondini malformation with recurrent meningitis. *Radiology* 1982; 144:335–341.

30. Lloyd TV, Van Aman M, Johnson JC: Aberrant jugular bulb presenting as a middle ear mass. *Radiology* 1979; 131:139–141.

31. Stern J, Goldenberg M: Jugular bulb diverticula in medial petrous bone. *AJR* 1980; 134:959–961.

32. Swartz JD, Bazarnic ML, Naidich TP, et al: Aberrant internal carotid artery lying within the middle ear. High resolution CT diagnosis and differential diagnosis. *Neuroradiology* 1985; 27:322–326.

33. Lo WWM, Solti-Bohman LG, McElveen JT Jr: Aberrant carotid artery: Radiologic diagnosis with emphasis on high-resolution computed tomography. *Radiographics* 1985; 5:985–993.

34. Guinto FC Jr, Garrabrant EC, Radcliffe WB: Radiology of the persistent stapedial artery. *Radiology* 1972; 105:365–369.

35. Sinnreich AI, Parisier SC, Cohen NL, et al: Arterial malformations of the middle ear. *Otolaryngol Head Neck Surg* 1984; 92:194–206.

36. Mafee MF, Singleton EL, Valvassori GE, et al: Acute otomastoiditis and its complications: Role of CT. *Radiology* 1985; 155:391–397.

37. Lenz RP, McDonald GA: Otitic hydrocephalus. *Laryngoscope* 1984; 94:1451–1454.

38. Swartz JD, Goodman RS, Russell KB, et al: High-resolution computed tomography of the middle ear and mastoid. Part II: Tubotympanic disease. *Radiology* 1983; 148:455–459.

39. Swartz JD, Wolfson RJ, Marlowe FI, et al: Postinflammatory ossicular fixation: CT analysis with surgical correlation. *Radiology* 1985; 154:697–700.

40. Swartz JD, Berger AS, Zwillenberg S, et al: Ossicular erosions in the dry ear: CT diagnosis. *Radiology* 1987; 163:763–765.

41. Swartz JD: Cholesteatomas of the middle ear. Diagnosis, etiology and complications. *Radiol Clin North Am* 1984; 22:15–35.

42. Jackler RK, Dillon WP, Schindler RA: Computed tomography in suppurative ear disease: A correlation of surgical and radiographic findings. *Laryngoscope* 1984; 94:746–752.

43. Stamm AC, Pinto JA, Coser PL, et al: Nonspecific necrotizing petrositis: An unusual complication of otitis in children. *Laryngoscope* 1984; 94:1218–1222.

44. Chole RA, Donald PJ: Petrous apicitis. Clinical considerations. *Ann Otol Rhinol Laryngol* 1983; 92:544–551.

45. Hoffman RA, Brookler KH, Bergeron RT: Radiologic diagnosis of labyrinthitis ossificans. *Ann Otol Rhinol Laryngol* 1979; 88:253–257.

46. Swartz JD, Mandell DM, Faerber EN, et al: Labyrinthine ossification: Etiologies and CT findings. *Radiology* 1985; 157:395–398.

47. Mendez G Jr, Quencer RM, Post MJD, et al: Malignant external otitis: A radiographic-clinical correlation. *AJR* 1979; 132:957–961.

48. Curtin HD, Wolfe P, May M: Malignant external otitis: CT evaluation. *Radiology* 1982; 145:383–388.

49. Chandler JR: Malignant external otitis: Further considerations. *Ann Otol Rhinol Laryngol* 1977; 86:417–428.

50. Strashun AM, Nejatheim M, Goldsmith SJ: Malignant external otitis: Early scintigraphic detection. *Radiology* 1984; 150:541–545.

51. Mendelson DS, Som PM, Mendelson MH, et al: Malignant external otitis: The role of computed tomography and radionuclides in evaluation. *Radiology* 1983; 149:745–749.

52. Shaffer KA: Comparison of computed tomography and complex motion tomography in the evaluation of cholesteatoma. *AJR* 1984; 143:397–400.

53. Mafee MF, Kumar A, Yannias DA, et al: Computed tomography of the middle ear in the evaluation of cholesteatomas and other soft-tissue masses: Comparison with pluridirectional tomography. *Radiology* 1983; 148:465–472.

54. Silver AJ, Janecka I, Wazen J, et al: Complicated cholesteatomas: CT findings in inner ear complications of middle ear cholesteatomas. *Radiology* 1987; 164:47–51.

55. Phelps PD, Lloyd GAS: The radiology of cholesteatomas. *Clin Radiol* 1980; 31:501–512.

56. Johnson DW, Hinshaw DB, Hasso AN, et al: Computed tomography of local complications of temporal bone cholesteatomas. *J Comput Assist Tomogr* 1985; 9:519–523.

57. Swartz JD, Goodman RS, Russell KB, et al: High-resolution computed tomography of the middle ear and mastoid. Part III: Surgically altered anatomy and pathology. *Radiology* 1983; 148:461–464.

58. Johnson DW, Voorhees RL, Lufkin RB, et al: Cholesteatomas of the temporal bone: Role of computed tomography. *Radiology* 1983; 148:733–737.

59. Chakeres DW, Mattox DE: Computed tomographic evaluation of nonmetallic middle-ear prostheses. *Invest Radiol* 1985; 20:596–600.

60. Swartz JD, Berger AS, Zwillenberg S, et al: Syn-

thetic ossicular replacements: Normal and abnormal CT appearance. *Radiology* 1987; 163:766–768.

61. Freeman J: Temporal bone fractures and cholesteatoma. *Ann Otol Rhinol Laryngol* 1983; 92:558–560.

62. Brookes GB, Graham MD: Post-traumatic cholesteatoma of the external auditory canal. *Laryngoscope* 1984; 94:667–670.

63. Chakeres DW, Kapila A, LaMasters D: Soft-tissue abnormalities of the external auditory canal: Subject review of CT findings. *Radiology* 1985; 156:105–109.

64. Naiberg J, Berger G, Hawke M: The pathologic features of keratosis obturans and cholesteatoma of the external auditory canal. *Arch Otolaryngol* 1984; 110:690–693.

65. Derlacki EL: Congenital cholesteatoma today. *Am J Otol* 1985; 6:19–21.

66. McDonald TJ, Cody DTR, Ryan RE Jr: Congenital cholesteatoma of the ear. *Ann Otol Rhinol Laryngol* 1984; 93:637–640.

67. Latack JT, Graham MD, Kemink JL, et al: Giant cholesterol cysts of the petrous apex: Radiologic features. *AJNR* 1985; 6:409–413.

68. Lo WWM, Solti-Bohman LG, Brackmann DE, et al: Cholesterol granuloma of the petrous apex: CT diagnosis. *Radiology* 1984; 153:705–711.

69. Gentry LR, Jacoby CG, Turski PA, et al: Cerebellopontine angle–petromastoid mass lesions: Comparative study of diagnosis with MR imaging and CT. *Radiology* 1987; 162:513–520.

70. Griffin C, DeLaPaz R, Enzmann D: MR and CT correlation of cholesterol cysts of the petrous bone. *AJNR* 1987; 8:825–829.

71. DeLozier HL, Parkins CW, Gacek RR: Clinical records: Mucocele of the petrous apex. *J Laryngol Otol* 1979; 93:177–180.

72. Osborn AG, Parkin JL: Mucocele of the petrous temporal bone. *AJR* 1979; 132:680–681.

73. Behnke EE, Schindler RA: Dermoid of the petrous apex. *Laryngoscope* 1984; 94:779–783.

74. Latack JT, Kartush JM, Kemink JL, et al: Epidermoidomas of the cerebellopontine angle and temporal bone: CT and MR aspects. *Radiology* 1985; 157:361–366.

75. Swartz JD, Faerber EN, Wolfson RJ, et al: Fenestral otosclerosis: Significance of preoperative CT evaluation. *Radiology* 1984; 151:703–707.

76. Mafee MF, Henrikson GC, Deitch RL, et al: Use of CT in stapedial otosclerosis. *Radiology* 1985; 156:709–714.

77. Mafee MF, Valvassori GE, Deitch RL, et al: Use of CT in the evaluation of cochlear otosclerosis. *Radiology* 1985; 156:703–708.

78. Valvassori GE, Dobben GD: CT densitometry of the cochlear capsule in otosclerosis. *AJNR* 1985; 6:661–667.

79. Damsma H, deGroot JAM, Zonneveld FW, et al: CT of cochlear otosclerosis (otospongiosis). *Radiol Clin North Am* 1984; 22:37–43.

80. Swartz JD, Mandell DW, Berman SE, et al: Cochlear otosclerosis (otospongiosis): CT analysis with audiometric correlation. *Radiology* 1985; 155:147–150.

81. Swartz JD, Lansman AK, Berger AS, et al: Stapes prosthesis: Evaluation with CT. *Radiology* 1986; 158:179–182.

82. Applebaum EL, Valvassori GE: Effects of magnetic resonance imaging fields on stapedectomy prostheses. *Arch Otolaryngol* 1985; 111:820–821.

83. Resnick D: Paget disease of bone: Current status and a look back to 1943 and earlier. *AJR* 1988; 150:249–256.

84. Petasnick JP: Tomography of the temporal bone in Paget's disease. *AJR* 1969; 105:838–843.

85. Valvassori G, Potter G, Hanafee W, et al: *Radiology of the Ear, Nose, and Throat.* Philadelphia, WB Saunders Co, 1982, pp 12–126.

86. Barrionuevo CE, Marcallo FA, Coelho A, et al: Fibrous dysplasia and the temporal bone. *Arch Otolaryngol* 1980; 106:298–301.

87. Nager GT, Kennedy DW, Kopstein E: Fibrous dysplasia: A review of the disease and its manifestations in the temporal bone. *Ann Otol Rhinol Laryngol (Suppl)* 1982; 92:5–51.

88. Rhea JT, Weber AL, Deluca SA: Three cases of fibrous dysplasia of the temporal bone. *Appl Radiol* 1987; 16:66–71.

89. Nager GT, Holliday MJ: Fibrous dysplasia of the temporal bone. Update with case reports. *Ann Otol Rhinol Laryngol* 1984; 93:630–633.

90. Schrimpf R, Karmody CS, Chasin WD, et al: Sclerosing lesions of the temporal bone. *Laryngoscope* 1982; 92:1116–1119.

91. Levine PA, Wiggins R, Archibald RWR, et al: Ossifying fibroma of the head and neck: Involvement of the temporal bone—An unusual and challenging site. *Laryngoscope* 1981; 91:720–725.

92. Holland BA, Brant-Zawadzki M: High-resolution CT of temporal bone trauma. *AJR* 1984; 143:391–395.

93. Schubiger O, Valavanis A, Stuckmann G, et al: Temporal bone fractures and their complications. Examination with high resolution CT. *Neuroradiology* 1986; 28:93–99.

94. Wiet RJ, Valvassori GE, Kotsanis CA, et al: Temporal bone fractures. State of the art review. *Am J Otol* 1985; 6:207–215.

95. Kaseff LG: Tomographic evaluation of trauma to the temporal bone. *Radiology* 1969; 93:321–327.

96. Ghorayeb BY, Yeakley JW, Hall JW III, et al: Unusual complications of temporal bone fractures. *Arch Otolaryngol Head Neck Surg* 1987; 113:749–753.

97. Tennenbaum P: Ear trauma, in Vignaud J, Jardin

C, Rosen L (eds): *The Ear Diagnostic Imaging CT Scanner, Tomography, and Magnetic Resonance.* New York, Masson Publishers USA, Inc, 1986, pp 146–158.

98. Cannon CR, Jahrsdoerfer RA: Temporal bone fractures. Review of 90 cases. *Arch Otolaryngol* 1983; 109:285–288.

99. Swartz JP, Swartz NG, Korsvik H, et al: Computerized tomographic evaluation of the middle ear and mastoid for posttraumatic hearing loss. *Ann Otol Rhinol Laryngol* 1985; 94:263–266.

100. Mafee MF, Valvassori GE, Kumar A, et al: Pneumolabyrinth: A new radiologic sign for fracture of the stapes footplate. *Am J Otol* 1984; 5:374–375.

101. Lipkin AF, Bryan RN, Jenkins HA: Pneumolabyrinth after temporal bone fracture: Documentation by high-resolution CT. *AJNR* 1985; 6:294–295.

102. Zimmermann RA, Bilaniuk LT, Hackney DB, et al: Magnetic resonance imaging in temporal bone fracture. *Neuroradiology* 1987; 29:246–251.

103. Clemis JD, Ballad WJ, Baggot PJ, et al: Relative frequency of inferior vestibular schwannoma. *Arch Otolaryngol Head Neck Surg* 1986; 112:190–194.

104. Valvassori GE: Radiologic evaluation of eighth nerve tumors. *Am J Otolaryngol* 1984; 5:270–280.

105. Kanter WR, Eldridge R, Fabricant R, et al: Central neurofibromatosis with bilateral acoustic neuroma: Genetic, clinical and biochemical distinctions from peripheral neurofibromatosis. *Neurology* 1980; 30:851–859.

106. Egelhoff JC, Ball WS, Towbin RB, et al: Dural ectasia as a cause of widening of the internal auditory canals in neurofibromatosis. *Pediatr Radiol* 1987; 17:7–9.

107. Graham MK, Sataloff RT: Acoustic tumors in the young adult. *Arch Otolaryngol* 1984; 110:405–407.

108. Laasonen EM, Troupp H: Volume growth rate of acoustic neurinomas. *Neuroradiology* 1986; 28:203–207.

109. Nedzelski JM, Canter RJ, Kassel EE, et al: Is no treatment good treatment in the management of acoustic neuromas in the elderly? *Laryngoscope* 1986; 96:825–829.

110. Hernanz-Schulman M, Welch K, Strand R, et al: Acoustic neuromas in children. *AJNR* 1986; 7:519–521.

111. Barrs DM, Brackmann DE, Olson JE, et al: Changing concepts of acoustic neuroma diagnosis. *Arch Otolaryngol* 1985; 111:17–21.

112. Sortland O: Computed tomography combined with gas cisternography for the diagnosis of expanding lesions in the cerebellopontine angle. *Neuroradiology* 1979; 18:19–22.

113. Bird CR, Hasso AN, Drayer BP, et al: The cerebellopontine angle and internal auditory canal: Neurovascular anatomy on gas CT cisternograms. *Radiology* 1985; 154:667–670.

114. Robertson HJ, Hatten HP Jr, Keating JW: False-positive CT gas cisternogram. *AJNR* 1983; 4:474–477.

115. Larsson EM, Holtas S: False diagnosis of acoustic neuroma due to subdural injection during gas CT cisternogram. *J Comput Assist Tomogr* 1986; 10:1025–1026.

116. Barrs DM, Vedder JS: Problems in air cisternography. *Arch Otolaryngol Head Neck Surg* 1986; 112:769–772.

117. Curati WL, Graif M, Kingsley DPE, et al: MRI in acoustic neuroma: A review of 35 patients. *Neuroradiology* 1986; 28:208–214.

118. Mikhael MA, Ciric IS, Wolff AP: MR diagnosis of acoustic neuromas. *J Comput Assist Tomogr* 1987; 11:232–235.

119. Enzmann DR, O'Donohue J: Optimizing MR imaging for detecting small tumors in the cerebellopontine angle and internal auditory canal. *AJNR* 1987; 8:99–106.

120. Daniels DL, Millen SJ, Meyer GA, et al: MR detection of tumor in the internal auditory canal. *AJR* 1987; 148:1219–1222.

121. Breger RK, Papke RA, Pojunas KA, et al: Benign extraaxial tumors: Contrast enhancement with Gd-DTPA. *Radiology* 1987; 163:427–429.

122. Curati WL, Graif M, Kingsley DPE, et al: Acoustic neuromas: Gd-DTPA enhancement in MR imaging. *Radiology* 1986; 158:447–541.

123. Swartz JD: *Imaging of the Temporal Bone.* New York, Thieme Medical Publishers, Inc, 1986, p 103.

124. Davis JM, David KR, Hesselink JR, et al: Case report. Malignant glomus jugulare tumor: A case with two unusual radiographic features. *J Comput Assist Tomogr* 1980; 4:415–417.

125. Batsakis JG: *Tumors of the Head and Neck. Clinical and Pathologic Considerations*, ed 2. Baltimore, Williams & Wilkins, 1979, pp 369–380.

126. Spector GJ, Sobol S, Thawley SE, et al: Panel discussion: Glomus jugulare tumors of the temporal bone. Patterns of invasion in the temporal bone. *Laryngoscope* 1979; 89:1628–1639.

127. van Baars F, van den Broek P, Cremers C, et al: Familial non-chromaffinic paragangliomas (glomus tumors): Clinical aspects. *Laryngoscope* 1981; 91:988–995.

128. Som PM, Reede DL, Bergeron RT, et al: Computed tomography of glomus tympanicum tumors. *J Comput Assist Tomogr* 1983; 7:14–17.

129. Olsen WL, Dillon WP, Kelly WM, et al: MR imaging of paragangliomas. *AJR* 1987; 148:201–204.

130. Lo WWM, Solti-Bohman LG, Lambert PR: High-resolution CT in evaluation of glomus tumors of the temporal bone. *Radiology* 1984; 150:737–742.

131. Mafee MF, Valvassori GE, Shugar MA, et al: High resolution and dynamic sequential computed tomography. Use in the evaluation of glomus complex tumors. *Arch Otolaryngol* 1983; 109:691–696.

132. Chakeres DW, LaMasters DL: Paragangliomas of the temporal bone: High-resolution CT studies. *Radiology* 1984; 150:749–753.

133. Larson TC III, Reese DF, Baker HL Jr, et al: Glomus tympanicum chemodectomas: Radiographic and clinical characteristics. *Radiology* 1987; 163:801–806.

134. Neely JG: Neoplastic involvement of the facial nerve. *Otolaryngol Clin North Am* 1974; 7:385–396.

135. Pillsbury HC, Price HC, Gardiner LJ: Primary tumors of the facial nerve: Diagnosis and management. *Laryngoscope* 1983; 93:1045–1048.

136. Latack JT, Gabrielsen TO, Knake JE, et al: Facial nerve neuromas: Radiologic evaluation. *Radiology* 1983; 149:731–739.

137. Disbro MA, Harnsberger HR, Osborn AG: Peripheral facial nerve dysfunction: CT evaluation. *Radiology* 1985; 155:659–663.

138. Curtin HD, Wolfe P, Snyderman N: The facial nerve between the stylomastoid foramen and the parotid: Computed tomographic imaging. *Radiology* 1983; 149:165–169.

139. Kienzle GD, Goldenberg MH, Just NWM, et al: Facial nerve neurinoma presenting as middle cranial fossa mass: CT appearance. *J Comput Assist Tomogr* 1986; 10:391–394.

140. Daniels DL, Czervionke LF, Pojunas KW, et al: Facial nerve enhancement in MR imaging. *AJNR* 1987; 8:605–607.

141. Lo WWM, Horn KL, Carberry JN, et al: Intratemporal vascular tumors: Evaluation with CT. *Radiology* 1986; 159:181–185.

142. Curtin HD, Jensen JE, Barnes L Jr, et al: "Ossifying" hemangiomas of the temporal bone: Evaluation with CT. *Radiology* 1987; 164:831–835.

143. Salama N, Stafford N: Meningiomas presenting in the middle ear. *Laryngoscope* 1982; 92:92–97.

144. Rietz DR, Ford CN, Kurtycz DF, et al: Significance of apparent intratympanic meningiomas. *Laryngoscope* 1983; 93:1397–1404.

145. Denia A, Perez F, Canalis RR, et al: Extracanalicular osteomas of the temporal bone. *Arch Otolaryngol* 1979; 105:706–709.

146. Beale DF, Phelps PD: Osteomas of the temporal bone: A report of three cases. *Clin Radiol* 1987; 38:67–69.

147. Gellad FE, Hafiz MA, Blanchard CL: Osteoblastoma of the temporal bone: CT findings. *J Comput Assist Tomogr* 1985; 9:577–579.

148. Potter C, Conner GH, Sharkey FE: Benign osteoblastoma of the temporal bone. *Am J Otol* 1983; 4:318–322.

149. Tanohata K, Noda M, Katoh H, et al: Chondroblastoma of temporal bone. *Neuroradiology* 1986; 28:367–370.

150. Komisar A, Som PM, Shugar JMA, et al: Benign chondroma of the petrous apex. *J Comput Assist Tomogr* 1981; 5:116–118.

151. Crumley RL, Wilson C: Schwannomas of the jugular foramen. *Laryngoscope* 1984; 94:772–777.

152. Vernick DM, Graham MD, McClatchey KD: Intralabyrinthine schwannoma. *Laryngoscope* 1984; 94:1241–1243.

153. Pulec JL: Glandular tumors of the external auditory canal. *Laryngoscope* 1977; 87:1601–1612.

154. Valvassori GE: Benign tumors of the temporal bone. *Radiol Clin North Am* 1974; 12:533–542.

155. Chen KTK, Dehner LP: Primary tumors of the external and middle ear. I. Introduction and clinicopathologic study of squamous cell carcinoma. *Arch Otolaryngol* 1978; 104:247–252.

156. Conley J, Schuller DE: Malignancies of the ear. *Laryngoscope* 1976; 86:1147–1163.

157. Wagenfeld DJH, Keane T, van Nostrand AWP, et al: Primary carcinoma involving the temporal bone: Analysis of twenty-five cases. *Laryngoscope* 1980; 90:912–919.

158. Bird CR, Hasso AN, Stewart CE, et al: Malignant primary neoplasms of the ear and temporal bone studied by high-resolution computed tomography. *Radiology* 1983; 149:171–174.

159. Olsen KD, DeSanto LW, Forbes GS: Radiographic assessment of squamous cell carcinoma of the temporal bone. *Laryngoscope* 1983; 93:1162–1167.

160. Phelps PD, Lloyd GAS: The radiology of carcinoma of the ear. *Br J Radiol* 1981; 54:103–109.

161. Cannon CR, McLean WC: Adenoid cystic carcinoma of the middle ear and temporal bone. *Otolaryngol Head Neck Surg* 1983; 91:96–99.

162. Glasscock ME III, McKennan KX, Levine SC, et al: Primary adenocarcinoma of the middle ear and temporal bone. *Arch Otolaryngol Head Neck Surg* 1987; 113:822–824.

163. Eden AR, Pincus RL, Som PL, et al: Primary adenomatous neoplasm of the middle ear. *Laryngoscope* 1984; 94:63–67.

164. Pallanch JF, Weiland LH, McDonald TJ, et al: Adenocarcinoma and adenoma of the middle ear. *Laryngoscope* 1982; 92:47–52.

165. Adam W, Johnson JC, Paul DJ, et al: Primary adenocarcinoma of the middle ear. *AJNR* 1982; 3:674–676.

166. McKenna EL Jr, Holmes WF, Harwick R: Primary melanoma of the middle ear. *Laryngoscope* 1984; 94:1459–1460.

167. Kagan AR, Steckel RJ: Diagnostic oncology case study. Cancer of the middle ear. *AJR* 1982; 138:943–944.

168. McCaffrey TV, McDonald TJ: Histiocytosis X of the ear and temporal bone: Review of 22 cases. *Laryngoscope* 1979; 89:1735–1742.

169. Jones RO, Pillsbury HC: Histiocytosis X of the head and neck. *Laryngoscope* 1984; 94:1031–1035.

170. Nolph MB, Luikin GA: Histiocytosis X. *Otolaryngol Clin North Am* 1982; 15:635–648.

171. Kimmelman CP, Nielsen E, Snow JB Jr: Histiocytosis X of the temporal bone. *Otolaryngol Head Neck Surg* 1984; 92:588–590.

172. Appling D, Jenkins HA, Patton GA: Eosinophilic granuloma in the temporal bone and skull. *Otolaryngol Head Neck Surg* 1983; 91:358–365.

173. Dehner LP, Chen KTK: Primary tumors of the external and middle ear. III. A clinicopathologic study of embryonal rhabdomyosarcoma. *Arch Otolaryngol* 1978; 104:399–403.

174. Feldman BA: Rhabdomyosarcoma of the head and neck. *Laryngoscope* 1982; 92:424–440.

175. Schwartz RH, Movassaghi N, Marion ED: Rhabdomyosarcoma of the middle ear: A wolf in sheep's clothing. *Pediatrics* 1980; 65:1131–1132.

176. Chasin WD: Rhabdomyosarcoma of the temporal bone. *Ann Otol Rhinol Laryngol (Suppl)* 1984; 112:71–73.

177. Carrol R, Miketic LM: Ewing sarcoma of the temporal bone: CT appearance. *J Comput Assist Tomogr* 1987; 11:362–363.

178. Berlinger NT, Koutroupas S, Adams G, et al: Patterns of involvement of the temporal bone in metastatic and systemic malignancy. *Laryngoscope* 1980; 90:619–627.

179. Coppola RJ, Salanga VD: Metastatic prostatic adenocarcinoma to the temporal bone. *Neurology* 1980; 30:311–315.

30

Nose, Paranasal Sinuses, and Facial Bones

Hugh D. Curtin, M.D.

Ellen K. Tabor, M.D.

The nasal passages and paranasal sinuses are a complex system of bone and soft tissue abutting a labyrinth-like airway. Computed tomography (CT) and magnetic resonance imaging (MRI) are both used for evaluation, each having advantages and disadvantages.[1-5]

With a "bone algorithm" CT can visualize the small bony septations and thin bony walls and provide excellent definition of air–soft-tissue interfaces. MRI can have trouble with small erosions of bone. Neither air nor bone gives significant signal and so have a similar appearance on MRI. Normally the bone and air in the sinuses are separated by a very thin layer of mucus that may be undetectable on MRI. However, pathology thickens the "mucosal line" or puts soft tissue where there should be air or bone and therefore signal where there should be none. Thus the pathology can be detected, and the excellent tissue discrimination of MRI comes into play to allow MRI to demonstrate a margin quite precisely. MRI has the advantage of multiple slice orientation, which is crucial in evaluation of the nasal/paranasal region.

Several concepts will be stressed in this chapter. Although one always tries to separate benign from malignant or inflammatory from neoplastic, often the more important role of the radiologist is to define the precise limit of the disease. The radiologist must be familiar with the anatomy as well as the pathways most often following as pathology progresses. By evaluating the extent of a disease and some internal CT or MRI characteristics, the radiologist can often be fairly specific in diagnosis. However, this opinion is often of secondary impor-

tance because most suspicious lesions will come to biopsy.

Bone forms the major boundaries of the sinuses, and so various bone changes visible on imaging will be discussed before proceeding with descriptions of various diseases. The opaque sinus will be discussed in light of the ability of CT and MRI to more precisely characterize the contents.

Finally, the section on the use of imaging in various disease states will begin with neoplasm, and it is in this section that routes of spread will be emphasized. Detection of spread necessitates knowledge of the anatomy as well as potential pathologic pathways. It is here that the anatomic landmarks important in evaluation of the sinuses will be presented. The specific anatomic landmarks that are important in surgery for chronic inflammation will be mentioned in the section on this disease process.

This chapter is not a complete description of individual pathologic entities but stresses general principles of MRI and CT evaluation. Some areas where MRI and CT are useful in the sinus area, such as encephaloceles and congenital defects, are discussed elsewhere in this book.

BONE CHANGES

As in plain radiography and tomography, bone changes are very important parameters of disease. Currently, the findings in CT or MRI are often an extrapolation of the findings on plain films or tomography.

Bone Destruction

Destruction of a bony wall is very significant in an aggressive process such as malignancy, mycotic infection, or granulomatous disease. In definition of bone destruction, CT is competitive with tomography. Very thin bone may have density lower than typical bone because of partial volume effect, especially if the slice orientation is slightly oblique to the bone (see Figs 30–5 and 30–17). Care must be taken when there is tissue on both sides of a thin septation. The very thin bone may "disappear," and one might think the bone has been destroyed; this phenomenon commonly occurs in the ethmoid air cells. Another frequent offender is the posterior portion of the medial wall of the maxillary sinus. One can be helped by looking at the

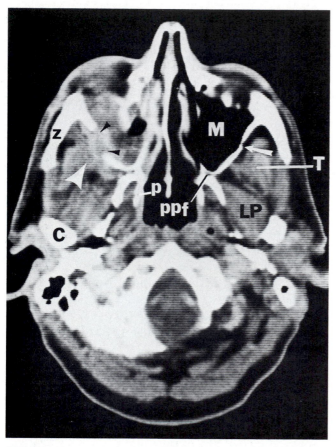

FIG 30–1.
Squamous cell carcinoma involving the maxillary sinus and infraorbital nerve. Note the destruction of the posterolateral wall of the sinus *(small arrowheads)* and tumor obliterating the fat plane just outside the sinus *(large arrowhead)*. Compare with normal structures on opposite side (M = maxillary sinus; the *arrow* denotes the fat plane outside the wall of the maxillary sinus; z = zygomatic arch; p = pterygoid plate; LP = lateral pterygoid muscle; C = mandibular condyle; ppf = pterygopalatine fossa; T = temporalis muscle).

contralateral side and determining whether the bone in the analogous region is dense enough to register as bone or is actually close to soft-tissue density. The correct interpretation of bone destruction is aided by the appearance of the soft tissues on the outer (nonsinus) side of the bone. A fat plane is often conveniently present on the outer side of the bony wall, and obliteration of this fat plane is a very sensitive indication of progression of pathology through the bone (Fig 30–1). Fat is an ideal subject for CT or T1-weighted MRI. When a fat plane is not present, it is more difficult to detect minimal extension through the bone. There is still often enough CT density difference or MR signal difference between the pathologic process and the soft tissues on the outer side of the bone that some assessment can be made. This will be further discussed in the section on direct extension of tumors.

Bowing of a Bony Wall

Bowing of key structures implies slow growth, remodeling occurring as the bone reacts to the presence and pressure of the lesion. Classically seen in mucocele formation, this phenomenon can also be seen in benign neoplasms. All too often, however, the "bowing" of bone occurs in malignancy, which makes the sign nonspecific (Figs 30–2 and 30–3).[6] Bowing therefore does not necessarily mean that a lesion is benign. For instance, the posterolateral wall of the maxillary sinus can be bowed but retain the cortical margin even in malignancy.

Enlargement of a Foramen or Neural Canal

Enlargement of a neural foramen demonstrated during the workup of a malignancy very strongly suggests extension of tumor along the nerve.[7, 8] In such a case, the radiologist must carefully evaluate the more central segments of the involved nerve to properly stage a tumor. Again, the advantage of CT or MRI lies in the ability to demonstrate the soft tissues both at the entrance and the exit of the various neural foramina. Benign lesions such as neuromas can also enlarge neural foramina.

Sclerotic Walls

Thickening of the bony wall is the bone's natural reaction to any stress or insult. This sclerotic change indicates a chronic lesion and is most com-

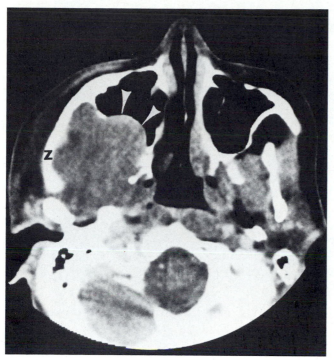

FIG 30–2.
Undifferentiated small-cell carcinoma in the infratemporal fossa (deep to the zygoma) that is bowing but not completely destroying the posterolateral wall of the maxillary sinus *(arrowheads)*. The tumor obliterates fat planes in the infratemporal fossa (z = zygoma).

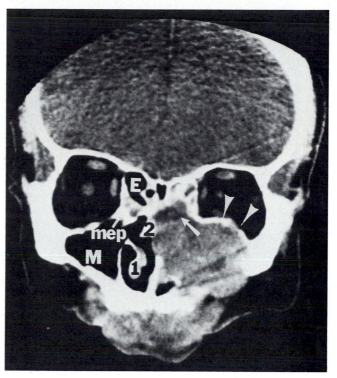

FIG 30–3.
Coronal scan showing fibrous histiocytoma of the maxillary sinus bowing the orbital floor superiorly *(arrowheads)* and pushing up the inferior rectus muscle. There is also destruction of the maxilloethmoidal plate *(arrow)* and lateral wall of the maxillary sinus as tumor extends into the ethmoid sinus and cheek respectively. The upper ethmoid may be opacified by obstruction rather than actual tumor involvement as evidenced by residual septation. Compare with the normal side (M = maxillary sinus; E = ethmoid sinus; *mep* = maxillary ethmoid plate; 1 = inferior turbinate; 2 = middle turbinate).

monly seen in inflammatory disease (Fig 30–4) such as chronic sinusitis but has also been described in association with tumors. Bony sclerosis and bone thickening can also be seen as a reaction to surgery or after radiation therapy (Fig 30–5).

Hyperostosis and sclerosis can be associated with meningioma and rarely will affect walls of the sinuses. This usually occurs in the region of the sphenoid sinus but can affect the maxillary sinus (see the discussion of meningioma in Chapter 17 of this book).

Bone Enlargement

Fibrous dysplasia represents abnormal formation and mineralization of bone. The bone is increased in size and can be very dense, resembling cortical bone, or can have a somewhat lower density depending on the degree of mineralization of the matrix. Descriptions of the CT appearances of fibrous dysplasia are somewhat limited (Fig 30–6).[9]

Other bony dysplasias can result in thickening and increased density in the bones of the skeleton.[10–12] These include osteopetrosis, craniometa-

physeal dysplasia, sclerosteosis, cortical hyperostosis, and Engelmann's disease (Figs 30–7 and 30–8). Although the abnormalities can be detected by CT, they are often evaluated by plain films. The radiologist may, however, see these changes incidently on CT when evaluating the patient for another problem.

CT has become useful in some of these dysplasias through the use of three-dimensional imaging for surgical planning. The appearance of the bony structures and relationships to overlying soft tissues are much more clearly shown than on plain-film representation.

A patient with an increased blood cell turnover, such as in thalassemia, can have grossly enlarged marrow spaces that may result in an increase in bony thickness without necessarily an increase in bony density (Fig 30–9). This represents an increase in the patient's marrow as it ex-

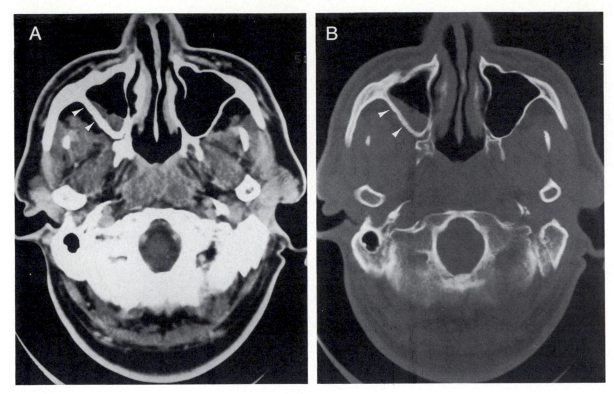

FIG 30-4.
Chronic right maxillary sinusitis. **A,** the bony wall is thickened and sclerotic *(arrowheads).* Compare to the normal side. **B,** bone detail is enhanced on CT with a bony algorithm.

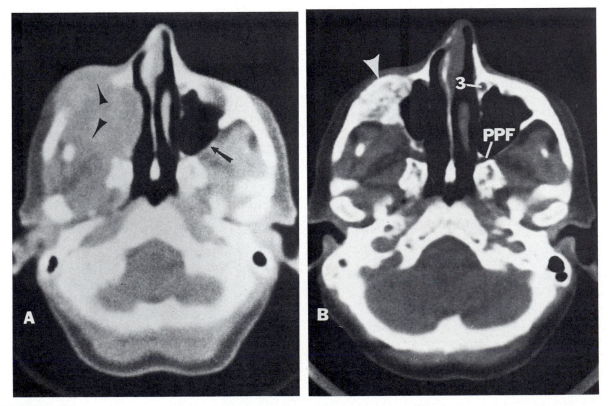

FIG 30-5.
Squamous cell carcinoma preradiation. Tumor of the maxillary sinus is "destroying" the anterior and posterior walls *(arrowheads).* Note, however, how the posterolateral wall of the maxillary sinus on the opposite side is indistinct because the bone is very thin. **B,** postradiation therapy. Note the thickened sclerotic bone of the malar eminence *(arrowhead)* (*PPF* = pterygopalatine fossa; *3* = nasolacrimal duct).

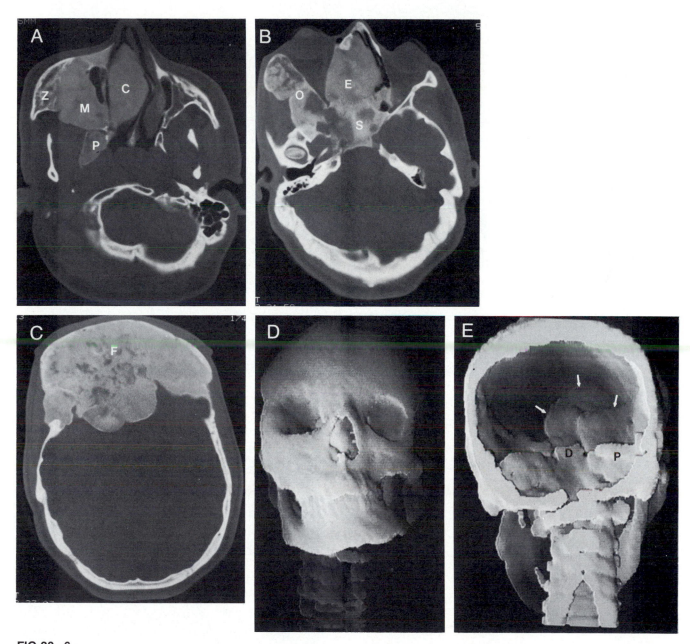

FIG 30–6.
Fibrous dysplasia. **A,** the process involves the right zygoma *(Z),* maxilla *(M),* pterygoid plates *(P),* and middle concha *(C).* **B** and **C,** the dysplasia extended superiorly to involve the lateral wall of the orbit *(O),* ethmoid *(E),* sphenoid sinus *(S),* and frontal bones *(F).* **D,** a three-dimensional image in the anteroposterior (AP) projection demonstrates the facial deformity. The mandible was not involved but is asymmetrical secondary to the mass effect. **E,** three-dimensional image, posterior view. The occiput has been removed, and the anterior and middle cranial fossa are viewed from behind. *Arrows* denote involvement of the frontal bones *(D* = dorsum sella; *P* = petrous ridge).

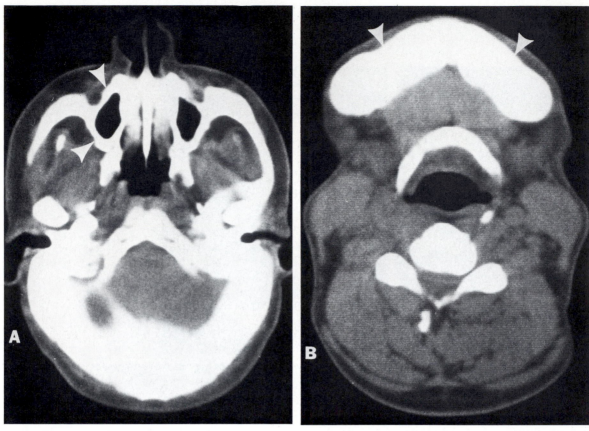

FIG 30–7.
Van Buchem's disease (hyperostosis corticalis generalisata). **A,** the skull base is thickened, as are the walls of the maxillary sinus *(arrowhead).* **B,** the mandible shows considerable hyperostosis also *(arrowheads).*

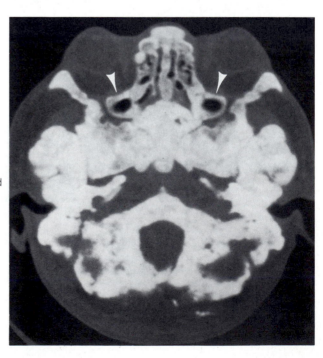

FIG 30–8.
Engelmann's disease (progressive diaphyseal dysplasia)—CT bone algorithm. There is diffuse involvement of the ethmoid, sphenoid, and skull base. The bony walls of the upper maxillary sinuses are also thickened *(arrowheads).*

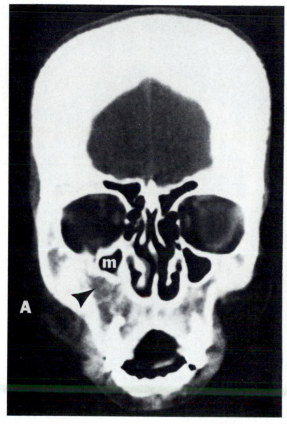

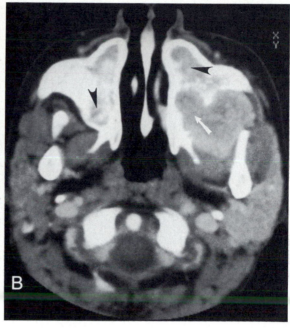

FIG 30–9.
Thalassemia major. **A,** CT coronal cut shows the marrow spaces in the maxilla and zygoma are enlarged *(arrowhead),* with resultant thickening of bone and a decrease in size of the maxillary sinuses *(m).* Note also the thickening of the skull. **B,** axial slice showing widened marrow spaces *(arrowheads).* The patient has juvenile angiofibroma extending into the infratemporal fossa and into the maxillary sinus *(arrow).*

tends into the bony walls of, for instance, the maxillary sinus. This results in a decrease in the size of the sinus but an increase in the size of the maxilla.

Paget's disease can thicken the facial bones and encroach upon the sinuses.

THE "OPAQUE SINUS"

Opacity of a sinus can be due to inflamed mucosa, cyst, tumor, retained secretions, blood, or occasionally the result of a bony obliteration or maldevelopment. When malignancy is present, the opaque sinus becomes an even more significant diagnostic problem. The opacity can be due to extension of tumor into the sinus itself or can be related to obstruction of the outflow of the sinus. When outflow from the sinus is compromised, there is retention of secretions that eventually may lead to mucocele formation. The earliest radiographic finding is opacification without any bony change.

A low uniform density in the sinus on an enhanced CT scan suggests retained secretions. The mucosa may enhance with intravenous contrast, and this combined with a uniform low density is quite reassuring (Fig 30–10). The mucosal enhancement is, however, not always visualized. Often, with rapid infusion of contrast, a tumor will enhance, and the ability to see the tumor margin bordered by the low density of retained secretions allows the radiologist to define how much of an opaque sinus is tumor (Fig 30–11).

If, however, the sinus does not have a uniformly low CT density, the problem is more difficult. Tumor and inflamed mucosa can have very similar appearances on intravenously enhanced CT scans. When an obstructed sinus develops infection and the mucosa is enlarged and inflamed, it is very difficult to differentiate where the neoplasm stops and the inflammatory mucosa begins. In the large maxillary sinus, this is not usually a problem because the mucosa is usually separated

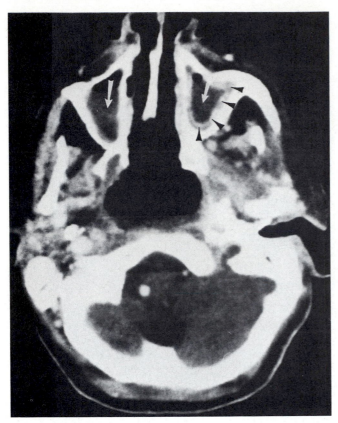

FIG 30–10.
Opaque sinuses. Note the retention of secretions that have low CT attenuation *(arrows)*. The mucosa presumed to be inflamed enhances *(arrowheads)* and outlines the sinus. The patient had undergone previous radiation therapy for a nasopharyngeal lesion.

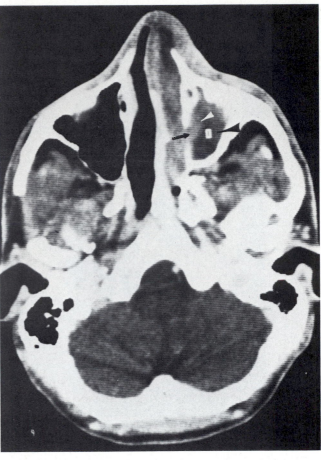

FIG 30–11.
Tumor (histiocytic lymphoma) in the nasal cavity is extending through the maxillary ostium *(arrow)* and causing obstruction. The lesion enhances and differentiates tumor *(small arrowhead)* from the retained secretions *(large arrowhead)*.

FIG 30–12.
Inverting papilloma and squamous cell carcinoma. Tumor of the nasal cavity and maxillary sinus is extending into the lower ethmoid sinus *(arrow)*. The upper ethmoids were not aerated. The septae *(black arrowhead)* are intact, which suggests obstruction rather than tumor extension, but tumor cannot be definitely excluded. Tumor also extends through the anterior wall of the maxillary antrum *(white arrowhead)*.

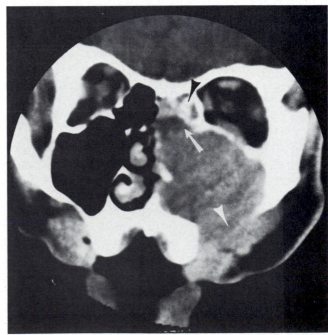

from the tumor by low-density secretions. It is, however, a major problem in smaller air cells such as in the ethmoid sinus, where minimal swelling of the mucosa may virtually occlude the space so that the entire sinus enhances and mimics tumor. In such a case, one hopes to demonstrate intact bony septations, which suggest obstruction of the outflow of the sinus and perhaps subsequent infection rather than actual extension of tumor throughout the air cells (Fig 30–12). More investigation with correlation of pathologic specimens and CT findings is necessary before firm conclusions can be made with respect to the opacified sinus.

MRI may offer an advantage in differentiating problem cases. Although experience is still somewhat limited, some authors have shown that inflammatory tissue can be separated from neoplasm, especially when using T2-weighted images (long repetition time [TR] long echo time [TE]).[13] Most neoplasms (including squamous cell carcinoma) have an intermediate signal intensity at this sequence, while inflammatory tissue or an obstructed sinus has a brighter higher signal intensity. Some neoplasms can have a relatively high signal intensity, and then differentiation would be difficult. These lesions include neural lesions, minor sali-

vary gland tumors, and hemangiomas. The tissue type is often known before the MRI results, so the radiologist would know when to expect problems differentiating tumor from inflammation.

TUMOR AND TUMORLIKE CONDITIONS

To evaluate neoplasm in the region of the nose and sinuses, one must have a knowledge of the anatomy and routes of spread of neoplastic processes.[2–4] The important methods of tumor spread are direct extension, extension along nerves, lymphatic spread to the nodes, and hematogenous spread. Hematogenous spread is less common.

Routes of Spread

Direct Extension

While tumor extension through a bony margin of a sinus can be detected by destructive changes in the bone itself, visualizing the pathology in the soft tissue on the other (outer) side of the bone is the true advantage of CT or MRI. The appearance of the tissue on the outer side of the bony wall of

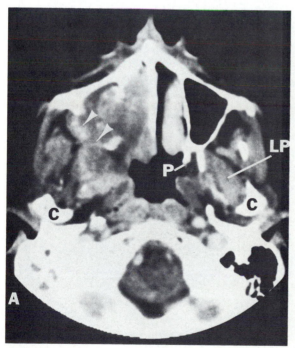
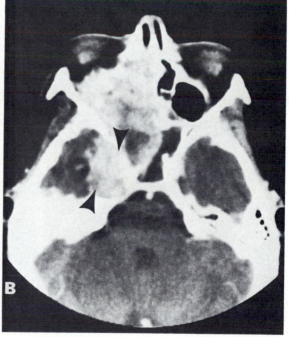

FIG 30–13.
Adenocystic carcinoma of the nasal cavity and maxillary sinus. **A,** tumor is extending through the posterolateral wall into the infratemporal fossa *(arrowheads)*. The pterygoid plates are destroyed and pterygoid muscle involved (normal side: *P* = pterygoid plates;

LP = lateral pterygoid muscle; *C* = mandibular condyles). **B,** tumor eroded through the skull base into the middle cranial fossa *(arrowheads)*.

the sinus determines the ease of detection of this transosseous spread of tumor.

Maxillary Sinus.—The maxillary sinus is perhaps the easiest to evaluate because its bony margins are oriented perpendicularly to either axial or coronal planes and the tissues or spaces on the outer side of the bone lend themselves to CT or MRI investigation. Tumor can progress in any direction.

Posterior and Posterolateral Extension.—Tumor extending through the posterolateral wall spreads into the infratemporal fossa. A well-defined fat plane borders the bony wall of the sinus and separates it from the temporalis muscle (Figs 30–13 and 30–14). The fat can be excellently imaged by using either CT or T1-weighted MRI. The pterygoid muscles are well seen, and involvement of the muscles themselves is of great importance in the determination of treatment.

Direct posterior extension gives tumor access to the pterygopalatine fossa and its cluster of nerves and vessels (Figs 30–13 and 30–14). There is almost always enough fatty tissue in the pterygo-

palatine fossa itself to allow visualization in both axial and coronal projections. Obliteration of this fat indicates extension into the area, but bone destruction is almost always present in cases of direct extension of malignancy. The pterygopalatine fossa can also be involved as tumor spreads along a nerve, especially the infraorbital nerve, as discussed in a later section.

Superior Extension.—Superiorly, tumor spreads from the maxillary sinus into the orbit where obliteration of the fat near the inferior rectus is a good indicator of tumor extension (Fig 30–15). Superomedial extension is through the bony maxilloethmoid plate into the ethmoid sinus (Fig 30–16). Again, the difficulty in attempting to differentiate tumor involving the ethmoid sinus from an obstructive process must be emphasized. The maxilloethmoid plate is usually thick enough to allow evaluation of destruction.

Coronal scans are used to evaluate subtle changes in the orbital floor and extension into the ethmoid sinuses. On axial scans, the superior recess of the maxillary sinus is often seen at the same level as the orbital contents, and tumor involvement of this recess should not be confused with ex-

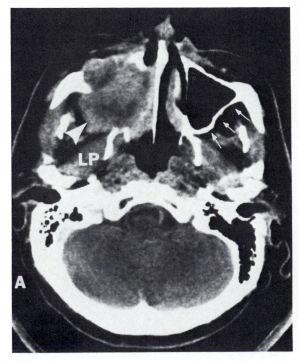
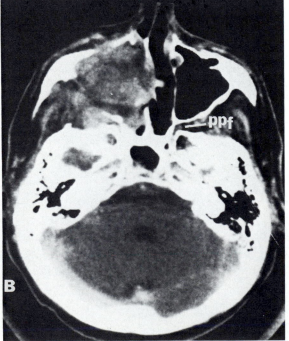

FIG 30–14.
Tumor extension. **A,** tumor eroding the posterolateral wall of the maxillary sinus and extruding into fat of the infratemporal fossa. An *arrowhead* denotes the tumor margin. The pterygoid muscle *(LP)* is not involved. Note the intact fat plane *(arrows)* behind the maxillary sinus on the normal side. **B,** higher slice showing involvement of the pterygopalatine fossa. Note the fat density in the pterygopalatine fossa *(ppf)* on the normal side.

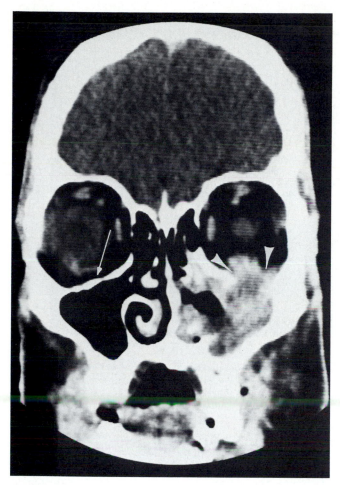

FIG 30–15.
Orbital extension. Tumor involving the upper maxillary sinus with destruction of the orbital floor and involvement of the orbit. The lesion obliterates the fat just above the floor *(arrowheads)*. Note the normal fat plane *(arrow)* just above the orbital floor on the normal side.

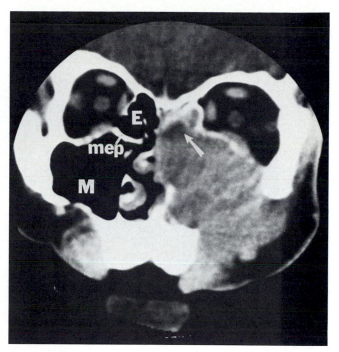

FIG 30–16.
Coronal CT section through a tumor of the maxillary sinus that is extending through the maxilloethmoid plate into the lower ethmoid *(arrow)* (normal side: *mep* = maxillary ethmoid plate; *M* = maxillary sinus; *E* = ethmoid sinus.)

tension into the orbit. The bony floor of the orbit is angled at this level and so is often not visible on axial CT (Fig 30–17). Coronal views can be used to make the differentiation.

Medial, Anterior, and Inferior Extension.—Medial extension from the maxillary sinus is into the nasal cavity and destroys the common wall between the nasal cavity and the sinus (Fig 30–18). This wall can be thin, which makes assessment of its integrity difficult. Anterior extension can be readily seen as tumor encroaches on the fat planes of the cheek (Fig 30–19).

Inferiorly, the tumor can destroy the alveolar ridge and form a mass in the oral cavity. Performing a scan with the mouth slightly open can be helpful because air bordering the palate will act as

a natural contrast agent. Extension by this route is, however, often detectable clinically (Fig 30–20).

Ethmoid Sinuses.—Extension from the ethmoid can be inferiorly into the maxillary sinus through the maxilloethmoid plate or into the nasal cavity. Tumor destroys the bone, and the mass is seen to encroach on the airspaces.

Evaluation of the extension into the orbits from the ethmoid is also quite accurate as tumor extends into the orbital fat, this time medial to the medial rectus (Fig 30–21).

Superior extension is indicated by destruction of the cribiform plate and roof of the ethmoid. Tumor extending through the dura involves the frontal lobe, and the tumor margin can usually be identified on a coronal CT scan with contrast enhancement (Figs 30–22 and 30–23).

CT is better than MRI in determining small erosions of bone in the superior and medial ethmoid at the borders of the cribiform plate. However, MRI tends to give better definition of the inferior aspect of the frontal lobe in relation to the tumor. As tumor erodes the thin bony plates at the upper medial limit of the ethmoid (fovea ethmoidalis), one would expect that the signal void (bone)

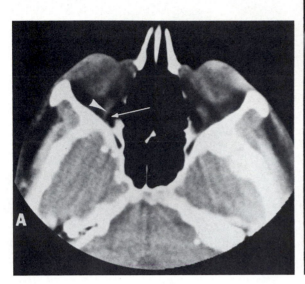

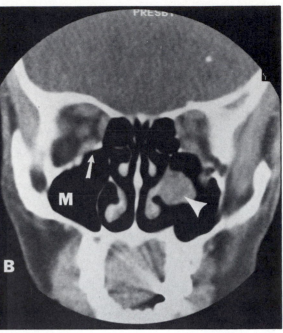

FIG 30–17.
False impression of tumor extension. **A,** axial scan through the superior recess of the maxillary sinus *(arrow)* at the level of the lower orbit. Tumor extending into this region can be confused with involvement of the orbit, especially as in this case, when the bony wall is indistinct *(arrowhead).* **B,** coronal scan showing the relationship of the superior recess *(arrow)* of the maxillary sinus *(M)* to the orbit. Tumor of the maxillary sinus is indicated by an *arrowhead.*

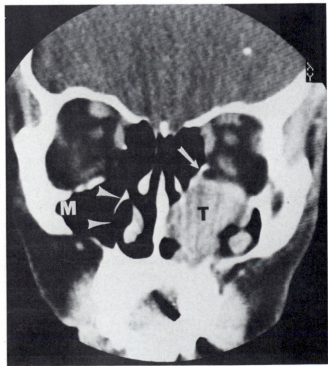

FIG 30–18.
Adenocystic carcinoma. Tumor *(T)* of the maxillary sinus and nasal cavity is destroying the medial wall of the maxillary sinus. Compare with the opposite side. The medial wall is indicated by *arrowheads* (*M* = maxillary sinus); the maxillary ethmoid plate is intact *(arrow).*

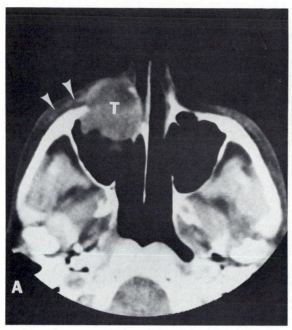

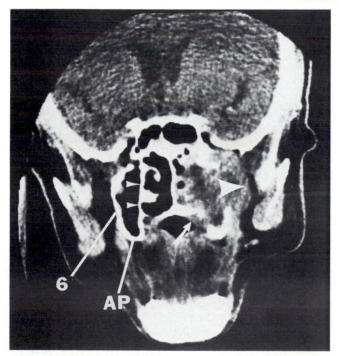

FIG 30–19.
Tumor extension. **A,** tumor *(T)* involving the anterior maxillary sinus wall and anterior cheek with destruction of the anterior wall of the maxillary sinus. The superficial muscle of the face is indicated by *arrowheads.* **B,** coronal scan with tumor extending into the fat planes of the cheek *(arrow).* Also note erosion of the orbital rim.

FIG 30–20.
Tumor extension. Coronal CT slice of tumor of the maxillary sinus that is destroying the medial and lateral walls. Tumor extends into fat planes of the infratemporal fossa *(large arrowhead).* The tumor breaks through into the mouth *(arrow).* On the normal side, the medial wall of the maxillary sinus is indicated by *small arrowheads,* the lateral wall by *6,* and the alveolar process by *AP.*

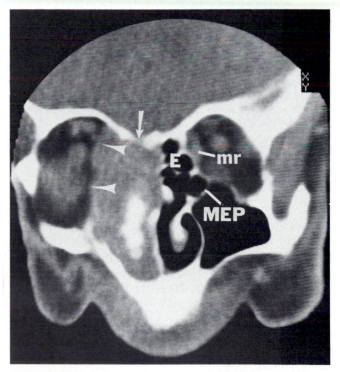

FIG 30–21.
Adenocystic carcinoma of the ethmoid is extending laterally into the orbit and obliterating fat planes near the medial rectus. The tumor margin is indicated by *arrowheads.* There is erosion of but not extension through the roof of the ethmoid *(arrow)* (normal side: *E* = ethmoid; *MEP* = maxillary ethmoid plate; *mr* = medial rectus).

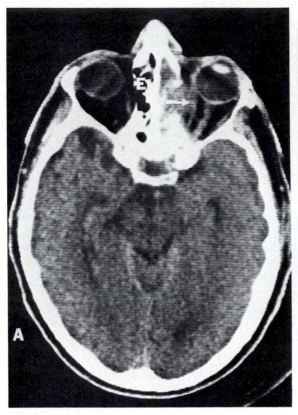

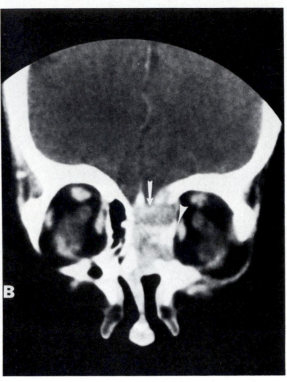

FIG 30–22.
Tumor of the ethmoid. An axial CT scan **(A)** shows tumor extending laterally and deviating the medial rectus *(arrow)* (*E* = ethmoid). **B,** a coronal view shows early lateral extension, but the fat plane is intact *(arrowhead),* which suggests that the lesion is limited by periosteum at this level. The cribriform plate is eroded *(arrow).*

would be replaced by signal from neoplastic tissue. However, even a small amount of normal mucosa or the normal intracranial tissue above "erases" the signal void of the extremely thin bone. Again, visualization of tissue above the expected level of the fovea ethmoidalis/cribiform plate becomes the key finding.

Posterior extension leads the tumor into the sphenoethmoidal recess and sphenoid sinus (Fig 30–24). The sphenoethmoidal recess is a narrow extension of the nasal cavity that partially indents the ethmoid and sphenoid sinuses. More laterally, only a bony wall separates the two sinuses. Bone destruction indicates tumor extension. Because of the position of the draining ostium of the sphenoid, tumor extending posteriorly from the ethmoid into the sphenoethmoid recess may obstruct the sphenoid sinus.

Sphenoid Sinus.—Tumors arising in the sphenoid are quite rare in our experience, and the problem is more commonly one of nasopharyngeal or ethmoid tumor extending into and at times through the sphenoid. Bone destruction is the key

to demonstrating extension, but again, CT or MRI can effectively visualize the structures outside the sinus. It may be very difficult to determine whether a tumor is extending into the brain or is limited by dura.

Superiorly, tumor extends into the pituitary fossa and suprasellar cisterns; posteriorly, it extends into the prepontine and crural cisterns. These areas normally are filled with cerebrospinal fluid and can be evaluated well by using coronal and axial scans respectively. Sagittal MRI scans are very helpful.

Tumor extends laterally into the cavernous sinus and eventually into the region of the temporal lobe.

CT examination performed with intravenous enhancement will show lateral bowing of the lateral margin of the cavernous sinus and can differentiate tumor from normal brain quite well (Fig 30–25). Without displacement of the cavernous sinus or extension into the temporal lobe, however, emphasis is placed again on the difficulty in differentiating bone loss resulting from tumor extension from that caused by early mucocele formation sec-

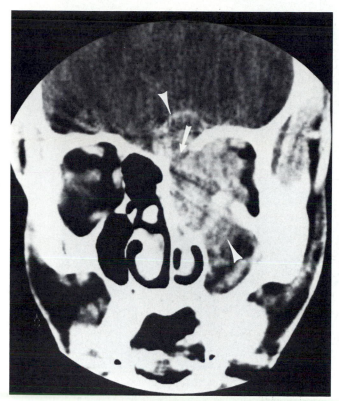

FIG 30–23.
Rhabdomyosarcoma of the ethmoid and orbit is extending through the roof of the ethmoid. Also note extension into the maxillary sinus. The tumor margin is indicated by *arrowheads*. The *arrow* denotes a defect in the roof of the ethmoid.

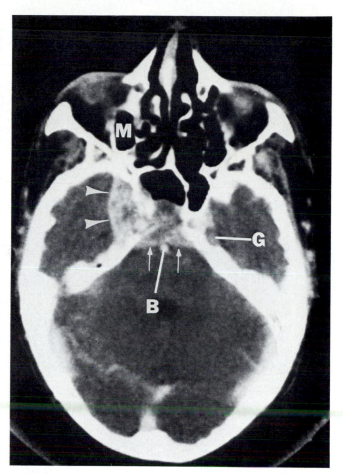

FIG 30–25.
Nasopharyngeal tumor involving the posterior and lateral walls of the sphenoid. Laterally, tumor extends through the gasserian ganglion and cavernous sinus and abuts on the temporal lobe *(arrowheads)*. Posteriorly, tumor extends into prepontine cistern *(arrows)* and pushes the basilar artery *(B)* (G = gasserian ganglion [normal]; M = superior recess of the maxillary sinus).

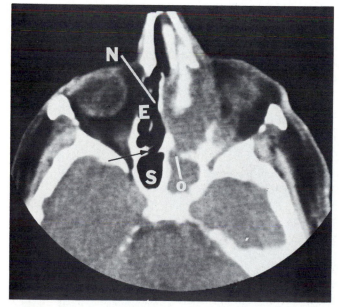

FIG 30–24.
Tumor of the ethmoid is extending posteriorly into the sphenoethmoid recess and sphenoid sinus as well as into the orbit (normal side: *E* = ethmoid; *S* = sphenoid; *arrow* = sphenoethmoid recess; *o* = ostium of the sphenoid sinus; *N* = upper nasal cavity).

ondary to sinus obstruction. Low density in the sinus can suggest mucocele formation, but central necrosis in the tumor will also produce an area of low density.

MRI has several advantages here. The sagittal orientation clearly defines the curving anterior wall and floor of the sella as well as the floor of the sphenoid sinus. The cavernous sinus is better evaluated on MRI than on CT not only because tumor can more readily be differentiated from the normal cavernous sinus but also because the carotid artery can be readily seen as a flow void in relation to the tumor or the cavernous sinus.

Frontal Sinus.—The frontal sinus is rarely a site of primary malignancy but may be along the route of spread of another malignancy (Fig 30–26). Detection of tumor spread posteriorly into the dura

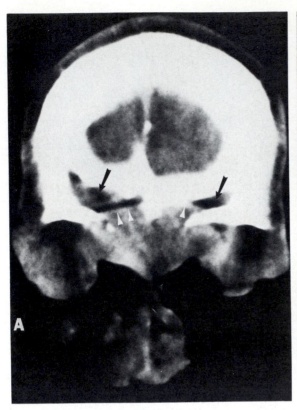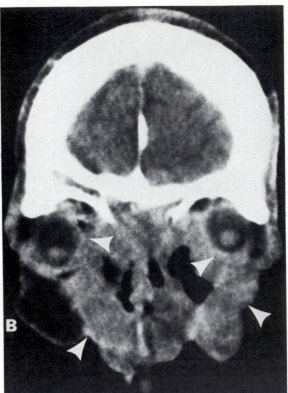

FIG 30–26.
Basal squamous cell carcinoma. **A,** tumor of the face is extending through the anterior wall of the frontal sinus. The tumor margin is indicated by *arrowheads*. The position of the tumor would prevent drainage of the sinuses through the nasofrontal ducts and cause mucus retention *(arrows)*. **B,** a more posterior slice shows involvement of the orbits with deviation of the eyes. The tumor margin is indicated by *arrowheads*.

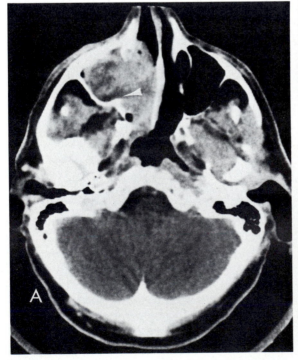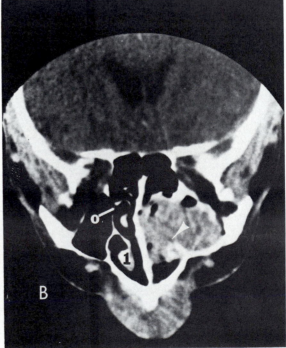

FIG 30–27.
Inverting papilloma. **A,** tumor of the nasal cavity is extending into the maxillary sinus. The tumor passes through the natural ostium but also destroys a portion of the medial wall of the maxillary sinus and turbinate *(arrowhead)*. **B,** coronal scan. Tumor erodes bone minimally *(arrowhead)* (normal side: *o* = maxillary ostium; *1* = inferior turbinate).

and brain can be detected both by the bone destruction and by the differential density between tumor and brain on an intravenously enhanced scan. MRI has the advantage of the sagittal orientation ideal for assessment of the curving junction where the floor of the anterior cranial fossa meets the posterior plate of the frontal sinus. The margin of the brain is usually more precisely seen on MRI than CT.

Nasal Cavity.—Tumors of the nasal cavity tend to extend into the sinuses where they can be seen in contrast to the air in the sinuses. Obstruction of the sinus ostium by the tumor is also quite common, which returns us to the problem of the opaque sinus (Fig 30–27).

Coronal imaging is key to evaluation of extension inferiorly through the palate or superiorly through the cribiform plate.

Lymphatic Spread

Lymphatic spread from sinus and nasal cavity lesions is relatively infrequent. The nodal groups most commonly involved should be included in the radiologic examination. They include the lateral pharyngeal nodes, the jugulodigastric nodes, and the deep cervical nodes.[14–16] The lymphatics of the most superior regions of the nasal cavity can travel on both sides of the cribiform plate and can also drain to the retropharyngeal nodes. A superficial lesion of the face or the vestibule of the nose can drain to the submandibular and parotid nodes. A common CT appearance of a node involved with metastatic disease is a low-density center with peripheral enhancement (Fig 30–28).

Perineural (Transforaminal) Spread

Tumor spread along a nerve trunk is an ominous sign (Fig 30–29).[7, 8, 17–19] Adenocystic carcinoma is well known for extending along nerves, but other malignancies can also metastasize in this manner. Tumor following the infraorbital nerve spreads to the pterygopalatine fossa (Fig 30–30). The alveolar and palatine nerves can also carry a malignancy to the pterygopalatine fossa (Fig 30–31). Involvement of this fossa is demonstrated by obliteration of the normal fat density within the fossa. The foramen rotundum connects the pterygopalatine fossa with the middle cranial fossa, and therefore, tumor can follow the maxillary division of the trigeminal nerve through the foramen rotundum to the region of the gasserian ganglion, cav-

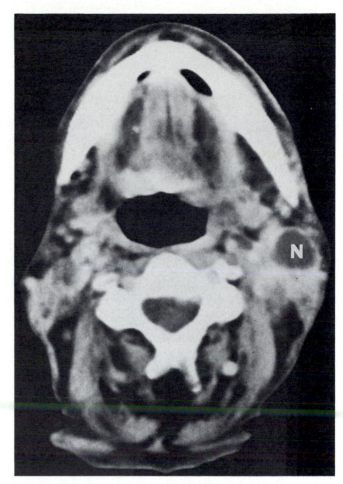

FIG 30–28.
Typical appearance of an involved jugulodigastric lymph node with an enhancing margin and low-density center (squamous cell carcinoma) (*N* = node).

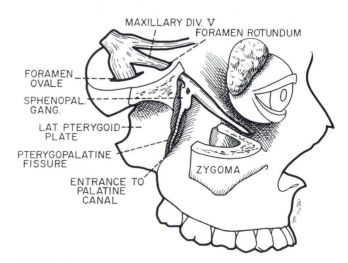

FIG 30–29.
Diagram of the maxillary division of the trigeminal (infraorbital) nerve, which is seen along the floor of the orbit.

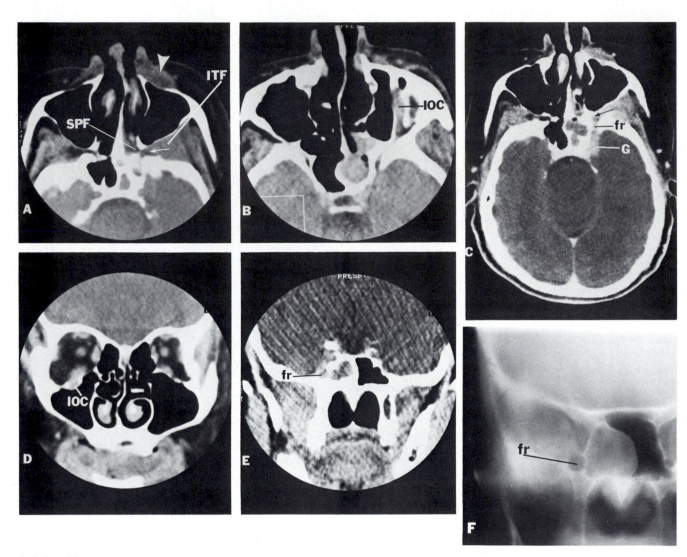

FIG 30–30.
Mixed histiocytic lymphocytic lymphoma. **A,** CT axial view, tumor of the cheek *(arrowhead)* and infratemporal fossa *(ITF)* obliterates the fat plane in the pterygopalatine fossa *(arrow)*. Tumor extends through the sphenopalatine foramen *(SPF)* into the posterior nasal cavity. **B,** axial view. The infraorbital canal is enlarged as it passes along the orbital floor *(IOC = infraorbital canal)*. **C,** tumor in the pterygopalatine fossa *(arrow)*. Tumor extends through and enlarges the foramen rotundum *(fr)*. Enhancement is seen in the gasserian ganglion region *(G)*. **D,** coronal slice through an enlarged infraorbital canal *(IOC)*. **E,** coronal slice showing an enlarged foramen rotundum *(fr)*. **F,** confirmatory tomogram of an enlarged foramen rotundum *(fr)*.

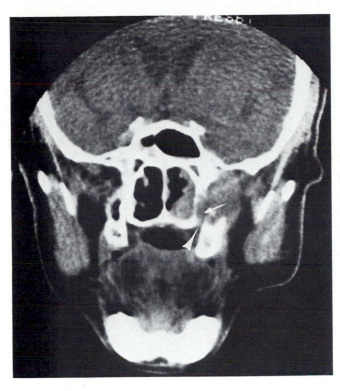

FIG 30–31.
Adenocystic carcinoma of the maxillary sinus has eroded into the lower portion of the pterygopalatine canal *(arrow)* just above the greater palatine foramen *(arrowhead)*. The pterygopalatine canal (palatine nerve) carried the tumor to the pterygopalatine fossa and eventually to the gasserian ganglion.

ernous sinus, and middle cranial fossa (Fig 30–32). The basal foramina, including their entrances and exits, can be well evaluated with CT or MRI using both axial and coronal projections.

Although enlargement of a foramen is a good indication of transforaminal spread, a word of caution must be added that demonstration of a normal foramen may not exclude extension through a foramen. So-called perineural extension may not enlarge a nerve and, therefore, may not enlarge the foramen. Distant recurrences, however, may be present, so the most common destination of this type of spread should still be radiographically evaluated.

Pterygopalatine Fossa Involvement

Before leaving our discussion of the types of spread of tumor, special emphasis should be made of the importance of the pterygopalatine fossa.[7, 8] This small area is situated between the posterior wall of the maxillary sinus and the anterior cortex of the pterygoid plate (Fig 30–33).

Axial imaging sections show definite fat density (or fat signal) within the fossa in normal situations. Visualization is optimal when slices are perpendicular to the posterior wall of the maxillary sinus (Fig 30–34). Coronal scans show the fat, which extends slightly toward midline in its superior portion. Small densities within the fat are neu-

ral and vascular structures. The importance of tumor spread into the pterygopalatine fossa relates not so much to any vital structures contained within the fossa as to the ease with which tumor can spread from the fossa to involve local or distant structures. Tumor extends into the fossa either directly or by transneural (perineural) spread along the infraorbital or palatine nerves.

From the pterygopalatine fossa, tumor has easy access to contiguous structures by way of the numerous foramina and fissures with which it connects. Superiorly, tumor extends through the inferior orbital fissure into the orbit.[20] Laterally, the fossa opens into the infratemporal fossa beneath the zygoma (Fig 30–35). Medially, the sphenopalatine foramen leads to the nasal cavity. These routes are important but not quite as ominous as spread posteriorly through the foramen rotundum, which gives access to the cavernous sinus and middle cranial fossa as mentioned in the previous section.

Evaluation of the pterygopalatine fossa and its connections should be considered as an important part of a CT or MRI study of the sinuses.

Types of Tumors

Neoplasms

Squamous cell carcinoma represents about 80% of malignant tumors of the sinuses and nasal cavity.

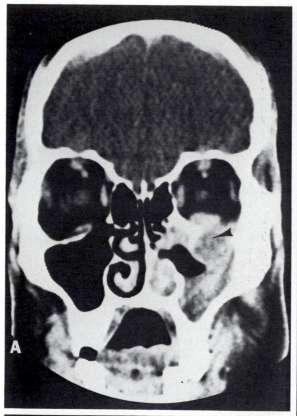

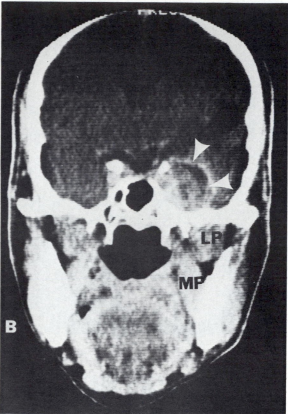

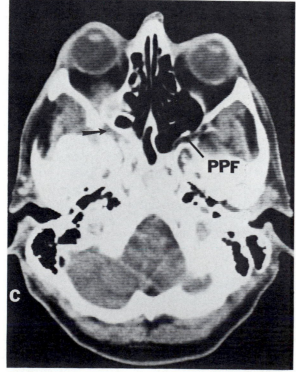

FIG 30–32.
Squamous cell carcinoma. **A,** tumor involves the cheek, sinus, and infraorbital nerve *(arrowhead)*. **B,** a coronal slice through the middle cranial fossa shows large tumor involving the gasserian ganglion and temporal lobe *(arrowheads)* (*LP* = lateral pterygoid muscle; *MP* = medial pterygoid muscle). **C,** an axial slice through the upper pterygopalatine fossa shows obliteration of fat planes *(arrow);* compare with the opposite side (*PPF* = upper pterygopalatine fossa). No destruction of the base of the skull around the foramen rotundum was seen.

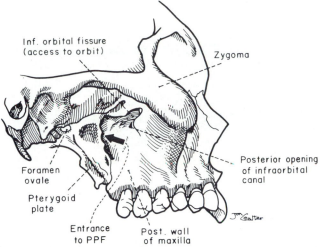

FIG 30–33.
Pterygopalatine fossa *(PPF)* between the posterior wall of the maxillary sinus and the anterior surface of the pterygoid plates.

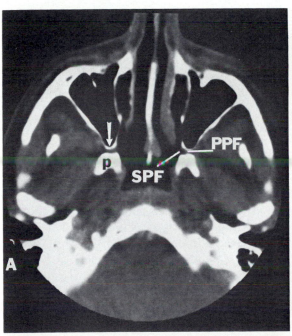

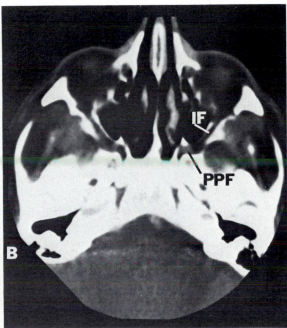

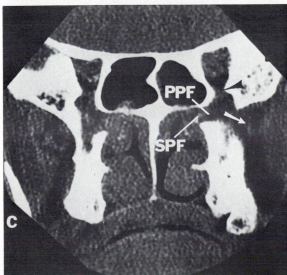

FIG 30–34.
Normal anatomy of pterygopalatine fossa *(PPF)*. **A,** normal axial slice low in the PPF (*p* = pterygoid plate; *arrow* = posterior wall of the maxillary sinus; *SPF* = sphenopalatine foramen). **B,** higher axial slice. The PPF meets the inferior orbital fissure *(IF)*. **C,** coronal slice through the PPF, which communicates medially with the nasal cavity through the sphenopalatine foramen *(SPF)* and laterally with the infratemporal fossa *(arrow)*. Superiorly, the fossa connects with the orbital apex *(arrowhead)*.

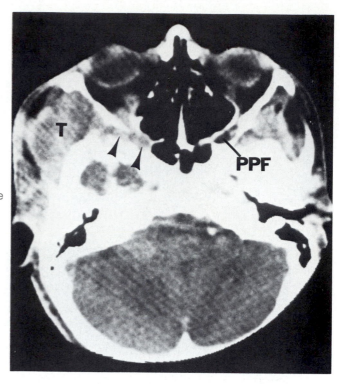

FIG 30–35.
Tumor *(T)* of the infratemporal fossa extending directly into the pterygopalatine fossa and obliterating the fat *(arrowheads).* Compare with the opposite normal side *(PPF* = pterygopalatine fossa).

Glandular tumors are less common, accounting for 10% to 14% of malignancies, and are broken down into adenocystic carcinoma, adenocarcinoma, mucoepidermoid, undifferentiated carcinoma, and pleomorphic adenoma. Rarer still are melanomas, lymphomas, plasmocytomas, and sarcomas. Olfactory neuroblastoma (esthesioneuroepithelioma) arises high in the nasal cavity. These tumors frequently extend through the cribiform plate (Fig 30–36). Even if apparently clear preoperatively, recurrence on the intracranial side of the cribiform plate is very frequent. This is best evaluated with coronal CT or MRI. At the time of this writing, a tissue-specific diagnosis of sinus and nasal cavity tumors cannot be made by CT or MRI, but the radiologist can estimate the aggressiveness of the tumor by the extent of the lesion and by how much bone is destroyed or remodeled. In some cases, bone or cartilage formation in the tumor can indicate an osteomatous or chondromatous lesion, but these represent a minority of cases (Fig 30–37). Osteomas (compact bone) may be single or multiple in Gardner's syndrome and be associated with colon polyps and skin lesions. Calcifications can be seen in some odontogenic tumors also.[21–23]

Other tumors arising in the bony skeleton of the sinuses are very rare. Giant-cell tumors have been described, although most authors conclude that almost all of these are giant-cell reparative granulomas. Giant-cell tumor may be seen in older patients in association with Paget's disease.[24–26]

Special note should be made of adenoid cystic carcinoma. This insidious tumor often exhibits perineural tumor spread and passes through the foramina to escape intracranially. Adenoid cystic carcinoma can also extend through a bone without causing a definite hole.[18, 19] Apparently passing through small defects in the bone, the tumor appears on the opposite side where the lesion is seen to contrast against the soft tissues.

Polyps and Papillomas

Benign lesions such as polyps and papillomas can be confused with malignancies because they are seen as masses causing obstruction and with some bone changes.

So-called polyps are inflammatory rather than neoplastic. They are translucent and smooth. The histologic picture is one of stromal edema and inflammatory cells. True papillomas are nontranslucent benign growths without the inflammatory edematous histologic appearance of polyps. Their etiology is most likely neoplastic, although the etiology remains unclear.

Polyps may or may not obstruct a sinus (Figs 30–38 and 30–39). They tend to cause bony remodeling rather than destruction if any bone change is present at all. Polyps can often be bilat-

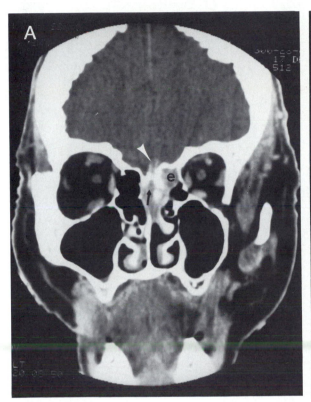

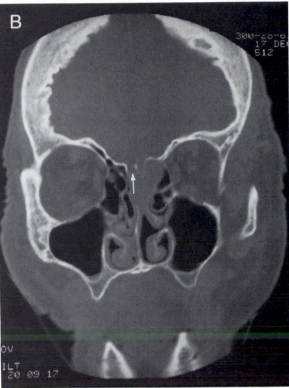

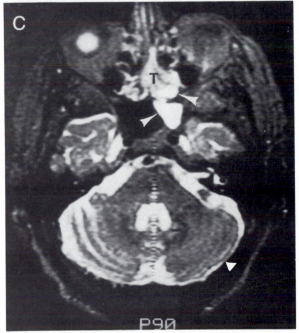

FIG 30–36.
Esthesioneuroblastoma. **A,** a coronal CT image shows an enhancing tumor in the high nasal cavity *(arrow)* extending into the ethmoid *(e)* and intracranially *(arrowhead)* through the cribiform plate. **B,** destruction of the cribiform plate is best demonstrated on a coronal CT with bony algorithm *(arrow)*. **C,** T2-weighted MRI showing tumor *(T)* obstructing the posterior ethmoid and sphenoid sinuses *(arrowheads)*.

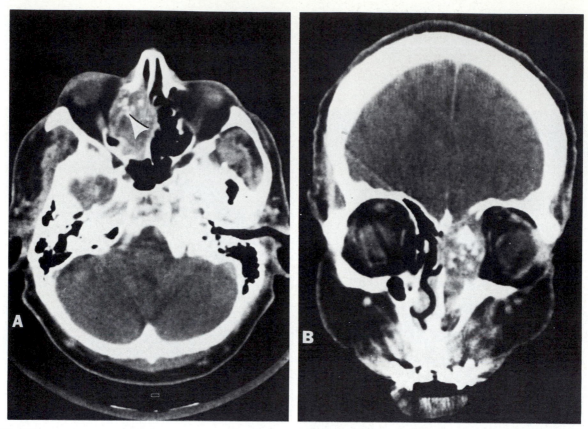

FIG 30–37.
Chondrosarcoma. An axial slice **(A)** through an ethmoid tumor shows calcification of the organic matrix *(arrowhead)*. **B,** coronal slice.

FIG 30–38.
Polyp. Axial CT slice through the maxillary sinus shows a polyp in the sinus *(arrowhead)* protruding through the ostium of the nasal cavity *(arrow)*.

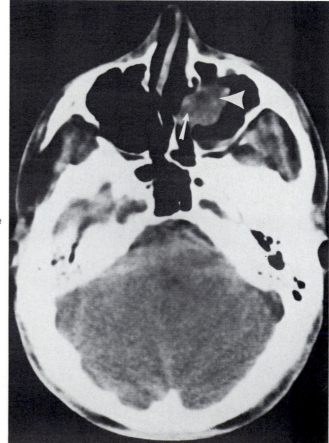

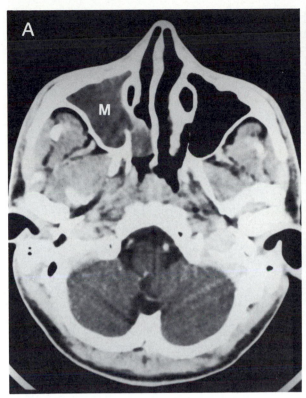

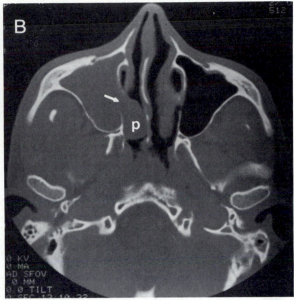

FIG 30–39.

Antrochoanal polyp. Axial CT slice **(A)** shows low-density soft tissue opacifying the maxillary sinus *(M)*. **B,** bone algorithm. The polyp *(P)* protrudes through a widened ostium *(arrow)* into the nasal cavity. The polyp extends posteriorly to the choana as marked by the pterygoid plates.

eral, especially when related to allergy, and can obstruct multiple sinuses without destroying large segments of bone (Fig 30–40). If a malignant tumor obstructs multiple sinuses, especially on both sides of the midline, there is almost always considerable bone destruction.

An inverting papilloma, although benign, is locally invasive and can cause bone destruction (Fig 30–41). Although the diagnosis may be suggested from the extent of the lesion and the position (almost all are unilateral and arise from the lateral wall of the nasal cavity), the diagnosis must be established by biopsy. Again, imaging is used to define the extent of the tumor and postoperatively to exclude recurrence.

Juvenile Angiofibroma of the Nasopharynx

Although not actually of the nasal cavity or sinus, this tumor can present with nasal obstruction and often affects the sinuses and nasal airway secondarily.[27] Producing epistaxis in adolescent males, the tumor has imaging findings that are usually characteristic. There is enlargement of the pterygopalatine fossa, with anterior displacement of the posterior maxillary wall (Fig 30–42). The tumor enhances intensely when the CT scan is performed with intravenous enhancement. The ptery-

gopalatine fossa normally can be unusually large when there is a hypoplastic maxillary sinus. In this case, the pterygopalatine fossa should contain the usual fat density.

Dental-Related Neoplasms and Cysts

Lesions arising in dental structures are seen during CT evaluation of the paranasal sinuses either as the primary pathology or as an incidental finding. Odontogenic tumors, benign or malignant, develop from cells that are related to formation of the tooth. These must be considered in evaluation of lesions of the alveolar process and floor of the maxillary sinus as well as of the mandible. Scans can define the extent of the lesion and suggest the nature of the central matrix of the abnormality.

The appearance of an odontogenic neoplasm is variable, depending on its cell origin and degree of differentiation. It can have a purely cystic appearance or may have varying amounts of calcification resembling a chondromatous lesion (Figs 30–43 and 30–44). Teeth in or bordering a lesion are also indicative of a dental origin, but the finding is not present in all cases.

The appearance of odontogenic tumors is well described in literature dealing with plain films. When a lesion is seen by CT or MRI, correlation

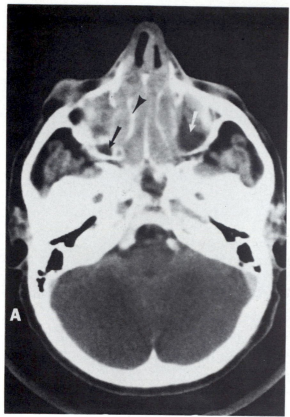

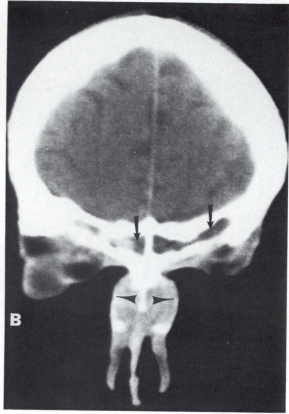

FIG 30–40.

Multiple polyps. Axial CT slice **(A)** shows diffuse enhancement filling the air spaces of the nasal cavity, but the bony turbinates are not destroyed *(arrowhead)*. Note the obstructed areas of the max-illary sinus, which shows characteristic low density *(arrows)*. **B,** a coronal slice shows obstructed frontal sinuses *(arrows)*. There is remodeling of the nasal bones *(arrowheads)*.

FIG 30–41.

Inverting papilloma with minimal destruction of the inferior turbinate *(arrow)*. Compare with the inferior turbinate *(1)* on the opposite side.

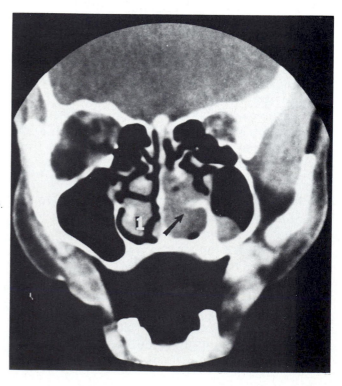

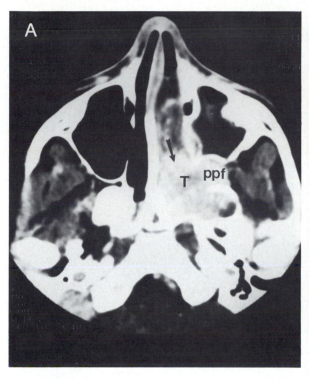

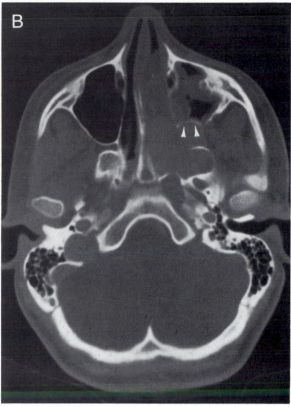

FIG 30–42.
Juvenile angiofibroma. Axial CT slice **(A)** shows enhancing tumor *(T)* in the posterior portion of the nasal cavity *(arrow)* with enlargement of the pterygopalatine fossa *(PPF)*. **B,** a bony algorithm demonstrates characteristic anterior bowing of the posterior wall of the maxillary sinus *(arrowheads)*.

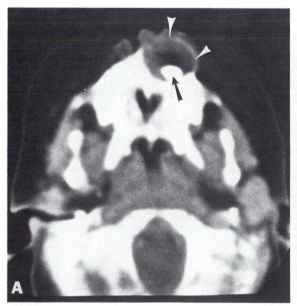

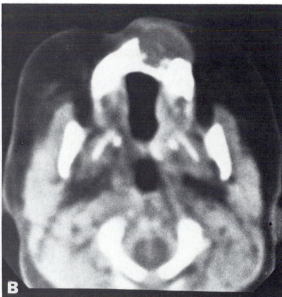

FIG 30–43.
Ameloblastic fibro-odontoma. **A,** axial CT shows a hypodense odontogenic tumor of the anterior maxilla *(arrowheads)*. The *arrow* indicates a tooth remnant. **B,** lower section showing a small amount of calcification in the lower part of the lesion.

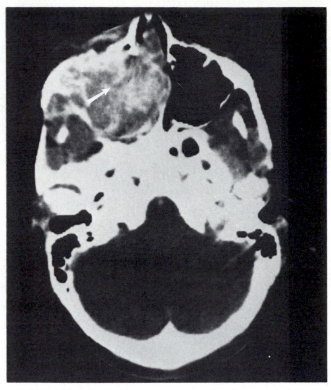

FIG 30–44.
Cemento-ossifying fibroma enlarging the maxillary sinus with central calcifications *(arrow).* The pterygopalatine fossa is "pushed" posteriorly, but the footplates are maintained.

with plain films, including dental films, is very important.[28] Little has been written about the CT findings in odontogenic neoplasms, but as further experience is accumulated, the ability of CT and MRI to give useful diagnostic information about the internal characteristics of these odontogenic neoplasms may allow for a more precise preoperative diagnosis.

Odontogenic and nonodontogenic cysts are also seen during evaluation of the sinuses. Odontogenic cysts can be recognized by the retained crown of the tooth (Fig 30–45). Some odontogenic tumors that do not calcify, such as ameloblastoma, odontogenic myxoma, and ameloblastic fibroma, can give a similar low-density appearance.

Nonodontogenic epithelial-lined cysts such as globulomaxillary or nasopalatine cysts do not arise from the tooth elements but from an epithelial remnant near the teeth. The incisive canal cyst (nasopalatine cyst) arises in the midline and widens or shortens the incisive canal between the central incisors (Fig 30–46). Most are small incidental findings, but very rarely one can grow large enough to present as a mass in the floor of the nose. The globulomaxillary cyst arises between the lateral incisor and the canine tooth.

Dentally related cysts arise within the bone of the alveolar process. Thus these lesions push the floor of the maxillary sinus or palate superiorly. A bony cortex passing along the superior aspect of a cyst, which represents the displaced floor of the maxillary sinus (or palate), is strong evidence that the lesion arises in the alveolar process and thus is of dental origin.

This brief description of some of the more common odontogenic entities that can occasionally be seen on CT or MRI is far from complete. Perhaps the most important thing to remember is how helpful correlation with dental films as well as with routine sinus views can be in these cases. An excellent description of the plain-film findings correlated with Pindborg's classification may be found in *Oral Roentgenographic Diagnosis* by Stafne and Gibilisco.[28]

Post-therapy Scanning

A brief note should be made about the role of imaging in the post-therapy patient. Familiarity with the various types of partial and total maxillectomy and ethmoidectomy as well as Caldwell-Luc defects can be helpful when trying to detect destruction from recurrent tumor (Fig 30–47).[29–31] The best method, however, is to obtain a scan in

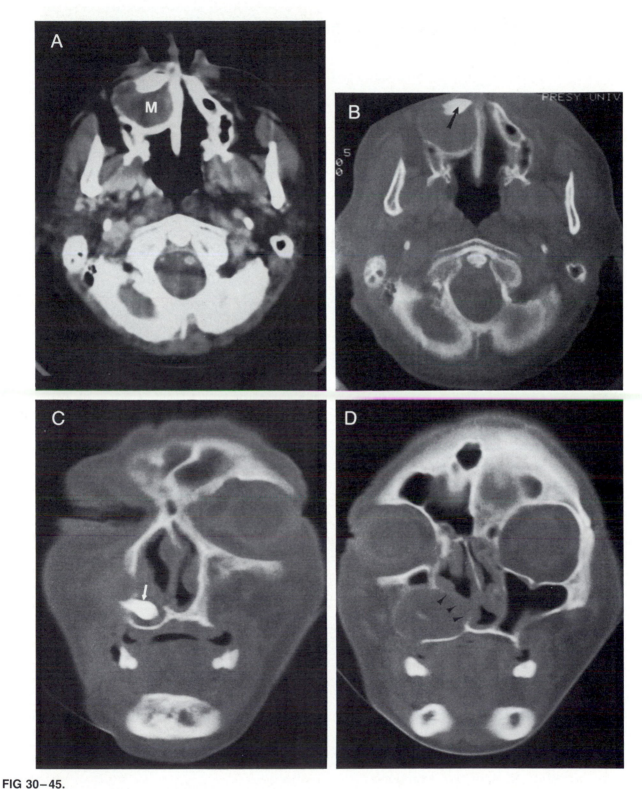

FIG 30–45.
Odontogenic cyst. **A,** a low-density lesion on a CT soft-tissue window is expanding into the maxillary sinus *(M)*. The cyst actually arises in the alveolar ridge. **B,** the *arrow* denotes a tooth remnant on the bone algorithm. **C,** a coronal slice shows the cyst and tooth remnant *(arrow)*. **D,** the superior margin represents the superior cortex of the bony alveolar process *(arrowheads)*.

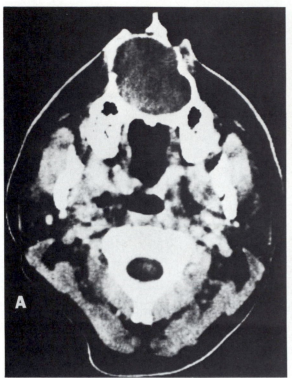 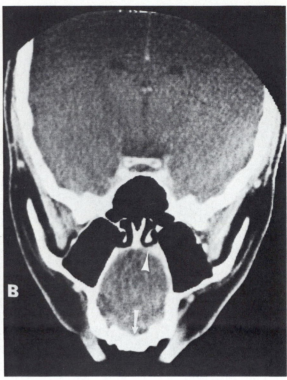

FIG 30–46.
Nasopalatine cyst (exceptionally large). **A,** this hypodense expansile lesion involves the anterior alveolar ridge and hard palate. **B,** coronal slice (angled because of metal fillings). The lesion is in the midline and extends into the septum. The upper bone margin *(ar-* *rowhead)* represents the superior cortex of the palate. The cyst arose in the nasopalatine canal between the central incisors *(arrow).*

the postoperative period so as to allow further comparison and detection of subtle recurrences. This postoperative scan should be done after 6 to 8 weeks to allow swelling to decrease.

INFECTION AND INFLAMMATORY PROCESSES

Sinusitis

Routine sinusitis is not usually evaluated with CT or MRI. When a secondary problem occurs such as orbital cellulitis or intracranial extension from frontal sinusitis, the secondary problem is evaluated by using the same principles for detection of spread as are used in staging tumors. In the same way that imaging shows the extension of tumor into the fat bordering the outer side of a bony wall, so too will imaging show extension of infection into the orbit. Most of our experience has been with CT. The infection may remain confined by the periosteum or can break through into the orbital fat. Precise localization can be made by CT as

the infection progresses, proptosis occurs, and the optic nerve is jeopardized.

Mucormycosis and Aspergillosis

Sinusitis can break through the lamina papyracea or follow the vessels to extend to tissues outside the sinuses. *Mucor* and other fungal infections, however, can destroy significant amounts of bone, enough so that they may be mistaken for malignancy (Fig 30–48).[32] Again, the radiologist must define as precisely as possible the extent of the lesion by using the same principles as in malignancies. Especially dangerous is extension through the orbital apex into the cavernous sinus. Here the invasive nature of the microorganism can cause occlusion of the ophthalmic and even the internal carotid arteries. Evaluation of the brain for evidence of infarction should also be performed during evaluation.

Aspergillosis can have a characteristic appearance on CT and MRI.[32] On CT the mycetoma is hyperdense. On MRI there is very little or no sig-

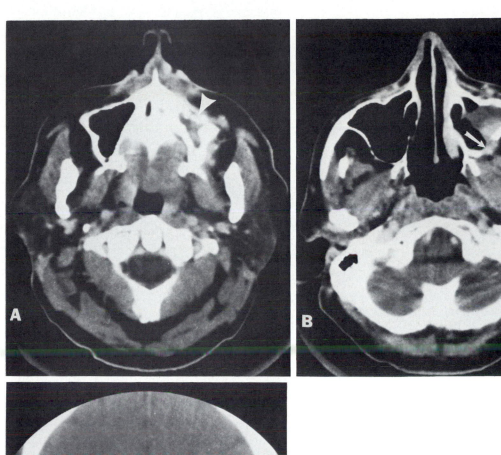

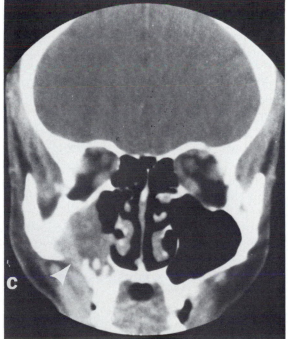

FIG 30–47.
Inverting papilloma with carcinoma in situ. An axial slice **(A)** shows irregular bone destruction of the anterior alveolar ridge *(arrowhead)*. This is the usual position of a Caldwell-Luc defect. **B,** higher slice showing a defect in the posterolateral wall *(arrow)* with slight impingement on the fat plane just outside the wall. This is not the usual defect and so underwent biopsy to show an inverting papilloma with carcinoma in situ. **C,** coronal slice through a defect from surgery just above the alveolar ridge. The defect is indicated by an *arrowhead*.

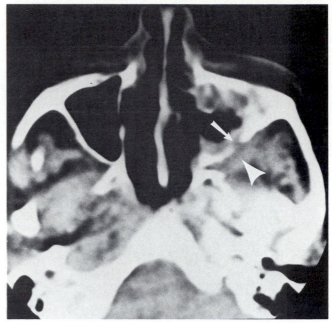

FIG 30–48.
Mucormycosis. An axial CT slice shows a defect in the posterolateral wall and obliteration of the normal fat plane outside the maxillary sinus. The defect is indicated by an *arrow*. Soft-tissue involvement in the infratemporal fossa is indicated *(arrowhead)*. Compare with the normal side.

nal mimicking an air-filled sinus. This is thought to be caused by certain paramagnetic properties of metallic constituents of the mycetoma itself (Fig 30–49).

Granulomatous Disease

Wegener's granulomatosis can cause bony changes, as can midline lethal granuloma. The bone destruction may suggest malignancy on CT scan. Bony replacement of the sinuses has been recently described in Wegener's granulomatosis.[33] At this time, however, more experience is needed to determine the imaging findings in this disease.

Mucocele

A mucocele forms when an entire sinus is obstructed.[34] The obstruction is usually related to sinusitis and inflammatory change but can also be associated with tumor. The bony walls of the sinus are remodeled as pressure builds behind the obstruction. In the usual case, this results in ballooning of the bony wall with some associated thinning (Fig 30–50). We have seen thinning of the bony wall without definite enlargement of the sphenoid sinus in obstruction by malignant neoplasm (Fig 30–51). Presumably, the more rapid course of the malignancy led to evaluation of the sinus before considerable expansion could occur.

Usually, the mucocele has a uniformly low density on CT, but this is not universal. With concurrent infection, a mucopyocele is formed that often shows enhancement on the postinfusion scan.

Any sinus can be affected. Involvement of the frontal and ethmoid sinuses is most common, followed by the sphenoid, which is less common, and the maxillary antrum, which is quite rare. In the ethmoid, one air cell may be grossly enlarged with isolated expansion, or the entire ethmoid can be enlarged with intact cell walls.[35, 36] This latter situation is usually seen in association with multiple polyps (Fig 30–52).

CT is ideally suited for defining the margin of the mucocele and also in detecting any complications related to "breakout" of the mucocele, be it into the orbit or into the anterior cranial fossa. Perhaps the most often asked question about a mucocele is in regard to its separation from the cranial contents. An intact bony cortex is reassuring to the surgeon, whereas detection of defects in the cortex, especially with enhancement of the dura, can forewarn the surgeon of a more difficult surgical problem (Fig 30–53).

Brief mention is made here of the retention cyst, which like a mucocele can have a uniform internal density, but unlike a mucocele does not involve the entire sinus. Rather, it has a smooth-domed margin and usually presents in the maxillary antrum (Fig 30–54).

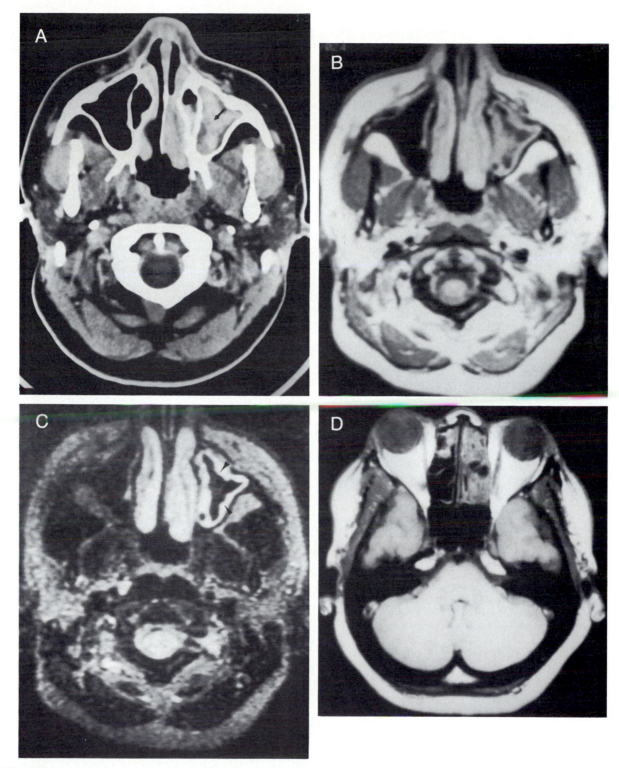

FIG 30–49.
Aspergillosis. **A,** an axial CT image with intravenous contrast shows enhancement centrally *(arrow)* within the left maxillary sinus. **B,** T1-weighted MRI demonstrates areas of low signal intensity that correspond to the enhancement on CT. **C,** a T2-weighted slice at the same level shows almost no signal from the mycetoma. The high signal intensity peripherally *(arrowheads)* represents inflammatory mucosa. **D,** a T1-weighted slice at a higher level shows involvement of the ethmoid sinus.

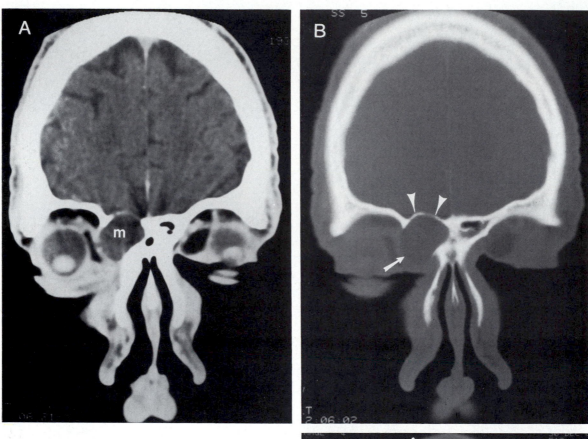

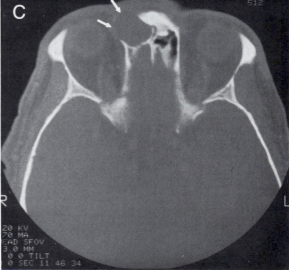

FIG 30–50.
Frontoethmoid mucocele. **A,** coronal CT slice through an expanded mucocele with displacement and actual defects in the bony wall. Note the low density within the mucocele *(m)* and the displaced globe. **B,** outward bowing of bone is indicated by *arrowheads* and the defect in bone by an *arrow*. **C,** axial slice with expansion of the frontoethmoid complex *(arrows).*

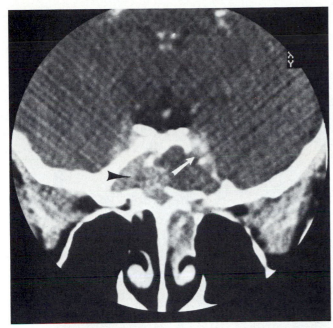

FIG 30–51.
Coronal CT in a patient with an obstructed sphenoid and tumor in the region of the ostium. Note the loss of the lateral bony wall of the sphenoid *(arrow)* and hypodense opacification of the sinus on that side. There is some enhancement on the opposite side *(arrowhead)*. At surgery, there was no tumor in the sphenoid, and the erosion of the lateral wall was from early mucocele formation. It was not clear whether the opposite side represented inflamed mucosa or slight extension of tumor into the anterior sphenoid on that side.

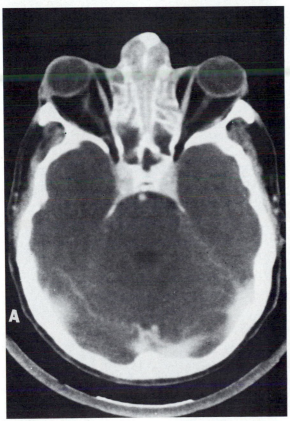

FIG 30–52.
Multiple polyps and diffuse opacification of the ethmoids and sphenoid. **A,** there is apparent expansion of the ethmoids, although the shape of the lateral wall of the ethmoids may be quite variable. **B,** coronal slice showing opacification of the nasal cavity and ethmoids. Note also a mucocele of the orbital roof *(arrow)*, which was a continuation of a mucocele involving the frontal sinus.

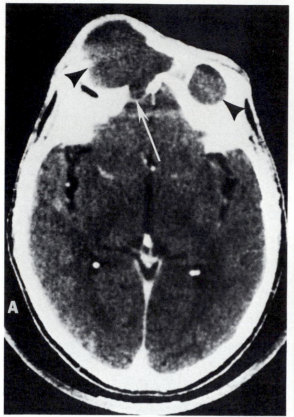

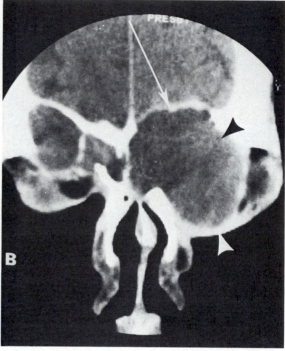

FIG 30–53.
Huge bilateral mucocele *(arrowheads)*. **A,** axial CT shows there is "breakthrough" of the posterior wall, with enhancement of the dura or wall of the mucocele *(arrow)*. At surgery, the dura and wall of the mucocele were adherent. **B,** coronal CT showing the mucocele *(arrowheads),* loss of bony margin, and enhancement of the wall of the mucocele or dura *(arrow)*.

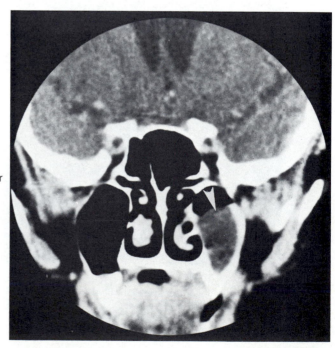

FIG 30–54.
Retention cyst in the maxillary sinus. Note the low density and upper "domed" margin *(arrowhead)*.

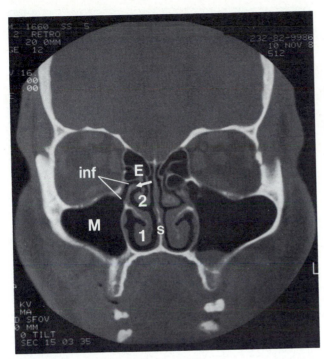

FIG 30–55.
Normal coronal anatomy of the middle meatus. The infundibulum *(inf)* is the groove between the lateral nasal wall/ethmoid bulla *(E)* and the uncinate process *(arrow)*. The infundibulum is continuous posteriorly with the middle meatus (1 = inferior turbinate; 2 = middle turbinate; S = nasal septum; M = maxillary sinus).

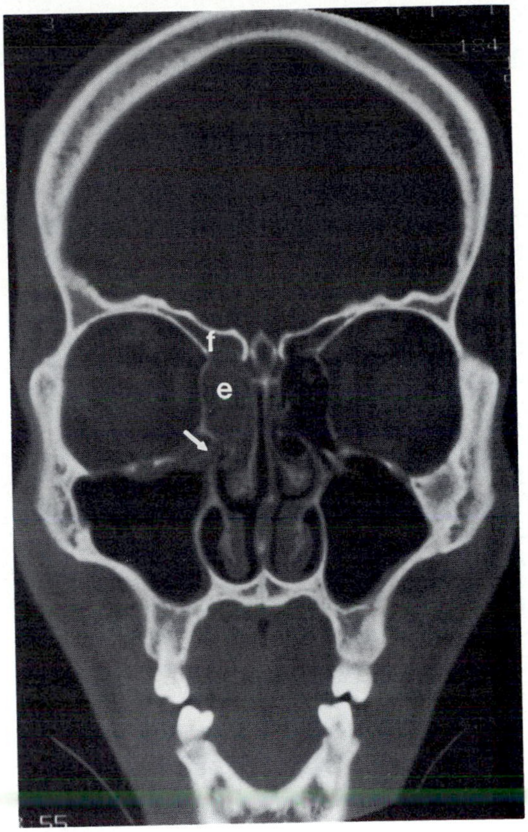

FIG 30–56.
Mucosal thickening occludes the infundibulum *(arrow)* and results in opacification of the frontal *(F)* and ethmoid *(e)* sinuses.

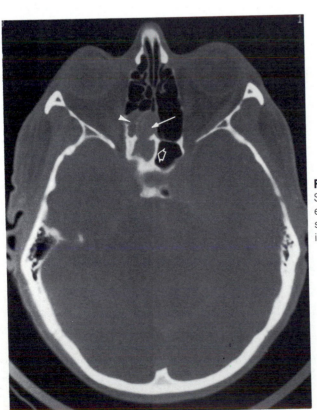

FIG 30–57.
Soft tissue in the sphenoethmoid recess *(arrow)* obstructs the posterior ethmoid air cells *(arrowhead)* and sphenoid sinus. The bony walls of the sphenoid sinus are thickened and sclerotic, thus indicating a chronic inflammatory process *(open arrow)*.

Endoscopic Surgery

The anatomy of the middle meatus has become increasingly important to the otolaryngologist because of recent developments in endoscopic nasal surgery.[37–40] The key landmarks during nasal endoscopy are the uncinate process and the infundibulum. CT in the direct coronal projection with bony algorithms is ideal for demonstrating these anatomic structures (Fig 30–55). Microscopic nasosinus surgery is aimed at relieving obstruction at the anterior end of the middle meatus. Either polyps are removed, or an infundibulotomy is performed by removing the uncinate process. Thus drainage is maintained through the natural ostium. Conventional surgical procedures create an artificial opening between the sinus and the nasal cavity.

Inflammatory mucosa, polyps, and tumors can occlude the middle meatus and result in characteristic opacification on CT. The frontal, anterior, and middle ethmoid air cells and the maxillary sinus drain into the middle meatus (Fig 30–56).

The posterior ethmoid air cells and the sphenoid sinus drain into the sphenoethmoid recess (Fig 30–57).

BONE DYSPLASIAS

These are briefly covered in the section on bone changes that was presented earlier in this chapter.

CRANIOFACIAL ANOMALIES

CT more than MRI has been used to stage congenital anomalies of the face and facial skeleton. Many anomalies can be appreciated on axial or coronal scans. For example, the bony defect in cleft palate patients can be appreciated in coronal images and usually axial images. Asymmetry of the sinuses or orbits or misalignment of the facial bones is easily visualized.

Patients with choanal atresia show convergence of the lateral wall of the nasal cavity toward the posterior nasal septum (Fig 30–58). Usually there is a small membranous area between the septum and the lateral wall of the nasal cavity rather than complete bony fusion.

In patients with craniofacial syndromes, the diagnosis is usually known, and the clinician wants

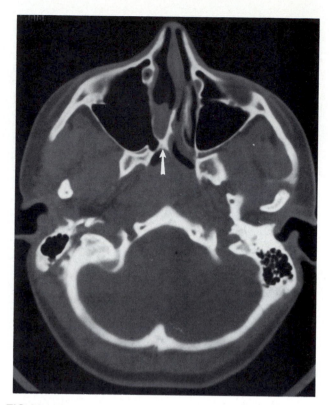

FIG 30–58.
Choanal atresia: bony fusion of the lateral nasal wall and the posterior nasal septum *(arrow)*. Retained secretions are present anterior to the atresia.

to know the relationship of the various bony structures. Recently three-dimensional imaging has been helpful in preoperative planning.[41] The relationship of the soft tissues to the bones as well as of one bone to another can be determined by using various computer programs (Fig 30–59). Measurements can be made in an attempt to determine how far a certain bone must be moved to achieve a more normal or symmetrical appearance.

An additional benefit of using three-dimensional CT is that the axial images that are used to generate the three-dimensional pictures also can be used to assess deeper structures. The temporal bone (especially the external and middle ears) may have an associated anomaly that can be assessed.

Facial Trauma

Facial fractures are routinely evaluated at this institution by plain films. If further information is needed, CT is done with coronal views as well as axial views. Fracture lines are best seen if the slice orientation is perpendicular to the surface of the bone fractured. Fractures in the same plane as the

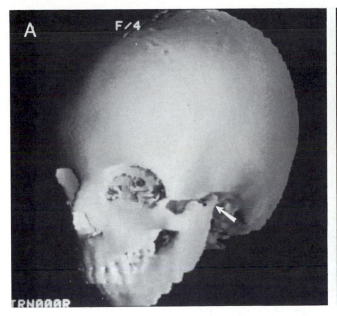

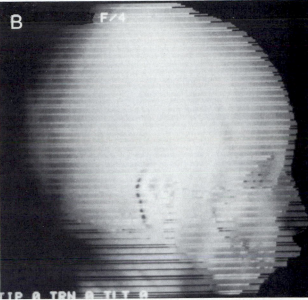

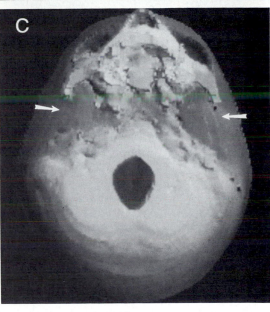

FIG 30–59.
Treacher Collins syndrome. **A,** an oblique three-dimensional image shows the absent zygomatic arch and hypoplastic mandible with shortening of the condyle *(arrow).* **B,** a lateral three-dimensional view with superimposition of the soft tissues demonstrates the posterior sloping of the anterior maxilla and micrognathia. **C,** base view after removal of the mandible. Note the absent zygomatic arches *(arrows).*

slice may be very difficult to assess. Fracture of the inferior orbital rim, orbital floor, lamina papyracea, palate, pterygoid plate as well as the roof of the ethmoid/cribiform plate area are all best seen in the coronal plane.

Axial plane images give good visualization of the anterior wall of the maxilla, posterolateral walls of the orbit and maxilla, zygomatic arch, and the anterior and posterior plates of the frontal sinus.

A blowout fracture is assessed in the coronal view whether it involves the lamina papyracea or the orbital floor (Fig 30–60). In the more significant floor fracture, the amount of herniated orbital

contents is important. Large fractures with significant amounts of fat herniation result in enophthalmos. The inferior rectus muscle can be "trapped" as a fracture opens and then closes. This can occur with very small fractures with little displacement. Lamina papyracea blowout fractures are less clinically significant unless they are very large.

Tripod fractures are most easily diagnosed by plain films. The zygomatic arch and frontozygomatic process fractures can be visualized in axial and coronal planes respectively. The third fracture line crosses from the inferior orbital rim to the lateral maxillary wall. This can be visualized directly on coronal CT. On axial CT this fracture line can

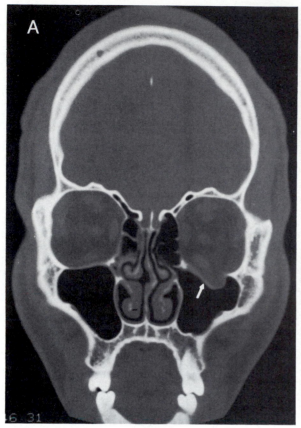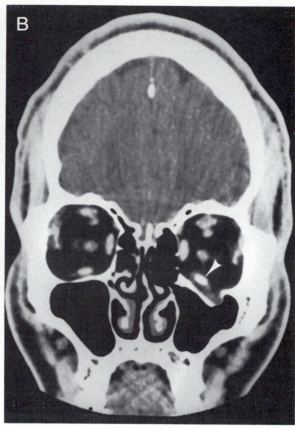

FIG 30–60.
Blowout fracture. **A,** coronal CT bony algorithm with an orbital floor fracture and inferior displacement *(arrow).* **B,** a soft-tissue window shows to better advantage herniation of fat through the fracture. The inferior rectus muscle *(arrowhead)* is not entrapped.

be seen to cross the orbital floor to the inferior orbital fissure and then along the posterolateral wall of the maxillary sinus (Fig 30–61). The posterolateral wall of the orbit is fractured as well and is seen in the axial image.

LeFort fractures represent separation of a portion of the face from the skull base. LeFort I crosses the lower maxilla and is actually in the axial plane. Coronal imaging is needed to visualize this fracture. LeFort II and III pass higher. Both cross the upper nose or bridge of the nose. LeFort II passes down over the inferior orbital rim and along the lateral maxillary sinus wall to exit through the pterygoid plate; LeFort III crosses higher through the lateral wall of the orbit and inferior orbital fissure. The zygomatic arch is spared in LeFort II, fractured in LeFort III.

All LeFort fractures eventually cross through the pterygoid plates. The fracture lines are in a horizontal or axial plane and thus are best visualized in the coronal plane.

The LeFort system has been less strenuously applied in recent times. The whole idea of imaging is to find a stable position to which the unstable fragment can be attached. For instance, attempted stabilization of a lower maxillary fracture to a zygomatic arch will fail if the zygomatic arch is free floating because of a subtle fracture that may be only slightly displaced.

The alveolar process may be crossed by a comminuted fracture and leave several free-floating fragments. This may be seen with sagittal split fractures of the palate. Each fragment must be identified and stabilized by sutures or intermaxillary fixation if the fragments are to heal correctly with good dental occlusion.

Fractures of the nasal bridge and frontal sinus are frequently associated with cribiform plate fracture and fracture of the posterior plate of the frontal sinus (Fig 30–62). Cerebrospinal fluid leak or hematoma may result and can be assessed by using axial and coronal CT.

Two- and three-dimensional reformatted images can be done from axial CT data and provide

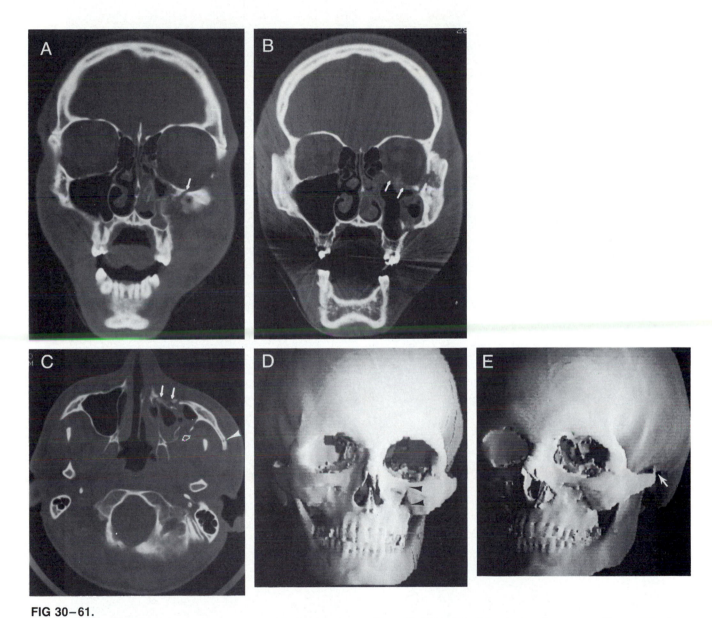

FIG 30–61.
Tripod fracture. **A** and **B,** coronal sections show fractures of the orbital rim and floor *(arrows).* **C,** fracture involves the zygomatic arch *(arrowhead).* Note the fractures through the anterior *(double arrows)* and posterolateral walls *(open arrow)* of the maxillary sinus.

D and **E,** AP and 45-degree left oblique views. Three-dimensional images show the fracture lines *(arrowheads)* and spatial relationships. Note the buckling of the zygomatic arch *(arrow).*

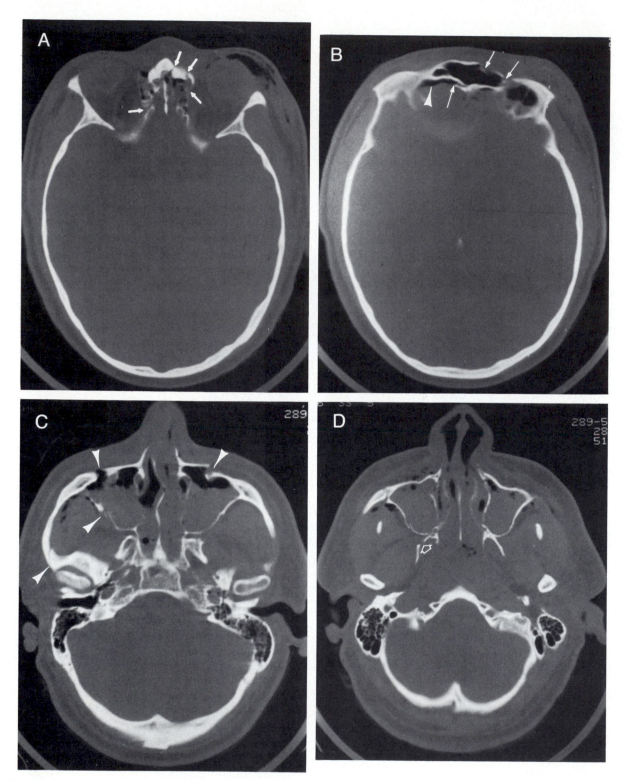

FIG 30–62.
Lefort fracture. **A,** comminuted fracture *(arrows)* through the ethmoid and bridge of the nose with posterior displacement. Fracture lines cross through the region of the crista galli and cribiform plate. **B,** the anterior and posterior walls of the frontal sinus are fractured *(arrow).* Pneumocephalus is present *(arrowhead).* **C,** a fracture involves the right zygomatic arch and both maxillary sinuses *(arrowheads).* **D,** the pterygoid plate is fractured on the right *(open arrow).*

good information about relationships of fracture fragments. Small fracture lines can easily be missed, and direct coronal imaging gives better resolution. Scans done acutely may be inappropriate for two-dimensional and three-dimensional reformats because any patient motion can significantly degrade the image.

Three-dimensional images have the added advantage that they can be rotated into any position to optimally view the relationship of a displaced bone. The surfaces are opaque, so superimposition of skull base shadows is not a problem as, for instance, in a plain radiograph.

Finally, hematoma of the soft tissues, especially in the orbit, can be seen on CT. Foreign bodies can be evaluated in reference to crucial structures such as the globe.

SUMMARY

Scanning by CT and MRI has become a very important mode of investigation in the region of the paranasal sinuses. In our institution, almost all lesions undergo biopsy, and the ability of CT or MRI to define the precise extent of the lesion has been more helpful than our ability to make a specific diagnosis. As experience increases, more definitive diagnoses may be made as MRI characteristics become more specific. The improved soft-tissue contrast and multiplanar imaging capability of MRI are distinct advantages over CT for tumor evaluation. CT with bone algorithms provides better detail of bony structures and therefore remains the imaging procedure of choice for craniofacial anomalies and facial trauma.

REFERENCES

1. Valvassori GE, Mafee MF (eds): Diagnostic imaging. *Otolaryngol Clin North Am*, May 1988.
2. Mancuso AA, Hanafee WN: *Computed Tomography and Magnetic Resonance Imaging of the Head and Neck*, ed 2. Baltimore, Williams & Wilkins, 1985.
3. Bergeron RT, Osborn AG, Som PM (eds): *Head and Neck Excluding the Brain*. St Louis, CV Mosby Co, 1984.
4. Valvassori GE, Potter GD, Hanafee WN, et al: *Radiology of the Ear, Nose and Throat*. Philadelphia, WB Saunders Co, 1982.
5. Brant-Zawadzki M, Norman D (eds): *Magnetic Resonance Imaging of the Central Nervous System*. New York, Raven Press, 1987.
6. Som PM, Shugar JMA, Cohen BA, et al: The non-specificity of the antral bowing sign in maxillary sinus pathology. *J Comput Assist Tomogr* 1981; 5:350–352.
7. Dodd GD, Dolan PA, Ballantyne AJ, et al: The dissemination of tumors of the head and neck via the cranial nerves. *Radiol Clin North Am* 1970; 8:445–461.
8. Curtin HD, Williams R, Johnson J: CT of perineural tumor extension: Pterygopalatine fossa. *AJNR* 1984; 5:731–737.
9. Higashi T, Iguchi M, Shimura A, et al: Computed tomography and bone scintigraphy in polyostotic fibrous dysplasia. *Oral Surg* 1980; 50:580–583.
10. Beighton P, Durr L, Hamersma H: Clinical features of sclerosteosis—a review of the manifestations in twenty-five affected individuals. *Ann Intern Med* 1976; 84:393–397.
11. Beighton P, Hamersma H, Horan F: Craniometaphyseal dysplasia: Variability of expression within a large family. *Clin Genet* 1979; 15:252–258.
12. Hamersma H: Facial nerve paralysis in the osteopetroses, in Fisch V (ed): *Proceedings of the 3rd Symposium on Facial Nerve Surgery*. Zurich, Switzerland, 1976, p 555.
13. Som PM, Shapiro M, Biller HF, et al: Sinonasal tumors and inflammatory tissues: Differentiation with MR imaging. *Radiology* 1988; 167:803–808.
14. Mancuso AA, Maceri D, Rice D, et al: CT of cervical lymph node cancer. *AJR* 1981; 136:381–385.
15. Som PM: Lymph nodes of the neck. *Radiology* 1987; 165:593–600.
16. Mancuso AA, Harnsberger HR, Muraki AS, et al: Computed tomography of cervical and retropharyngeal lymph nodes: Normal anatomy, variants of normal, and applications in staging head and neck cancer. Part I: Normal anatomy. *Radiology* 1983; 148:709–714.
17. Ballantyne AJ, McCarten AB, Ibanez ML: The extension of cancer of the head and neck through peripheral nerves. *Am J Surg* 1963; 106:651–667.
18. Conley J, Dingham DL: Adenoid cystic carcinoma in the head and neck (cylindroma). *Arch Otolaryngol* 100:81–90.
19. Spiro RH, Huvos AG, Strong EW: Adenoid cystic carcinoma of salivary origin: A clinicopathologic study of 242 cases. *Am J Surg* 1974; 128:512–520.
20. Hesselink JR, Weber AL: Pathways of orbital extension of extraorbital neoplasms. *J Comput Assist Tomogr* 1982; 6:593–597.
21. Batsakis JG: *Tumors of the Head and Neck: Clinical and Pathological Considerations*, ed 2. Baltimore, Williams & Wilkins, 1979.
22. Sisson GA, Becker SP: Cancer of the nasal cavity and paranasal sinuses, in Suen JY, Myers EN (eds): *Cancer of the Head and Neck*. New York, Churchill Livingstone, Inc, 1981, pp 242–279.
23. Barnes L: *Surgical Pathology of the Head and Neck*, New York, Marcel Dekker, Inc, 1985.
24. Handler SD, Savino PJ, Peyster RG, et al: Giant

cell tumor of the ethmoid sinus: An unusual cause of proptosis in a child. *Otolaryngol Head Neck Surg* 1982; 90:513–515.

25. Jaffe HL: Giant cell reparative granuloma, traumatic bone cyst and fibrous (fibro-osseous) dysplasia of the jaw bones. *Oral Surg* 1953; 6:159–175.

26. Spjut HJ, Dorfman HD, Fechner RE, et al: *Tumors of Bone and Cartilage.* Washington, DC, Armed Forces Institute of Pathology, 1970.

27. Bryan RN, Sessions RB, Horowitz BL: Radiographic management of juvenile angiofibroma. *AJNR* 1981; 2:157–166.

28. Stafne EC, Gibilisco JA: *Oral Roentgenographic Diagnosis,* ed 4. Philadelphia, WB Saunders Co, 1975.

29. Lore JM: Partial and radical maxillectomy. *Otolaryngol Clin North Am* 1976; 9:255–267.

30. Som PM, Shugar JMA, Billar HF: The early detection of antral malignancy in the post maxillectomy patient. *Radiology* 1982; 143:509–512.

31. Som PM, Lawson W, Biller HF, et al: Ethmoid sinus disease: CT evaluation in 400 cases, Part II. Postoperative Findings. *Radiology* 1986; 159:599–604.

32. Centeno RS, Bentson JR, Mancuso A: Ct scanning in rhinocerebral mucormycosis and aspergillosis. *Radiology* 1981; 140:383–389.

33. Paling MR, Roberts RL, Fauci AS: Paranasal sinus obliterations in Wegener's granulomatosis. *Radiology* 1982; 144:539–543.

34. Hesselink JR, Weber AL, New PFJ, et al: Evaluation of mucoceles of the paranasal sinuses with computed tomography. *Radiology* 1979; 133:397–400.

35. Jacobs M, Som P: The ethmoidal "polypoid mucocele." *J Comput Assist Tomogr* 1982; 6:721–724.

36. Som PM, Shugar JA: CT classification of ethmoid mucoceles. *J Comput Assist Tomogr* 1980; 4:199–203.

37. Kennedy DW, Zinreich SJ, Rosenbaum AE, et al: Functional endoscopic sinus surgery. *Arch Otolaryngol* 1985; 3:576–582.

38. Stammberger H: Endoscopic endonasal surgery—Concepts in treatment of recurring rhinosinusitis. Part I. Anatomic and pathophysiologic considerations. *Otolaryngol Head Neck Surg* 1986; 94:143–146.

39. Stammberger H: Endoscopic endonasal surgery—Concepts in treatment of recurring rhinosinusitis. Part II. Surgical technique. *Otolaryngol Head Neck Surg* 1986; 94:147–156.

40. Hollinshead WH: The nose and paranasal sinuses, in *Anatomy for Surgeons, vol 1. The Head and Neck, ed 3.* Philadelphia, Harper & Row Publishers, Inc, 1982, pp 223–267.

41. Marsh JL, Vannier MW, et al: *Comprehensive Care for Craniofacial Deformities.* St Louis, CV Mosby Co, 1985.

31

Selected CT and MRI Examinations of the Maxilla, Mandible, and Temporomandibular Joints

George A. Carr, D.D.S.

Charles E. Seibert, M.D.

Glen E. Burmeister, M.D.

Techniques for conventional dental intraoral roentgenographic examinations have experienced minimal modification as compared with extraoral assessment of the dental arches and surrounding structures. Intraoral radiographic examinations will vary from complete to partial evaluation of the individual dental units and consist of periapical films, bite-wing films, and occasionally an occlusal film for larger alveolar and soft-tissue structures. Extraoral radiographic examinations consist of a variety of panoramic, cephalometric, transcranial studies, tomography, computerized tomography (CT), magnetic resonance imaging (MRI), and arthrography to assess the maxilla, mandible, temporomandibular joints (TMJs), salivary glands, and other related cranial anatomy. With the introduction of computer software for computer-generated reformation, CT and MRI have become extremely valuable in the evaluation of dental structures.

Through computer-assisted design (CAD) and computer-assisted manufacturing (CAM), a CT scan of either the maxilla and/or mandible can be acquired and reformatted and a synthetic bone model manufactured. From this model a subperiosteal framework is designed by the dentist, and a subperiosteal dental implant is custom fabricated. The procedure eliminates bone impression surgery and results in one surgery for placement.

Another CT scanning technique is the assessment of the dental arches for the placement of a dental endosseous implant. Computer software programmed to create various oblique cross sections from axial images provides location of essential anatomic structures, cross-sectional measurements for implant length and width determination, and various bone densities. Maximum utilization of available bone is now incorporated into the plan for the location of an endosseous dental implant, thereby improving the success of the implant procedure.

MRI of the TMJ and surrounding areas has benefitted the diagnosis of TMJ dysfunction by its ability to demonstrate soft-tissue anatomy significantly better than CT or arthrography. This noninvasive technique accurately demonstrates meniscus morphology as it relates to internal derangement and degeneration. Dynamic motion studies of the TMJ during function may further enhance meniscus examination vs. the single or bilateral, closed or open views alone.

SUBPERIOSTEAL DENTAL IMPLANT FABRICATION FROM CAD-CAM MULTIPLANAR DIAGNOSTIC IMAGING

The first subperiosteal dental implant was designed by a Swedish dentist, Gustav Dahl, in

1941.[1] In 1948, the Americans Gershoff and Goldberg visited Dahl and incorporated this form of implant into their armamentarium.[2] Their first implants were made by utilizing soft-tissue impressions and a full series of periapical radiographs. The stone models from the impressions were then scraped according to the mucosal thickness estimated from the individual periapical radiographs to simulate the underlying bony topography.[3, 4] Narrow strips of Vitallium (a chromium-cobalt alloy from Howmedica, Inc., Chicago) were constructed, based on the models. These strips rested only on the top of the crest of the alveolar ridge and were held in place by Vitallium screws.[5]

Subperiosteal Methodology

The sophistication of diagnostic as well as surgical advancement has enhanced clinical implementation of this procedure, which has undergone important revisions. For over 20 years, the conventional method of subperiosteal implant placement has required two surgical procedures.[6, 7] The first procedure is to surgically expose the residual bony ridge and make an impression. A model is then fabricated in dental stone. Upon this model a surgical Vitallium framework is constructed in the laboratory. The second surgical procedure involves placing the custom framework on the bony surface and covering it with the existing mucoperiosteum. This technique has the following disadvantages: (1) the patient must undergo two surgical procedures, (2) it is time-consuming, and (3) impression of the residual structures is technique sensitive due to the surgical field.

In the mid-1980s, Truitt, James, and Boyne introduced a technique by which a presurgical three-dimensional model of a patient's mandible was fabricated by incorporating CT scanning.[8, 9] This revolutionized the technique since it eliminated the first surgical procedure, the bone impression. Modifications of scanning and protocol technique were reported by Benjamin for 38 cases in 1987.[10] Currently, Calcitek, Inc. (Carlsbad, Calif.) and Cemax, Inc. (Fremont, Calif.) supply technical information and protocols to the dentist and radiologist for CT scanning and CAD-CAM fabrication.

Consequently, the subperiosteal dental implant procedure has undergone further revisions. The framework still seats directly on the residual atrophic maxillary and/or mandibular alveolar ridge below the oral soft tissues. Four abutment posts protrude through the remaining attached gingiva bilaterally in the region of the patient's cuspids and first molars (Fig 31–1). A new design in subperiosteal framework utilizes increased surface area on the lateral aspects of the rami of the mandible and two posterior struts for stress distribution (Fig 31–2).[11] The final removable implant prosthesis is completely supported by the subperiosteal implant superstructure and, therefore, has no contact with the patient's residual ridge.

CT Scanning of the Patient

A multidisciplinary approach to patient preparation and treatment is planned prior to the CT

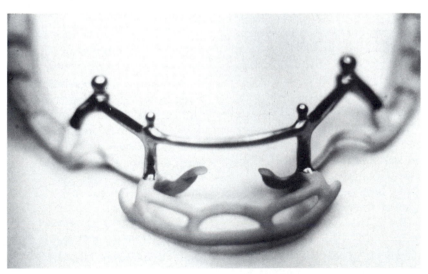

FIG 31–1.
Superstructure of CT subperiosteal implant illustrating post placement in areas of cuspids and first molars. (Courtesy of Calcitek, Inc., Carlsbad, Calif.)

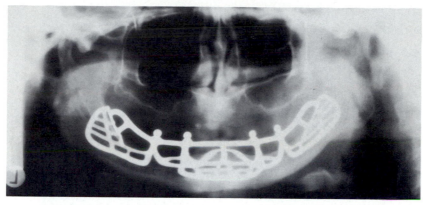

FIG 31–2.
Panorex radiograph of mandibular subperiosteal implant showing extensions of lateral framework onto both lateral rami of the mandi- ble and two posterior struts attached to ascending rami. (Courtesy of Dr. Carl R. Misch, Dearborn, Mich.)

scan. The patient is evaluated medically, dentally, and psychologically to assess patient acceptability for the subperiosteal implant. During this acquisi- tion of information, the patient should be informed of the CT scan format and be given comprehensive instructions concerning the implant placement. As with any CT scan, the possibility exists that the scan may not be adequate for model fabrication, and a bone impression would be an alternate methodology.

It is necessary that the patient's maxilla and/or mandible be immobilized during the scanning pro- cedure. This is accomplished by the fabrication of nonradiopaque self-curing acrylic resin intraoral stents. The stents also represent the proper vertical dimension of occlusion and centric relation for that patient, which the dentist records at an appoint- ment prior to stent fabrication. Consideration must be given to the possibility of saliva accumulation during scanning, and an access portal can be incor- porated in a stent to utilize a nonmetallic saliva ejector. The dentist supplies this equipment to the CT scanning personnel along with denture adhe- sive for fixation of the stents. It may be necessary to premedicate the patient with an antisialagogue to decrease saliva. The decision to use this form of medication will depend in part on the patient's medical history.

A Panorex radiograph of the patient must ac- company the stents to indicate the vertical extent of the ascending ramus of the mandible and/or maxilla to be included in the CT scan. The radio- graph is an excellent screening modality for metal restorations present at or near the edentulous ar-

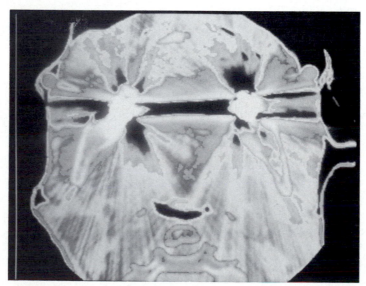

FIG 31–3.
Image of a metal artifact. (Courtesy of Calcitek, Inc., Carlsbad, Calif.)

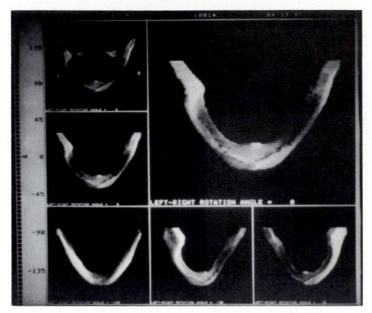

FIG 31–4.
Three-dimensional reconstruction of the mandible from CT scan image data. (Courtesy of Calcitek, Inc., Carlsbad, Calif.)

eas. These dental restorations can create image artifact (Fig 31–3) and should be replaced with composite resin material.

During the CT scan, the patient is secured on the CT scan table, and the head is positioned at the proper angle. At the beginning of the scan, the patient must be evaluated for proper stent placement and adequate saliva control and be verbally assured of the procedure so that there is no movement of the head. Slice thickness should be 2 mm or less, spaced every 1 mm for good three-dimensional (3-D) reformations. Dynamic scanning should be used to decrease motion; scan times may vary according to the particular machine used. Equipment requirements for the CT scan are straightforward, and many machines may be used. The technical settings for recommended CT scan machines can be requested from the subperiosteal consulting company.

CAD-CAM Methodology

Once the CT scan is completed, the image data are transferred to magnetic tape. These data are reformatted by computer, and a (3-D) image is constructed (Fig 31–4). From this image the computer interfaces with a computer numerically controlled (CNC) milling device (Fig 31–5) to fabricate a synthetic bone model (Fig 31–6). The bone model is utilized by the dentist to design a custom subperiosteal dental implant (Fig 31–7).

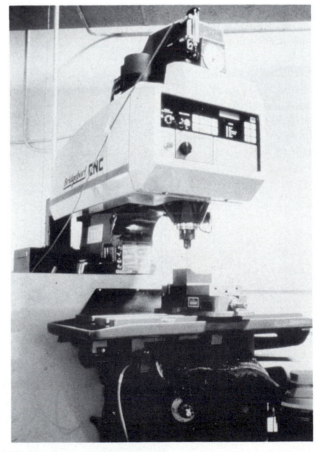

FIG 31–5.
CNC milling device for the fabrication of the synthetic bone model. (Courtesy of Calcitek, Inc., Carlsbad Calif.)

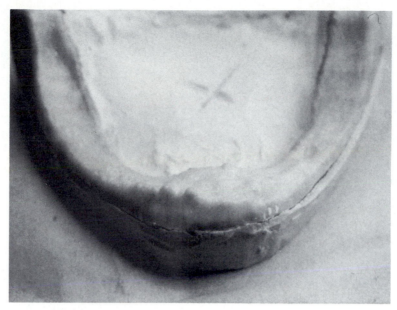

FIG 31–6.
Synthetic bone model in a stone base for framework design. (Courtesy of Calcitek, Inc., Carlsbad Calif.)

Summary

With the advances of computer imaging, both dentistry and medicine are experiencing rapid growth in bone reconstruction techniques. Although the implant procedure previously described concentrates on only two anatomic structures, the mandible and the maxilla, various protocols are available to replicate other head and neck structures (Fig 31–8). Consequently, various bony defects and anomalies can be visualized, an appropriate surgical plan can be formulated, and essential prostheses can be manufactured prior to surgical correction.

CAD-CAM multiplanar diagnostic imaging has removed clinical barriers encountered in the treatment of the subperiosteal implant patient. This technique has eliminated the bone impression surgery, which has allowed for a less traumatic implant procedure. The CT-derived bone model has allowed for extension of the subperiosteal framework into areas limited by direct bone impression. Vital structures can be outlined on the CT reconstruction, thereby decreasing possible injury during surgical placement of the subperiosteal implant.

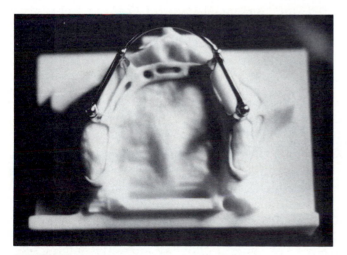

FIG 31–7.
Maxillary subperiosteal implant constructed on the synthetic bone model coated with hydroxylapatite. (Courtesy of Calcitek, Inc., Carlsbad, Calif.)

CT ASSESSMENT OF THE MANDIBLE AND MAXILLA FOR DENTAL OSSEOINTEGRATED IMPLANTS

Forty-two percent of Americans over 65 years of age and 4% of those 34 to 65 are totally edentulous. It is estimated that as many as 300,000 dental implants will be used in the United States by 1992. The availability and application of osseointegrated dental implants for the mandible and maxilla have expanded interest in preoperative imaging assessment of potential implant receptor sites.[12] The traditional Panorex-type film of the mandible or maxilla can demonstrate the general architectural appearance of the maxilla and mandible *en face*

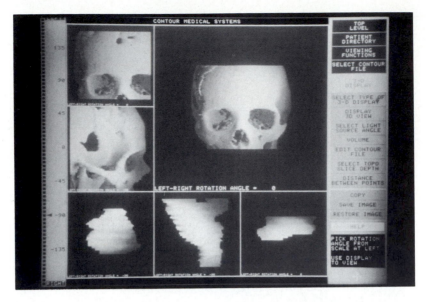

FIG 31–8.
Three-dimensional reconstruction of a gunshot wound to the cranium and three-dimensional reconstruction of lost temporal and frontal bones for cranial implant fabrication. (Courtesy of Calcitek, Inc., Carlsbad, Calif.)

but does not depict the shape, width, and contour of the alveolar ridge, the exact position of the mandibular canal, nor its buccal-lingual location and relationships. The precise position and location of the mandibular canal that contains the inferior alveolar nerve is of fundamental importance in planning endosseous implant procedures for the mandible. The inferior alveolar nerve, a branch of the fifth cranial nerve, enters the mandible at the medial midramus and supplies the teeth of the jaw from the alveolar canal. Its mental branch exits at the mental foramen to supply sensation to the skin of the chin and mucous membrane and skin of the lower lip. Damage to the nerve can result in unacceptable anesthesia to the chin and lip.

Computer software programs are now available for use in CT scanning to allow the use of CT scan data generated in the axial projection to create not only Panorex-type views of the maxilla and mandible but also true oblique cross sections along the maxilla or mandible perpendicular to the alveolar ridge. These images, generated through computer software reformations, not only provide the location of essential anatomic structures, including the location of the mandibular canal, but also define the degree of bone atrophy and potential cortical bone availability. Armed with this knowledge, the surgical implant team can design implants with advanced knowledge of the bone quality and shape and contour of the alveolar ridge so that the maximum available bone is used to support the implant. The surgeon can optimize the size of available implant materials and diminish risk to underlying structures.

The original dental CT multiplanar reformation approach was designed and implemented by Schwarz et al.[13, 14] at Multiplanar Diagnostic Imaging (MPDI) as a software package addition for conventional CT scanners. Recently, other vendors (e.g., Cemax, Columbia Scientific Incorporated, General Electric) have produced similar dental programs and packages available either as add-on software to existing CT units or as software additions to three-dimensional work stations that utilize previously generated CT data.[15] An appealing feature of the updated programs is that all of the generated images may be life size, thus allowing direct measurement for implant sizing directly off the film without having to calculate magnification/minification factors.

CT Methodology

The technique utilizes a high-resolution CT scanner (such as a General Electric 9800), a bone algorithm, and a set of axial 1.5-mm-thick sections at 1-mm intervals for the mandible or at 1.5-mm intervals for the maxilla. Approximately 35 sections are used for the mandibular study and 25 for the maxillary study, following an initial lateral scout for slice location selection. The dynamic scanning mode provides quality images at a low x-ray dose and a rapid examination with data acquisition within 5 minutes by using a 15-cm field of view, head calibration file, and 512 × 512 matrix.

The mandible and maxilla are examined separately, with positioning of the head and face to allow optimum position of the alveolar ridge relative to the scanning plane. For the mandible, the alveolar ridge or ramus of the mandible should be perpendicular to the table top and parallel to the gantry (Fig 31–9,A). Similarly, for the maxillary examination, the alveolar ridge should be perpendicular to the table top and parallel to the gantry, which requires slight flexion of the head relative to the mandibular examination (Fig 31–9,B). Conventional restraining tape and/or head-positioning Velcro aids are helpful, and a padded tongue depressor in the mouth limits swallowing artifacts.

Following the generation of a series of axial images, the technologist selects an appropriate axial image and draws a line through the midmandible or maxilla following the line of the alveolar ridge, upon which a series of oblique reformations will be generated (Fig 31–10,A). In addition, Panorex-type reformations in the plane of this central line and two on both the buccal and lingual sides of this central line are generated (Fig 31–10,B). Oblique reformatted images are generated at 2-mm intervals (Fig 31–10,C and D), with the position of the oblique images identified on the Panorex views by markers along the bottom of the images (Fig 31–10,B). The reformations require approximately 45 minutes of processing time, and this im-

age set is then available for hard copy reproduction, evaluation, and interpretation.

Mandible

Figure 31–10 shows summary images of a patient referred for mandibular and maxillary dental evaluation for osseointegrated implants. Figure 31–10,A shows the line drawn by the technologist along the path of the generated oblique reformations. These oblique images are 2 mm apart and one pixel size thick (tissue thickness of approximately 0.3 mm). The computer-generated Panorex-type image is shown in Figure 31–10,B, with the numbers of the oblique reformations identified by location on the lower scale. The oblique reformations are shown in Figures 31–10,C and D, with their number locations noted in the lower left-hand corner of each image. In viewing the images, it is important to note that the buccal side is on the viewer's left and the lingual side to the right (see Fig 31–10,C). The mental foramen can be identified and is a good starting point for the identification of basic anatomy (see Fig 31–10,D). The mandibular canal is seen in Figures 31–10,C and D. Although the mandibular canal can almost always be identified, atrophic changes can make identification of its entire course difficult. In Figure 31–11,A, although the mandibular canal can be seen in the area of normal dentition, it is lost in the area of atrophy and artifacts from dental amalgam. Its position, however, can be extrapolated by drawing a line parallel to the visualized canal. In prac-

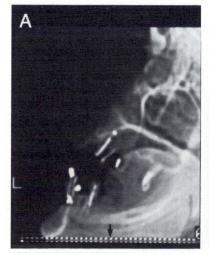
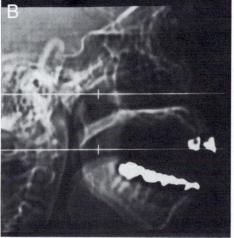

FIG 31–9.
Head positioning for CT scanning. **A,** mandible, lateral scout film. Note the gantry line *(arrow)* parallel to the alveolar ridge. **B,** max- illa, lateral scout film. Note the gantry lines parallel to the alveolar ridge—the head is more flexed on the neck than in **A.**

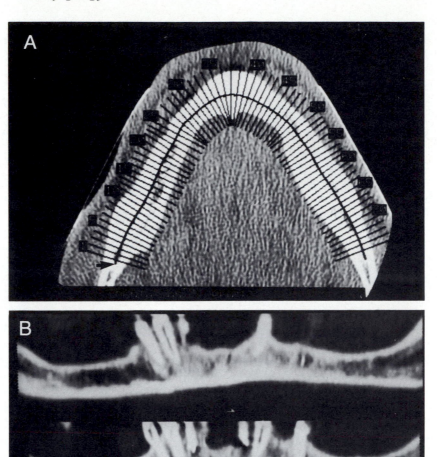

FIG 31–10.
CT-reformatted images of mandible. **A,** axial mandibular image with positions of oblique reformations indicated. Each image is 2 mm apart. **B,** Panorex-type CT-reformatted images. *Arrows* indicate markers that identify the location of each oblique reformatted image. **C** and **D,** *(facing page)* oblique reformations through the right side of the mandible. *Large arrows* (**C,** images 2 and 18; **D,** image 19) indicate the mandibular canal traversing to the mental foramen (**D,** image 24, *small arrow*). Oblique image numbers are in *lower left corners*. Note the buccal/lingual markers on images 2 of **C** and 20 of **D.** Available bone for an implant site is indicated by an *open arrow* in image 19 of **D.**

tice, the implant surgeon can decide, on the basis of the clinical examination, where to place the implants, correlate this with the Panorex-type views, and then move to the oblique reformations to see whether the bony anatomy is optimum.

Variable-sized implants are available, with the smallest being 3.5 × 7 mm. Larger implants provide more strength for subsequent dental prosthetics; thus the surgeon would prefer as large a size as possible. Recently, Jensen has classified sites for implants to assist in implant optimization.[16] A class A site for implantation has at least 10 mm of verti-

cal bone and 6 mm of horizontal bone present. A class B site has 7 to 10 mm of vertical bone and at least 4 mm of horizontal bone. A class C site has less than 7 mm of vertical bone or less than 4 mm of horizontal bone present. In class D sites there is an absent alveolar process (severe atrophy) or severe basal bone loss requiring bone graft reconstruction. Using this classification may help in communicating measurement information to the implant team (Fig 31–12).

Atrophy affects the apparent position of the inferior alveolar nerve (mandibular canal). There

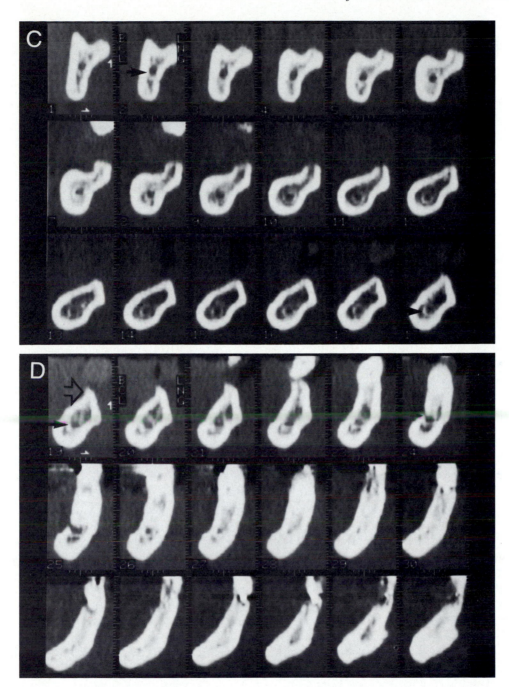

may be excellent bone above the nerve (see Fig 31–12,A), or in other cases the nerve appears to run on the surface (see Fig 31–12,B). The surgeon attempts to keep the implant cephalad to the projected level of the nerve to avoid injury. Potentially, implants can still be inserted if the nerve is in either an eccentric buccal or lingual location that allows enough space for implant insertion. This type of information is not available on regular Panorex x-ray films but is available on the CT-re-

formatted images. With the knowledge of the buccal/lingual location of the canal, many cases can still be salvaged for implant surgery.

An important variant of anatomy deserves emphasis. Occasionally, the alveolar nerve in its intramandibular course makes a loop medial to the mental foramen before branching into the sensory division that exits the foramen and the incisor division to the canine and incisor teeth. Usually the area medial to the mental foramen is considered a

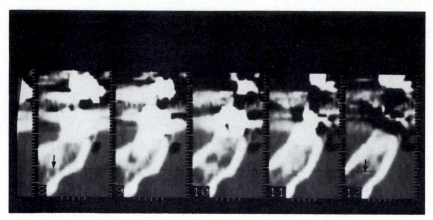

FIG 31–11.
Series of oblique reformations with less than optimal visualization of the mandibular canal *(arrows)* on every image, but its position can be reliably estimated by extrapolation.

safe zone by the implant surgeon; however, when this loop is present medially, this variant could predispose to nerve injury from a deep implant. Fortunately, this looping course can be identified on oblique reformatted images as a double-barrel canal instead of a single channel medial to the mental foramen.

Maxilla

The maxillary CT examination is similar to the mandibular one. As in the mandible, a line is drawn for the oblique reformatted series on an axial image, and reformatted views are generated as well as reformatted Panorex-type images (Fig 31–13). In the maxilla, however, the overlying anatomy changes emphasis. The shape and contour of the maxillary alveolar ridge is of great importance as well as the thickness and contour of available bone relative to the overlying maxillary sinus. An additional important feature is the attitude of the alveolar ridge and whether its axis is angulated or vertical. In order to utilize the optimum available bone, the implant follows the long axis of the alveolar ridge. If the alveolar ridge angle is significantly decreased, difficulty with prosthetic management may ensue (Fig 31–14).

In Figure 31–13, axial images demonstrate atrophy and diminished bone in the central and pericentral region on the left side, with Panorex and oblique reformations demonstrating potential sites for implantation. Figure 31–14 demonstrates a case in which the attitude of the alveolar ridge is quite flat (angulated forward); thus close coordination between the prosthodontist and the oral surgeon was necessary. Figure 31–15 shows a patient

with severe atrophy in which no standard implantation is possible. At surgery iliac donor bone grafts were seated and eight implants inserted. Figure 31–16 demonstrates excellent type B sites to implant, but an unexpected residual root socket changed the implant site selection.

Summary

The availability of osseointegrated dental implants has demanded accurate anatomic imaging of the mandible and maxilla to optimize results and diminish risk. A CT dental software program that utilizes axial-generated data for reformation of oblique images of the mandible and maxilla as well as Panorex-type views answers most of the questions for the implant team. These programs are becoming increasingly available and will undoubtedly be used with increased frequency when implant surgery is contemplated.

THE TEMPOROMANDIBULAR JOINT

As a relative newcomer to medical diagnosis, the TMJ has become a very popular and yet controversial subject. TMJ dysfunction affects from 15% to 28% of the American population[17] and has a strong predilection for females (female-to-male ratio, 9:1). The spectrum of TMJ dysfunction varies widely from painless clicking of the joint to incapacitating headache, chronic depression, and even suicide.

Headache is the most common presenting complaint, although symptoms commonly include earache, joint and jaw pain, neck and shoulder pain,

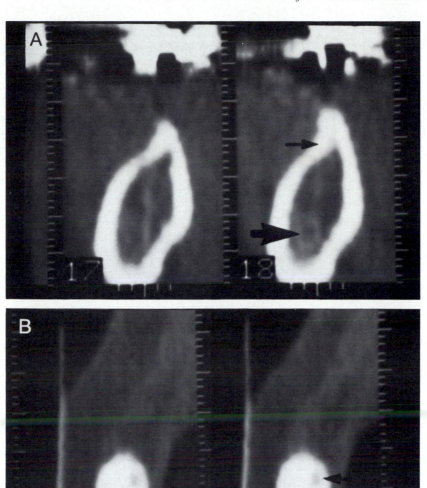

FIG 31–12.
Mandibular implantation sites. **A,** oblique reformation of an implantation site. The pointed top of the aveolar ridge *(small arrow)* will be removed, but a good implantation site is still present (5 × 8 mm; a class B site). The *large arrow* is at the mandibular canal. **B,** atrophic alveolar ridge, with the mandibular canal *(arrow)* almost on the surface; a class D site (*B* = buccal; *L* = lingual).

as well as tinnitus. Physical examination often reveals audible or palpable clicking in one or both joints. Crepitus is a late finding often associated with degenerative changes in the joint. During opening of the mouth, the mandible often deviates to one side and may remain deviated in the fully open position. Limited opening of the mouth is another common presenting complaint.

The most common form of TMJ dysfunction is internal derangement. This most often begins in the early teenage years when clicking of the joint is first noticed. This early stage of internal de-

rangement is often asymptomatic and discovered on routine dental examination. With time, patients experience "locking" of the jaw in the closed-mouth position. This symptom often occurs upon awakening in the morning and may take several minutes before full opening can be achieved. With progression, opening of the mouth may become even more restricted and painful.

The controversy surrounding the TMJ primarily centers around the wide variety of treatments available, which can be both expensive and prolonged. The primary goal of treatment is relief of

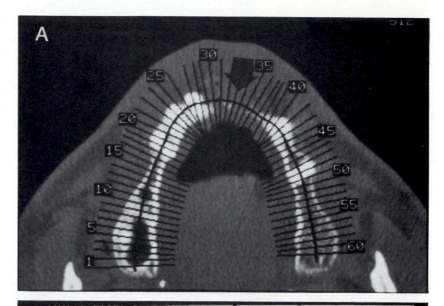

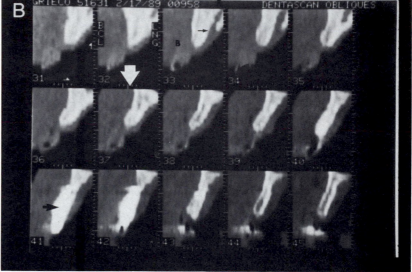

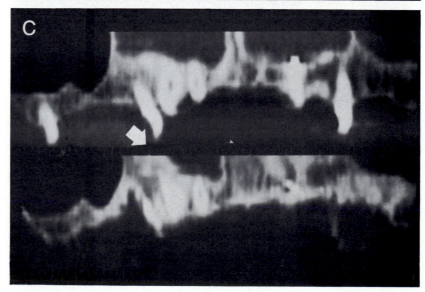

FIG 31–13.
CT-reformatted images of maxilla. **A,** axial maxillary image with a line drawn by a technologist and positions of oblique reformations indicated. The *arrow* denotes atrophic bone. **B,** series of oblique reformatted images of the maxilla. The incisive canal (midline) is indicated by a *small black arrow* on image 33. Bone available for implant on image 31 is 6 × 12 mm (class A site). Note that reformations are not ideal since they do not include soft tissue above bone; compare to Figure 31–16,B. The plane and position of Panorex-type views are indicated by a *wide white arrow* on image 32, oblique reformatted image location number by a *curved arrow* on image 34. A *large black arrow* (image 41) indicates a residual tooth. **C,** maxillary Panorex-type reformation views. The *white arrow* designates positions of oblique reformatted images.

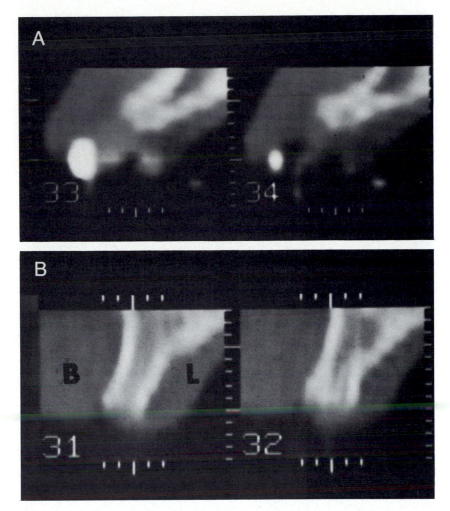

FIG 31–14.
Maxillary implantation sites. **A,** maxillary oblique reformatted image demonstrates a class C site, 3.8 × 8 mm available bone but a very flat angle of the alveolar ridge. This requires coordination of the prosthetic/implant team. **B,** relatively normal angle of the alveolar ridge of the maxilla—compare with **A** (*B* = buccal; *L* = lingual).

patient symptoms and stabilization of the joint. Occlusion changes considerably when the disk is displaced. While recapture of the disk may seem ideal, many patients are successfully treated "off the disk." The mainstay of therapy is often "unloading" the joint with use of a bite plate or splint placed in the mouth to reposition the condylar lead lower or more anterior in the articular fossa. This allows more space for the disk to return to its anatomic position and also allows for healing of the stretched and damaged posterior ligament. Ancillary treatment includes physical therapy, biofeedback, and medical management. There is a wide variety of surgical arthroplasties available as well as arthroscopy of the TMJ.

Accurate imaging techniques have greatly improved diagnosis because clinical findings and symptoms can often be misleading. For example, it is common for patients with bilateral internal derangement to have fewer symptoms in the joint where perforation of the ligament has occurred. Historically, perforation is clearly a more advanced stage in the natural history of internal derangement.

Improved diagnosis should certainly result in improved clinical results by clarifying the underlying pathology and providing a more rational approach for treatment planning.

Diagnostic Imaging

In the late 1970s, contrast arthrography of the TMJ became readily available as the "gold standard" of diagnosis.[18–23] This procedure allows in-

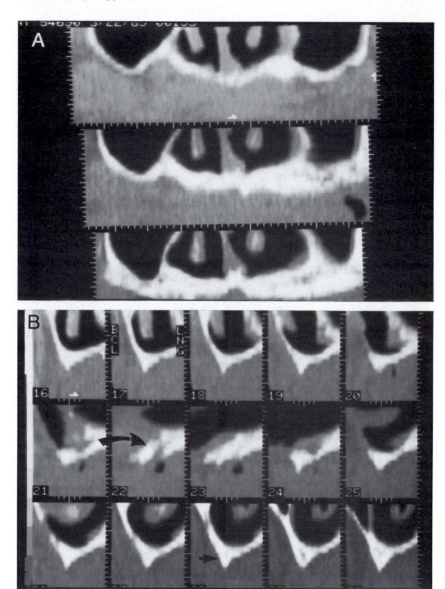

FIG 31–15.
Atrophy of maxillary alveolar ridge. **A,** Panorex-type reformation of a maxilla with profound atrophy of the alveolar ridge. **B,** oblique axial reformations confirm the atrophy and flat contour (*small arrow,* class D site); the *curved arrow* indicates the incisive canal.

direct visualization of the disk (meniscus) by injecting contrast material into the lower joint space. Major disadvantages of arthrography include the invasive, painful nature of the procedure as well as its technical difficulty.

CT application to the TMJ was then introduced as a noninvasive way to directly visualize the disk.[24, 25] This approach had limited success because of poor contrast resolution of the disk and difficulty in positioning patients for direct sagittal imaging.

With the introduction of MRI and the develop-ment of small surface coils, the soft-tissue anatomy of the TMJ is even better visualized.[26–28] For the first time, the junction of the posterior band of the disk with the posterior ligament (bilaminar zone) could be routinely demonstrated. The morphology of the disk as well as its position in the joint and relation to the condylar head could all be readily visualized.[29] Internal derangement is primarily a soft-tissue disease, and bone changes are a late manifestation. Degenerative changes of the joint are well demonstrated with this noninvasive imaging technique.

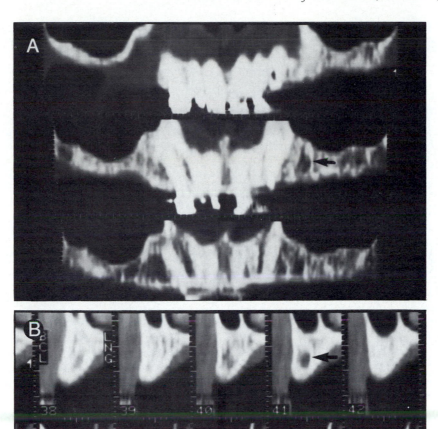

FIG 31–16.
Maxillary implantation sites. Panorex **(A)** and oblique **(B)** reformatted images of the maxilla in an implantation candidate. *Arrows* indicate an unsuspected residual root socket with inadequate bone. This location was noted and avoided when implants were performed.

MRI is clearly the procedure of choice for optimal imaging of the TMJ. Indications include initial patient evaluation, particularly for patients where the clinical diagnosis is unclear. Patients who have not responded to initial treatment may also benefit from more accurate diagnosis. Insurance carriers often require imaging studies to document the need of a proposed surgical procedure. Also, there is a growing number of workmen's compensation and other legal cases where the prognosis and associated expenses may be better predicted with MRI. Other indications include those patients with acute or previous trauma for evaluation of soft-tissue or bone injury, internal derangement, postoperative evaluation, and bone or soft-tissue tumors around the TMJ.

Physicians often include TMJ dysfunction very low in the differential diagnosis of headache, earache, tinnitus, or neck pain. In these patients, MRI may be the key to accurate diagnosis.

MRI Technique

Patients are placed in the scanner and advised to keep their back teeth gently closed while obtaining the axial localizer image. A small surface coil (10 cm or less) is the key to imaging the TMJ. Dual surface coils can reduce scanning time signif-

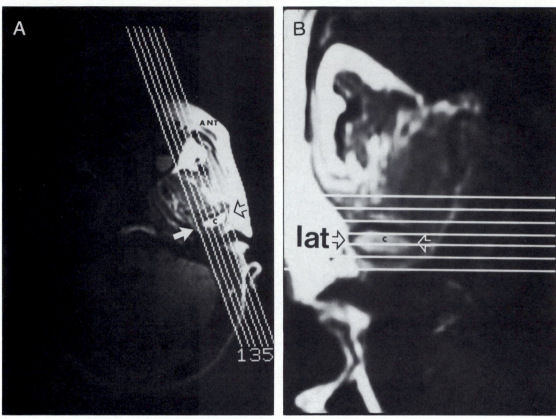

FIG 31–17.
TMJ MRI technique. A preliminary axial image is obtained through the level of the mandibular condyles. **A,** oblique sagittal images should be obtained perpendicular to the axis *(arrows)* of the condylar head *(c)*. **B,** coronal images *must* be obtained parallel to the long axis of the condylar head *(c)*. If coronal images are obtained "off axis," a false-positive interpretation of medial displacement or rotational displacement may be offered.

icantly by simultaneous scanning of both joints.

Once the condylar heads are visualized, sagittal images are obtained perpendicular to the condylar axis (Fig 31–17,A). T1-weighted images are then obtained with a field of view of 12 cm, a repetition time (TR) of 500 ms, an echo time (TE) of 20 ms, and 3-mm-thick contiguous slices with two acquisitions. Scanning time is 6.5 minutes, and therefore patient comfort is an important consideration in maintaining a steady position during scanning. MRI is not indicated in patients with metal implants in the joint or wire sutures near the joint. Orthodontic wires do not, however, interfere significantly with the image quality. The higher–field strength magnets offer better resolution, particularly when trying to characterize the morphology and structure of the disk.[30] Closed-mouth oblique sagittal images are then obtained with the mouth gently closed. Full open-mouth images can be obtained with the aid of a bite block or other suitable device. TMJ dysfunction patients can be quite un-comfortable in the fully open position, and a compromise position may be required to allow better patient cooperation.

Dynamic images can be obtained with fast-scan techniques, although this has limitations since it involves passive motion of the mandible as opposed to physiologic motion controlled by the muscles of mastication.[31]

Coronal images are obtained parallel to the axis of the condyle and in the closed-mouth position (see Fig 31–17,B). These are extremely helpful in patients with pure medial or lateral displacement of the disk. Since the predominant internal derangement involves anteromedial displacement of the disk, coronal imaging is not necessary in all patients.

T2-weighted images have been helpful in detecting joint effusion as well as other evidence of edema or inflammation within the joint.[32] Bilateral imaging of the TMJ has also proved quite helpful since a patient with proven internal derangement on one side has an 80% likelihood of internal derangement on the contralateral side even though symptoms and physical findings may be minimal or absent on the contralateral side.

The Normal Joint

The normal TMJ is composed of two synovial compartments separated by a fibrocartilage disk (meniscus). Capsular attachments are present laterally, medially, and anteriorly, while a very elastic posterior ligament (bilaminar zone) extends from the posterior margin of the disk to the posterior wall of the articular fossa. During full opening, the posterior ligament is stretched between three and four times its resting length. The elasticity of the posterior ligament helps to pull the disk back into the articular fossa during closing.

In the closed mouth position (Fig 31–18,A), the normal meniscus has a medium signal intensity, is biconcave in contour, and is interposed between the condylar head and the posterior slope of the articular eminence. The posterior band of the disk is somewhat thicker than the anterior band.

The junction of the posterior band and posterior ligament should be well demonstrated and lies at the 12 o'clock position in relation to the condylar head. Also, the thinner intermediate zone of the disk should be in close proximity to the anterior cortex of the condylar head. It is important to identify the disk in all of the sagittal images for complete evaluation of its position.

The disk may be of similar signal intensity to the cortex of the condylar head and therefore may be difficult to see, particularly on closed-mouth images. By placing your finger or thumb over the condylar head, you may be able to obscure the cortex of the condyle and improve visualization of the disk. This method can be utilized in most patients where the contour of the condyle is smooth.

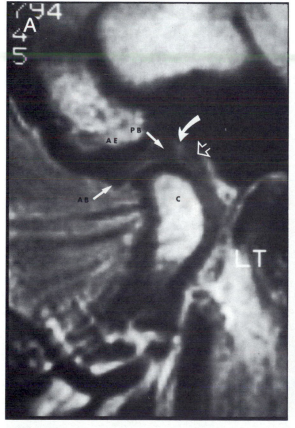 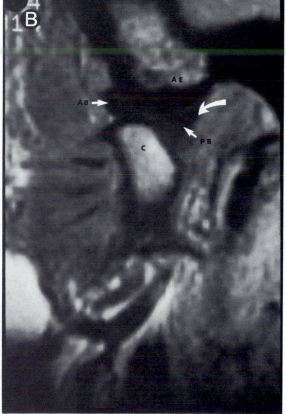

FIG 31–18.
MRI of a normal TMJ. **A,** closed-mouth position. Note that the junction *(curved arrow)* of the posterior band *(PB)* and the posterior ligament *(open arrow)* is located directly over the center of the condylar head *(C)*. Also labeled are the articular eminence *(AE)* and anterior band of the disk *(AB)*. **B,** open-mouth position. The condylar head *(C)* is now anterior to the apex of the articular eminence *(AE)*. The disk has migrated to the posterior cortex of the condyle but remains between the condylar head and articular eminence. The disk-ligament junction is marked with a *curved arrow*.

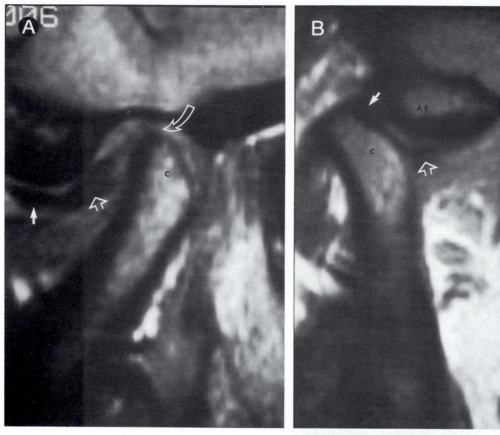

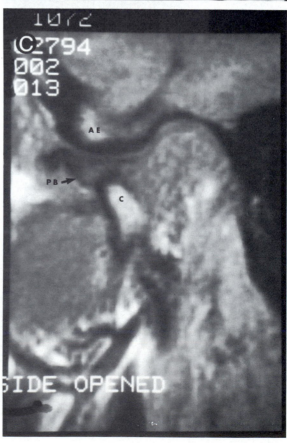

FIG 31–19.
Internal derangement. **A,** closed-mouth position. The entire disk is anterior to the condylar head, with the posterior band *(open arrow)* directly in front of the condyle *(c)* *(closed arrow on anterior band).* The fibers of the posterior ligament *(curved arrow)* are stretched over the condylar head and pinched between the cortex of the condyle and the cortex of the articular fossa. **B,** open-mouth view with reduction of the disk. The disk is recaptured and returns to a normal position *(closed arrow marks anterior band, open arrow marks posterior band).* Note the similarity with Figure 31–18,B. During opening, the condyle has moved under the disk, while there has been relatively little motion of the disk itself. **C,** open-mouth view without reduction. In a different patient, the entire disk remains anterior to the condyle in spite of a normal degree of translation of the condylar head *(c).* The posterior band *(PB)* is thickened, and the disk is folded. Note the increased signal in the center of the posterior band in this abnormal disk.

The posterior ligament (bilaminar zone) parallels the posterior cortex of the condylar head and attaches to the posterior band of the disk. With a 1.5-tesla scanner, the posterior ligament has a layered appearance with a medium signal intensity in the central zone and higher signal intensity above and below the central zone.

Muscle fibers of the superior belly of the lateral pterygoid muscle extend anterior from the condylar head. Some of these fibers may insert directly into the anterior band of the disk.

In the open-mouth view (see Fig 31–18,B), the condyle has translated and rotated anteriorly and usually rests near or just beyond the apex of the articular eminence. The disk has migrated over the apex of the condyle and has a more horizontal axis.

Internal Derangement

The most common internal derangement of the TMJ is anteromedial displacement of the disk (Fig 31–19,A). In the classic form of anterior displacement, the posterior band of the disk is well anterior to the condylar head. Some patients, however, may demonstrate 1 to 2 millimeters of anterior displacement from the 12 o'clock position, and it may be difficult to determine whether this is a normal variation or clinically significant anterior displacement. Positioning of the patient with flexion of the neck during scanning may result in the appearance of mild anterior displacement when the joint is actually normal.

With opening, the disk is frequently recaptured and is again interposed between the condyle and articular eminence (see Fig 31–19,B). Patients most often feel a clicking sensation in the joint during opening when the disk returns to the normal position. This process is termed anterior displacement of the disk with reduction. Morphology of the disk is usually normal, and there is seldom any associated degenerative change of the bone.

Patients who go untreated will often progress

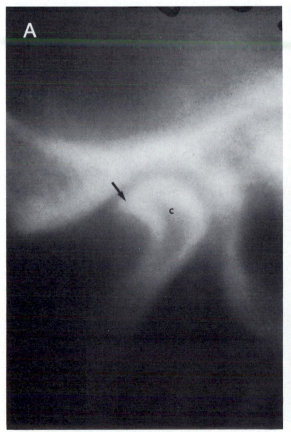 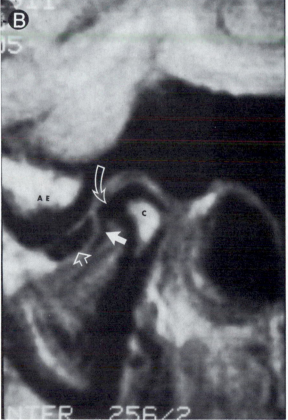

FIG 31–20.
Degenerative changes. **A,** a tomogram demonstrates moderate osteophyte formation projecting anteriorly from the condylar head *(arrow).* **B,** Sagittal MRI provides significant additional information. The osteophyte is clearly seen *(curved arrow),* and the bright mar- row signal of the condylar head *(c)* is preserved. The deformed disk *(open arrowhead)* is displaced anteriorly. There is associated thickening of the tendon of the lateral pterygoid muscle *(solid arrow)* as it inserts on the tip of the osteophyte.

to "acute closed lock,"[33] where they frequently wake in the morning unable to open their mouth more than a few millimeters. Sagittal MRI in these patients demonstrates persistent anterior displacement of the disk in the open-mouth view. This finding is associated with a decrease in translation of the condyle. Degenerative changes are again uncommon at this stage.

With further progression of internal derangement, the disk is pushed more and more anterior by the condyle during opening (see Fig 31–19,C). Translation may actually return to a normal range. Sagittal images show a deformity of the disk that is frequently folded or globular in contour. Diagnosis at this time is anterior displacement of the disk without reduction.

Internal derangement is a common cause of malocclusion and should be thoroughly evaluated and accurately diagnosed before orthodontic treatment is instituted.

Degenerative Change

Without the cushioning effect of the disk interposed between the condyle and articular eminence, the tremendous forces generated across the joint eventually damage the posterior ligament. This can cause fibrosis or "hyalination"[34, 35] of the posterior ligament and result in areas of decreased signal intensity on T1 images.

Although seldom confirmed on MRI, perforation of the posterior ligament occurs commonly with chronic anterior displacement of the disk. Since the posterior ligament is richly innervated, anterior displacement without reduction can be a very painful stage of internal derangement that is commonly associated with headache, muscle spasm, and joint pain. Perforation of the posterior ligament may actually decrease the patient's symptoms but is also associated with the onset of degenerative changes in the joint. Flattening of the

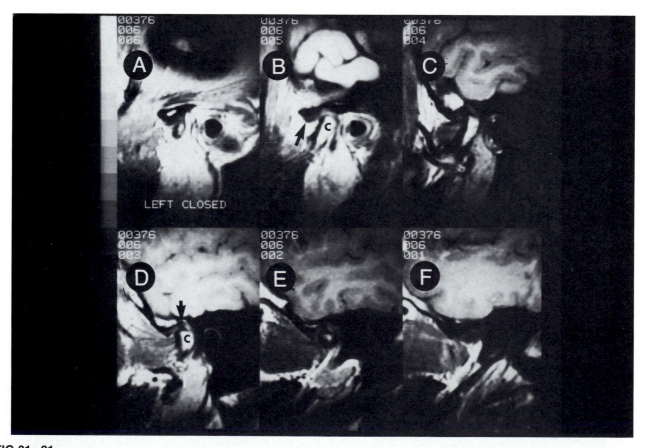

FIG 31–21.
Rotational displacement. A series of sagittal images through the entire TMJ with 3-mm slice thickness and the closed-mouth position. **A,** a sagittal image through the lateral pole of the condyle; **E,** obtained through the very medial aspect of the joint space. **D,** the position and contour of the disk *(arrow)* appears normal; **B,** a crescent-shaped disk *(arrow)* that is anterior to the condyle. Thus the lateral aspect of the disk is displaced, while the medial aspect is not indicating rotational displacement.

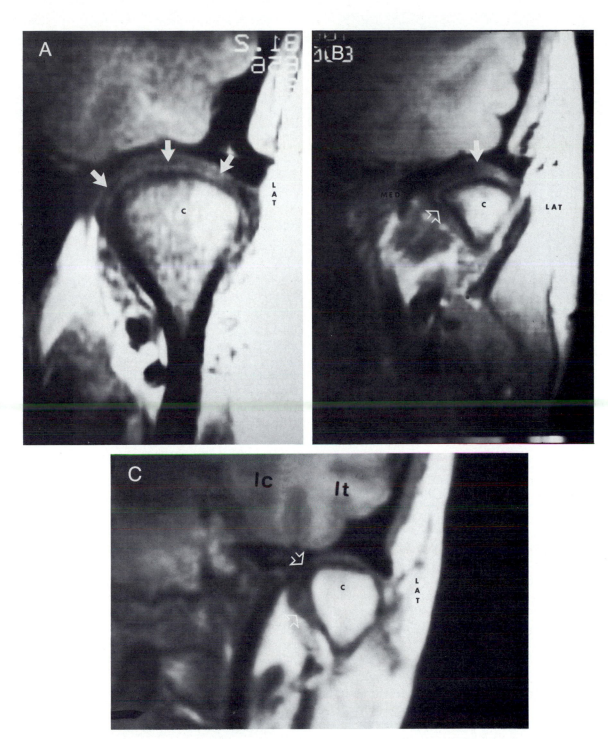

FIG 31–22.
Coronal MRI. **A,** normal coronal image demonstrates a uniformly thick joint space. The disc *(arrows)* is seen to cover the condylar head from the medial to the lateral pole. **B,** medial displacement of the disk is demonstrated in another patient. Note the narrowing of the lateral joint space. The lateral margin of the disk *(solid arrow)* is now in the center of the joint space, with the remainder of the disk wrapping around the medial pole of the condyle *(open arrow).* **C,** more advanced medial displacement in a different patient where the entire disk *(open arrows)* has slipped into the medial recess of the joint space. It should be noted that precise coronal imaging parallel to the long axis of the condyle is required to avoid false-positive interpretation.

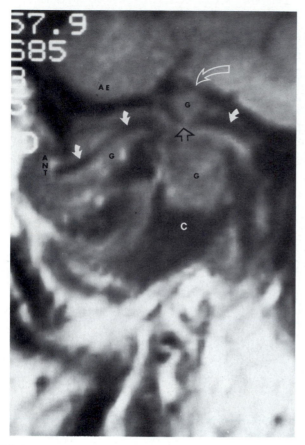

FIG 31–23.
Postoperative MRI of a 24-year-old female who is 4 years earlier had placement of a synthetic implant *(solid white arrows)* into the TMJ. The central portion of the implant is perforated *(open black arrow),* and there are multiple areas of granulation tissue *(G)* that surround the implant. The neck of the condyle *(C)* is black due to replacement of the fatty marrow. The condylar head, meanwhile, has been almost totally eroded by granulation tissue. The floor of the articular fossa *(curved open arrow)* has been eroded by the inflammatory reaction.

condylar head and osteophyte formation along the anterior cortex of the condylar head are common manifestations of early degenerative change (Fig 31–20).

The articular eminence may also become flattened, particularly along the posterior slope. Crepitus is a common physical finding at this time and usually indicates perforation of the posterior ligament. Unfortunately, adhesions within the joint space tend to be microscopic and are seldom resolved with MRI.

Rotational Displacement

With the development of thin-section sagittal MRI, the diagnosis of rotational displacement has

become commonplace.[36] In these patients (Fig 31–21) sagittal closed-mouth images through the medial portion of the condyle demonstrate the disk in normal position, while more lateral sagittal images show classic anterior displacement of the disk. Open-mouth images appear normal with complete reduction (recapture) of the entire disk. The disk again rotates into an abnormal position during closing of the mouth. Rotational displacement probably represents a very early stage of internal derangement.

Medial Displacement

While anteromedial displacement of the disk is common, pure medial displacement of the disk is much less common. If routine sagittal imaging in the closed-mouth position demonstrates a normal position of the disk in the medial aspect of the joint but poor visualization or thinning of the disk laterally, medial displacement should be suspected.[29, 36] In these patients, coronal imaging is invaluable (Fig 31–22). It is important for accurate diagnosis that coronal images be parallel to the long access of the condyle.

Postoperative Examination

There is a wide variety of surgical procedures available for internal derangement. MRI is helpful in patients who have had plication surgery with repositioning of the disk to determine whether the disk has remained in its anatomic position. Although no longer utilized, permanent implants of Teflon and Silastic are well visualized with MRI (Fig 31–23). In addition to evaluation of the integrity and position of the implant, the osseous anatomy is well seen along with any granulation tissue that might occur with the breakdown of the implant.[37, 38]

Other Indications

MRI can be used in acute trauma of the TMJ to look for occult condylar fractures as well as assessment of disk integrity and position.

Multiplanar imaging can be utilized for osseous and soft-tissue tumor imaging (Fig 31–24) to aid in surgical planning.

The clinical benefit of T2-weighted imaging of inflammatory disease of the TMJ is currently being evaluated.[32]

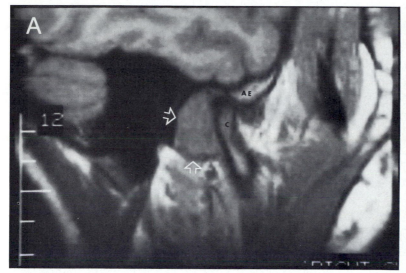

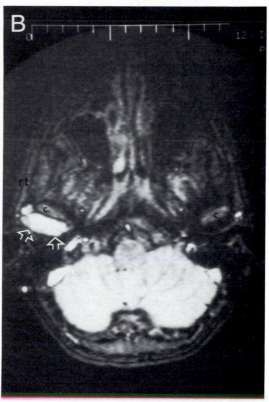

FIG 31–24.
Intra-articular tumor in a 17-year-old male with progressive lateral deviation of the mandible. A nodule was palpable in the region of the right condylar head. **A,** a sagittal image show homogeneous tumor *(arrowheads)* in the posterior joint space. The condyle *(C)* is displaced anteriorly, but there is no internal derangement. **B,** an axial image of a different patient was done with fat-suppression technique (short inversion time inversion recovery sequence) and shows very bright signal *(arrowheads)* from the area of the reactive fibrosis. Based on histology, this reactive fibrosis was presumably caused by previous trauma and/or hemorrhage (Picker 0.5-tesla Vista MRI).

REFERENCES

1. Dahl GSA: Subperiosteal implants and superplants. *Dent Abstr* 1957; 2:685.
2. Linkow LI: Evolutionary design trends in the mandibular subperiosteal implant. *J Oral Implantology* 1984; 11:402.
3. Gershoff A, Goldberg N: Implant lower dentures. *Dent Digest* 1949; 55:490.
4. Gershoff A, Goldberg N: Further report on the full lower implant denture. *Dent Digest* 1950; 56:11.
5. Goldberg N, Gershoff A: Implants: Biologic or mechanical. *NYJ Dent* 1950; 16:397.
6. Leh I: Full upper and lower denture implants. *Dent Concepts* 1952; 4:17.
7. Berman N: Implant technique for full lower dentures. *Wash Dent J* 1950; 19:15.
8. Truitt H, James R, Boyne PJ: Non-invasive technique for mandibular subperiosteal implants: A preliminary report. *J Prosthet Dent* 1986; 55:494.
9. James RA: Complete mandibular subperiosteal implant fabrication from model generated from computer tomography data. *Implantologist* 1986; 13:35.
10. Benjamin LS: Versatility of the subperiosteal implant utilizing CAD-CAM multiplanar diagnostic imaging. *J Implantology* 1987; 13:282–295.
11. Misch CE: Misch Implant Institute, Dearborn, Mich Personal communication, Jan 1990.
12. Branemark PI, Hansson BO, Adell R, et al: Osseointegrated implants in the treatment of edentulous jaw: Experience from a 10-year period. *Scand J Plast Reconstr Surg* 1977; 11:suppl 16.
13. Schwarz MS, Rothman SLG, Rhodes ML, et al: Computed tomography. I. Preoperative assessment of the mandible for endosseous implant surgery. *Int J Oral Maxillofac Implant* 1987; 2:137–141.
14. Schwarz MS, Rothman SLG, Rhodes ML, et al: Computed tomography. II. Preoperative assessment of the maxilla for endosseous implant surgery. *Int J Oral Maxillofac Implant* 1987; 2:143–148.
15. Golee TS: CAD-CAM multiplanar imaging for subperiosteal implants. *Dent Clin North Am* 1986; 30:85–95.
16. Jensen O: Site classification for the osseointegrated implant. *J Prosthet Dent* 1989; 51:228–234.
17. Katzberg RW, Dolwich MF, Helms CA, et al: Arthrotomography of the temporomandibular joint. *AJR* 1980; 134:995–1003.
18. Norgaard F: *Temporomandibular Arthrography* (thesis), University of Copenhagen, 1947.
19. Farrar WB, McCarty WJ Jr: Inferior joint space arthrography and characteristics of condylar paths in internal derangements of the TMJ. *J Prosthet Dent* 1979; 41:548–555.
20. Wilkes CH: Arthrography of the temporomandibular joint. *Minn Med* 1978; 61:645–652.
21. Katzberg RW, Dolwick MF, Helms CA, et al: Arthrotomography of the temporomandibular joint: New technique and preliminary observations. *AJR* 1979; 132:949–955.

22. Westesson P-L, Bronstein BL, Liedberg J: Temporomandibular joint: Correlation between single-contrast videoarthrography and postmortem morphology. *Radiology* 1986; 160:767–771.

23. Kaplan PA, Tu HK, Sleder PR, et al: Inferior joint space arthrography of normal temporomandibular joints: Reassessment of diagnostic criteria. *Radiology* 1986; 159:585–589.

24. Helms CA, Morrish RB, Kircos LT, et al: Computed tomography of the meniscus of the temporomandibular joint: Preliminary observations. *Radiology* 1982; 145:719–722.

25. Thompson JR, Christiansen E, Hasso A, et al: Temporomandibular joint high resolution computed tomography. *Radiology* 1984; 150:105–110.

26. Harms SE, Wilk RM, Wolford LM, et al: The temporomandibular joint: Magnetic resonance imaging using surface coils. *Radiology* 1985; 157:133–136.

27. Katzberg R, Bessette RW, Tallents RH, et al: Normal and abnormal temporomandibular joint: MR imaging with surface coil. *Radiology* 1986; 158:183–189.

28. Harms SE, Wilk RM: Magnetic resonance imaging of the temporomandibular joint. *Radiographics* 1987; 7:521–542.

29. Westesson P-L, Katzberg RW, Tallents RH, et al: Temporomandibular joint: Comparison of MR images with cryosectional anatomy. *Radiology* 1987; 164:59–64.

30. Hansson L-G, et al: MR imaging of the temporomandibular joint: Comparison of images of autopsy specimens at 0.3T and 1.5T with anatomic cryosection. *AJR* 1989; 152:1241–1244.

31. Burnett KR, Davis CL, Read J: Dynamic display of the temporomandibular joint by using "fast-scan" MR imaging. *AJR* 1987; 149:959–962.

32. Schellhas K, Wilkes C: Temporomandibular joint inflammation: Comparison of MR fast scanning with T1 and T2 weighted imaging techniques. *AJR* 1989; 153:93–98.

33. Farrar W, McCarty W: *Outline of Temporomandibular Joint Diagnosis and Treatment*, ed 6. Montgomery, Ala, The Normandie Study Group, 1980.

34. Isberg A, Isacsson G, Johansson AS, et al: Hyperplastic soft-tissue formation in the temporomandibular joint associated with internal derangement. *Oral Surg Oral Med Oral Pathol* 1986; 61:32–38.

35. Shira R: Histologic features of the temporomandibular joint disk and posterior disk attachment: Comparison of symptom-free persons with normally positioned diseased patients with internal derangement. *Oral Surg Oral Med Oral Pathol* 1989; 67:635–643.

36. Katzberg WR, et al: Temporomandibular joint: MR assessment of rotational and sideway disk replacement. *Radiology* 1988; 169:741–748.

37. Shellhas KP, Wilkes CH, El Deeb M, et al: Permanent proplast emporomandibular joint implants: MR imaging of destructive complications. *AJR* 1988; 151:731–735.

38. Kneeland JB, Ryan DE, Carrera GF, et al: Failed temporomandibular joint prothesis: MR imaging. *Radiology* 1987; 165:179–181.

32

The Nasopharynx and Paranasopharyngeal Space

Hugh D. Curtin, M.D.

Ellen K. Tabor, M.D.

The parapharyngeal region is inaccessible to the clinician's physical examination. Computed tomography (CT) and magnetic resonance imaging (MRI) both offer excellent visualization and have become essential in tumor diagnosis.[1–10] The mucosal surface is best evaluated by direct inspection, but the deeper areas have become the domain of the radiologist.

Tumor diagnosis relies primarily on the relationship between the tumor and various fascial planes, so knowledge of the pertinent anatomy is obligatory. Recently MRI has determined internal characteristics in some lesions, which permits further narrowing of the differential diagnosis.

ANATOMY

The nasopharynx extends from the choana to the level of the soft palate.[1, 2, 6, 11] The most prominent landmark of the lateral wall is the torus tubarius, which with the salpingopharyngeal fold surrounds the opening of the eustachian tube on three sides (Fig 32–1). The fossa of Rosenmüller is a recess that parallels the outer circumference of the torus. In the midline, the mucosa and submucosa of the roof of the nasopharynx are closely applied to the base of the skull (sphenoid). More posteriorly (posterior wall of the nasopharynx), the mucosa and submucosa are separated from the basiocciput by the prevertebral muscles. The posterior wall and the roof may form a smooth curve or may form a right angle.

The structures below the mucosa can be grouped according to muscle and fat planes, which are well seen on CT (Figs 32–2 and 32–3).

The deglutitional muscles make up the soft-tissue densities immediately lateral to the nasopharynx airway. Low in the nasopharynx, according to some authors, the superior pharyngeal constrictor muscles merge with fibers from the palatal muscles to form a complete ring around the nasopharynx called Passavant's ring (see Fig 32–3,A). Above the ring, the superior constrictors are absent along the lateral wall of the nasopharynx but do continue up to the base of the skull posteriorly. The "gaps" in the lateral wall are closed by the pharyngobasilar fascia, a thin but very tough fibrous sheath that attaches to the base of the skull. The fascia holds the nasopharynx open. At this level, the levator and tensor veli palatini muscles as well as the wall of the eustachian tube are the soft-tissue densities lateral to the airway on CT (see Fig 32–3,B).

The area lateral to the deglutitional ring can be organized into three compartments: masticator space, prestyloid parapharyngeal space, and poststyloid parapharyngeal space.[1, 7, 8] These are separated by fairly dense fascial layers.

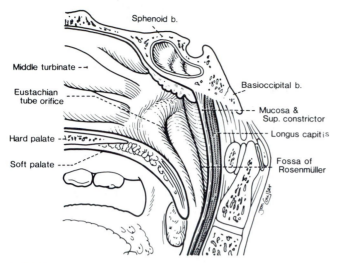

FIG 32–1.
Lateral wall of the nasopharynx viewed from the midline. The fossa of Rosenmüller is the crease paralleling the outer margin of the torus tubarius, which partially surrounds the eustachian tube orifice. The prevertebral musculature inserts on the base of the skull, roughly separating the roof from the posterior wall of the nasopharynx. (From Curtin HD: Infratemporal fossa, nasopharynx, and parapharyngeal spaces, in Carter B (ed): *Computed Tomography of the Head and Neck.* New York, Churchill Livingstone, Inc, 1984. Used by permission.)

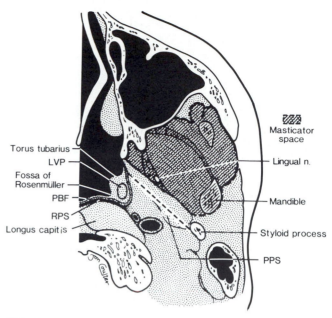

FIG 32–2.
Horizontal section depicting the nasopharynx and related deeper structures. Only one side is shown. The parapharyngeal space *(PPS)* is between the pharyngobasilar fascia and the masticator space. The *dotted line* approximates the separation between the prestyloid and poststyloid compartments. The structures in the poststyloid compartment represent the carotid artery and jugular vein *(LVP* = levator veli palatini; *PBF* = pharyngobasilar fascia; *RPS* = retropharyngeal space). (From Curtin HD: Intratemporal fossa, nasopharynx, and parapharyngeal spaces, in Carter B (ed): *Computed Tomography of the Head and Neck.* New York, Churchill Livingstone, Inc, 1984. Used by permission.)

The masticator muscles (pterygoids, masseter, and temporalis) are enveloped in a continuous fascial layer.[12] The fascial layer attaches to the angle and inferior margin of the mandible. Laterally the fascial layer covers the lateral surface of the masseter muscle. The medial layer is important because this layer represents the separation between the masticator space and the more medial parapharyngeal space. This layer is thin as it covers the medial surface of the medial pterygoid muscle. At the superior margin of the medial pterygoid muscle, the layer fuses with the interpterygoid fascia, and the combined layer continues to the skull base. Immediately beneath the skull base, the lateral pterygoid and the third division of the fifth cranial nerve (V_3) are totally within the masticator space.[8]

The space between the masticator space margin and the deglutitional ring is divided into two major compartments: the prestyloid and poststyloid parapharyngeal spaces (see Fig 32–2). These compartments are separated by the layer of fascia stretching between the tensor veli palatini muscle and the muscles that attach to the styloid process. This separating line extends obliquely from the styloid process to the small sulcus between the pterygoid plates. The prestyloid and poststyloid

compartments are actually anterolateral and posteromedial, respectively. The superior attachment of the fascial layers is such that the masticator space is open to the foramen ovale, the prestyloid parapharyngeal space is closed, and the poststyloid parapharyngeal space is open to the jugular and carotid canals.

Inferiorly the poststyloid space continues along with the great vessels and has been called the vascular space by some authors.[11, 13]

The retropharyngeal space (posterior to the nasopharynx) is a potential space between the pharyngobasilar fascia and the prevertebral musculature. According to some authors, this space can be separated into two compartments by an extra fascial layer called the alar fascia. This separation is not currently as useful to the radiologist as the separation of the parapharyngeal area.

On CT done with intravenous contrast an enhancing line is often seen following the mucosal surface (see Fig 32–25). This line is thought to represent the submucosal venous plexus, which

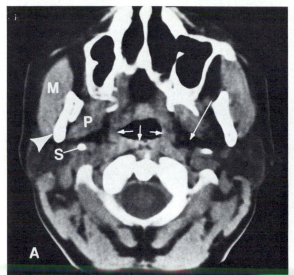

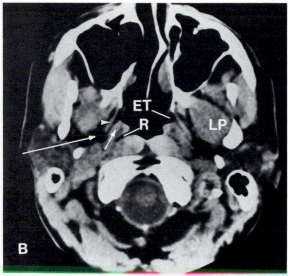

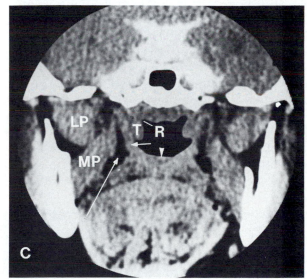

FIG 32–3.
A, axial slice through the nasopharynx at the level of
Passavant's ring. *Small white arrows* depict Passavant's
ring (*P* = medial pterygoid; *M* = masseter; *S* = styloid).
The mandibular ramus is indicated by the *large white
arrowhead* and the parapharyngeal space by the *long
white arrow.* **B,** higher slice through the nasopharynx
(*LP* = lateral pterygoid; *R* = fossa of Rosenmüller; *ET* =
eustachian tube orifice). The tensor veli palatini
is indicated by an *arrowhead,* the levator veli palatini by
the *short white arrow,* and the parapharyngeal space by
the *long white arrow.* **C,** coronal view through the
nasopharynx (*T* = torus tubarius; *R* = fossa of
Rosenmüller). Deglutitional muscles are represented by
the levator veli palatini *(short white arrow).* This extends
into the soft palate *(white arrowhead).* The masticator
muscles are represented by the lateral pterygoid *(LP)*
and the medial pterygoid *(MP).* The parapharyngeal
space *(long white arrow)* separates the deglutitional
muscles from the masticator muscles. The image was
taken during a metrizamide cisternogram done for unrelated problem. (From Curtin HD: Intratemporal fossa, nasopharynx, and parapharyngeal spaces, in Carter B (ed): *Computed Tomography of the Head and Neck.* New York, Churchill
Livingstone, Inc, 1984. Used by permission.)

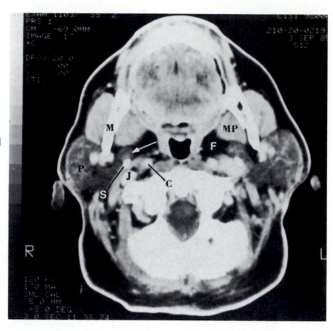

FIG 32–4.
Axial CT through the parapharyngeal space at the level of the medial pterygoid muscle. The parapharyngeal process of the parotid gland *(arrow)* can be seen squeezing between the styloid process *(S)* and the mandible *(M)* (*MP* = medial pterygoid; *P* = parotid; *F* = parapharyngeal fat; *C* = carotid artery; *J* = jugular).

passes along the pharyngeal surface of the torus tubarius and extends into the fossa of Rosenmüller. Lesions limited to the pharyngeal side of this line are usually related to the lymphoid (adenoid) tissue or from the mucosal surface itself. A lesion crossing this line can be assumed to have invaded the deeper soft tissues.

The contents of the various fascial compartments are important because types of tumor found in a given area tend to reflect the tissues within. As stated, the poststyloid compartment (posteromedial to the tensor veli palatini fascia) contains the important vascular structures, the carotid artery, and jugular vein. Cranial nerves IX, X, and XII parallel the vessels. Cranial nerve XI exits the skull into the poststyloid parapharyngeal space but immedi-

ately travels laterally toward the neck. The masticator space contains the pterygoid, temporalis, and masseter muscles as well as the mandible. The third division of the trigeminal nerve exiting the foramen ovale passes into the masticator space and is separated from the prestyloid parapharyngeal space by the combined fascial layer forming the medial boundary of the masticator space.

The prestyloid parapharyngeal space is anterolateral to the tensor veli palatini fascia and is squeezed between the poststyloid parapharyngeal space and the masticator space. The prestyloid parapharyngeal space is almost totally filled with fat. The only important structure present is a small process of the parotid gland that squeezes behind the ramus of the mandible to reach the prestyloid

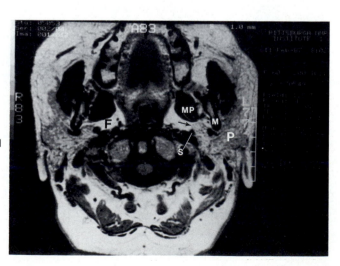

FIG 32–5.
MRI, T1-weighted image. The parapharyngeal process *(arrow)* squeezes between the styloid *(S)* and mandible *(M)* (*MP* = medial pterygoid; *F* = parapharyngeal fat; *P* = parotid).

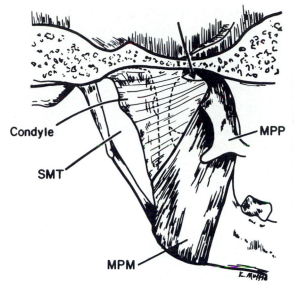

FIG 32–6.
Drawing of the medial wall of the masticator space (*MPM* = medial pterygoid muscle; *MPP* = medial pterygoid plate; *SMT* = stylomandibular tunnel through which the parapharyngeal process of the parotid gland passes). The masticator space is closed above the medial pterygoid muscle by the fascial layer extending up to the skull base. Note how the stylomandibular tunnel is closed off inferiorly by the stylomandibular ligament. The *arrow* marks a very small gap between the upper margin of the fascial layer and the skull base. Small neural twigs pass through this very small gap. (From Curtin HD: *Radiology* 1987; 163:195–204. Used by permission.)

parapharyngeal space compartment (Figs 32–4 and 32–5).

This process of the parotid extends through the stylomandibular tunnel between the styloid process and mandible. The "tunnel" is closed off inferiorly by the stylomandibular ligament (Fig 32–6).

Whether the deep process of the gland is actually separated from the prestyloid parapharyngeal space fat is controversial. Some authors refer to a separating fascial layer; others say there is no layer. This does not make a big difference to the radiologist. Tumors arising in the deepest part of the parotid extend into the parapharyngeal fat.

PATHOLOGY

Tumors

The effect of a tumor on the parapharyngeal fat is key to determination of the origin of a tumor.

Nasopharynx

Nasopharyngeal tumors can obliterate the airway.[1, 2, 6, 9, 14, 15] Lateral extension first widens the deglutitional ring and then impinges on the parapharyngeal fat from the medial side (Fig 32–7). Involvement of the eustachian tube orifice causes a middle-ear effusion. Fluid in the middle ear appearing for the first time in an older individual should direct the physician's attention to the na-

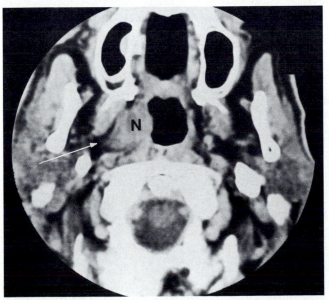

FIG 32–7.
Neurilemoma *(N)* involving the nasopharyngeal wall and pushing laterally into the parapharyngeal space on the normal side. The parapharyngeal space is indicated by a *long white arrow*. (From Curtin HD: Infratemporal fossa, nasopharynx, and parapharyngeal spaces, in Carter B (ed): *Computed Tomography of the Head and Neck*. New York, Churchill Livingstone, Inc, 1984. Used by permission.)

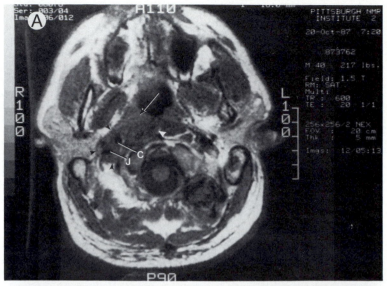

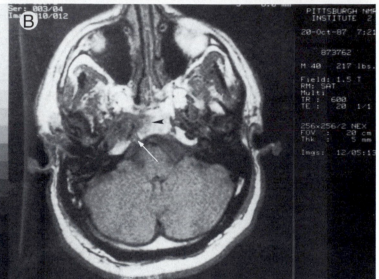

FIG 32–8.
A, a small cell lesion of the nasopharynx shows thickening of the nasopharyngeal wall *(arrow)* and lesion extending posterolaterally to surround the carotid and jugular. The lesion involves the retropharyngeal musculature *(arrowheads = limits of the tumor; C = carotid; J = jugular).* **B,** a slightly higher slice at the level of the hypoglossal canal *(arrow)* shows the lesion with minimal involvement of the skull base *(arrowhead).* **C,** a sagittal section shows the lesion invading the skull base *(arrow).* The normal high signal intensity of the fatty marrow of the clivus *(arrowhead)* is replaced by the intermediate signal of the tumor. (From Curtin HD, Tabor EK: Radiologic evaluation, in Suen JY, Myers EN (eds): *Cancer of the Head and Neck,* ed 2. New York, Churchill Livingstone, Inc, in press. Used by permission.)

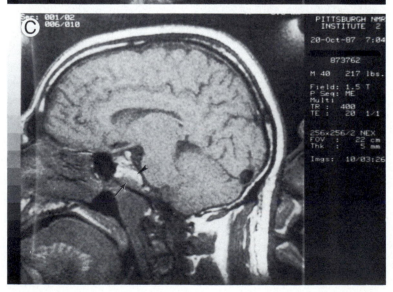

sopharynx. On CT or MRI, obstruction of the eustachian tube can be suspected when there is fluid in an otherwise normally developed mastoid (normal number of air cells). Deeper involvement results in cranial nerve palsies and in skull base erosion (Figs 32–8 and 32–9).

Masses in the lumen of the nasopharynx, including choanal polyps and adenoidal tissue, may obliterate the airway but do not compromise the parapharyngeal fat or erode bone (Fig 32–10). With rapid infusion of intravenous contrast during the scan, the submucosal plexus may blush, and thus an intraluminal location of a lesion can be confirmed. Adenoid tissue, although usually in midline, can be quite asymmetrical.

Nasopharyngeal Carcinoma.—Approximately 90% of nasopharyngeal malignancies are squamous cell carcinoma.[16] Early lesions may efface the fossa of Rosenmüller and eustachian tube or widen the deglutitional muscle ring. Small asymmetries can be normal and should be evaluated by direct visualization and biopsy.

Deeper involvement deforms the parapharyngeal space from the medial aspect, and if the direction of extension is posterior or superior, the skull base can be eroded (see Fig 32–10).

Erosion of the skull base can be detected on CT by using bone algorithms, and at the time of this writing CT is considered more sensitive than MRI is. On MRI the black line of cortical bone may show a defect because tumor gives signal where there should be none. Once the medullary space has been reached, the tumor replaces fat containing yellow marrow and is seen as a low-signal area against the usual bright signal of marrow on T1 images (see Fig 32–8).

Nasopharyngeal tumor can spread through fissures or suture lines, which can be considered weaker barriers to tumor spread. Tumor can spread along the eustachian tube sulcus to reach the middle ear.[9] The eustachian tube passes through a gap in the pharyngobasilar fascia to reach the middle ear. This gap between the skull base and the upper margin of the pharyngobasilar fascia is called the hiatus of Morgagni. The gap also represents a potential pathway of spread for extension of tumor

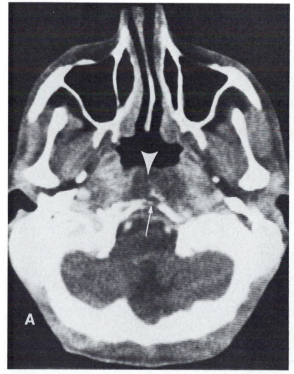 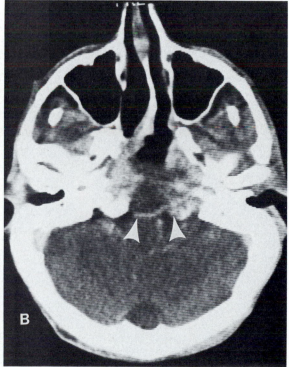

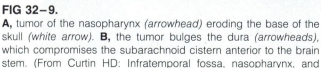

FIG 32–9.
A, tumor of the nasopharynx *(arrowhead)* eroding the base of the skull *(white arrow).* **B,** the tumor bulges the dura *(arrowheads),* which compromises the subarachnoid cistern anterior to the brain stem. (From Curtin HD: Infratemporal fossa, nasopharynx, and parapharyngeal spaces, in Carter B (ed): *Computed Tomography of the Head and Neck.* New York, Churchill Livingstone, Inc, 1984. Used by permission.)

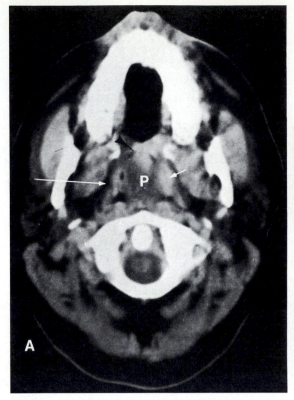

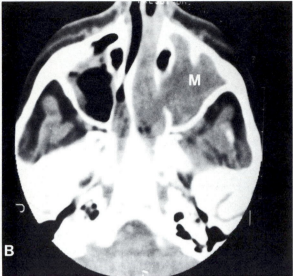

FIG 32–10.

A, intraluminal mass (choanal polyp). The polyp *(P)* appears to blend in with the deglutitional muscles *(small white arrow)*. The parapharyngeal spaces are, however, not deformed *(long white arrow)*. A small amount of air is seen between the polyp and the soft palate *(arrowhead)*. **B,** higher cuts show obliteration of the nasal cavity and involvement of the maxillary sinus *(M)*. (From Curtin HD: Intratemporal fossa, nasopharynx, and parapharyngeal spaces, in Carter B (ed): *Computed Tomography of the Head and Neck*. New York, Churchill Livingstone, Inc, 1984. Used by permission.)

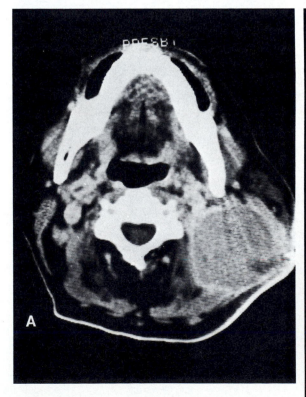

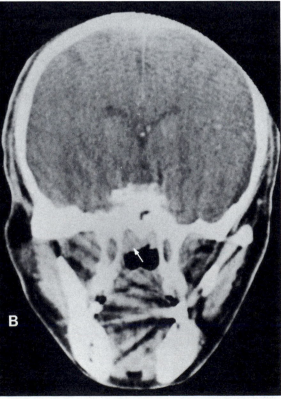

FIG 32–11.

A, large mass with peripheral enhancement and a central hypodense area, which represents a spinal accessory node involved with squamous cell carcinoma. **B,** a coronal scan shows asymmetry of the soft tissues in the nasopharynx. Biopsy of the abnormal side *(small white arrow)* revealed nasopharyngeal carcinoma. No bone erosion was identified. (From Curtin HD: Intratemporal fossa, nasopharynx, and parapharyngeal spaces, in Carter B (ed): *Computed Tomography of the Head and Neck*. New York, Churchill Livingstone, Inc, 1984. Used by permission.)

into the extreme superior aspect of the parapharyngeal region.

Tumor reaching the intracranial side of the skull base either by eroding directly through bone or by passing through a suture line (for instance, the petro-occipital suture) involves first the dura and then the subarachnoid space. On CT, involvement of the dura first causes an enhancing bulge abutting the subarachnoid space anterior to the brain stem. MRI appears to have a slight advantage in assessing extension into the cistern.

Anterior extension involves the ethmoid sinuses and nasal cavity.

Nasopharyngeal carcinoma can spread to several nodal groups.[17–19] The upper spinal accessory nodes high in the posterior triangle of the neck are particularly important, and enlargement of these nodes is highly suggestive of squamous cell carcinoma of the nasopharynx (Fig 32–11). The jugulo-digastric and retropharyngeal nodes may also be involved. Nodes involved with squamous cell carcinoma often show low-density centers (necrotic areas) and peripheral enhancement.[17–19]

Other Malignancies.—Rhabdomyosarcoma occurs in children, and by the time of presentation it may involve the ear and skull base as well as the nasopharynx. The point of origin may therefore be unclear. Lymphoma is also a likely diagnosis in children but can occur at any age. Adenoid cystic carcinoma, melanoma, plasmacytoma, and other rarer lesions can also arise in this area.

Tumor may extend into the nasopharynx from the skull base or nasal area. Tumors of the oral cavity and soft palate can extend superiorly to involve the submucosal area of the nasopharynx[20] (Fig 32–12). The fossa of Rosenmüller may be effaced without actual involvement of the mucosa.

Benign Lesions.—Juvenile angiofibromas are discussed in Chapter 30.

Tornwaldt's cyst can form in the pharyngeal bursa and present in the second or third decade. The cyst would be in the midline high in the nasopharynx. Small cysts may be seen inadvertently as small bright structures on a T2-weighted image.

Choanal polyps protrude into the nasopharynx. They do not disturb the parapharyngeal spaces. The nasal cavity is involved on one side, and the maxillary sinus is usually opacified (see Fig 32–10).

Chordomas arise from notochordal remnants. They usually arise in the clivus, but occasionally

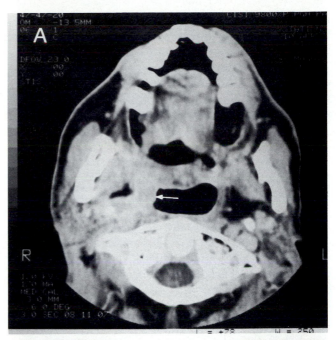

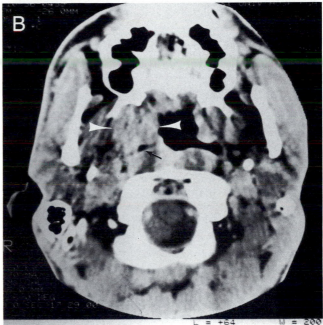

FIG 32–12.
Patient with a lesion of the tonsil extending by submucosal spread to the nasopharynx. **A,** the lesion is seen to extend submucosally along the pharyngeal wall and thicken the deglutitional ring *(arrow)* at the level of Passavant's ring. Lower slices showed a large tumor of the tonsillar pillar. **B,** at the level of the nasopharynx there is thickening of the pharyngeal wall between *arrowheads* at the level of the fossa of Rosenmüller *(arrow)*. This lesion was completely submucosal at the level of the nasopharynx and thus impossible to appreciate endoscopically.

remnants of the notochord can be found in the posterior wall of the nasopharynx.[21] Chordomas can therefore arise rarely in the nasopharyngeal wall.

Rathke's pouch tumors (craniopharyngiomas) can occur high in the nasopharyngeal vault but are much more commonly intracranial than extracranial. Calcification is very common.

Encephaloceles can extend into the nasopharynx. They are covered elsewhere in this volume.

Neuromas and other benign lesions are uncommon in the wall of the nasopharynx itself (see below) (see Fig 32–7).

Parapharyngeal Space

Prestyloid Lesions.—If a lesion is totally within the prestyloid compartment, that is, does not violate the fascial boundaries of the space, it is almost always of salivary gland origin.[8, 22–25] The classic appearance is the "dumbbell" tumor squeezing through the stylomandibular tunnel (Fig 32–13). A parapharyngeal component is seen medial to the mandible, and a more lateral portion of the lesion is seen posterior to the mandible. A lesion that does not extend through the tunnel but is totally within the prestyloid space is still probably a salivary gland tumor arising either from a salivary gland rest or from the extreme medial tip of the parapharyngeal process of the parotid (Fig 32–14,A). On CT or MRI the radiologist should define the relationship of the lesion to the stylomandibular tunnel because this relationship makes a difference in the preferred surgical approach (see Fig 32–14). If a lesion has a component lateral to the stylomandibular tunnel, the approach must be chosen to protect the facial nerve.

The CT or MRI findings that indicate the prestyloid parapharyngeal space location are displacement of the parapharyngeal space fat medially and passage through or to the stylomandibular tunnel. Usually there is a fat line separating the lesion from the deglutitional ring (see Figs 32–13 and 32–14).

Prestyloid lesions tend to spare a small amount of fat between the lesion and the lateral pterygoid muscles. The fat can be compressed but is not often obliterated. Benign lesions of the prestyloid parapharyngeal space do not go through the foramen ovale. They are anterior to the carotid artery and jugular vein.

Most lesions are benign. Pleomorphic adenomas are the predominant cell type. These should be removed completely without disturbing the tumor wall. If biopsied through the pharyngeal

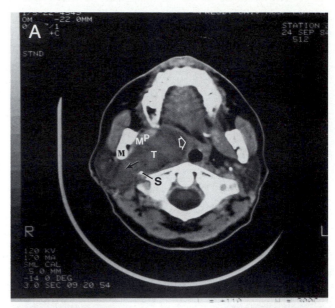

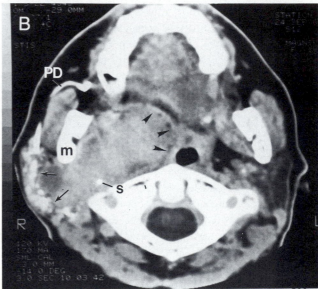

FIG 32–13.
Dumbbell lesion (pleomorphic adenoma of the parotid). **A,** an axial slice shows the tumor *(T)* extending medially and laterally *(arrow)* between the styloid *(S)* and mandible *(M).* The lateral margin of the lesion blends with the remainder of the parotid gland. The deglutitional ring *(open arrow)* is pushed medially. The medial pterygoid muscle *(MP)* does not appear to be invaded. **B,** after a sialogram, the lateral margin *(small arrows)* can be more clearly defined. A small "cap" of fat *(small arrowheads)* is seen separating the lesion from the pharyngeal wall (S = styloid; M = mandible; PD = parotid duct.) (From Heeneman H, Johnson JT, Curtin HD, et al: SIPac, the parapharyngeal space: Anatomy and pathologic conditions with emphasis on neurogenous tumors. Washington, DC, The American Academy of Otolaryngology-Head and Neck Foundation, Inc, 1987. Used by permission.)

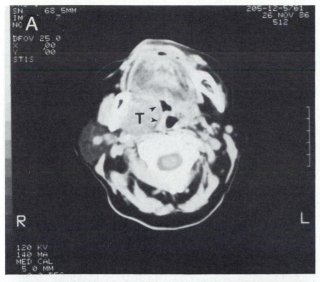

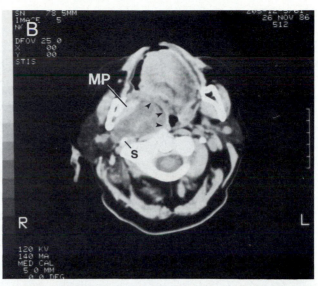

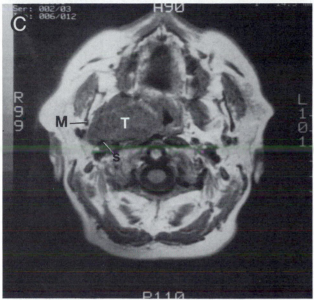

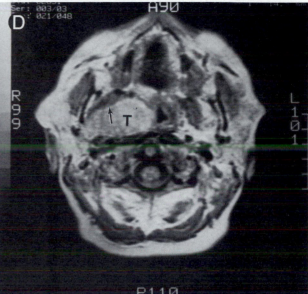

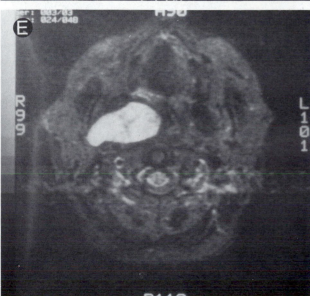

FIG 32–14.
CT and MRI of a prestyloid parapharyngeal space mass: pleo-morphic adenoma. **A,** a low slice shows the tumor *(T)* within the parapharyngeal space. The fat is compressed medially *(arrowheads)* but is not completely obliterated. At this level, the lesion does not pass through the stylomandibular tunnel. If this were the only slice available, one would still think the le-sion is of salivary gland origin but perhaps arising from an em-bryonic rest. **B,** a slightly higher slice again shows the com-pressed fat *(arrowheads)*. The lesion at this level partly squeezes between the styloid *(S)* and the mandible, thus indi-cating its parotid origin *(MP = medial pterygoid muscle)*. **C,** an axial T1-weighted image shows the tumor *(T)* squeezing between the mandible *(M)* and the styloid *(S)*. The tumor can-not be separated clearly from the medial pterygoid muscle on this pulse sequence. **D,** proton spin density (long repetition time [TR] short echo time [TE]). The tumor *(T)* can now be clearly separated from the medial pterygoid muscle *(arrow)*, but its lateral margin is less well defined relative to the parotid gland. **E,** a T2-weighted image (long TR, long TE) shows poor definition of surrounding structures but precise definition of the margins of the tumor. (From Curtin HD: Assessment of sali-vary gland pathology, in Valvassori GE, Mafee HF (eds): *Otolaryngologic Clinics of North America, Diagnostic Imaging in Otolaryn-gology—I: The Ear.* Philadelphia, WB Saunders Co, 1988. Used by permission.)

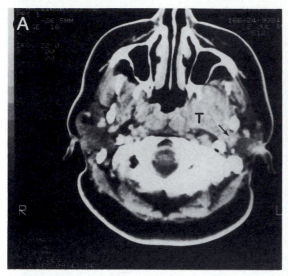
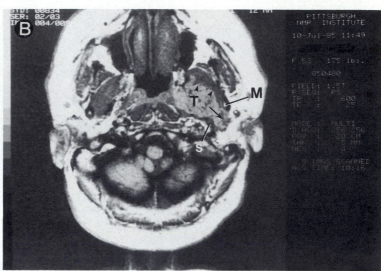

FIG 32–15.

Patient with metastatic thyroid carcinoma to the parapharyngeal space. **A,** a CT scan through the lesion *(T)* showed a small extension *(arrow)* between the styloid and the mandible that suggested a parotid lesion. The tumor blended inperceptibly with the pterygoid muscle. **B,** MRI precisely defines the irregular margin *(arrowheads)* between the tumor and the pterygoid muscle. An irregular margin is thought to represent invasion. The lesion is therefore not a benign pleomorphic adenoma. Malignancy is suspected *(T* = tumor; *M* = mandible; *S* = styloid; *short arrow* = tumor extending laterally into the parotid). (From Curtin HD: Assessment of salivary gland pathology, in Valvassori GE, Mafee MF (eds): *Otolaryngologic Clinics of North America, Diagnostic Imaging in Otolaryngology—I, The Ear.* Philadelphia, WB Saunders Co, 1988. Used by permission.)

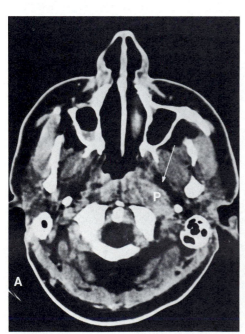
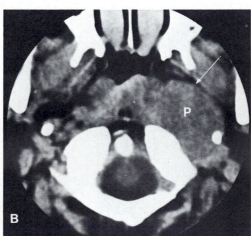
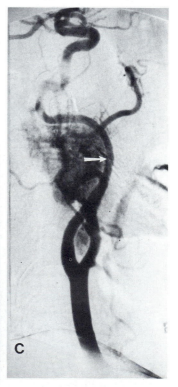

FIG 32–16.

A, axial slice through the paraganglioma *(P)*. The parapharyngeal space *(arrow)* is pushed anteriorly and laterally. **B,** a slightly lower cut shows the bulk of the paraganglioma *(P)*, further displacing the parapharyngeal fat *(arrow)*. **C,** an arteriogram shows tumor blush pushing the carotid anteriorly *(arrow)*.

wall, pleomorphic adenomas often recur. This phenomenon is responsible for the interest in parapharyngeal space scanning. The radiologist can reliably state whether or not the lesion is a pleomorphic adenoma. If totally confined to the prestyloid parapharyngeal space, the pleomorphic adenoma is by far the most likely diagnosis. A lesion extending out of the prestyloid space into the masticator or poststyloid space is very unlikely to be a benign salivary gland lesion (Fig 32–15). A malignant lesion would still be considered. Salivary gland neoplasms do not arise in the poststyloid compartment or the masticator space.

Currently we prefer MRI to CT because of the ease of definition of the tumor margins. The relationship to the carotid is easily determined. Coronal images may help visualize the relationship of a lesion to the skull base.

CT sialography (see Fig 32–13) was used in the past to better define a lesion poorly seen on CT. This procedure is almost never needed now because of the sensitivity of high-resolution CT and MRI.

Poststyloid Lesions.—Poststyloid (posteromedial) tumors are related to the neurovascular elements associated with the jugular vein and carotid artery. Lesions arising here push the parapharyngeal fat anteriorly and slightly laterally (Figs 32–16 and 32–17). A fat plane may separate the tumor from the nasopharyngeal mucosa (see Fig 32–17). As the tumor expands and is limited posteriorly by the bony elements, the bulk of the tumor may actually be located further anteriorly than is the styloid process. A tumor that enlarges laterally tends to press behind the styloid process rather than passing anterior to the process through the stylomandibular tunnel.

Paragangliomas.—Paragangliomas (glomus tumors) (Figs 32–16 and 32–18) arise in the poststyloid compartment and enhance prominently with rapid-flow contrast administration. Glomus vagale tumors arise in the vagal ganglion inferior to the temporal bone. Glomus jugulare tumors can extend from the jugular fossa inferiorly into the poststyloid space. Differentiation is made by looking for destruction of the jugular foramen. The glomus vagale pushes the carotid artery anteriorly on arteriography. Paragangliomas may be multiple but are rarely malignant.

MRI shows a so-called salt-and-pepper appear-

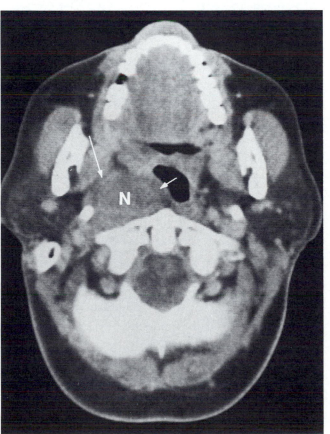

FIG 32–17.
Neurilemoma *(N)* arising in the poststyloid parapharyngeal space. The parapharyngeal fat *(long arrow)* is pushed anteriorly and laterally. A small fat plane *(short arrow)* is seen between the tumor and the pharyngeal mucosa. (From Curtin HD: Infratemporal fossa, nasopharynx, and parapharyngeal spaces, in Carter B (ed): *Computed Tomography of the Head and Neck.* New York, Churchill Livingstone, Inc, 1984. Used by permission.)

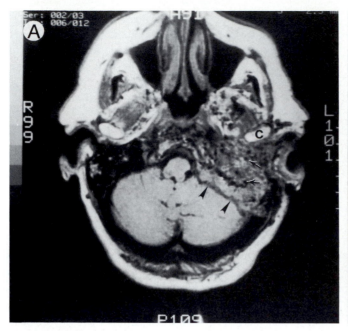

FIG 32–18.
Large erosive glomus tumor eroding the skull base. The lesion extends from the posterior fossa *(arrowheads)* to the mandibular condyle *(C)*. Note the typical "salt-and-pepper" appearance of the tumor with numerous small flow voids *(arrows)* within the lesion. **B,** a slightly inferior slice shows the poststyloid location of the tumor *(T)* pushing the parapharyngeal fat *(arrow)* anteriorly. The parapharyngeal process of the parotid *(arrowhead)* is seen to be anterolateral to the tumor.

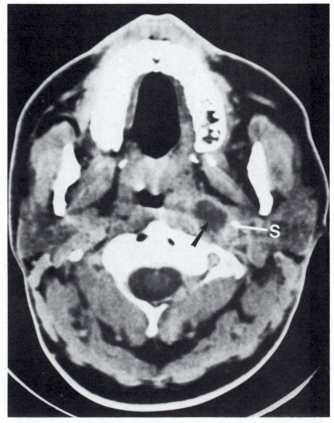

FIG 32–19.
Squamous cell carcinoma involving the retropharyngeal node *(arrow)*. The parapharyngeal fat is pushed anteriorly. The bulk of the lesion is medial to the styloid process. Note the necrotic center *(S = styloid)*. (From Curtin HD: Infratemporal fossa, nasopharynx, and parapharyngeal spaces, in Carter B (ed): *Computed Tomography of the Head and Neck.* New York, Churchill Livingstone, Inc, 1984. Used by permission.)

ance with small black holes representing a flow void phenomenon of large vessels (see Fig 32–18). This phenomenon is unusual in neurilemoma, which represents the major differential possibility. The "salt-and-pepper" appearance may not be as obvious in small paragangliomas.[26]

Neuromas.—Neuromas often enhance and can be confused with paragangliomas. They have a different appearance on angiography. Neuromas involving the jugular foramen tend to involve the more medial part (pars nervosa) than the lateral ones (pars vasculare).

Lateral Retropharyngeal Nodes.—Lateral retropharyngeal nodes arise just medial to the carotid and behave as poststyloid masses.[18] They usually have a necrotic center that is hypodense on CT scans (Fig 32–19).

Meningiomas.—Meningiomas may involve the prestyloid or poststyloid spaces as well as the mas-

ticator area. They cause hyperostosis of the bone and may calcify (Fig 32–20).

Masticator Space (Infratemporal Fossa)

Tumors involving the masticator space are usually extensions from primaries in the surrounding areas.[8] The most common is probably from the maxillary sinus, retromolar trigone, and pharyngeal wall (Fig 32–21) (see Chapter 30). Primary tumors may arise in the mandible or in the associated musculature.

A lesion expanding in the masticator space pushes the parapharyngeal fat posteromedially.[21, 22] A lesion confined to the masticator space respects the upper attachment of the medial fascial boundary (fused medial pterygoid fascia and interpterygoid fascia). This fascial boundary attaches to the skull base along a line extending roughly from the midpoint between the pterygoid plates to the spine of the sphenoid (Fig 32–22). This line thus passes medial to the foramen ovale and spinosum. The line then curves laterally toward the posterior margin of

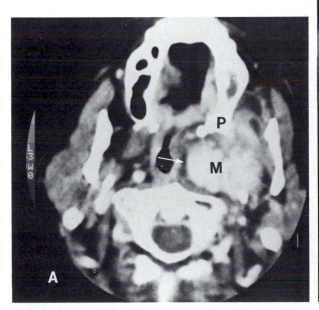

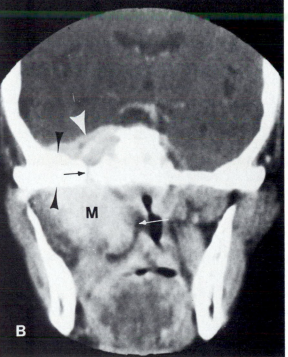

FIG 32–20.
A, axial slice through a meningioma *(M)*. This involves the masticator space and prestyloid space. The parapharyngeal fat *(arrow)* is pushed medially. Note the hyperostosis of the lower part of the pterygoid *(P)*. **B,** a coronal slice shows the meningioma *(M)*. The parapharyngeal fat *(white arrow)* is pushed medially. The tumor extends through the foramen ovale *(black arrow)* and also involves the middle cranial fossa *(large white arrowhead)*. Note the hyperostosis of the skull base *(black arrowheads)*. (From Curtin HD: Infratemporal fossa, nasopharynx, and parapharyngeal spaces, in Carter B (ed): *Computed Tomography of the Head and Neck.* New York, Churchill Livingstone, Inc, 1984. Used by permission.)

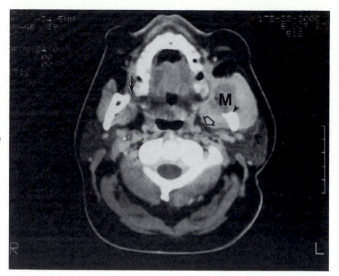

FIG 32–21.
Carcinoma of the retromolar trigone extends into the masticator space. The mass *(M)* expands the masticator space and obliterates the fat planes and tissues anterior to the mandible. Compare with the normal retromolar trigone *(arrow)* on the opposite side. There is erosion of the mandible *(arrowhead)*. Note how the parapharyngeal fat is pushed posteriorly and medially *(open arrow)*.

the mandible. Tumors of the masticator space will obliterate the normal fat planes within the masticator space.

Tumors may leave the masticator space by extending into the middle cranial fossa via the foramen ovale or into the pterygopalatine fossa. Extension into these areas can be detected because of the difference in CT density or MRI signal between the tumor and the normal soft tissue (fat in the pterygopalatine fossa and brain in the middle cranial fossa).

Primary tumors of the masticator space may be sarcomas or undifferentiated carcinomas. Neural lesions and meningiomas occur. Notably, salivary gland tumors do not.

Mandibular and lingual nerves pass through the masticator space and can be enlarged by perineural extension (see Chapter 30). This would be very rare as an initial finding, and other manifestations of the tumor would certainly be present.

Hematogenous metastasis can reach the mandible usually from the breast, kidney, lung, colon, or prostate (Fig 32–23).

Tumor Workup

At the time of this writing, we prefer MRI as the initial step. The boundaries of the lesion are usually more obvious with MRI than CT. This is especially true where the tumor abuts muscle (see Fig 32–15). The relationship of the tumor to the great vessels can be more easily appreciated on MRI than CT, especially in the case of a glomus tumor where vessel and tumor blend together on CT. The ease of coronal imaging is also an advantage.

When a lesion involves the poststyloid parapharyngeal space, arteriography is performed to help differentiate the various tumors and define the relationship of tumor to the great vessels. Arteriography is not usually necessary in prestyloid masses.

Infection

The fascial planes of the area may direct the spread of an infectious process. The infection may be of dental or tonsillar origin. Infection may also drain into the retropharyngeal nodes where an abscess can form in the retropharynegal or the poststyloid parapharyngeal space.

Infection of the masticator space can spread easily into the temporal space, which is actually the superior extension of the masticator space (Fig 25–24). The buccal space, lateral to the buccinator muscle, can be involved anterior to the masticator space. Retropharyngeal infection can spread down into the mediastinum. The spaces are not impervious but may limit the spread of infection to some extent.

Malignant external otitis is a persistent *Pseudomonas* infection, usually in an elderly diabetic patient. There is usually bone destruction. Disease may extend down into the soft tissues beneath the temporal bone. This usually involves the area just beneath the external auditory canal, but occasionally the disease can extend medially into

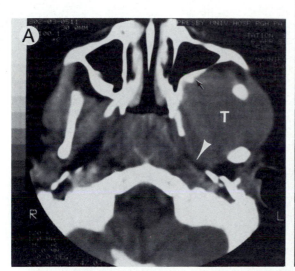

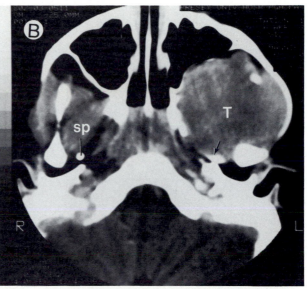

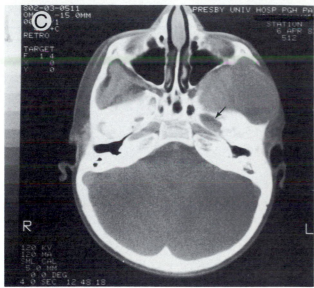

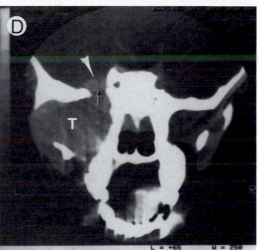

FIG 32–22.

Large sarcoma (synovial) of the masticator space. **A,** tumor *(T)* fills the masticator space and impinges on surrounding structures. The parapharyngeal fat is pushed posteriorly and medially *(arrowhead)*. The posterior wall of the maxillary sinus is remodeled anteriorly *(arrow)*. **B,** slightly higher slice. Tumor *(T)* pushes on the posterolateral wall of the maxillary sinus anteriorly and the zygomatic arch laterally. The medial margin of the tumor does not cross the attachment of the medial wall of the masticator space, which attaches to the spine of the sphenoid *(short arrow),* and continues anteriorly toward the anterior plate *(arrowhead). (sp* = spine of the sphenoid on the normal side. This should not be confused with the more inferior styloid process.) **C,** a slightly higher slice shows enlargement of the foramen ovale *(arrow).* Compare with the opposite side. **D,** a coronal image shows the tumor *(T)* extending through the foramen ovale *(arrow)* with a very small intracranial component *(arrowhead).* (From Curtin HD: Infratemporal fossa, nasopharynx, and parapharyngeal spaces, in Carter B (ed): *Computed Tomography of the Head and Neck.* New York, Churchill Livingstone, Inc, 1984. Used by permission.)

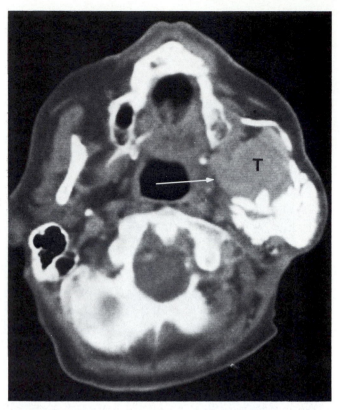

FIG 32–23.
Metastatic tumor from the lung to the mandible (*T* = tumor). The tumor replaces the coronoid process. The tumor was thought to represent a parotid tumor, but is actually deep with respect to it. The tumor pushes into the parapharyngeal fat *(arrow)* and pushes it medially (parotid sialogram). (From Curtin HD: Infratemporal fossa, nasopharynx, and parapharyngeal spaces, in Carter B (ed): *Computed Tomography of the Head and Neck.* New York, Churchill Livingstone, Inc, 1984. Used by permission.)

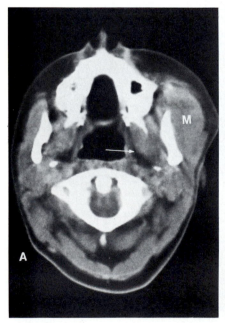 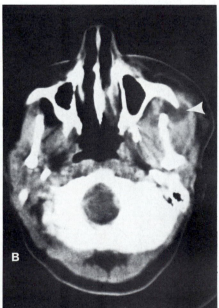 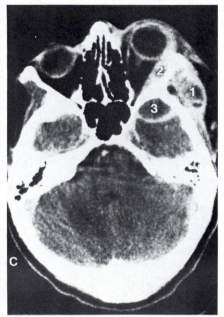

FIG 32–24.
A, infection from a molar extraction. The masseter muscle appears to be enlarged because of the abscess in the masticator space (*M* = enlarged masseter). The parapharyngeal space *(arrow)* is normal. **B,** a higher slice shows an abscess just beneath the zygomatic arch *(arrowhead).* This represents the junction of the masticator and temporalis spaces. **C,** a higher slice shows an abscess in the temporal space *(1)* and orbit *(2).* There is also an epidural abscess *(3).*

the region of the nasopharynx and obliterate the fat planes.[27]

MISCELLANEOUS

Atrophy of the muscles bordering the nasopharynx can accentuate the normal recesses in the elderly. If cranial nerve V is destroyed, the muscles of mastication atrophy (Fig 32–25). When atrophy is seen, the more central connections of the trigeminal nerve should be evaluated.

In a patient undergoing hemimandibulectomy, the condyle and part of the ramus may be left on the resected side. Because there are no teeth to

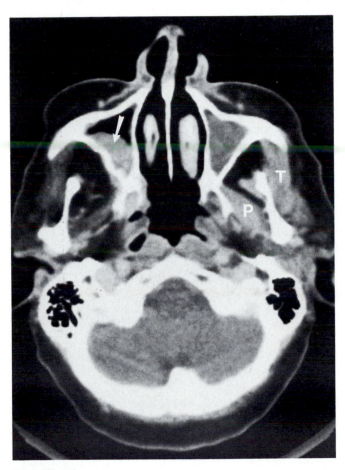

FIG 32–25.
Adenoid cystic carcinoma of the maxillary sinus *(arrow)*. Tumor involves the maxillary division of the trigeminal nerve and is causing atrophy of the masticator muscles. Compare with the opposite normal side (*P* = normal pterygoid; *T* = normal temporalis muscle). The maxillary sinus on the uninvolved side showed an obstructive phenomena with mucous retention. Note the enhancing line following the surface of the nasopharynx, especially as it dips into the fossa of Rosenmüller. This is thought to be due to a submucosal venous plexus.

limit the motion of the fragment, the pterygoid muscles pull the bone anteriorly. This may result in a pseudoenlargement of the muscle when compared with the opposite side. This apparent enlargement is due to shortening of the muscle and may mimic tumor recurrence.

SUMMARY

The symmetrical muscles and fat planes make the nasopharynx and surrounding structures ideal for CT or MRI. The effect of a tumor on the parapharyngeal space is especially important in definition of tumor origin. The radiologist's primary role is to determine the location and extent of the disease.

Perhaps the most important concept is that the radiologist tries to determine which lesions are salivary gland tumors and which are not. This determination is made by defining whether or not a lesion arises in and is limited to the prestyloid parapharyngeal space. This determination strongly influences the surgical approach as well as the need for further radiologic workup.

REFERENCES

1. Mancuso AA, Hanafee WN: *Computed Tomography and Magnetic Resonance Imaging of the Head and Neck*, ed 2. Baltimore, Williams & Wilkins, 1985.
2. Bergeron RT, Osborn AG, Som PM (eds): *Head and Neck Excluding the Brain*. St Louis, CV Mosby Co, 1984.
3. Valvassori GE, Potter GD, Hanafee WN, et al: *Radiology of the Ear, Nose and Throat*. Philadelphia, WB Saunders Co, 1982.
4. Brant-Zawadzki M, Norman D (eds): *Magnetic Resonance Imaging of the Central Nervous System*. New York, Raven Press, 1987.
5. Som PM, Shapiro M, Biller HF, et al: Sinonasal tumors and inflammatory tissues: Their MR differentiation. *Radiology*, in press.
6. Teresi LM, Lufkin RB, Vinuela F, et al: MR imaging of the nasopharynx and floor of the middle cranial fossa. Part I. Normal anatomy. *Radiology* 1987; 164:811–816.
7. Som PM, Biller HF, Lawson W: Tumors of the parapharyngeal space: Preoperative evaluation, diagnosis and surgical approaches. *Ann Otol Rhinol Laryngol* 1981; 90 (suppl 80):3–15.
8. Curtin HD: Separation of the masticator space from the parapharyngeal space. *Radiology* 1987; 163:195–204.

9. Teresi LM, Lufkin RB, Vinuela F, et al: MR imaging of the nasopharynx and floor of the middle cranial fossa. Part II. Malignant tumors. *Radiology* 1987; 164:817–821.
10. Carter B: Computed tomography, in Valvassori GE, Potter GD, Hanafee WN, et al (eds): *Radiology of the Ear, Nose and Throat.* Philadelphia, WB Saunders Co, 1982.
11. Silver AJ, Mawad ME, Hilal SK, et al: Computed tomography of the nasopharynx and related spaces: I. Anatomy. *Radiology* 1983; 147:725–731.
12. Grodinsky M, Holyoke EA: The fascia and fascial spaces of the head, neck and adjacent regions. *Am J Anat* 1938; 63:367–408.
13. Silver AJ, Mawad ME, Hilal SK, et al: Computed tomography of the nasopharynx and related spaces: II. Pathology. *Radiology* 1983; 147:733–738.
14. Barnes L: *Surgical Pathology of the Head and Neck.* New York, Marcel Dekker, Inc, 1985.
15. Bohman L, Mancuso A, Thompson J, et al: CT approach to benign nasopharyngeal masses. *AJR* 1981; 136:173–180.
16. Choa G: Cancer of the nasopharynx, in Suen JY, Myers EN (eds): *Cancer of the Head and Neck.* New York, Churchill Livingstone, Inc, 1981.
17. Som PM: Lymph nodes of the neck. *Radiology* 1987; 165:593–600.
18. Mancuso AA, Maceri D, Rice D, et al: CT of cervical lymph node cancer. *AJR* 1981; 136:381–385.
19. Mancuso AA, Harnsberger HR, Muraki AS, et al: Computed tomography of cervical and retropharyngeal lymph nodes: Normal anatomy, variants of normal, and applications in staging head and neck cancer. Part I: Normal anatomy. *Radiology* 1983; 148:709–714.
20. Mancuso AA, Hanafee WN: Elusive head and neck cancers beneath intact mucosa. *Laryngoscope* 1983; 93:133–139.
21. Bonneville J, Belloir A, Mawazini H, et al: Calcified remnants of the notochord in the roof of the nasopharynx. *Radiology* 1980; 137:373–377.
22. Bass R: Approaches to the diagnosis and treatment of tumors of the parapharyngeal space. *Head Neck Surg* 1982; 4:281–289.
23. Doubleday LC, Jing B, Wallace S: Computed tomography of the infratemporal fossa. *Radiology* 1981; 138:619–624.
24. Som PM, Braun IF, Shapiro MD, et al: Tumors of the parapharyngeal space and upper neck: MR imaging characteristics. *Radiology* 1987; 164:823–829.
25. Som PM, Biller HF, Lawson W, et al: Parapharyngeal space masses: An updated protocol based upon 104 cases. *Radiology* 1984; 153:149–156.
26. Olsen WL, Dillon WP, Kelly WM, et al: MR imaging of paragangliomas. *AJNR* 1986; 7:1039–1042.
27. Curtin HD, Wolfe P, May M: Malignant external otitis: CT evaluation. *Radiology* 1982; 145:383–388.

33

The Normal and Abnormal Neck

R. Nick Bryan, M.D., Ph.D.

Charles W. McCluggage, M.D.

Barry L. Horowitz, M.D.

David Jenkins, M.D.

CROSS-SECTIONAL IMAGING OF THE CERVICAL REGION

Newer cross-sectional techniques are significantly changing and increasing the value of imaging evaluations of the neck. This is primarily a consequence of two factors: (1) the relative ease of the examinations and (2) the vastly superior information available as compared with that from earlier imaging techniques.[1, 2] The neck, which extends from the inferior border of the mandible and foramen magnum to the thoracic inlet, is a relatively small, thin area that is amenable to direct clinical observation and palpation externally and direct endoscopic observation internally. Most masses within this area are clinically detectable while relatively small in size. However, this is not to say that additional morphologic information is not needed by the clinician.

While the neck is a small anatomic area, it is very complex, with many small critical structures and tissues closely approximated. While lesions might be easily detectable, their precise anatomic location and relationships are not always obvious by clinical means alone. Unfortunately, prior radiographic techniques usually did not provide the necessary anatomic and pathologic resolution that the clinician wanted. In fact, traditional radiographic techniques often mimicked or duplicated clinical observations. Plain x-ray films of the neck demonstrated little beyond the air-contrasted res-

piratory tract, the bone of the cervical spine, and to a lesser degree, the cartilaginous anatomy of the larynx. For most lesions, the plain x-ray films offered only gross, indirect anatomic information. Even the more invasive techniques such as laryngography, air-contrast pluridirectional tomography, and barium studies of the digestive tract yielded only information concerning gross displacements or the appearance of the mucosal surfaces, which in most cases could be obtained by direct and indirect endoscopy. In only a limited number of cases did contrast opacification of visceral structures by lymphangiography, angiography, or sialography provide direct information about internal soft tissues. In selected cases, high-resolution ultrasound provided some intrinsic information, particularly about the thyroid gland. On the other hand, cross-sectional techniques now allow very high resolution anatomic images that display the major muscles, viscera, vessels, and associated intervening spaces. Indeed, computed tomography (CT) and now magnetic resonance imaging (MRI) provide far more information concerning the anatomy and even occasionally the pathology of lesions than can be obtained by clinical examination.[3] Furthermore, these examinations are essentially noninvasive and easy to perform.

Unfortunately, clinical application of these techniques has been relatively slow. One of the main reasons has been the lack of knowledge and hence interest in this area by many radiologists.

Now that the usefulness of the techniques is becoming obvious, it is imperative that the imaging physician refamiliarize himself with the fine anatomy of this area and reacquaint himself with the important pathology.

This chapter will concentrate on the anatomy of the neck and attempt to relate the traditional topographic and surgical anatomy of the neck with the cross-sectional anatomy as displayed by CT and MRI. This correlation is extremely important because many clinicians remain traditional anatomically oriented and do not easily correlate cross-sectional anatomy with the clinical, gross anatomic situation. Subsequently, a few of the major pathologic processes in the neck will be discussed and correlated with appropriate cross-sectional images. Because one cannot attempt to cover all of the widely diverse pathologic conditions of the neck in a single chapter, we will concentrate on lesions involving the salivary glands, larynx, and lymphatic system, as well as a few other miscellaneous topics.

While the cervical spine is obviously a large and important component of the neck, its anatomy and pathology are basically a different topic that will be covered elsewhere. In addition, the dorsal aspect of the neck (to be defined later) will be minimally discussed in this section because it contains the relatively simple anatomy of the paraspinal muscles and is involved with little pathology independent of the cervical spine. Therefore, we will concentrate on the soft tissues of the anterior two thirds of the neck.

ANATOMY

Cervical Triangles

The anterior portion of the neck has traditionally been divided into triangular regions that are defined and separated by major muscles (Fig 33–1). This descriptive subdivision of the neck has been of great clinical usefulness because (1) various regions can usually be defined by observation and palpation, (2) the regions are related to relatively consistent underlying anatomy that allows postulation of the location and origin of contained lesions, and (3) important surgical approaches are suggested.[4]

The posterior extent of the "triangular" neck is the anterior border of the trapezius muscle. Anything posterior to this plane is in the dorsal portion of the neck and will not be discussed in this section. Each right and left half of the neck has symmetrical and essentially identical triangular regions.

The major division is into an anterior and a posterior triangle, which are separated by the sternocleidomastoid (SCM) muscles. These large, easily palpable muscles that extend from the mastoid process to the medial end of the clavicle and adjacent manubrium define the posterior border of the anterior triangle, which extends to the ventral midline, and the anterior border of the posterior triangle, which extends back to the trapezius muscle. The posterior triangle is subdivided into a subclavian and occipital triangle by the intervening posterior belly of the omohyoid muscle. The omohyoid muscle has two bellies, the posterior of which originates from the area of the suprascapular notch of the scapula and extends to an intermediate tendon that is attached to the medial clavicle and first rib. The anterior belly then proceeds superiorly to insert on the body of the hyoid bone. The occipital triangle lies between the trapezius muscle posteriorly, the SCM muscle anteriorly, and the posterior belly of the omohyoid inferiorly. The subclavian triangle lies inferior to the posterior belly of the omohyoid muscle, posterior to the SCM muscle, and rostral to the clavicle.

The large anterior cervical triangle can be subdivided into an upper and lower portion separated by the hyoid bone. The upper portion contains two triangular regions. The digastric triangle lies below the inferior border of the mandible and between the anterior and posterior bellies of the digastric muscle. Anteriorly, the digastric muscle is attached to the inner surface of the mandibular symphysis. The anterior belly then passes posterolaterally to a tendinous sling attached by an aponeurosis to the lateral aspect of the body of the hyoid bone. The posterior belly extends posteriorly to the base of the skull at the digastric notch just medial to the mastoid tip. The smaller submental triangle lies between the anterior belly of the digastric muscle and the midline, below the symphysis of the mandible, and above the hyoid bone.

The lower portion of the anterior cervical triangle is subdivided into an upper carotid triangle and a lower muscular triangle, which are separated from each other by the anterior belly of the omohyoid muscle. The carotid triangle is bounded by the posterior belly of the digastric muscle superiorly, the SCM muscle posteriorly, and the anterior belly of the omohyoid muscle anteroinferiorly. The muscular triangle lies between the anterior belly of the

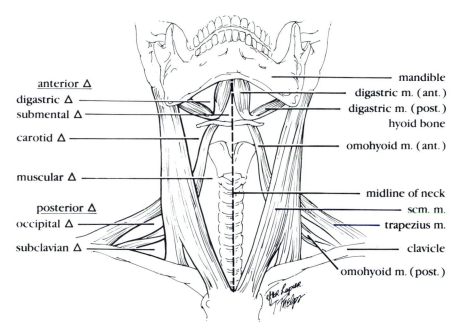

FIG 33–1.
Anatomic triangles of the neck.

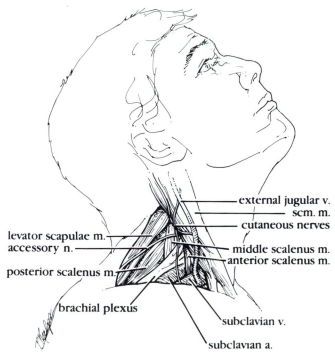

FIG 33–2.
Contents of the posterior cervical triangle.

omohyoid muscle superiorly, the SCM muscle posteriorly, and the midline anteriorly.

Each of the cervical triangles contains certain critical structures (Figs 33–2 to 33–4). The posterior triangle has a deep floor of muscles, which are basically the anterior and lateral paravertebral muscles and are contained within the tough prevertebral fascia. From anterior to posterior, these muscles are the anterior, middle, and posterior scalene and levator scapula muscles. This is a relatively continuous sheath of muscles, except for a gap between the anterior and middle scalene through which pass the cervical and upper brachial nerve plexuses and the subclavian artery. The subclavian vein passes anterior to the anterior scalene muscle at the medial aspect of the clavicle. In the occipital triangle, the floor then consists of the above muscles and the cervical plexus. The branches of the cervical plexus (which supply essentially all of the muscles of the cervical region as well as the overlying skin) loop about the posterior border of the SCM before they course to their respective muscles and cutaneous territories. Only a few superficial cervical lymph nodes are located in the occipital triangle. The 11th cranial nerve crosses the midaspect of the occipital triangle as it passes from behind the SCM muscle to the undersurface of its termination in the trapezius muscle. Crossing the anterior aspect of the occipital triangle and extending down across the subclavian triangle is the external jugular vein, which lies outside of the investing layer of the deep cervical fascia.

Within the subclavian triangle, the subclavian vein lies just anterior to the anterior scalene mus-

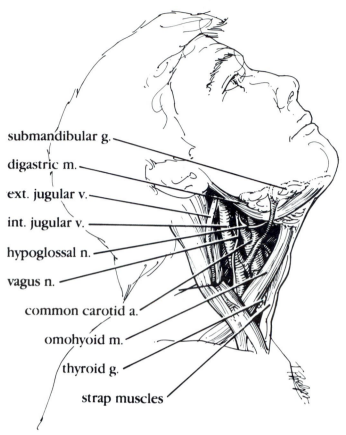

FIG 33–3.
Contents of the anterior cervical triangle, lateral view.

submandibular g.
digastric m.
ext. jugular v.
int. jugular v.
hypoglossal n.
vagus n.
common carotid a.
omohyoid m.
thyroid g.
strap muscles

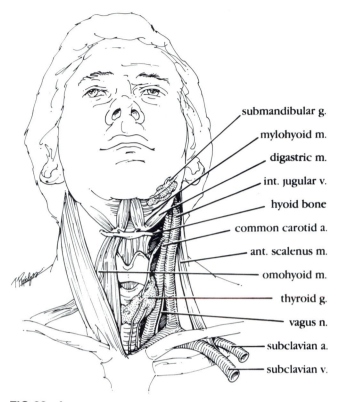

FIG 33–4.
Contents of the anterior cervical triangle, frontal view.

submandibular g.
mylohyoid m.
digastric m.
int. jugular v.
hyoid bone
common carotid a.
ant. scalenus m.
omohyoid m.
thyroid g.
vagus n.
subclavian a.
subclavian v.

cle, while the subclavian artery and brachial plexus proceed laterally between the anterior and middle scalene muscles.

The digastric triangle has as its floor the mylohyoid muscle anteriorly, while lateral pharyngeal wall structures form the floor more posteriorly. Within the triangle lies the superficial portion of the submandibular gland, submandibular lymph nodes, and the facial artery. The small submental triangle has the mylohyoid muscle as its floor and contains only a few submental lymph nodes. The carotid triangle has the middle and inferior constrictor muscles of the pharynx and the pretracheal strap muscles as its floor. It contains the carotid artery, cervical sympathetic plexus, vagus nerve, internal jugular vein, and deep cervical lymph nodes.

The muscular triangle has the inferior portion of the carotid sheath, pretracheal fascia, and pretracheal strap muscles as its floor. It contains the inferior portions of the internal jugular vein, common carotid artery, vagus nerve, cervical sympathetic plexus, inferior thyroidal vessels, inferior laryngeal nerve, and inferior deep cervical lymph nodes.

Visceral Columns

Another conceptual approach to the anatomy of the neck is that of a concentric columnar structure (Fig 33–5). The neck can be viewed as consisting of a median visceral column, lateral visceral column, and surrounding musculofacial sheath. The median visceral column primarily consists of pharyngeal derivatives, including the hypopharynx, larynx, trachea, and esophagus. It is a concentrically tight, facially isolated compartment, but is open superiorly and inferiorly.

Anterolateral to the median visceral column is the lateral visceral column, which is an intermediate fascial space that consists primarily of the major vascular structures of the neck and components of pharyngeal arch derivatives. This column includes the carotid sheath (which contains the internal jugular vein, carotid arteries, and vagus nerve), deep cervical lymph nodes, and in a subdivided anterior inferior compartment, the thyroid and parathyroid glands. The salivary glands, particularly the parotid and submandibular glands, might also be included in this compartment, although in a somewhat artificial manner.

Enveloping the central columns is a strong V-shaped musculofacial sheath consisting primarily

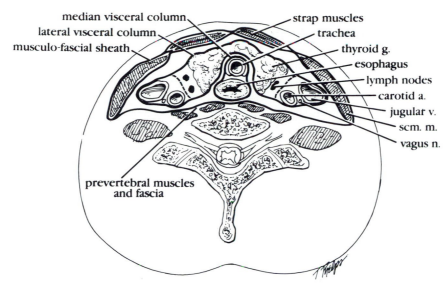

FIG 33–5.
Columnar organization of the neck.

of the deep cervical fascia and the SCM and trapezius muscles, which this strong fascia envelopes. Posterolaterally, the deep cervical fascia is continuous with the prevertebral fascia, which basically separates the posterior aspect of the neck. The anatomic boundaries between these three anatomic columns are relatively strong, and therefore lesions external to the deep cervical fascia or posterior to the prevertebral fascia tend to be excluded from the deeper spaces. The lateral visceral column, while effectively separated from the median visceral column and the overlying musculofacial sheath, is relatively open throughout its length, including the top and bottom. This forms a potential conduit for disease to spread throughout the length of the neck and beyond.

Lymphatic System

With respect to spread of disease in the cervical region, one must also consider the lymphatic system of this area, which may be subdivided into four main groups: (1) superficial cervical nodes, (2) deep cervical nodes, (3) junctional nodes, and (4) anterior cervical nodes (Fig 33–6). The superficial cervical nodes are relatively few in number and lie external to the deep cervical fascia, primarily over the parotid region and along the external jugular vein. The deep cervical nodes are more numerous and are far more important. They basically all lie along the carotid sheath–jugular vein region and hence are sometimes called jugular nodes. They may be subdivided into an upper group, which is above the anterior belly of the omohyoid muscle,

and an inferior group caudal to that plane. The upper group includes jugulodiagastric nodes near the middle tendon of the digastric muscle, which receive lymph from the tonsillar region; the jugulo-omohyoid nodes, which drain the anterior tongue

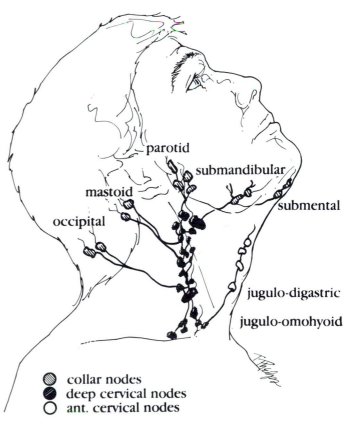

collar nodes
deep cervical nodes
ant. cervical nodes

FIG 33–6.
Cervical lymph nodes.

and submental nodes; the retropharyngeal nodes near the base of the skull, which drain the nasopharynx and the eustachian region; and the deep parotid nodes, which lie within the parotid gland. The inferior group of deep cervical nodes receive efferent vessels from the superior deep cervical channels as well as apical axillary nodes.

Junctional nodes lie at the junction of the head and neck and include one or two occipital nodes, several mastoid nodes, the nodes in relationship to the parotid gland, approximately five nodes near the submandibular gland, and one to four submental nodes.

The anterior cervical nodes generally lie along the ventral midline and include infrahyoid nodes on the thyrohyoid membrane, prelaryngeal nodes near the cricothyroid membrane, and pretracheal and paratracheal nodes. It is important that one not only remember the general location of these nodes but also note their usual drainage patterns.

Salivary Glands

While only part of the salivary glands are in the cervical region, we will include a discussion of these structures because they do relate to the upper portion of the neck and are seen and evaluated on scans of this region. Only the parotid and submandibular glands are well demonstrated by common imaging modalities, and descriptive anatomy

and pathology will be limited to these salivary structures (Figs 33–7 and 33–8).

The parotid gland is the largest of the major salivary glands and is roughly triangular in shape both in the lateral and axial projections. It is a fatty glandular tissue that is encased in a dense capsule. Because of this, the parotid gland on CT is consistently more lucent than surrounding muscles are and likewise is distinctly more radiodense than adjacent fat is in the subcutaneous tissues, infratemporal fossa, and lateral pharyngeal space. On T1-weighted MRI the gland appears hyperintense relative to surrounding muscles, yet relatively hypointense to most fat. The parotid duct is not routinely visualized without intraductal contrast opacification.

The gland is arbitrarily and indistinctly divided into a medial and lateral portion by the facial nerve. The facial nerve enters the gland posteriorly as it exits from the stylomastoid foramen. The nerve then passes lateral to the styloid process and anteriorly through the gland lateral to the external carotid artery and retromandibular vein to break up into its major trunks lateral to the mandible. One can routinely define the styloid process and retromandibular vein. The facial nerve itself cannot be seen passing through the gland.

The medial portion of the parotid extends behind the mandible to occupy the retromandibular space. More medially, it abuts the pterygoid mus-

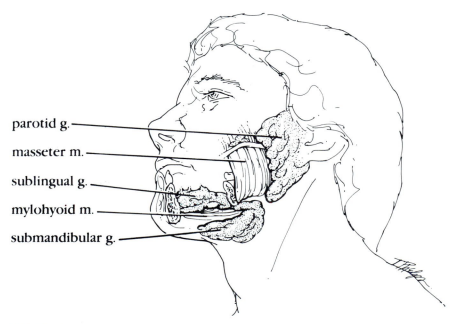

FIG 33–7.
Major salivary glands, lateral view.

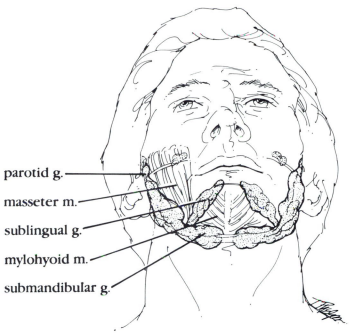

FIG 33–8.
Major salivary glands, frontal view.

cles anteriorly and the lateral pharyngeal space medially. The deep portion of the gland is separated posterolaterally from the major neurovascular bundle by the styloid diaphragm and stylopharyngeus ligament. Because of the tough fascial, ligamentous, and membranous capsule, lesions of the parotid tend to remain localized within the gland.

The parotid gland is intimately related to two groups of lymph nodes. The superficial group lies along the surface of the gland, while the deep nodes lie scattered within the gland itself.

The submandibular gland is approximately one half the size of the parotid gland. It is a hockey stick–shaped structure, with the larger superficial portion of the gland covered by platysma and lying below the mylohyoid muscle, which is the major muscle supporting the floor of the mouth. The gland then passes around the back of the mylohyoid muscle where its smaller deep portion lies on top of the mylohyoid muscle. The submandibular duct passes forward from this deep portion beneath and adjacent to the sublingual gland to its opening in the papilla in the anterior portion of the floor of the mouth. The submandibular gland is adjacent to numerous lymph nodes throughout its course but contains no nodes within its capsule.

On CT and MRI, the bulk of the superficial portion of the gland is seen as a lobular soft-tissue structure along the superolateral aspect of the hyoid bone. The submandibular glands are more radiodense (or hypointense) than the parotid glands are and are approximately the same as adjacent muscles. The deeper portions and the ducts of the submandibular glands are best seen on coronal scans.

Larynx

The larynx is obviously one of the most important structures in the neck. Because of its relatively small and complex structure, it deserves a few specific comments. Both from a gross anatomic as well as imaging viewpoint, the larynx can best be understood by first appreciating its bony and cartilaginous skeleton (Fig 33–9). This consists, superiorly to inferiorly, of the hyoid bone and the major cartilages—thyroid, arytenoid, and cricoid. The hyoid bone is the U-shaped bone suspended from the floor of the mouth mainly by the geniohyoid, mylohyoid, styloid, and digastric muscles. Suspended from it by the thyrohyoid membrane is the V-shaped thyroid cartilage, with broad lateral laminae extending from the midline anteriorly to the free posterior borders where the smaller superior and inferior cornua arise. The superior cornu ascends to near the hyoid bone, while the inferior cornu extends inferiorly to articulate with the cricoid cartilage. The thyroid cartilage calcifies in

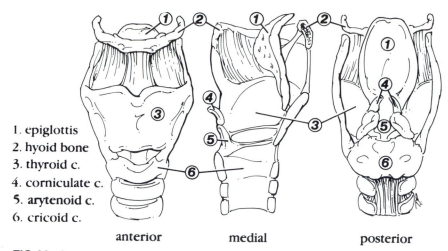

1. epiglottis
2. hyoid bone
3. thyroid c.
4. corniculate c.
5. arytenoid c.
6. cricoid c.

anterior   medial   posterior

FIG 33–9.
Osseous and cartilaginous skeleton of the larynx.

an extremely variable fashion, usually its internal and external cortices first, with the central medullary portion last.

The signet ring–shaped cricoid cartilage is the foundation of the larynx. It is suspended anteriorly from the thyroid cartilage by the thyrocricoid ligament, but posteriorly the lamina ascends to reach the level of the midthyroid cartilage where the two small L-shaped arytenoid cartilages articulate with the upper surface of the cricoid cartilage. The vocal ligament extends from the thyroid cartilage anteriorly just below the thyroid notch to the anteriorly projecting vocal processes of the arytenoids posteriorly. The superior processes of the arytenoids extend to the posteroinferior aspects of the aryepiglottic folds. The cricoid cartilage tends to calcify earlier and more intensely than the thyroid cartilage does. All of the laryngeal skeletal structures may be identified on CT and MRI. On CT, the cartilages are bright due to radiodense calcium, especially in the cortex, while they appear bright on MRI due to medullary fatty marrow. The hyaline cartilage of the epiglottis is musclelike in density and signal.[5]

The soft tissue of the larynx may be simplified by considering it to be a suspended stockinglike sheath open superiorly at its attachment to the posterior inferior epiglottis and aryepiglottic folds and inferiorly where it is continuous with the tracheal mucosa (Fig 33–10). This relatively simple column of mucosa and underlying submucosal areolar tissue has a lateral tuck or fold near its midportion at the level of the glottis between the false and true vocal cords. This lateral fold is the laryngeal ventricle, which lies just superior to the true vocal

cords and beneath the false vocal cords. The true and false vocal cords then bulge toward the midline above and below the ventricle itself. The false vocal cord lies at the plane of the superior-most portion of the arytenoid cartilage and extends anteriorly to the inferior-most aspect of the epiglottis and pre-epiglottic space just above the thyroid notch. It contains relatively loose areolar tissue as well as mucous glandular tissue and has a relatively distinctive fatty triangular appearance on CT and MRI. The true vocal cord, on the other hand, lies at the plane of the cricoarytenoid joint and the anteriorly projecting vocal process of the arytenoid. The vocal cord itself is relatively dense by CT and MRI (as compared with the false cord) because it consists of the relatively solid vocal muscle and the vocal ligament that extends forward to attach to the posterior aspect of the thyroid cartilage just below the thyroid notch. This junctional area between the two true vocal cords and the thyroid cartilage is the anterior commissure, which is little more than a thin layer of mucosa and perichondrium.

The false vocal cord is approximately 6 mm in vertical height, while the true vocal cord is 5 to 6 mm. There is a fairly sharp transition from true vocal cord to subglottic space at the level of the midcricoid cartilage. It must be remembered that the true vocal cord is at the plane of and closely related to the upper cricoid cartilage posteriorly. However, the true vocal cord is well above the more inferiorly positioned anterior portion of the cricoid ring. The pre-epiglottic space anterior to the epiglottis and behind the thyrohyoid ligament

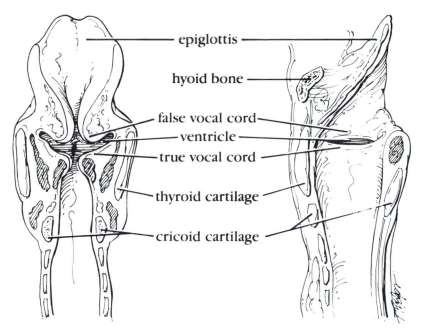

FIG 33–10.
Pharyngeal soft tissues.

is primarily filled with fat and is therefore relatively lucent on CT and hyperintense on T1W MRI.

An abbreviated atlas of normal cross-sectional anatomy of the neck is presented in Figure 33–11.

PATHOLOGY

Developmental

Developmental anomalies of the cervical region are not common, although one, the branchial cyst, is not rare. It, like other anomalies, is best understood by review of the embryology of the cervical region. This, of course, is basically the story of the pharyngeal pouch system (Fig 33–12).[6] The most striking developmental structures in the cervical region are the mesodermal pharyngeal arches. These solid, bilaterally symmetrical, horizontal pillars of soft tissue develop in relationship to the original six pharyngeal arch arteries as the adjacent mesodermal tissues differentiate and coalesce about the vessels. Between the solid-tissue arches, entodermal pouches of the primitive pharynx extend laterally to approach but not reach shallow depressions of the superficial ectodermal surface of the embryo. These early ectodermal depressions are termed pharyngeal clefts. Important structures develop in relationship to ectodermal pharyngeal clefts, mesodermal arches, and entodermal pouches.[7] During later development, the pharyngeal pouches become pinched off and discontinuous with the final central pharyngeal derivatives. They may evolve into tubular structures such as the middle ear and eustachian tube from the first and second pouches, solid lymphatic structures such as the palatine tonsil from the second pouch, or glandular structures such as the parathyroid glands from the third and fourth branchial pouches.

There may be a persistent epithelial-lined tract in the developmental course of a pharyngeal pouch that can become a branchial cyst in the adult. Approximately 95% of such branchial cysts are remnants of the second branchial pouch. They may be a continuous fistula from skin to pharyngeal wall or anything in between, including a small cutaneous fistula, internally isolated cyst, or sinus tract of the pharyngeal wall. At any rate, the lesion will lie somewhere along a path from the anterior border of the SCM, inferior to the hyoid and above the sternum, through the deep cervical fascia just beneath the SCM muscle, along the carotid sheath—between the external carotid artery and the more posterior internal carotid artery—to the pharyngeal wall near the tonsillar region or into the tonsillar fossa itself.[8, 9]

Most of these cysts present as painless fluctu-

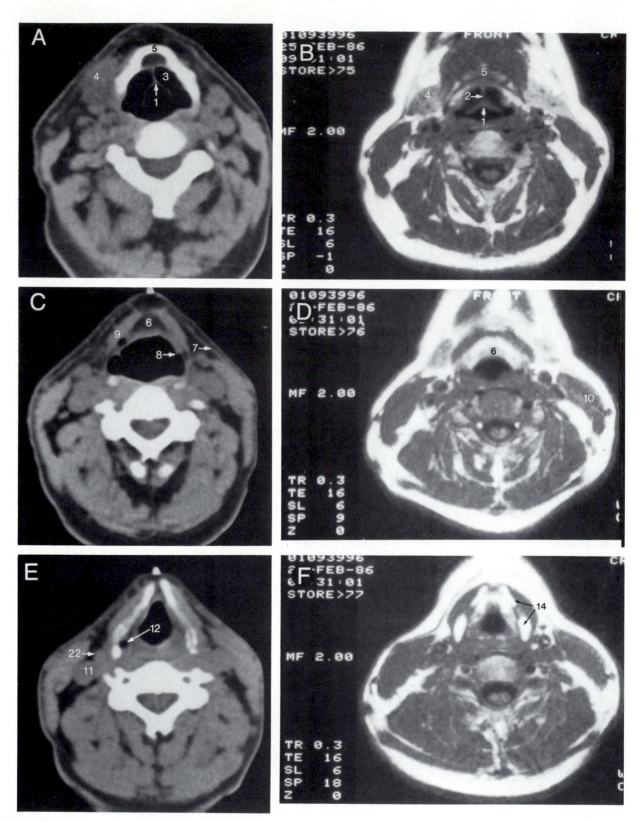

FIG 33–11.
Normal cervical CT **(A, C, E, G, I,** and **K)** and MRI scans **(B, D, F, H, J,** and **L).** Levels of the slices are the hyoid bone **(A** and **B),** pyriform sinuses **(C** and **D),** vestibule **(E** and **F),** false vocal cord **(G** and **H),** true vocal cord **(I** and **J),** and lower cricoid cartilage **(K** and **L).** Anatomic legend: *1* = epiglottis; *2* = glossoepiglottic ligament; *3* = vallecula; *4* = submandibular gland; *5* = hyoid bone; *6* = pre-epiglottic space; *7* = platysma muscle; *8* = aryepiglottic fold, *9* = infrahyoid strap muscle; *10* = sternocleidomastoid muscle; *11* = jugular vein; *12* = pyriform sinus; *13* = false vocal cord; *14* = thyroid cartilage; *15* = true vocal cord; *16* = anterior commissure; *17* = arytenoid cartilage; *18* = cricoid cartilage; *19* = cricothyroid articulation; *20* = levator muscle of the scapulae; *21* = inferior cornu of the thyroid cartilage; *22* = carotid artery; and *23* = trapezius muscle.

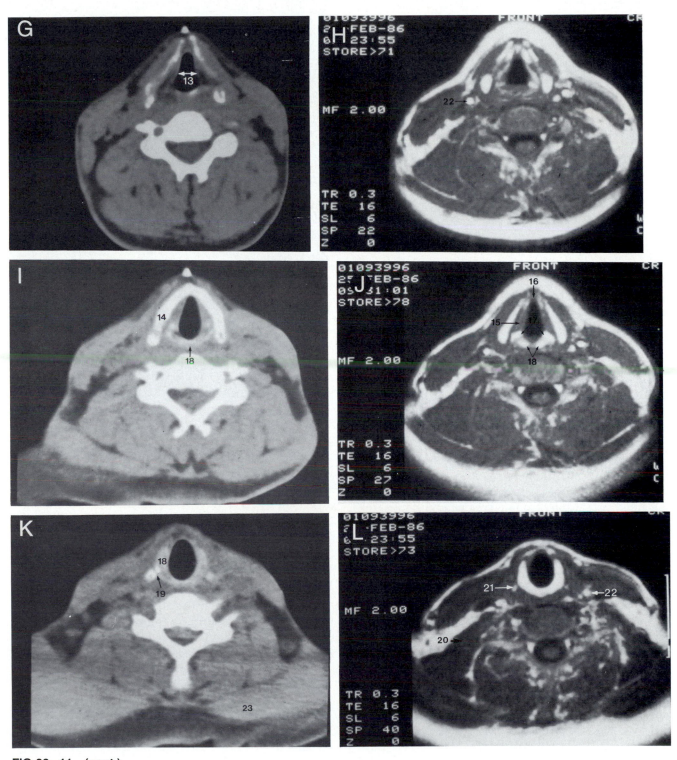

FIG 33–11   (cont.).

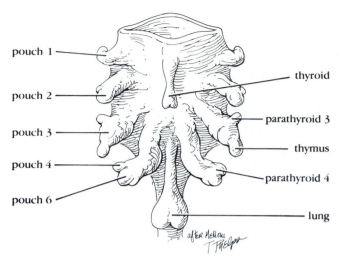

FIG 33–12.
Branchial pouch embryogenesis.

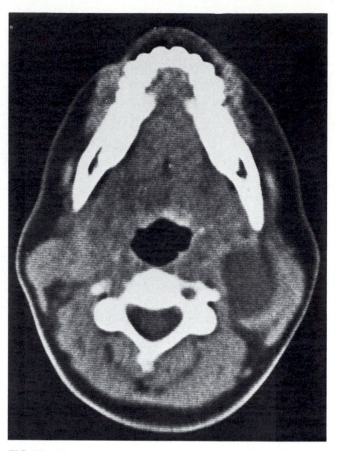

FIG 33–13.
Branchial cyst. A well-defined, thin-walled, cystlike mass lies directly beneath the left SCM.

ant swellings just below the angle of the mandible along the anterior border of the SCM muscle. They may become infected, with signs of inflammation. They are relatively distinct from adjacent structures, thin walled, filled with yellowish fluid, and lined by squamous epithelium. If of sufficient size, they are well demonstrated by cross-sectional scans (Fig 33–13). They are usually sharply marginated, centrally lucent masses with some enhancement of the adjacent capsule. On MRI, they are hypointense on T1-weighted images, and hyperintense on T2-weighted images. The primary radiographic differential diagnosis is abscess, but the history usually suggests a more chronic course.

One of the most common congenital tumors of the neck is cystic hygroma. This is a benign but often large, locally insinuating lesion that usually occurs in the posterior triangle of the neck. Pathologically, cystic hygroma is of lymph vessel origin and is dominated by large cysts with lesser parts of discrete lymph vessels. It usually originates in the subclavian triangle and extends superiorly, posterior to the SCM. If it occurs higher in the neck, it usually involves the region of the tail of the parotid gland. These tumors appear as irregularly marginated, lucent masses on CT, with internal meshlike soft-tissue densities (Fig 33–14). The appearance is fairly characteristic because most other tumors are more radiodense and simple cysts and abscesses lack this internal architecture. On MRI, their morphologic features are similar to those seen on CT but appear hypointense on T1-weighted images and hyperintense on spin-density (SD) and T2-weighted images. Other congenital vascular tumors with mass are not common in the

neck except in relationship to the inferior portion of the face and mouth.

Salivary Glands

While many patients with diseases of the major salivary glands can be easily evaluated clinically because of the superficial location of the glands, there remains a significant number of cases where radiologic consultation is required to establish and define the pathologic process. Until recently, imaging of the major salivary glands has primarily involved plain-film demonstration of calcification, radionuclide scanning for evidence of "hot or cold" masses, angiography for delineation of rare vascular lesions, and most importantly, sialography for definition of intraductal lesions and demonstration of masses within the parotid or submandibular gland. Sialography has been shown to be highly accurate in demonstrating intraductal lesions, relatively accurate in demonstrating masses, but poorly predictive of histology, except in certain

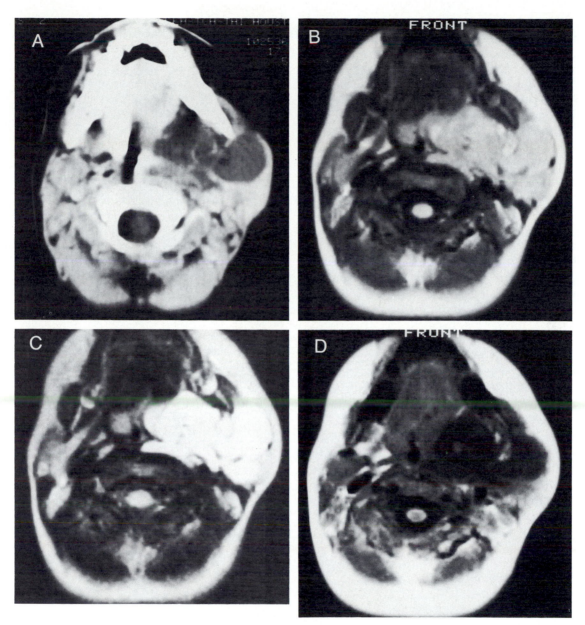

FIG 33–14.
Cystic hygroma in an 8-month-old child with difficulty swallowing. CT **(A)** shows a multiloculated parapharyngeal and parotid region mass that is more fully delineated by SDW **(B),** T2-weighted **(C),** and T1-weighted **(D)** MRI scans.

types of chronic inflammatory lesions such as sialectasis.[10] Sialography, however, may be tedious to perform, associated with some patient discomfort, and difficult to interpret with precision.

We have used CT to evaluate over 100 patients for possible salivary gland lesions.[11] When those patients who had surgical exploration, biopsy, or an obvious clinical diagnosis were analyzed, the overall sensitivity of CT in detecting salivary gland lesions was over 95%. In addition, the anatomic relation of the lesion to adjacent crucial structures such as the facial nerve was excellent. More recent MRI reports indicate similar clinical sensitivity.[12, 13]

While their sensitivity is quite good, the specificity of the scans alone, without clinical information, is only approximately 75% when categorizing lesions as to benign neoplasia, malignant neoplasia, or diffuse or focal inflammatory disease with or without calculi.[14] When combined with clinical information and laboratory findings, the overall specificity was 90%. The main diagnostic difficulty is differentiating focal sialoadenitis, without calculi, from malignant neoplasia. The clinical history of acute swelling, fever, and tenderness aids in the differentiation. Extension of the disease beyond the capsule of the gland indicates neoplasm rather than inflammatory disease. Although not systematically evaluated, intense contrast enhancement seems to suggest inflammatory disease.

We believe that conventional sialography is seldom if ever needed in neoplastic disease and probably not often necessary in inflammatory processes except to show obstructive lesions, although others disagree.[14–16] A conventional sialogram is not as anatomically precise as a cross-sectional image in showing the size and location of tumors or demonstrating extension beyond the gland. In nonobstructive inflammatory disease, the sialogram may give more precise anatomic information concerning ductal sialectasis; however, CT and the history can usually differentiate this disease from neoplasia and normal glandular tissue. It is probably unnecessary to demonstrate the sialectasis. In fact, it is preferable to avoid the irritating sialogram. In cases of obstructive inflammatory disease, the sialogram is clearly superior in anatomic detail, and if demonstration of ductal anatomy is clinically necessary, sialography is indicated.

Based on our experience, CT or MRI with a high-resolution scanner is the initial radiographic procedure of choice in evaluating salivary gland masses, particularly if neoplasia is the prime consideration. Only in selected patients with inflammatory disease is sialography necessary.

A complete detailed classification of diseases of the salivary glands may be found in Work and Batsakis[17]; however, these detailed classification systems are not particularly practical for the radiologist because they include many clinical lesions that require no radiographic imaging and many rare lesions without distinctive radiographic findings. An abbreviated and more workable classification is from Work and Hecht and is included in Table 33–1. Even this simplified outline includes numerous conditions that do not require radiographic diagnosis such as mumps and metabolic atrophy of the salivary glands. A summary of the salivary gland lesions that we have evaluated by CT is contained in Table 33–2 and provides a reasonable statistical approximation of the most common salivary gland lesions that are amenable to image analysis.

Approximately three fourths of salivary gland tumors will occur in the parotid gland and approximately 20% in the submandibular gland. In the

TABLE 33–1.

Salivary Gland Diseases*

I. Nonneoplastic disorders
  A. Acute inflammatory disorders
    1. Mumps (epidemic parotitis)
    2. Sialodochitis fibrinosa (Kussmaul's disease)
    3. Acute abscess (acute suppurative sialadenitis)
  B. Chronic inflammatory disorders
    1. Recurrent
      a. Nonobstructive
        (1) Chronic recurrent sialadenitis
        (2) Chronic sialectasis (sialodochitis)
      b. Obstructive
        (1) Sialolithiasis
        (2) Duct stricture
    2. Progressive
      a. Granulomatous
      b. Lymphoepithelial sialadenopathy
  C. Metabolic and endocrine disorders
    1. Benign hypertrophy
    2. Benign atrophy
    3. Gouty parotitis
  D. Congenital disorders
  E. Traumatic disorders
  F. Cystic disorders
II. Neoplastic disorders
  A. Neoplasms of supporting tissue origin
    1. Benign
      a. Lymphangioma
      b. Hemangioma
      c. Lipoma
      d. Neuroma
    2. Malignant (sarcomas)
  B. Neoplasms of epithelial tissue origin
    1. Benign
      a. Mixed tumors
      b. Mucoepidermoid "tumor"
      c. Adenomas
        (1) Papillary cystadenoma lymphomatosis (Warthin's tumor)
        (2) Acidophilic cell adenoma (oncocytoma)
        (3) Serous cell adenoma (acinic cell)
    2. Malignant
      a. Squamous cell carcinoma
      b. Gland cell carcinoma
        (1) Adenoid cystic adenocarcinoma
        (2) Acinic cell adenocarcinoma
        (3) Acidophilic cell adenocarcinoma
      c. Mucoepidermoid "tumor"
      d. Unclassified

*From Work WP, Hecht DW: Congenital malformations and trauma of the salivary glands, in Paparella MM, Shumrick DA (eds): *Otolaryngology*. Philadelphia, WB Saunders Co., 1973, vol 3, pp 253–257.

parotid gland, approximately three fourths of the tumors will be benign, while this 3:1 benign/malignant ratio is reversed in the submandibular gland. By far and away the most common benign tumor of the parotid gland is the mixed tumor (Fig 33–15), which accounts for approximately 60% of

TABLE 33–2..

Salivary Gland Lesions Demonstrated by CT*

Lesion	No.
Neoplastic	
Benign	
Mixed tumor	8
Warthin	5
Other	2
Subtotal	15
Malignant	
Mixed tumor	2
Adenocarcinoma	4
Squamous carcinoma	2
Mucoepidermoid carcinoma	1
Lymphoma	1
Metastasis	2
Subtotal	12
Inflammatory	
Obstruction with calculus	6
Localized sialadenitis	9
Diffuse sialectasis	2
Sarcoid	1
Inflammatory nodes	2
Subtotal	20
Trauma: hematoma	1

*From Bryan RN, Miller RH, Ferreyro RI, et al,: Computed tomography of the major salivary glands. *AJR* 1982; 139:547.

neoplasms of the parotid. Approximately 90% of mixed tumors are benign, with the remainder being malignant, the latter fact being determined more by tumor behavior than by histology. No more than 30% of these tumors occur in the submandibular gland. The other common benign tumor of the major salivary glands is the Warthin's tumor (papillary cystadenoma lymphomatosis). This tumor accounts for between 5% and 10% of parotid tumors and rarely occurs elsewhere. These benign tumors are readily demonstrable by CT and MRI. On CT, they appear as hyperdense (in comparison with the relatively lucent parotid tissue), sharply marginated masses within the gland (Fig 33–16). MRI demonstrates the tumors as hypointense relative to the normal gland on T1-weighted images, isointense on spin-density–weighted (SDW) images, and hyperintense on T2-weighted images. Essentially all benign neoplasms have this same appearance and cannot be differentiated from each other by CT or MRI. An exception to this statement is when multiple lesions are seen, in which case the diagnosis is usually Warthin's tumor. These tumors are frequently multiple and bilateral in older males.

In most pathologic series, the most frequent malignant tumor of the salivary glands is mucoepi-

dermoid carcinoma, followed by various types of adenocarcinoma including adenocystic carcinoma and squamous cell carcinoma. The typical CT image of any malignant salivary gland tumor is a poorly defined area of increased density within the gland, often with obscuration of the fatty-fascial planes about the gland (Fig 33–17). The loss of the glandular margins suggests extension of the disease into adjacent structures. Very small, low-grade malignancies of the salivary glands may, however, have a very similar appearance to benign tumors (Fig 33–18).

Of clinical importance in any parotid tumor is the relationship to the facial nerve and involvement of the deep lobe of the parotid. Deep-lobe involvement is perhaps better shown by MRI than any other method due to its multiplanar capabilities (Fig 33–19). However, involvement of the facial nerve can only be inferred because the nerve itself cannot be identified by CT or MRI.

Any disease process that results in lymph node enlargement may mimic benign salivary neoplasm by CT because the nodes, either on the surface or within the parotid gland, are usually hyperdense and well marginated. Both inflammatory as well as neoplastic nodal enlargement can result in discrete CT masses (Fig 33–20).

In children, the differential diagnosis of salivary neoplasms is different in that they have a far higher percentage of congenital vascular neoplasms such as hemangioma, lymphangioma, and cystic hygroma. These benign lesions account for approximately one third of the total childhood salivary neoplasms. Benign mixed tumor remains the most common tumor after those of developmental origin, with mucoepidermoid carcinoma being the most common malignant neoplasm.

Inflammatory disease of the salivary glands is clinically far more common than neoplasia but less frequently requires radiographic evaluation. The more common inflammatory conditions may be subdivided into those that are noninfectious or infectious, with the latter being subdivided into acute and chronic conditions. The most common noninfectious condition that the radiologist may be asked to investigate is sialectasis from a benign lymphoepithelial sialadenopathy. This occurs in Sjögren's syndrome in which the salivary disease occurs in conjunction with keratoconjunctivitis sicca and often a rheumatoid-type arthritis. Pathologically, there is a periductal infiltrate of lymphocytes with subsequent replacement of glandular tissue by lymphoepithelial collections, ductal dila-

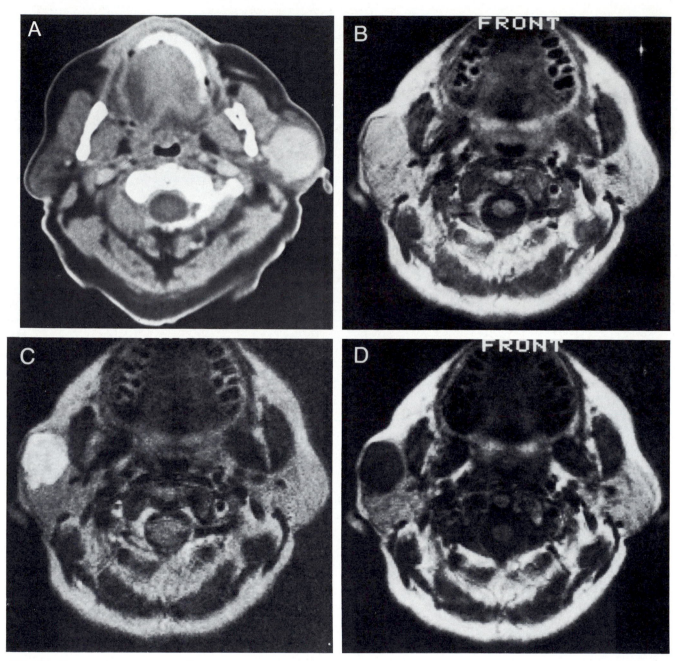

FIG 33–15.
Benign mixed tumors. A CT scan **(A)** shows a hyperdense, sharply marginated lesion within the left parotid gland. An SDW MRI scan **(B)** reveals isointense signal of tumor relative to normal right pa- rotid, but increased signal on T2W **(C)** and decreased signal on T1W **(D)** images.

tation, and finally replacement of the gland by lymphoid and fibrous tissue surrounding large dilated cysts. The disease commonly occurs in middle-aged females and is usually bilateral. The CT appearance is that of a diffusely increased radiodense gland with many small lucent cystic collections (Fig 33–21). MRI is less sensitive to these small, diffuse changes. Sarcoid also frequently involves the parotid gland and has the opposite appearance of chronic sialectasis in that there are many small focal hyperdense collections scattered throughout the normal relatively lucent gland.[14]

Acute infections of the salivary glands, either viral or bacterial in origin, seldom require radio-

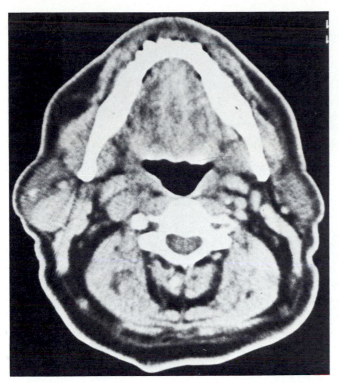

FIG 33–16.
Warthin's tumor. Note the hyperdense, multicentric neoplasm of the right parotid gland on CT scan.

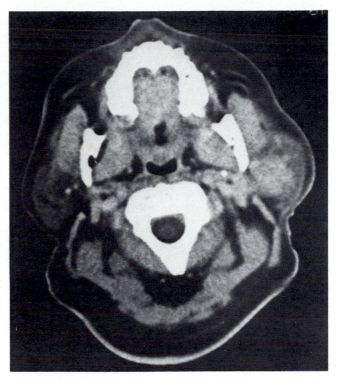

FIG 33–18.
Adenocarcinoma of left parotid gland. A moderately well-defined, slightly hyperdense mass with slightly irregular lateral borders suggests malignancy on this CT scan.

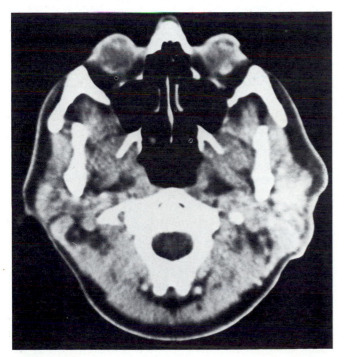

FIG 33–17.
Malignant parotid neoplasm. Note on the axial CT scan the poorly defined, hyperdense left parotid mass with violation of the capsule of the gland and invasion of the surrounding tissues.

graphic diagnosis, which is required only when the inflammatory condition becomes more chronic or clinically confusing. Chronic sialoadenitis is usually bacterial in origin and usually is associated with some ductal obstruction. By CT, the involved region is a poorly defined hyperdense area. It may be confused with malignant neoplasia of the gland; however, it oftentimes enhances after contrast injection much more intensely than do neoplasms, and it also assiduously observes the glandular boundaries (Fig 33–22).

Sialolithiasis is both the cause and consequence of chronic recurring sialadenitis and can be a cause of acute disease. The stones, composed of inorganic calcium and sodium phosphate, are far more common in the submandibular gland (90%) than in the parotid gland. Because of its increased sensitivity to calcium, CT can be very accurate in detecting these stones. It also can demonstrate the associated sialadenitis (Fig 33–23). MRI is not as sensitive to small calcifications and should not be used for these purposes. While CT may demonstrate many inflammatory lesions, sialography may still be important because it demon-

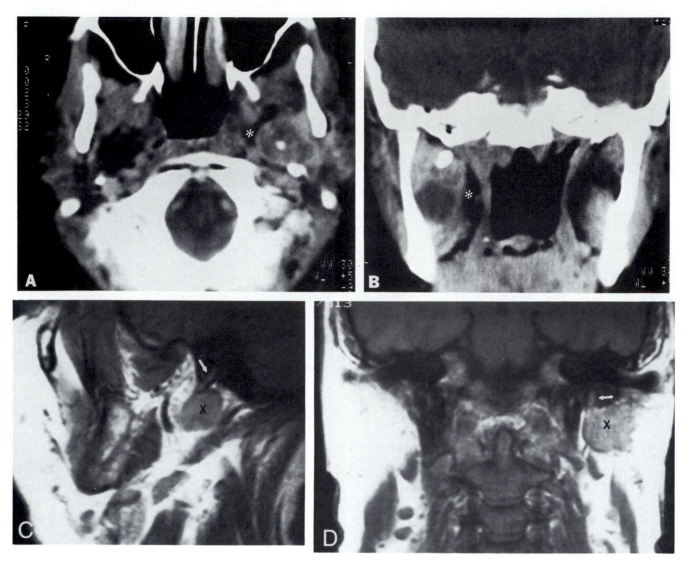

FIG 33–19.
Deep-lobe parotid tumors. **A** and **B,** Malignant mixed tumor in a deep lobe of the left parotid gland: cystic, inhomogeneous, and partially calcified mass lateral to the lateral pharyngeal space *(asterisk)* in a 31-year-old woman with a 4-month history of left sev-

enth nerve palsy. **C** and **D,** Acinic cell carcinoma (X) extending into facial nerve canal *(arrow)* on parasagittal **(C)** and coronal **(D)** T1W MRI scans.

strates the fine ductal anatomy and location of strictures and obstructions far more accurately than CT does.

Larynx

For practical purposes, imaging of the larynx—MRI, CT, laryngography, etc.—is primarily for evaluation of carcinoma of the larynx. At least 90% of "tumors" of the larynx that require radiographic aid are squamous cell carcinomas. Furthermore, diagnosis of this tumor is clinical, and the radiologist is merely helping to stage the tumor for subsequent treatment. Therefore, it is important to un-

derstand the basic concepts of squamous cell carcinoma of the larynx.

First, one must understand the staging of larynx cancer. The lesions are anatomically divided into infraglottic, glottic, supraglottic, and transglottic lesions. The lesions are then subcategorized as to their extent as shown in Table 33–3. The purpose of this classification is to statistically organize them for determination of the optimum treatment modality. It should be remembered that there are really two major types of larynx cancer. The first and most common is glottic cancer with or without supraglottic or infraglottic extension. These tumors are clinically diagnosed relatively early, because

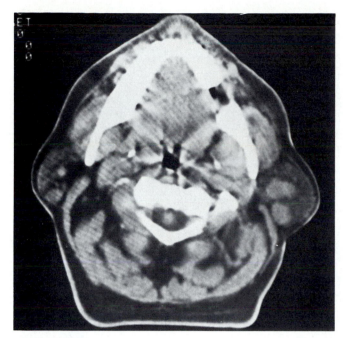

FIG 33–20.
Enlarged parotid lymph nodes. Two hyperdense, well-demarcated masses within the left parotid gland are shown on CT in a patient with lymphoma.

involvement of true vocal cords results in early symptoms (such as hoarseness) that precipitate the initial clinical visit. Most of these tumors are relatively small and are stage I·or II tumors. On the other hand, supraglottic tumors do not involve crit-

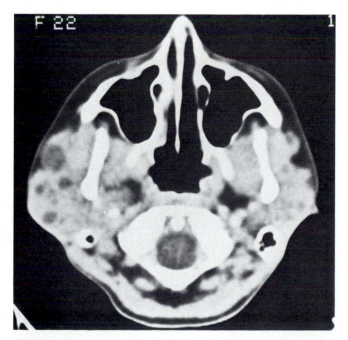

FIG 33–21.
Sjögren's syndrome. Bilateral multicystic degeneration of the parotid glands with greater involvement on the right.

TABLE 33–3.

Tumor Classification: Larynx*

Supraglottis	
TIS	Carcinoma in situ
T1	Tumor confined to region of origin with normal mobility
T2	Tumor involving adjacent supraglottic site(s) or glottis without fixation
T3	Tumor limited to larynx with fixation and/or extension to involve postcricoid area, medial wall of pyriform sinus, or preepiglottic space
T4	Massive tumor extending beyond the larynx to involve oropharynx, soft tissues of neck, or destruction of thyroid cartilage
Glottis	
TIS	Carcinoma in situ
T1	Tumor confined to vocal cords(s) with normal mobility (including involvement of anterior or posterior commissures)
T2	Supraglottic and/or subglottic extension of tumor with normal or impaired cord mobility
T3	Tumor confined to the larynx with cord fixation
T4	Massive tumor with thyroid cartilage destruction and/or extension beyond the confines of the larynx
Subglottis	
TIS	Carcinoma in situ
T1	Tumor confined to the subglottic region
T2	Tumor extension to vocal cords with normal or impaired cord mobility
T3	Tumor confined to the larynx with cord fixation
T4	Massive tumor with cartilage destruction, extension beyond the confines of the larynx, or both

*Reproduced in part from Paparella MM, Shumrick DA: *Otolaryngology.* Philadelphia, WB Saunders Co, 1973, vol 3, p 2514.

ical structures that lead to early presentation. As a result of this, they tend to be much larger tumors, less well restricted, and stage III and IV when diagnosed. These patients do not present with hoarseness, but rather with symptoms of a mass in the hypopharynx. There is likewise a great difference in the metastatic behavior in that glottic tumors have a relatively low percentage of nodal metastasis at the original diagnosis while supraglottic tumors have a high percentage of nodal metastasis primarily to the prelaryngeal and jugular nodes.[18]

In general, stage I tumors are treated with radiation therapy, stage II tumors are treated with local surgery with voice preservation, while stage III and IV tumors usually require extensive surgery including laryngectomy and loss of voice function.

The role of radiographic evaluation of carcinoma of the larynx is to precisely define its extent and optimally define those lesions that can be treated with conservative therapy vs. those that require more extensive resection. The mucosal surface of the lesion is of little importance to the radiologist because the endoscopist can usually

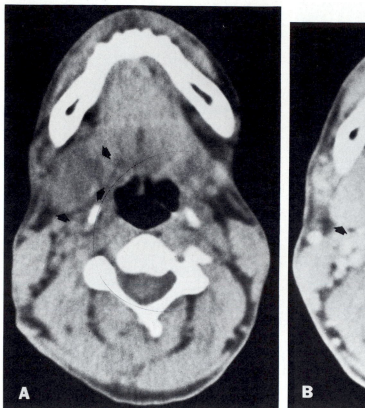
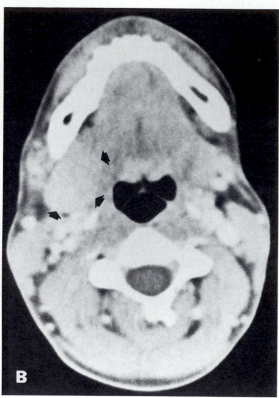

FIG 33–22.
Chronic submandibular sialadenitis. Unenhanced **(A)** and enhanced **(B)** CT scans show a well-defined, enhancing right submandibular mass *(arrows)* in a patient with chronic, recurrent sialadenitis who had a left submandibulectomy for the same disease.

visualize this aspect of the tumor. It is the deep extension that is of primary importance. While laryngography has been helpful in the past, it is rarely useful at the present time in evaluation of these tumors. It is primarily a duplication of the endoscopic evaluation because it primarily images the mucosa. On the other hand, MRI and CT much more adequately display the deeper components of the tumor, including the involvement of cartilage or the presence of adenopathy.[19–27]

Performing CT or MRI of the larynx is relatively easy because it simply involves thin sections of the larynx from the hyoid to the bottom of the cricoid cartilage. We routinely use 5-mm sections with the patient in quiet respiration. Occasionally, 3-mm slices are obtained. It is important that the patient not move during the examination and particularly that he not swallow or otherwise move his larynx. In general, it is best not to tell the patient anything during the procedure. An instruction to the patient to "hold your breath" usually results in a Valsalva maneuver and motion on the scan. Contrast injection is very important for CT in the eval-

uation of lymph nodes and may be helpful in evaluation of the boundaries of the lesion, although the tumors tend not to enhance in any clinically useful fashion. One of the advantages of MRI is its natural contrast between vessels and soft tissue, thereby making added intravenous (IV) contrast unnecessary.

Stage I lesions are focal mucosal lesions that diagnostically lie in the realm of the clinical endoscopist. These lesions are too small, shallow, and superficial to be reliably demonstrated by CT and MRI. The purpose of imaging in these patients is to make sure that they are indeed stage I lesions rather than more occult, higher-grade tumors. If at all demonstrated by CT or MRI, these tumors are seen as minimal asymmetry of the true and/or false vocal cords, where they usually occur (Fig 33–24). However, one must not overcall minimal laryngeal asymmetries. The verrucous-type carcinoma of the larynx may be stage I but is often demonstrable by CT because it tends to be a more discrete mass protruding off the vocal cord (Fig 33–25).

Stage II tumors, regardless of location, are usu-

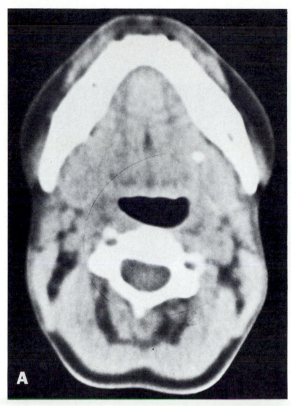

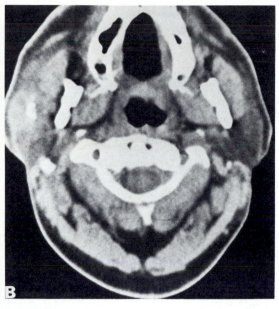

FIG 33–23.
Sialolithiasis demonstrated on CT scans. **A,** left submandibular stone. **B,** right parotid stone. Note the associated sialadenitis in **B,** which is characterized by swelling and increased radiodensity of the gland.

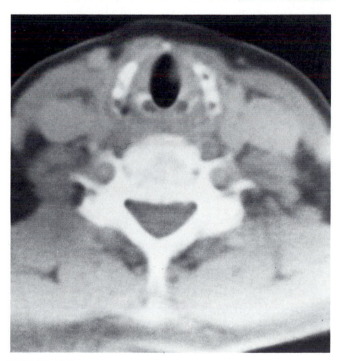

FIG 33–24.
Carcinoma of the left true vocal cord, stage I. A shallow nodular mucosal elevation is confined to the true vocal cord.

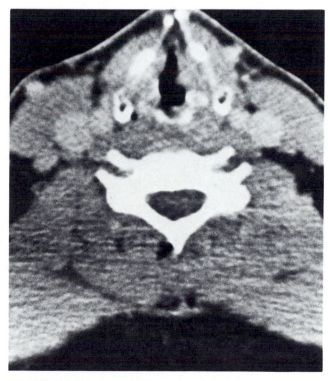

FIG 33–25.
Verrucous carcinoma of the left true vocal cord, stage I.

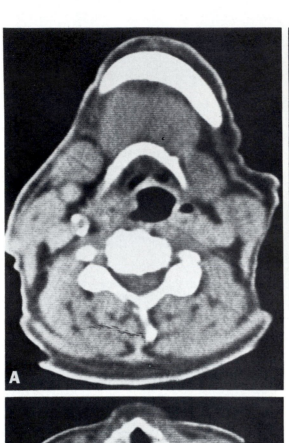

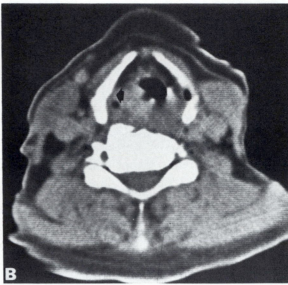

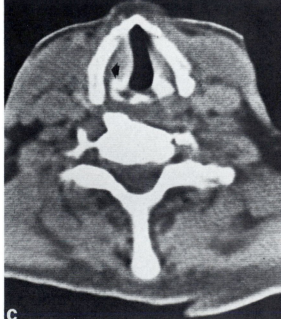

FIG 33–26.
Transglottic stage II carcinoma of the right true and false cords with pyriform sinus invasion. CT scans are at the levels of the epiglottis and vallecula **(A)**, supraglottis **(B)**, and true vocal cord **(C)**. Note the preservation of the lucent line adjacent to the inner margin of the thyroid cartilage (**B** and **C**, *arrows*).

ally demonstrable by CT and MRI, and it is the differentiation between these and the more invasive stage III tumors that is the challenge to the physician. When confined to the vocal cord, the lesion is seen as increased bulk in the cord and occasionally has slightly increased density, although this is not consistent (Fig 33–26). Due to its T2 relaxation times, the lesion usually has increased signal on T2W images. One must closely evaluate its anterior extent in relationship to the anterior commissure, which is normally the thinnest soft-tissue density behind the thyroid notch. In looking for deep extension of the tumor and thyroid destruction, one should carefully note the usually present thin lucent band on CT right along the inner surface of the cartilage. Obliteration of this line (which is presumably perichondrium) raises the possibility of cartilage invasion and therefore a stage III or IV tumor. However, for a definitive diagnosis of cartilage destruction, there must be obvious, frank destruction of the thyroid lamina or other cartilage (Fig 33–27). One cannot rely on asymmetry of calcification within the thyroid cartilage for this diagnosis because there is significant normal asymmetry from side to side.[28]

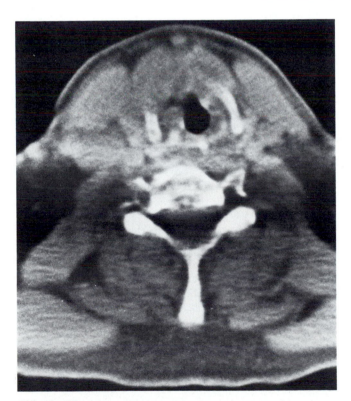

FIG 33–27.
Carcinoma of the larynx, stage IV, with bilateral invasion and destruction of the thyroid lamina.

Subglottic extension of these tumors is also critical. While radiologists have often used a "magic number" for subglottic extension, i.e., 10 mm, of far more importance is the relationship of the inferior extension to the cricoid cartilage. For voice conservation surgery, the skeletal base of the larynx—the cricoid—must be preserved. Because the cricoid cartilage lies at a much higher level posteriorly than anteriorly, subglottic extension should be evaluated in terms of cricoid involvement rather than absolute millimeters below the true cord. Scans by CT or MRI can accurately delineate subglottic extension to 5 mm or less, and for practical purposes this is adequate, although thinner sections can increase this accuracy. In general, more than 5-mm subglottic extension posteriorly and 10-mm subglottic extension anteriorly may obviate conservation surgery (Fig 33–28).

Supraglottic spread of glottic tumor is reflected by obliteration of the ventricular cavity and invasion of the false cord with loss of its normally lucent interior densities and increased bulk (Figs 33–29 and 33–30). While subtle supraglottic spread of tumor into the ventricle might seem very difficult to determine, MRI can delineate craniocaudal extension nicely with coronal imaging, and we have found it to be feasible in most cases.

Contralateral spread of disease is also critical in evaluation of these tumors. As classified in Table 33–3, T1 and T2 true vocal cord lesions can be conservatively treated as long as there is no significant contralateral spread. This means that no more than one fourth to one third of the opposite true cord may be involved with tumor. These anatomicosurgical conditions are a function of the basic types of conservative laryngectomy that can be performed. Either vertical or horizontal partial laryngectomies may be performed. Horizontal or supraglottic laryngectomies involve resection of tumor above the true vocal cords at the plane of the ventricle, while vertical laryngectomies are hemilaryngectomies with resection of one side of the larynx. The vertical hemilaryngectomy can only minimally cross the midline to the side opposite the tumor.

In general then, T2 tumors are mucosal and submucosal tumors with minimal deep extension that do not cross the important anatomic boundaries that would be the margins of partial laryngectomies.

Tumors classified as T3 are larger tumors that extend deep into underlying muscle with fixation of adjacent tissue and often metastatic nodal

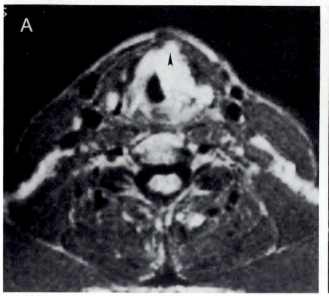

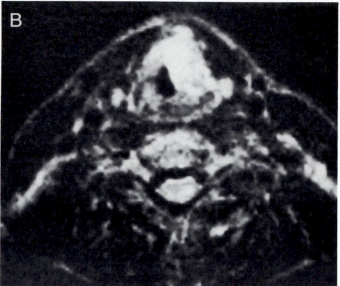

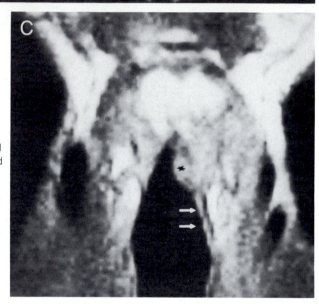

FIG 33–28.
Transglottic carcinoma of the larynx, stage IV. Axial SDW **(A)** and
T2-weighted **(B)** scans show involvement of the left false and true vocal
cords with extralaryngeal extension *(arrowhead)*. A coronal T1-weighted
scan **(C)** shows a large supraglottic mass (*) with thin subglottic
extension *(arrows)*.

spread. They and the larger, more invasive T4 lesions are not particularly common at the glottic
level except in patients who have neglected them,
whereas they are quite common in the supraglottic
region. Conservative therapy, as a rule, cannot be
done, but laryngectomy with or without additional
radiation therapy may still be curative, although in
a lower percentage. The use of CT and MRI is
very helpful in defining the margins of these larger
tumors so that the surgeon can better anticipate the
extent of resection. This is particularly important
in lesions in the supraglottic region that are related
to the tongue base. The larger tumors also have a
high percentage of occult nodes that can often be
detected by CT and MRI, although radical neck
dissection may be performed on clinical grounds.

Supraglottic cancers rostral to the false vocal
cords are basically hypopharyngeal cancers and
may be subdivided into posterior pharyngeal wall,
pyriform sinus, and hypopharyngeal tumors (see
Fig 33–30).[29, 30] The latter primarily involve the
epiglottis and are the most likely to involve the
tongue base. Tumors that present on the laryngeal
surface of the epiglottis without anterior extension
into the fatty pre-epiglottic space have a much better prognosis than do those with anterior extension
and those that extend down to the anterior commissure near the petiole, which is the base of the
epiglottis just superior to the thyroid notch.

In our experience, CT or MRI of the larynx has
replaced laryngography because of its greater ease
and convenience as well as its greater diagnostic

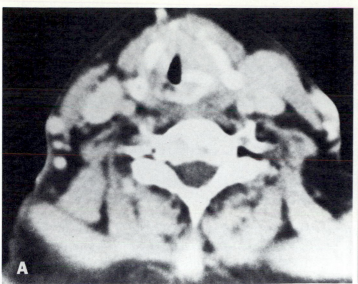

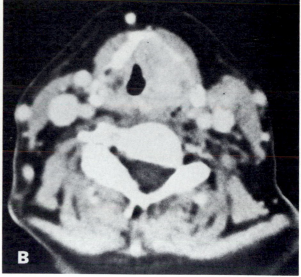

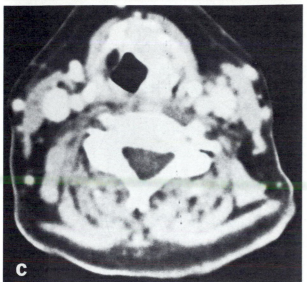

FIG 33–29.
Supraglottic invasive carcinoma of the larynx with cartilage destruction and extension above the plane of the glottis. Scans are at the levels of the arytenoid **(A),** 1 cm above **(B),** and 2 cm above the arytenoid **(C).**

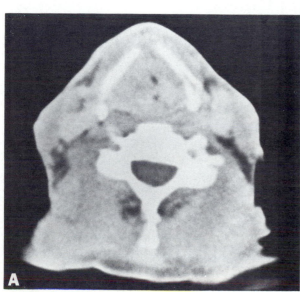

FIG 33–30.
Stage IV carcinoma of the larynx with bilateral involvement and supraglottic extension into the epiglottis. There is almost total oblitera-tion of the glottis **(A).** Numerous nodal metastases are present with a large, centrally CT-lucent necrotic node obvious on the left **(B).**

usefulness. It must, however, be carefully performed with close clinical correlation for optimum results. One must also remember that the scan is not histologically specific and 10% of cases will not be squamous carcinoma (Fig 33–31). With superior contrast resolution, improved spatial resolution with surface coils, and multiplanar capabilities, MRI shows great promise in the evaluation of the larynx and other parts of the neck. In fact, in several studies that used surface coils, MRI was comparable to or better than CT.[31–33]

Lymph Nodes

An important use of scans in the cervical region is evaluation of the lymph nodes. With high-resolution cross-sectional scanning, one may see numerous small (less than 1 cm) densities scattered in the usual regions of nodal occurrence, particularly along the carotid sheath. According to Mancuso et al. and Harnsberger and Dillon,[34, 35] if the nodes are less than 1 cm in diameter, they are usually normal or not involved with malignancy. The nodes that are greater than 2 cm in diameter are usually malignant, although focal infectious disease can cause similar enlargement. Such inflammatory nodal enlargement is far more common in children than in adults, and the clinical history usually clarifies the situation. Lymph nodes between 1 and 2 cm in diameter are indeterminate, but in the presence of known malignancy they should be considered as suspicious. Several repre-

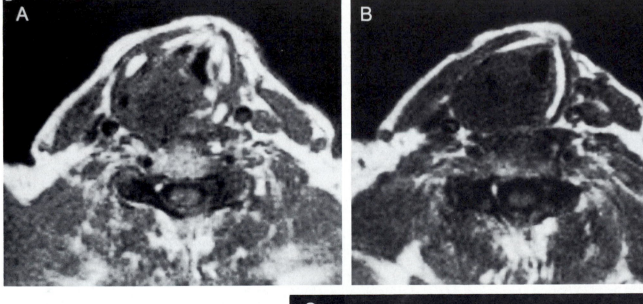

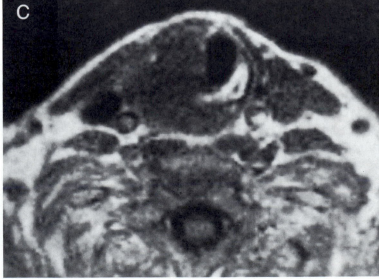

FIG 33–31.
Chondroma of cricoid cartilage. Contiguous axial T1-weighted MRI scans **(A–C)** show a well-marginated mass centered in the cricoid region, but of nonspecific appearance.

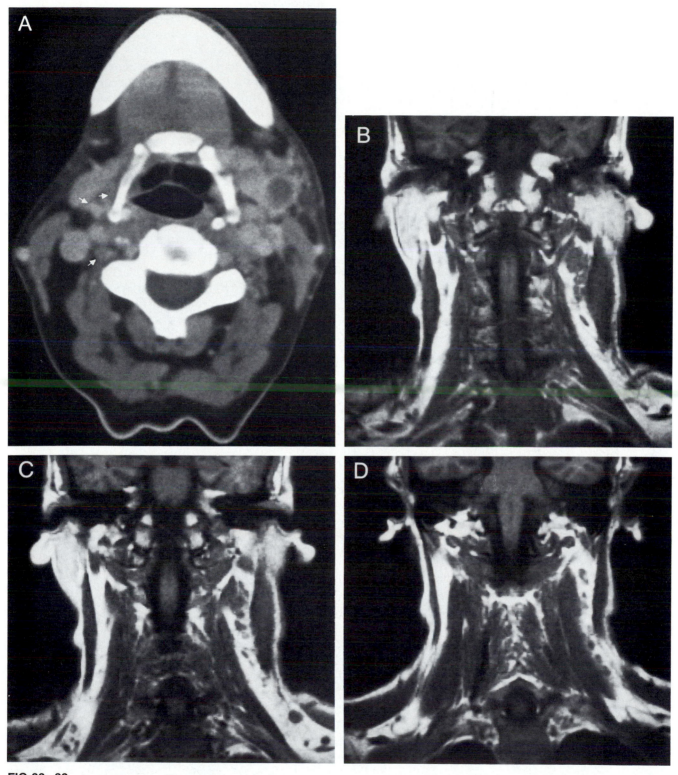

FIG 33–32.
Metastatic lymph nodes. CT examples **(A)** of both solid and ne-crotic enlarged lymph nodes are present in the left portion of the neck, while the contralateral side exhibits examples of normal nodes *(arrows)*. T1-weighted MRI scans **(B, C,** and **D)** show me-tastases to the superior and inferior jugular nodes.

sentative cases of normal lymph nodes, as well as nodes involved with metastatic disease, are shown in Figure 33–32. Lymph node disease in the parotid region has already been discussed, and one must remember the close relationship between the submandibular gland and submandibular lymph nodes, which can usually be well differentiated.

Miscellaneous

There are many additional lesions of the cervical region that can be displayed by cross-sectional imaging, of which only a few representative cases will be shown. Lipomas are one of the more distinctive lesions demonstrated by x-ray CT or MRI because of their negative Hounsfield units and short T1. Figure 33–33 shows two cases, and there

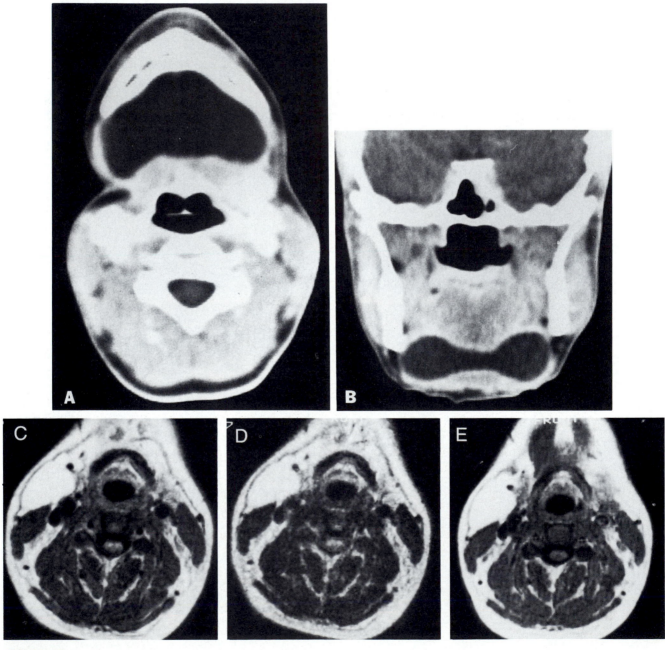

FIG 33–33.
Lipomas. Axial **(A)** and direct coronal **(B)** CT scans demonstrate the large well-circumscribed lesion with a density of fat. SDW **(C),** T2W **(D),** and T1W **(E)** MRI scans show a characteristic bright signal on all sequences.

is usually little difficulty in diagnosis. From a clinical viewpoint, these tumors may be more infiltrative or insinuating than is obvious, and CT can be quite helpful in preoperative evaluation.[36]

The classic vascular neoplasms of the cervical region include the nonchromaffin paragangliomas such as glomus tumors and carotid body tumors. They appear as relatively well marginated, intensely enhancing lesions, particularly if drip infusion is used. They occur primarily in the expected areas along the carotid sheath, and their clinical relationships at the skull base are well demonstrable but oftentimes require coronal scans (Fig 33–34). Gadolinium–diethylenetriamine pentaacetic acid (Gd-DTPA) enhancement is a critical adjunct for MRI of these high cervical and skull base lesions.

Hemangiomas also occur in the cervical region, although as previously mentioned, usually occur near the lower portion of the face and the oral region. In contrast to the vascular paragangliomas, hemangiomas may not enhance any more than adjacent tissue because the blood vessels within them are very slowly flowing vessels that may not contain any more contrast than normal muscle does. Because of this, they may be more difficult to see and their margins more indistinct.

In children, the various soft-tissue sarcomas occur in the neck and usually present as large, rapidly growing, ill-defined tumors obliterating fascial planes and destroying bone in the neighborhood. Small round-cell tumors such as neuroblastoma may appear as more well defined lesions (Fig 33–35). The scans often demonstrate greater extent of these tumors than is clinically appreciable.

While the upper part of the esophagus lies within the cervical region, it is less often evaluated by cross-sectional imaging because barium studies usually suffice and malignancies of the upper portion of the esophagus extending into adjacent tissues are not common. Figure 33–36 is a curiosity case—a Zenker's diverticulum incidentally found in a patient with a paralyzed right true vocal cord.

The thyroid gland and parathyroid glands occur in the lower cervical region and can be evaluated by CT or MRI.[37–43] On CT, the thyroid gland appears dense because of its increased iodine content. One can well demonstrate pathology of the thyroid gland, as shown in Figure 33–37. Doppman and coworkers[44] have discussed CT and MRI scanning for the parathyroid glands, which may be clinically useful in selected cases.

The thyroid gland develops from epithelial tis-

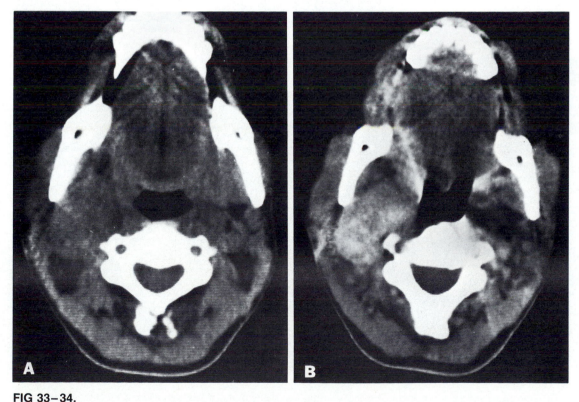

FIG 33–34.
Carotid body tumor. A homogeneously enhancing right parapharyngeal mass is obliterating details in the carotid sheath on unenhanced **(A)** and enhanced **(B)** CT scans.

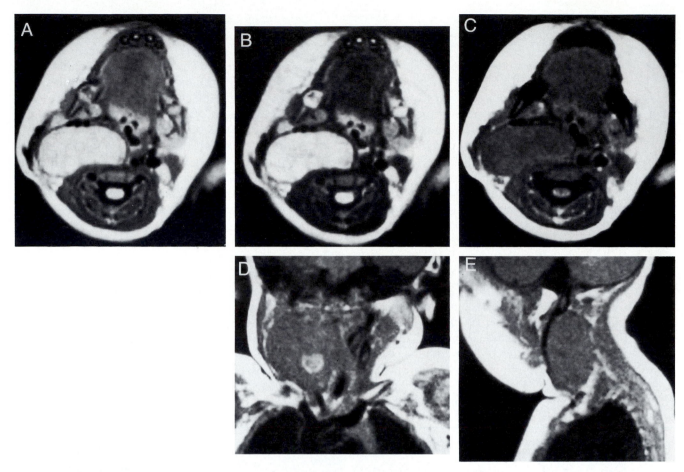

FIG 33–35.
Neuroblastoma in a 2-year-old with a large retropharyngeal mass on SDW **(A),** T2W **(B),** and T1W **(C, D,** and **E)** MRI scans.

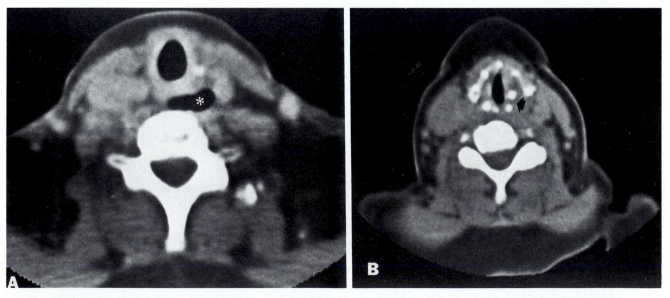

FIG 33–36.
Zenker's diverticulum (**A,** *asterisk),* an incidental finding in a patient examined for paralysis of the left vocal cord. Note the asymmetry of the glottis with slight adduction of the left true cord and cricoid-arytenoid separation (**B,** *arrow).*

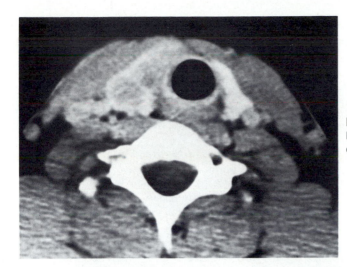

FIG 33–37.
Follicular adenoma, right thyroid lobe. Note the multicystic character of this well-defined lesion on CT scan.

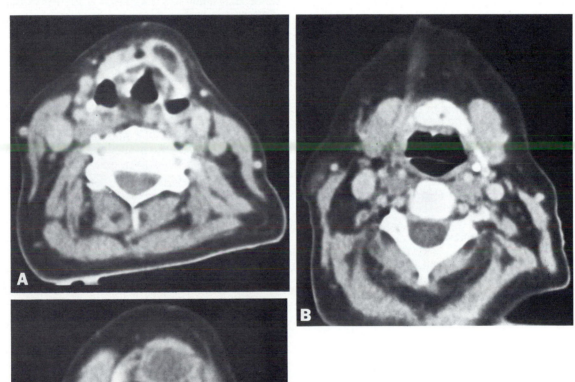

FIG 33–38.
Thyroglossal duct cyst. Note the extension of the lesion from the left lobe of the thyroid **(A)** through the hyoid bone **(B)** to the base of the tongue **(C).** The lesion is superficial to the thyroid cartilage and does not communicate with the larynx.

sue related to the site of the foramen cecum near the tongue base. The thyroid tissue descends in relation to the thyroglossal duct through or intimately near the hyoid bone to end anterior to the larynx in the paratracheal region of the lower portion of the neck. Ectopic tissue or remnant duct cysts may occur anywhere along this course, but two thirds occur just inferior to the hyoid bone and anterior to the thyrohyoid ligament with or without a fibrous connection to the foramen cecum (Fig 33–38).[45]

REFERENCES

1. Baker SR, Latack JT: Magnetic resonance imaging of the head and neck. *Otolaryngol Head Neck Surg* 1986; 95:82–89.

2. Dillon WP: Magnetic resonance imaging of head and neck tumors. *Cardiovasc Intervent Radiol* 1986; 8:275–282.

3. Stark DD, Moss AA, Gamsu G, et al: Magnetic resonance imaging of the neck. Part I: Normal anatomy. *Radiology* 1984; 150:447–454.

4. Paff GH: *Anatomy of Head and Neck.* Philadelphia, WB Saunders Co, 1973.

5. Castelijns JA, Doornbos J, Verbeeten B, et al: MR imaging of the normal larynx. *J Comput Assist Tomogr* 1985; 9:919–925.

6. Paparella MM, Shumrick DA (eds): *Otolaryngology,* vol 3. Philadelphia, WB Saunders Co, 1973.

7. Chandler JR, Mitchell BV: Branchial cleft cysts, sinuses, and fistulas. *Otolaryngol Clin North Am* 1981; 14:175–186.

8. Kreipke DL, Lingeman RE: Cross-sectional imaging (CT, NMR) of branchial cysts: Report of three cases. *J Comput Assist Tomogr* 1984; 8:114–116.

9. Mafee MF, Rasouli F, Spigos DG, et al: Magnetic resonance imaging in the diagnosis of nonsquamous tumors of the head and neck. *Otolaryngol Clin North Am* 1986; 19:523–536.

10. Gates GA: Sialography and scanning of the salivary glands. *Otolaryngol Clin North Am* 1977; 10:379–390.

11. Bryan RN, Miller RH, Ferreyro RI, et al: Computed tomography of the major salivary glands. *AJR* 1982; 139:547–554.

12. Schaefer SD, Maravilla KR, Close LG, et al: Evaluation of NMR versus CT for parotid masses: A preliminary report. *Laryngoscope* 1985; 95:945–950.

13. Teresi LM, Lufkin RB, Wortham DG, et al: Parotid masses: MR imaging. *Radiology* 1987; 163:405–409.

14. Som PM, Biller HF: The combined CT-sialogram. *Radiology* 1980; 135:387–390.

15. Carter BL, Karmody CS, Blickman JR, et al: Computed tomography and sialography: I. Normal anatomy. *J Comput Assist Tomogr* 1981; 5:42–45.

16. Rice DH, Mancuso AA, Hanafee WN: Computerized tomography and simultaneous sialography in evaluating parotid tumors. *Arch Otolaryngol* 1980; 106:472–473.

17. Work WP, Batsakis JG: Classification of salivary gland diseases. *Otolaryngol Clin North Am* 1977; 10:287–296.

18. Batsakis JG: *Tumors of the Head and Neck,* ed 2. Baltimore, Williams & Wilkins, 1979.

19. Archer CR, Yeager VL, Friedman W II, et al: Computer tomography of the larynx. *J Comput Assist Tomogr* 1978; 2:404–411.

20. Archer CR, Friedman W II, Yeager VL, et al: Evaluation of laryngeal cancer by computed tomography. *J Comput Assist Tomogr* 1978; 2:618–624.

21. Archer CRT, Sagel SS, Yeager VL, et al: Staging of carcinoma of the larynx: Comparative accuracy of CT and laryngography. *AJR* 1981; 136:571–575.

22. Mancuso AA, Hanafee WN, Julliard GJ, et al: The role of computed tomography in the management of cancer of the larynx. *Radiology* 1977; 124:243–244.

23. Mancuso AA, Hanafee WN: A comparative evaluation of computed tomography and laryngography. *Radiology* 1979; 133:131–138.

24. Scott M, Forsted DH, Rominger CJ, et al: Computed tomographic evaluation of laryngeal neoplasms. *Radiology* 1981; 140:141–144.

25. Glazer HS, Niemeyer JH, Balfe DM, et al: Neck neoplasms: MR imaging, Part I. Initial evaluation. *Radiology* 1986; 160:343–348.

26. Glazer HS, Niemeyer JH, Balfe DM, et al: Neck neoplasms: MR imaging, Part II. Posttreatment evaluation. *Radiology* 1986; 160:349–354.

27. Castelijns JA, Gerritsen GJ, Kaiser MC, et al: MRI of normal or cancerous laryngeal cartilages: Histopathologic correlation. *Laryngoscope* 1987; 97:1085–1093.

28. Lloyd GA, Michaels L, Phelps PD: The demonstration of cartilaginous involvement in laryngeal carcinoma by computerized tomography. *Otolaryngol Head Neck Surg* 1980; 88:726–733.

29. Gamsu G, Webb WR, Shallit JB, et al: CT in carcinoma of the larynx and pyriform sinus: Value of phonation scans. *AJR* 1981; 136:577–584.

30. Larsson S, Mancuso AA, Hoover L, et al: Differentiation of pyriform sinus cancer from supraglottic laryngeal cancer by computed tomography. *Radiology* 1981; 141:427–432.

31. Lufkin RB, Hanafee WN, et al: Larynx and hypopharynx: MR imaging with surface coils. *Radiology* 1986; 158:747–754.

32. Castelijns JA, Kaiser MC, Valk J, et al: MR imaging of laryngeal cancer. *J Comput Assist Tomogr* 1987; 11:134–140.

33. Hoover LA, Wortham DG, Lufkin RB, et al: Mag-

netic resonance imaging of the larynx and tongue base: Clinical applications, *Otolaryngol Head and Neck Surg* 1987; 97:245–256.

34. Mancuso AA, Maceri D, Rice D, et al: CT of cervical lymph node cancer. *AJR* 1981; 136:381–385.

35. Harnsberger HR, Dillon WP: Imaging tumors of the central nervous system and extracranial head and neck. *CA* 1987; 37:225–238.

36. Som PM, Braun IR, Shapiro MD, et al: Tumors of the parapharyngeal space and upper neck: MR imaging characteristics. *Radiology* 1987; 164:823–829.

37. Machida K, Yoshikawa K: Aberrent thyroid gland demonstrated by computed tomography. *J Comput Assist Tomogr* 1979; 3:689–690.

38. Wolf BS, Nakagawa H, Yeh HC: Visualization of the thyroid gland with computed tomography. *Radiology* 1977; 123:368.

39. Sekiya T, Tada S, Kawakami K, et al: Clinical application of computed tomography to thyroid disease. *Comput Tomogr* 1979; 3:185–193.

40. Stark DD, Moss AA, Gamsu G, et al: Magnetic resonance imaging of the neck, Part II: Pathologic findings. *Radiology* 1984; 150:455–461.

41. Higgins CB, McNamara MT, et al: MR imaging of the thyroid. *AJR* 1986; 147:1255–1261.

42. Noma S, Nishimura K, Togashi K, et al: Thyroid gland: MR imaging. *Radiology* 1987; 164:495–499.

43. Gefter WB, Spritzer CE, Eisenberg B, et al: Thyroid imaging with high-field-strength surface-coil MR. *Radiology* 1987; 164:483–490.

44. Doppman JL, Brennan MF, Koehler JO, et al: Computed tomography for parathyroid localization. *J Comput Assist Tomogr* 1977; 1:30–36.

45. Noyek AM, Friedberg J: Thyroglossal duct and ectopic thyroid disorders. *Otolaryngol Clin North Am* 1981; 14:187–201.

PART XII

The Spine

34

CT Anatomy of the Spine

Jeffrey M. Rogg, M.D.

Susan S. Kemp, M.D.

Computed tomography (CT) is frequently employed in the evaluation of the spine in spite of rapid development and acceptance of magnetic resonance imaging (MRI) techniques. Some investigators are advancing MRI as the procedure of choice, particularly for spinal cord lesions.[1] However, a sufficient number of controlled prospective studies have yet to be performed to determine the relative value and diagnostic accuracy of MRI as compared with CT in various spinal disorders.

The diagnostic accuracy of CT may be facilitated by the use of intravenous and/or intrathecal contrast media following standard myelography. Studies with intrathecal contrast can be routinely performed as outpatient procedures[2, 3] due to the low toxicity of newer nonionic contrast agents. CT myelography may provide information not apparent on myelography and may provide important additional information[4, 5] in comparison with plain CT when both methods are used for evaluation.[4, 6]

The following is a description of the normal anatomy and scanning techniques necessary for CT evaluation of the craniocervical junction and cervical, thoracic, and lumbar portions of the spinal column.

CRANIOCERVICAL JUNCTION

Technique

Basic evaluation of the craniocervical junction can be performed by axial scanning at 0-degree an-gulation to the orbitomeatal line with contiguous 1.5- or 3-mm-thick sections. If reconstructions are to be employed, i.e., for evaluation of the osseous articulations, 1.5-mm slice thickness is advisable. Scanning is performed from the superior aspect of the foramen magnum to the C2 vertebral body. Scans are imaged by standard and bone algorithms.

Osseous Anatomy and Articulations

The basiocciput is the first osseous structure imaged when scanning in a craniocaudal direction. This structure is formed from four components that surround the foramen magnum and are fused by approximately 6 years of age. The components are (1) the basilar portion, which forms the anterior margin of the foramen magnum; (2) the condylar portions, which form the two lateral margins of the foramen magnum; and (3) the squamous portion, which forms the posterior margin of the foramen magnum (Fig 34–1,A and B).

The occipital condyles extend caudally from the lateral condylar components. They are inferiorly convex protuberances on either side of the foramen magnum that provide the articular surfaces for the concave upper aspect of the superior articular facets (SAFs) of C1 (Fig 34–2). Posterior to each condyle is a condylar fossa containing the condylar canal, occasionally seen on CT,[7] which transmits an emissary vein that joins the suboccipital venous plexus to the transverse sinus.[8] Anterior and superior to the condyles are the hypoglos-

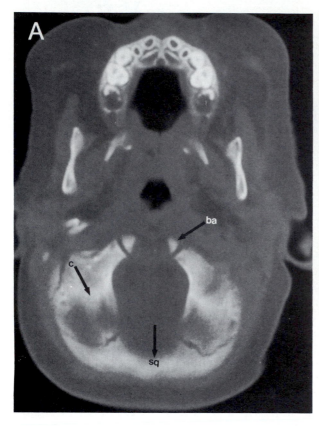

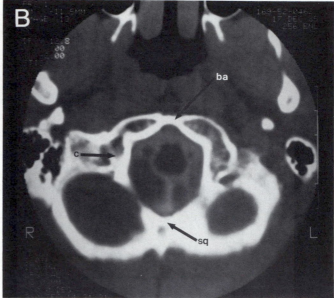

FIG 34–1.
A, the four unfused components of the basiocciput are demonstrated in this 1-year-old child. **B,** fusion generally occurs by approximately 6 years of age (*ba* = basilar portion; *ch* = condylar portion; *sq* = squamous portion).

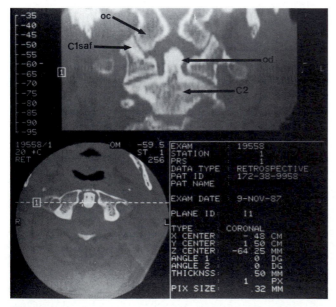

FIG 34–2.
The convex occipital condyles are seen to articulate with the concave superior articular facets of C1 *(C1 saf)* on this axial **(a)** and coronal **(b)** reconstruction (*oc* = occipital condyle; *od* = odontoid). The articulation of C1 with C2 is also shown.

sal canals, usually seen on CT (Fig 34–3), which transmit cranial nerve XII, the meningeal branch of the ascending pharyngeal artery, and rarely a persistent hypoglossal artery.[9]

The foramen magnum has an oval shape with the long axis in the midsagittal plane. The orientation of the foramen magnum in the axial plane is governed by the variable length of the clivus, which is formed inferiorly by the basiocciput.[10] Therefore, often only a portion of the foramen will be visualized on a single axial scan.[7]

The first cervical vertebra is next visualized as scanning continues inferiorly. This vertebra is named the atlas for a mythologic Greek Titan who was forced to bear the weight of the heavens on his shoulders. The atlas is recognized as a ring formed by fused anterior and posterior arches (Fig 34–4). The atlas has no vertebral body or spinous process. On 0-degree axial images the anterior arch will frequently be imaged cephalad to the posterior arch.[7] The bilateral sites of fusion of the arches form the lateral masses that are the support struts for the weight of the skull.

The SAFs of the lateral masses are concave and in the axial plain have a reniform shape. Coronal

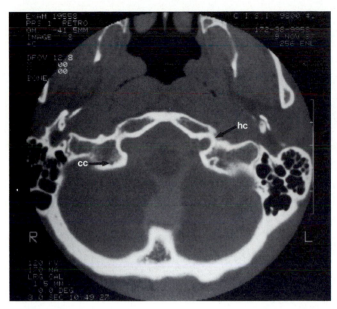

FIG 34–3.
The condylar canal *(cc)*, which transmits an emissary vein, and the hypoglossed canal *(hc)*, which transmits cranial nerve XII, are demonstrated.

imaging demonstrates the craniocaudal slope of the articulation from lateral to medial margins (see Fig 34–2). This angulation contributes to the lateral stability of the joint. The atlanto-occipital articulation is a synovial joint that permits flexion

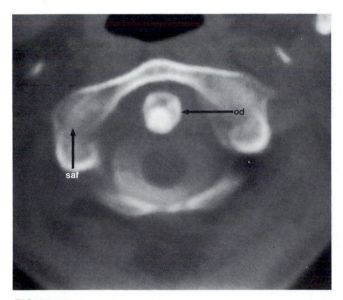

FIG 34–4.
The C1 vertebra is formed by fusion of anterior and posterior arches at the lateral mass. There is no vertebral body or spinous process. The superior articulating facet *(saf)* has a reniform shape on axial images. The odontoid *(od)* is seen to articulate with the anterior arch of C1.

and extension as well as slight bilateral tilting of the head.[11]

As scanning continues caudally, the inferior articular facets (IAFs) are demonstrated. These appear circular in the axial plane. They present a flat or slightly convex surface to C2. The inferior facets slope craniocaudally medially to laterally to articulate with the superior facets of C2 (Fig 34–2). This articulation opposes two convex surfaces and permits a sliding motion to occur during head rotation. There is no intervertebral disk at the C1–2 interspace.

The second cervical vertebra (Figs 34–2 and 34–5), named the axis for its role as the fulcrum around which the atlas and head rotate, is the most massive vertebrae of the cervical spine.[12] This vertebra body is identified on axial or coronal imaging by the odontoid process, a superiorly projecting tubercle that extends from the body of C2 through the anterior third of the C1 ring. This structure provides a pivot for the rotation of C1 and an attachment site for the multiple ligaments contributing to the stability of the craniocervical junction.

The pedicles and lamina of C2 are notably thick and strong. The spinal canal is large, but smaller than that of C1. The spinous process is massive and usually bifid.[12] Small transverse pro-

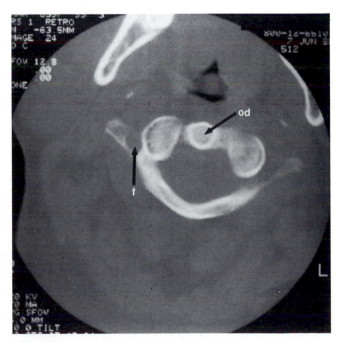

FIG 34–5.
The C2 vertebra is identified by the superiorly projecting odontoid process *(od)*, bifid spinous process, and foramina transversaria *(f)*.

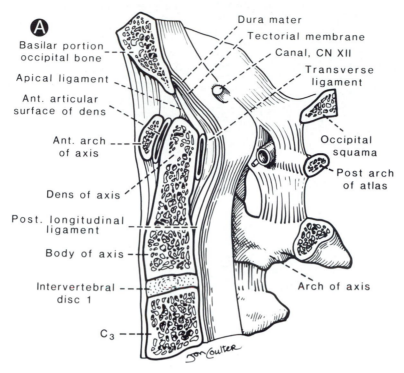

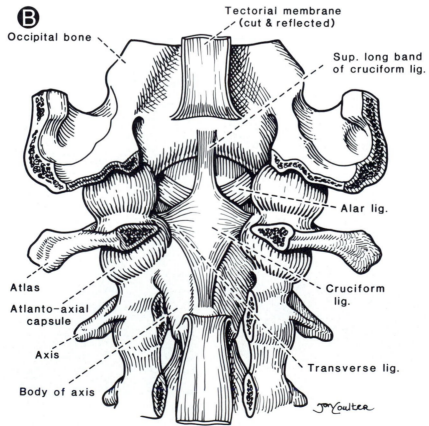

FIG 34–6.
Diagrams of craniocervical junction sagittal **(A)** and coronal **(B)** views.

cesses containing foramina transversaria are demonstrated on axial scanning. The IAFs slope caudally and ventrally, a pattern to be repeated at other cervical levels.

Spinal Canal Contents

The posterior longitudinal ligament (PLL) is demonstrated dorsal to the body of C2 as a broad soft-tissue density measuring approximately 1 mm in thickness (Fig 34–6,A and B). The ligament is contiguous superiorly with the tectorial membrane, which extends to the occiput. The tectorial membrane is imaged axially together with the closely approximated anterior dura as an enhancing soft-tissue density posterior to the odontoid, which is contained between the lateral masses of C1 (Fig 34–7).[13]

The cruciate ligament is anterior to the tectorial membrane and contiguous with the posterior margin of the odontoid. This ligament is T shaped in the coronal plane (see Fig 34–6,B). The long axis extends from the odontoid to the occiput. The short thick axis, or transverse ligament, extends between small medially facing tubercles that project from the lateral masses of C1.[11, 13] The transverse ligament can occasionally be identified on axial images as an enhancing curvilinear soft-tissue density of variable thickness that is adjacent to the dorsal margin of the odontoid (Figs 34–7 and 34–8).[13]

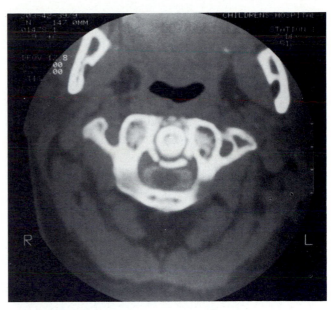

FIG 34–8.
Calcified transverse ligament.

Near the apex of the odontoid, small paramedian soft-tissue densities separated by epidural fat may be imaged on axial scans[13] (Fig 34–9). These are the alar ligaments, which extend from the odontoid to the medial inferior aspects of the occipital condyles. These ligaments may at times be seen on coronal CT images (see Fig 34–6,B). Also occasionally identified on coronal CT is the thin apical

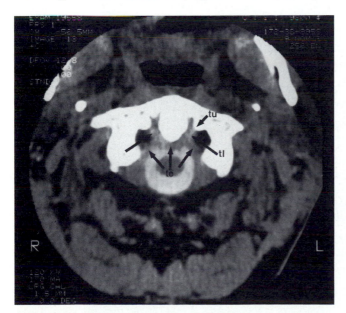

FIG 34–7.
An axial contrast-enhanced CT at the C1 level demonstrates the traverse ligament and tectorial membrane (*tu* = tubercle; *t1* = transverse ligament; *te* = tectorial membrane with dura).

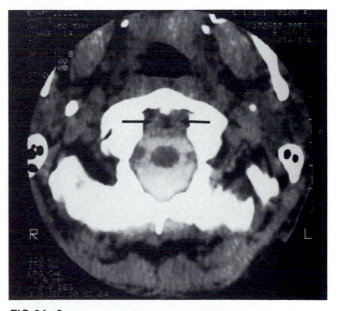

FIG 34–9.
A scan at the level of the superior aspect of C1 demonstrates the alar ligaments as they extend from the odontoid to the occipital condyles.

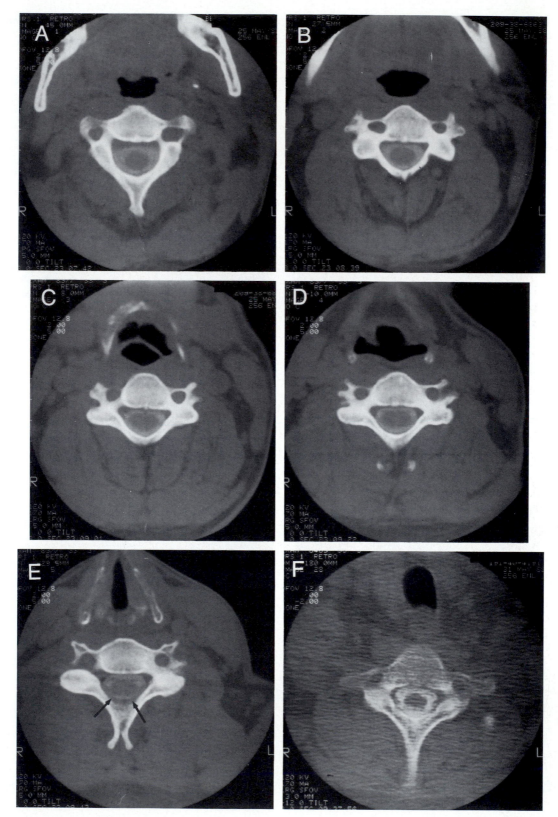

FIG 34–10.
Axial images of the C spine: C2 **(A)**, C3 **(B)**, C4 **(C)**, C5 **(D)**, C6 **(E)**. *Arrows* **(E)** demonstrate the ligamentum flava. The crab leg ap-

pearance of the ventral and dorsal nerve roots is well demonstrated with intrathecal contrast. **F,** C7.

ligament, which extends from the apex of the odontoid to the anterior rim of the foramen magnum (see Fig 34–6,A).[13]

A patulous subarachnoid space containing cerebrospinal fluid (CSF) generally provides adequate natural contrast for visualization of the spinal cord. However, the combined absence of epidural fat and the adherence of the dura to the osseous canal at this level make detailed analysis of neural structures difficult.[10,14–16] Intrathecal contrast provides the necessary background contrast for accurate CT evaluation.[17, 18]

The cervical cord is nearly circular on axial images at the C1 level. The cord then gradually flattens through the midcervical levels to again expand to become nearly circular at the C7–T1 level (Fig 34–10).[16] The position of the cord at the craniocervical junction is slightly anterior within the canal. If flexion and extension images are performed, approximately 1 mm of anteroposterior (AP) cord movement is demonstrated in the normal patient.[19] The cord has a homogeneous appearance, with slight indentations noted anteriorly and posteriorly representing the anterior and posterior median fissures.

Occasionally the C1 and C2 nerve roots will be imaged as they extend laterally to exit just posterior to the lateral masses. The first cervical nerve

exits between the occiput and posterior arch of C1. The second cervical nerve exits between the posterior arches of the atlas and the axis.

At the foramen magnum, a gradual expansion of the spinal cord occurs to form the medulla, which begins just rostral to the highest rootlet of the first cervical spinal nerve. The beginning of the medulla is roughly differentiated on CT from the spinal cord by the deep anterior median fissure that separates the pyramids and is variably interrupted by the pyramidal decussations. The vertebral arteries are seen at this level to ascend anterolateral to the medulla within the spinal canal. Also noted at approximately this plane are the cerebellar tonsils (Fig 34–11). The caudal extent of the tonsils may, in the normal patient, be identified at or above the level of the foramen magnum.[20, 21] Frequently the inferior vermis[20, 21] will also be partially imaged at approximately this level and defines the inferior extent of the body of the cerebellum.

CERVICAL SPINE

Technique

Imaging of the cervical spine by CT is best accomplished when the study is tailored to accomplish specific goals. Thin-section (1.5 mm) scanning will provide the best evaluation of disk and osseous detail, but cord evaluation may be improved when thicker sections are obtained.[22] A satisfactory compromise is to use a slice thickness of 3 mm. Occasionally thinner sections, as in fracture evaluation, or thicker sections, as in evaluation of syringomyelia, may be necessary.

Most studies are performed with intravenous contrast enhancement because of the increased anatomic detail that has been noted when compared with noncontrast CT.[23] A 150-cc drip infusion or a combination bolus and infusion technique may be used. The evaluation of disk disease in the cervical region is complicated by a relative paucity of low-density epidural fat and a relatively thin mid-density disk. Therefore, dural and epidural venous enhancement provide useful anatomic landmarks, especially for evaluation of the epidural space.

Intrathecal contrast is used when precise definition of the cord is necessary. It is also helpful to better define the extent and degree of subarachnoid space compromise by extradural disease as in metastatic carcinoma. Nonionic contrast material is

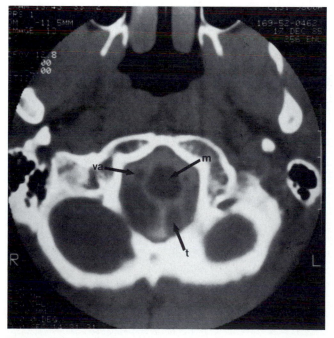

FIG 34–11.
An axial image at the level of the foramen magnum demonstrates the medulla *(m)*, vertebral arteries *(va)*, and cerebellar tonsils *(t)*.

administered via C1–2 puncture followed by myelographic filming and immediate postmyelogram focused CT scanning.

Osseous Anatomy and Articulations

The cervical spine comprises approximately 20% of the length of the spinal column.[12] The basic construction of the cervical vertebra is typical of other levels in the spinal column. A vertebral body serves as the principle structural foundation. Pedicles and laminae surround a central spinal canal. Transverse and spinous processes project dorsolaterally and dorsally, respectively, and provide insertion sites for the multiple ligaments and tendons that mobilize and stabilize the spinal column (see Fig 34–10).

The width of the cervical vertebral body increases from C2 to C7 as weight bearing increases. The bodies are oval shaped. The lateral aspects of the cranial surface of the vertebral body have superior projections called uncinate processes (Fig 34–12,A and B). Uncinate processes project into shallow concavities in the lateral margins of the inferior surface of the rostral vertebral body. This uncovertebral joint is unique to the cervical spine and has the effect of increasing the stability of the intervertebral joint.[11]

The cervical intervertebral disk is peculiar in that it is smaller laterally than is the vertebral body. The disk is also thicker ventrally than dorsally, which contributes to the lordosis of this region of the spine. Disk material accounts for a relatively large proportion of the length of the cervical spine and thus provides for increased flexibility.[11]

The vertebral canal at the cervical region is triangularly shaped and is spacious so that it can accommodate the cord through a large range of motion. The AP diameter varies from an average of 20 mm at C3 to 18 mm at C7.[24] The lower limit of normal is approximately 12 mm below C2.[25]

The articular facets of the cervical spine are flat and oval. SAFs are directed dorsally, cranially, and medially. The inferior facets face ventrally, caudally, and laterally. The articulation of the facets form the zygoapophyseal joints.

The transverse processes of the cervical spine are unique in that they contain foramina transversaria (see Fig 34–10), which transmit the vertebral artery, and the sympathetic nerve plexus. The foramina are generally seen on axial CT scans within the first 6 vertebrae. They are small, absent, or multiple at C7. C7 is also distinguished by having a long horizontal spinous process into which is inserted the ligamentum nuchae.

The osseous margins of the neural foramina are formed by the vertebral body and uncinate processes anteromedially and by the articular pillars posteriorly. The foramina are closely related to the uncovertebral joint medially and zygoapophyseal joint laterally. The foramina are oval in parasagittal

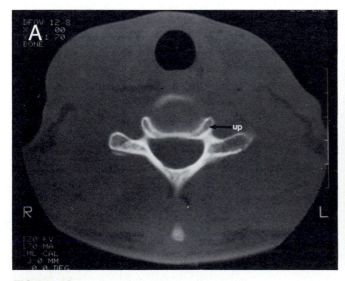 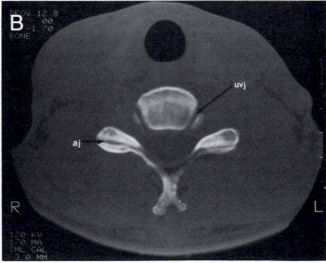

FIG 34–12.
A normal cervical vertebral body demonstrates the uncinate process **(A,** *up*) and uncovertebral joint **(B,** *uvj*). The apophyseal joint is also seen *(aj)*.

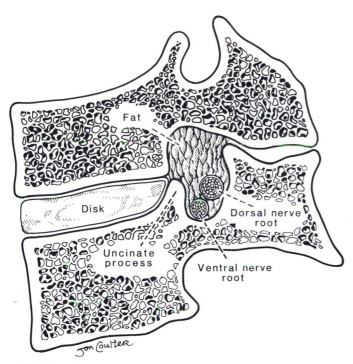

FIG 34–13.
A sagittal diagram of the cervical spine on CT demonstrates margins and contents of a typical neural foramina.

section and have a height of approximately 9 mm (Fig 34–13).[20]

Spinal Canal Contents

The PLL and the ligamentum flavum are frequently imaged on axial CT.[14] The PLL extends from the axis to the sacrum. It widens and becomes adherent at the disk level and at the posterior superior and posterior inferior margins of the vertebral body. The PLL may serve as a barrier to posterior disk herniation (see Fig 34–6,A).

The ligamenta flava are also seen on axial CT scanning. These ligaments, which extend from the axis to the sacrum, are thin and wide in the cervical region. They attach at the ventral surface of the lamina of the upper vertebra and at the dorsal superior surface of the lamina below (see Fig 34–10,C).

The spinal cord diameter enlarges between C5 and T1. This enlargement corresponds to the innervation of the upper extremities. The cord is elliptical at all levels, with the coronal-sagittal ratio being greatest at C4 and C5. At the T1 level the cord is nearly round (see Fig 34–10).[18]

Cervical nerve roots are identified following the administration of intrathecal contrast (see Fig 34–10,E). They are also frequently seen with in-

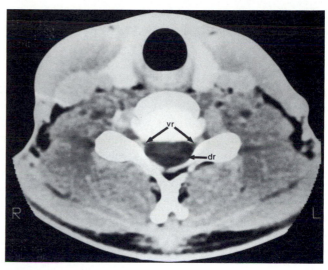

FIG 34–14.
This axial image with intravenous contrast demonstrates the ventral *(vr)* and dorsal *(dr)* nerve roots.

travenous contrast enhancement (Fig 34–14). Nerve root visualization has been noted in 87% of cases when using a high-volume intravenous contrast bolus technique.[23]

There are eight pairs of cervical spinal nerves that are formed from ventral (motor) and dorsal (sensory) nerve roots at each level. Fusion generally occurs just lateral to the dorsal sac (Fig 34–15). The dorsal root ganglion may occasionally be imaged near the point of fusion[27] within the spinal canal. Cephalad roots descend obliquely, while mid and lower cervical roots have a relatively horizontal course toward the neural foramen. Therefore, bilaterally paired roots can generally be seen on a single axial section. Both ventral and dorsal nerve roots lie in the inferior portion of the neural foramina. The dorsal root is found superior to the ventral root at or below the level of the disk (see Fig 34–13).

THORACIC SPINE

Technique

Successful imaging of the thoracic spine requires that the imaging technique be modified according to the interests of each examination. For example, thin-section scanning will improve resolution when looking for osseous lesions or disk disease, but the spinal cord is better seen when thicker sections are used.[28] Without intrathecal contrast, cord visualization is in large part governed by the size of the surrounding subarachnoid

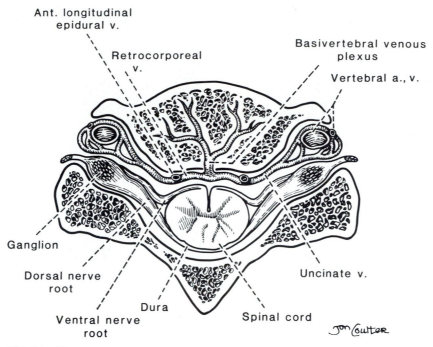

Ant. longitudinal
epidural v.

Retrocorporeal
v.

Basivertebral venous
plexus

Vertebral a., v.

Ganglion

Dorsal nerve
root

Ventral nerve
root

Dura

Uncinate v.

Spinal cord

FIG 34–15.
Axial diagram of the cervical spine demonstrating the relative positions of the spinal cord, the dorsal and ventral nerve roots, the dorsal root ganglion, and the epidural venous plexuses.

space, which serves as a natural contrast agent. Therefore, the lower thoracic region, where cord expansion occurs, is difficult to image without contrast in most cases. However, upper thoracic cord imaging is hampered by artifact arising from the shoulders. Overall, the thoracic cord is reasonably well visualized without intrathecal contrast approximately one third of the time.[28]

Intravenous contrast is generally used to take advantage of dural and epidural venous enhancement in circumstances where pathology would be expected to enhance (i.e., neoplasia or abscess). In the setting of a clinically apparent focal neurologic deficit, intrathecal contrast is employed for myelographic plain film and focused postmyelographic CT evaluation.

Osseous Anatomy and Articulations

The thoracic spine measures approximately 40% of the length of the vertebral column.[12] The vertebrae are midway in size between those of the cervical and lumbar spine, with a gradual transition in shape and mass occurring at either end.

The most distinguishing feature of the thoracic vertebral body is the presence of costal facets and, on axial scanning, of ribs seen in the plane of section (Fig 34–16,A and B). The vertebral bodies are "heart shaped" and are taller dorsally than ventrally, which accounts for the natural lordotic curvature of this portion of the spine. The intervertebral disk has a uniform thickness and is thin relative to the size of the vertebral body.

The laminae are thick and overlap from one level to the next. The spinous processes are long and oblique caudally. The spinal canal is relatively small and round, with little surrounding subarachnoid space or epidural fat.

The articulations of the thoracic spine are unusual in that they restrict motion, thereby protecting the volume of the thorax.[11] The superior articular processes project a flat, dorsally facing facet, and the inferior articular processes project a small tuberosity (Fig 34–16,B). The effect of this articulation is to restrict flexion. The long overlapping spinous processes and laminae restrict extension. Lateral motion is restricted by the rib cage.

Spinal Canal Contents

Descriptions of the soft-tissue structures within the vertebral canal at the thoracic level are not unlike those of the lower cervical cord. The PLL and ligamenta flava continue through this portion of the spine.

The spinal cord is nearly circular in the tho-

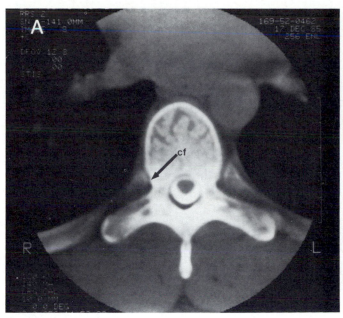
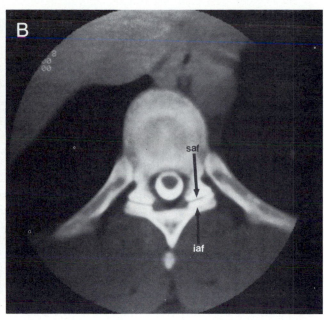

FIG 34–16.
Axial images of the thoracic spine (**A** and **B**) demonstrate the costal facets (*cf*), the thick laminae, the long spinous process, and articulations of the superior (*saf*) and inferior (*iaf*) articular facets. Canal contents are also clearly shown with intrathecal contrast.

racic region. The circumference is relatively constant from T2 to T9, at which point lumbar enlargement begins. This enlargement reaches a maximum circumference at the 12th thoracic vertebral level before tapering to the conus medullaris, which is generally located between T12 and L1–2 (Fig 34–17).[29]

The thoracic cord is surrounded by a small epi-dural space with little epidural fat. The thoracic nerve roots extend toward their respective neural foramina within the axial plane. Their configuration within the intravertebral canal and neural foramen mimics that of the mid and lower cervical nerve roots.

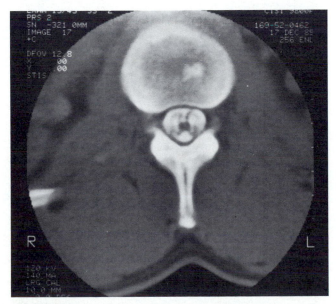

FIG 34–17.
Axial image following intrathecal contrast administration at the level of the conus medullaris. Dorsal and ventral nerve roots are seen to exit within the plane of section.

LUMBAR SPINE

Technique

Routine lumbar CT examination may be performed following intravenous contrast administration. Contiguous 5- or 3-mm-thick sections are performed parallel to the disk space to eliminate difficulties in interpretation created by volume averaging of the intervertebral disk (Fig 34–18 and 34–19).[30, 31] The images are performed from pedicle to pedicle, and locations are selected from an initially performed digital image. If sagittal or coronal reformations are necessary as in suspected spinal stenosis or spondylolisthesis, contiguous sections are obtained throughout the lumbosacral spine without gantry angulation. Thin sections (at least 3 mm) are necessary for satisfactory reformations. Imaging is performed with standard and bone algorithms.

Intrathecal contrast is used in preoperative evaluation or if noncontrast CT has been inconclusive. Contrast is introduced via lumbar puncture, and myelographic films are performed prior to CT.

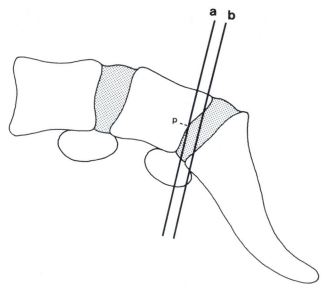

FIG 34–18.
Slice nonparallel to the disk space. When the scanning plane is nonparallel to the disk, there may be a false impression of the disk extending posterior to the vertebral body. In slice *a*, the posterior edge of the vertebral body appears to stop at point *p*. Slice *b* includes the posterior edge of S1.

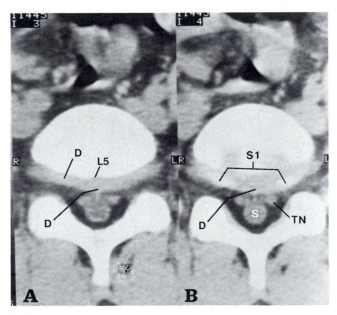

FIG 34–19.
Analysis of nonparallel slices through a normal L5–S1 disk. **A,** passing through the posterior part of the disk. **B,** a few millimeters lower to include the posterior edge of S1. In **A,** note the "flattening" of the back of *L5* and the symmetrical shape of the disk *(D)* ending at the posterolateral edges of *L5* and, most importantly, the normal relationship between the disk and the spinal canal contents with no encroachment on the dural sac or roots. In **B** part of the posterior edge of *S1* shows the true relationship of the disk to the vertebral body *(TN = traversing nerve; S = dural sac; D = disk).*

Adequate mixing of contrast is necessary, and the patient may need to be rolled several times prior to CT scanning.[4] CT should be performed within 6 hours of the introduction of intrathecal contrast. However, waiting 2 to 3 hours may provide optimal contrast density.[6] A prone positioning following intrathecal contrast may reduce lordosis and more satisfactorily outline the posterior disk margin with intrathecal contrast.[32] Breath holding is necessary to successfully execute this technique. Standard and bone algorithms are employed to image the lumbar spine with intrathecal contrast.

Osseous Anatomy and Articulations

The five lumbar vertebral bodies are larger in transverse than sagittal diameter.[33] The basivertebral venous plexus courses through the cancellous bone of the lumbar vertebral body[34] and exits to communicate with the anterior internal vertebral vein through a small bony depression in the posterior surface of the vertebral body (Fig 34–20). A complete bony ring is present at the level of the pedicles (Fig 34–21) and consists of the vertebral body anteriorly and the pedicles and laminae laterally and posteriorly.

The neural (intervertebral) foramen is bounded by the pedicles superiorly and inferiorly, the verte-

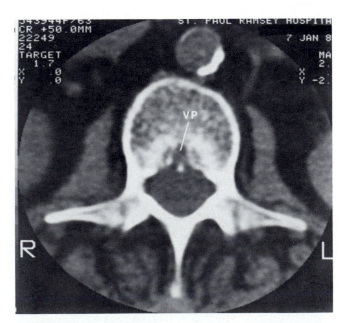

FIG 34–20.
Defect at the back of the vertebral body for the intravertebral venous plexus *(VP)*. At this level of the complete bony ring, there may be little epidural fat to aid in defining tissue planes; therefore, optimal soft-tissue resolution is very important.

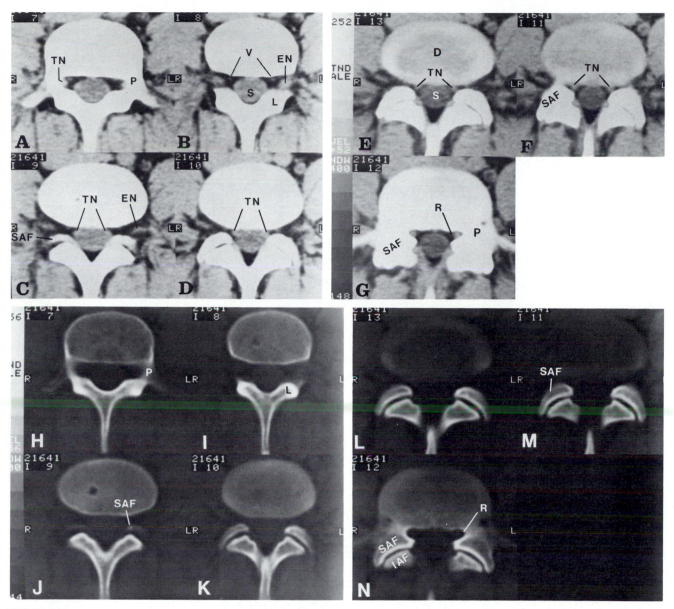

FIG 34–21.

Normal sequence of axial slices from pedicle to pedicle: **A** to **G,** soft-tissue setting; **H** to **N,** bone setting. **A** and **H,** lower aspect of the pedicle *(P)* with the traversing nerve *(TN)* about to become an exiting nerve. **B** and **I,** upper neural foramen. The exiting nerve *(EN)* is seen in this large part of the foramen. Note that the articular facets are not yet seen *(V* = anterior internal vertebral veins in the epidural space; *L* = lamina; *S* = dural sac). **C** and **J,** lower in the foramen. The exiting nerve *(EN)* is more lateral, and the top of the superior articular facet *(SAF)* has appeared. The traversing nerves *(TN),* which will exit below, have moved to the anterolateral part of the dural sac. They are slightly increased in density because they are not surrounded by as much CSF as when in the dural sac. **D** and **K,** larger SAF. The slice is still above the disk. The traversing nerves *(TN)* are a little more separated from the sac. **E** and **L,** disk level. The disk *(D)* is of higher attenuation than the dural sac *(S).* The traversing nerves *(TN)* have completely separated from the dural sac. They lie in this position when compressed by a classic posterolateral herniated nucleus pulposus. **F** and **M,** the *SAF* starting to merge into the pedicle below *(TN* = traversing nerve). **G** and **N,** upper pedicle. This is the level of the lateral recess *(R)* in which the traversing nerve is medial to the pedicle *(P)* and anterior to the superior articular facet *(SAF)* *(IAF* = inferior articular facet).

bral body anteriorly, the intervertebral disk antero-inferiorly, the pars interarticularis posterosuperiorly, and the facet joint posteroinferiorly. The exiting nerve root traverses the neural foramen superiorly, just beneath the pedicle (Fig 34–22).

The articular facets are seen at the midlevel of the intervertebral foramina. The SAF lies anterior and lateral to the IAF of the next cephalad vertebra. As the slices pass caudally through the neural foramen, the IAF becomes smaller, and the SAF

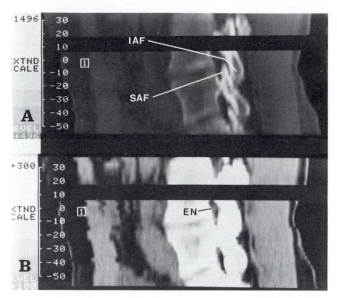

FIG 34–22.
Normal reformatted image through the neural foramen. **A,** bone; **B,** soft-tissue setting (*EN* = exiting nerve surrounded by fat in the neural foramen; *IAF* = inferior articular facet; *SAF* = superior articular facet).

enlarges. At the inferior border of the intervertebral foramen, the SAF becomes continuous with the pedicle (see Fig 34–21). The facet joints are synovial joints that are oblique to the sagittal plane and curved.[35] Axial images are useful in evaluation of facet joint disorders.

The intervertebral disk is composed of the gelatinous nucleus pulposis centrally and the dense fibrous annulus fibrosis peripherally, which is attached to the adjacent vertebral ring apophysis.[33] The intervertebral disk has greater CT density than does the CSF-containing thecal sac (Fig 34–23). The posterior margin of the intervertebral disk is concave at L2–3 and L3–4 (Fig 34–24) and flat or minimally convex at L4–5 and L5–S1 (Fig 34–25).

Spinal Canal Contents

Epidural fat surrounds and delineates structures within the spinal canal and neural foramina by acting as a natural contrast medium. Obliteration of epidural fat can occur with disk herniation, spondylotic changes, or previous surgery. Epidural fat is most prominent at L4–5 and L5–S1.[36] Fat is less prominent at the level of the pedicles and at upper lumbar levels. The lumbar thecal sac is round or oval in shape and tapers to end caudally at approximately the midsacrum. Intrathecal con-

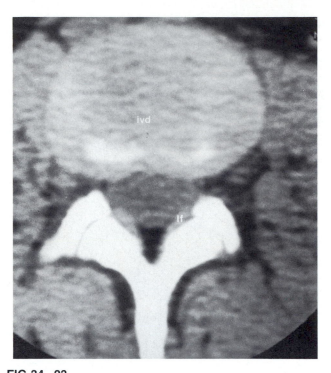

FIG 34–23.
The intervertebral disk *(ivd)* is of greater density than the thecal sac. The ligamentum flavum *(lf)* is obvious at this level.

trast is generally necessary to identify structures within the thecal sac.[14, 33, 37]

The normal conus medullaris is identified at approximately T12 to L1 in adults but may be identified as far caudally as L2.[29] The conus med-

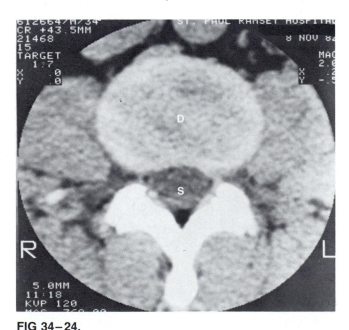

FIG 34–24.
Normal concave disk at L3–4. The disk is denser than the dural sac (*D* = disk; *S* = dural sac).

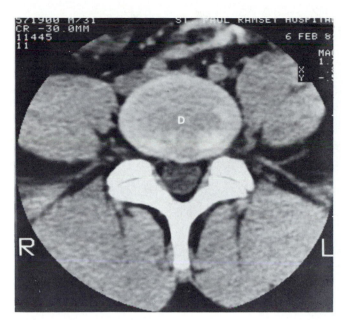

FIG 34–25.
Normal minimally convex disk at L4–5 (*D* = disk).

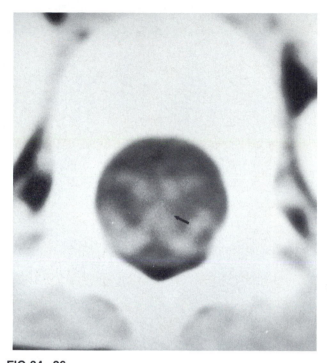

FIG 34–26.
The normal conus medullaris *(arrow)* and nerve roots of the cauda equina can occasionally be visualized without intrathecal contrast in a patulous thecal sac.

ullaris possesses an oval configuration and an anterior sulcus corresponding to the anterior median fissure.[38] A small posterior eminence may also be identified.[38] The nerve roots of the cauda equina are seen laterally and caudally as the conus gently tapers to its termination. This produces a spider-like configuration on axial CT performed with intrathecal contrast (Figs 34–17 and 34–26).

The nerve roots of the cauda equina lie in the posterior portion of thecal sac and proceed anteriorly as they approach the exiting sleeves.[33, 39] The nerve root sleeve surrounds the exiting nerve root and terminates proximal to the dorsal root ganglion[39] at approximately the level of the midpedicle (Fig 34–27).[14] Beyond this point, intrathecal contrast normally will not be seen, and the nerve root is identified by virtue of contrast produced by surrounding fat.

The lumbar and sacral nerve roots are best described as either "exiting" or "traversing" (Fig 34–28). The exiting root passes under the pedicle of the corresponding level and through the upper part of the neural foramen above the level of the disk. The traversing roots move anterolaterally within the thecal sac and, in fact, may be distinguished as separate from the sac at L5–S1. The traversing nerve roots approach the pedicle in the lateral recess and become exiting nerve roots as they pass laterally under the pedicle and through the neural foramen (see Fig 34–21).

The extra-arachnoid spaces may be seen by CT even when there is no evidence of extra-arachnoid injection on the myelogram. This may be due to leakage of contrast from the needle tract, or the needle may puncture the dura anteriorly (Fig 34–28).

The ligamenta flava are paired bilateral structures that are attached to the laminae and articular processes at each spinal level. They are seen as a thin strip of soft-tissue density in the posterolateral canal, anterior to the articular facets (see Fig 34–23). The anterior longitudinal ligament extends along the ventral surface of the vertebral bodies throughout the extent of the spine. It is generally not visualized on routine axial CT. The PLL has a more clinically significant relationship to the intervertebral disk than does the anterior longitudinal ligament. It is adherent to the annulus fibrosis posteriorly[14] but is not adherent to the concavity of the posterior surface of the vertebral body.[40] Vascular and connective tissues are located between the ligament and the posterior aspect of the vertebral body.

The lumbar epidural venous anatomy may be at least partially opacified by intravenous contrast (Fig 34–29). A communicating valveless network of veins constitute the vertebral venous system. The interosseous vertebral veins drain each verte-

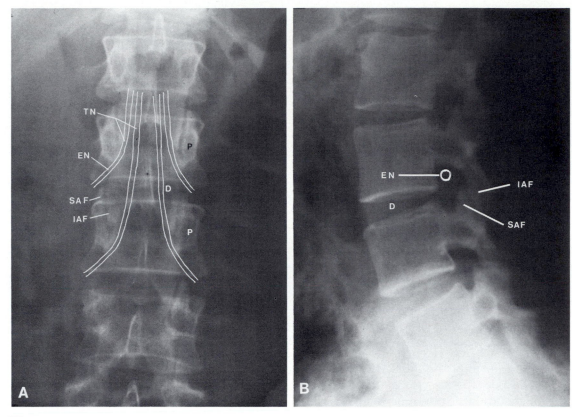

FIG 34–27.
Normal AP **(A)** and lateral **(B)** plain films. The intervertebral foramen extends from pedicle to pedicle. The exiting nerve *(EN)* is
high in the neural foramen, just below the pedicle. The disk *(D)* lies
at the level of the midforamen and below the exiting nerve. The
lower part of the foramen has a very narrow AP diameter *(TN =
traversing nerve; SAF = superior articular facet; IAF = inferior articular facet; P = pedicle).*

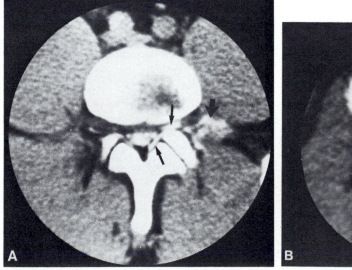
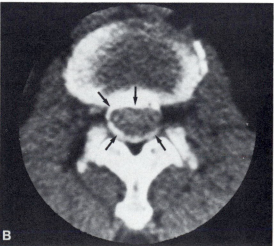

FIG 34–28.
Extra-arachnoid spaces. **A,** leakage of contrast material has occurred into the epidural space *(medial arrow)*. Contrast medium is
also noted in the intervertebral foramen *(middle arrow)* and is seen
in the extraspinal space laterally *(large arrow)*. In **B,** the myelogram revealed subdural contrast medium. A CT section obtained
after demonstrates a band of contrast medium *(arrows)* surrounding the thecal sac. No contrast medium was observed in the extradural location.

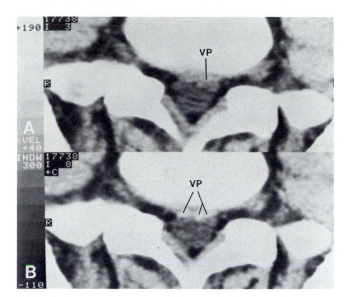

FIG 34-29.
Epidural venous plexus. **A,** without contrast, the high-density structure *(VP)* anterior to the dural sac could be confused with an L5–S1 midline herniated nucleus pulposus. **B,** after bolus intravenous contrast, marked enhancement confirms a normal venous plexus *(VP)*.

bral body and empty into a basivertebral vein that exits posteriorly, through the nutrient foramen of the vertebral body (see Fig 34–20).[41] This communicates with the anterior internal vertebral veins.[41] These structures are positioned close to the posterior aspect of the vertebral bodies and are seen as soft-tissue densities on axial CT immediately posterior to the vertebral body.[33] It is important not to confuse these for traversing nerve roots or disk material. The anterior internal vertebral veins communicate with the paravertebral veins via suprapedicular and infrapedicular veins coursing through the inferior and superior aspects of the neural foramen, respectively.[41]

Extraspinal abnormalities may be identified in more than 1% of lumbar spine CT cases.[43] Lesions that originate in the spine may extend to the paraspinal musculature, or the spine may be secondarily involved from an extrinsic process.[44] The choice of field of view and display format influence the amount of perispinal anatomy delineated.

REFERENCES

1. Haughton VM: MR imaging of the spine. *Radiology* 1988; 166:297–301.
2. Tate CF, Wilkovh R, Lestange, et al: Outpatient lumbar myelography: Initial results in 79 examinations using a low-dose metrizamide technique. *Radiology* 1985; 157:391–393.
3. Zinreich SJ, Wang H, Updike ML, et al: CT myelography for outpatients: An inpatient/outpatient pilot study to assess methodology. *Radiology* 1985; 157:387–390.
4. Dublin AB, McGahon JP, Reid MH, et al: The value of computed tomographic metrizamide myelography in the neuroradiologic evaluation of the spine. *Radiology* 1983; 146:79–86.
5. Barrow DL, Wood GH, Hoffman JC: Clinical indications for computer-assisted myelography. *Neurosurgery* 1983; 12:47–57.
6. Arnand AK, Lee BCP: Plain and metrizamide CT of lumbar disk disease: Comparison with myelography. *AJNR* 1982; 3:567–571.
7. LaMasters DL, deGroot J: Normal craniocervical junction, in Newton TH, Potts DG (ed): *Computed Tomography of the Spine and Spinal Cord.* St Anselmo, Calif, Clavadel Press, 1983, pp 31–52.
8. Gathier JC, Bruyn GW: The so-called condyloid foramen in the half axial view. *AJR* 1969; 107:515–519.
9. Shapiro R: Enlargement of the hypoglossal canal in the presence of a persistent hypoglossal artery. *Radiology* 1979; 133:395–396.
10. Gladstone RJ, Erichssen-Powell W: Manifestation of occipital vertebrae and fusion of the atlas with the occipital bone. *J Anat Physiol* 1915; 49:190–199.
11. Clemente CD: *Gray's Anatomy*, ed 30. Philadelphia, Lea & Febiger, 1985, pp 341–354.
12. Clemente CD: *Gray's Anatomy*, ed 30. Philadelphia, Lea & Febiger, 1985, pp 127–144.
13. Daniels DL, Williams AL, Haughton VM: Computed tomography of the articulations and ligaments at the occipito-atlanto axial region. *Radiology* 1983; 146:709–716.
14. Haughton VM, Syversten A, Williams AL: Soft-tissue anatomy within the spinal canal as seen by computed tomography. *Radiology* 1980; 134:649–655.
15. Drayer BP, Rosenbaum AE: Cerebrospinal fluid imaging using serial metrizamide CT cisternography. *Neuroradiology* 1977; 13:7–17.
16. Carpenter MB: *Core Text of Neuroanatomy.* Baltimore, Williams & Wilkins, 1972; pp 68–89.
17. DiChiro G, Schellinger D: Computed tomography of the spinal cord after lumbar intrathecal introduction of metrizamide (computer assisted myelography). *Radiology* 1976; 120:101–104.
18. Thijssen A, Keyser MW: Morphology of the cervical spinal cord on computed myelography. *Neuroradiology* 1979; 18:51–62.
19. Osborne D, Triolo P, Dubois B, et al: Assessment of craniocervical junction and atlantoaxial relation using metrizamide-enhanced CT in flexion and extension. *AJNR* 1983; 4:843–845.
20. Wickbom I, Hanafee W: Soft tissue masses immediately below the foramen magnum. *Acta Radiol* 1963; 1:647–658.

21. LaMasters D, Watanabe T, Chambers E, et al: Multiplanar metrizamide-enhanced CT imaging of the foramen magnum. *AJNR* 1982; 3:485–494.
22. Orrison WW, Johansen JG, Eldevik OP, et al: Optimal computed-tomographic techniques for cervical spine imaging. *Radiology* 1982; 144:180–182.
23. Heinz ER, Yeates A, Burger P, et al: Opacification of epidural venous plexus and dura evaluation of cervical nerve roots: CT technique. *AJNR* 1984; 5:621–624.
24. Boijsen E: The cervical spinal canal in intraspinal expansive processes. *Acta Radiol* 1954; 42:101–115.
25. Epstein BS: *The Spine. A Radiological Text and Atlas.* Philadelphia, Lea & Febiger, 1976.
26. Pech P, Daniels D, Williams AL, et al: The cervical neural foramina: Correlation of microtomy and CT anatomy. *Radiology* 1985; 155:143–146.
27. LaMasters D, deGroot J, Williams AL, et al: Normal cervical spine, in Newton TH, Potts DG (eds): *Computed Tomography of the Spine and Spinal Cord.* St Anselmo, Calif, Clavadel Press, 1983, pp 53–68.
28. Taylor A, Haughton VM, Doust BD: CT imaging of the thoracic spinal cord without intrathecal contrast medium. *J Comput Assist Tomogr* 1980; 4:223–224.
29. Shapiro R: Anatomy, in Shapiro R (ed): *Myelography,* ed 4. Chicago, Year Book Medical Publishers, Inc, 1984, p 102.
30. Hirschy JC, Leve WM, Berninger WH, et al: CT of the lumbosacral spine: Importance of tomographic planes parallel to vertebral and plate. *AJR* 1981; 126:47–52.
31. Braun IF, Lin JP, George AE, et al: Pitfalls in the computed tomographic evaluation of the lumbar spine in disc disease. *Neuroradiology* 1984; 26:15–20.
32. Tehranzadeh J, Gabriele OF: The prone position for CT of the lumbar spine. *Radiology* 1984; 152:817–818.
33. Haughton VM, Williams AL: CT anatomy of the spine. *CRC Crit Rev Diagn Imaging* 1981; 13:173–192.
34. Dorwart RH, DeGroot J, Sauerland EK, et al: Computed tomography of the lumbosacral spine: Normal anatomy, anatomic variants and pathologic anatomy. *Radiographics* 1982; 2:459–499.
35. Carrera GF, Haughton VM, Syversten A, et al: Computed tomography of the lumbar facet joints. *Radiology* 1980; 134:145–148.
36. Fries JW, Abodeely DA, Vijungco JG, et al: Computed tomography of herniated and extruded nucleus pulposis. *J Comput Assist Tomogr* 1982; 6:874–887.
37. Naidich TP, King DG, Moran CJ, et al: Computed tomography of the lumbar thecal sac. *J Comput Assist Tomogr* 1980; 4:37–41.
38. Grogan JP, Daniels DL, Williams AL: The normal conus medullaris: CT criteria for recognition. *Radiology* 1984; 151:661–664.
39. Williams AL, Haughton VM, Daniels DL, et al: CT recognition of lateral lumbar disk herniation. *AJR* 1982; 139:345–347.
40. Parke WW: Applied anatomy of the spine, in Rothman RH, Simeone FA (eds): *The Spine,* ed 2. Philadelphia, WB Saunders Co, 1982, p 33.
41. Gershater R: Lumbar epidural venography: Review of 1200 cases. *Radiology* 1979; 131:409–421.
42. Meijenhorst GCH: Computed tomography of the lumbar epidural veins. *Radiology* 1982; 145:687–691.
43. Frager DH, Elkin CM, Kansler F, et al: Extraspinal abnormalities identified on lumbar spine CT. *Neuroradiology* 1986; 28:58–60.
44. Osborn AG, Koehler PR, et al: Computed tomography of the paraspinal musculature: Normal and pathologic anatomy. *AJR* 1982; 138:93–98.

35

Magnetic Resonance Imaging of the Normal Spine

Louis Wener, M.D.

Stanley M. Perl, M.D.

The exquisite soft-tissue contrast of magnetic resonance imaging (MRI) presents vividly detailed images requiring a heightened appreciation of multi-planar anatomy. Pulse sequence selection determines these tissue contrasts, and to fully exploit the modality, one should have an understanding of the biophysical basis of proton MRI.[1] MRI studies are noninvasive, requiring no ionizing radiation or injection of iodinated contrast material. Intravenous administration of gadolinium-diethylene-triamine pentaacetic (DTPA) is often useful in studies of the postoperative lumbar spine and better characterization of other lesions of the entire spine.

The "ideal" field strength remains controversial, and the proponents of various manufacturers have attempted to make a case for their particular bias. Thin sections, essential for increased spatial resolution in spinal studies, result in a significant decrease in the signal-to-noise ratio (SNR). There is no argument that a higher–field strength magnet yields greater signal per unit time, which makes more signal available for these thinner sections. Other methods to improve the SNR are employing surface coils[2, 3] or increasing the number of excitations (NEX), which increases the imaging time.

Most patients with back complaints will not tolerate lengthy examination times, and therefore the unit that can accomplish the study with the highest SNR in the shortest study time has the best chance of producing superior images. The material in this chapter was acquired by using a superconducting magnet operating at 1.5 tesla (General Electric Medical Systems, Milwaukee). Imaging time is the product of repetition time (TR), NEX, and matrix size (e.g., 400 ms × 1 × 128 = 51 seconds).

A word should be said about claustrophobia. This is a real problem that affects approximately 10% of the patients scheduled for MRI studies (Wener L. and Strait C., unpublished data). The majority of these individuals will not be aware of their claustrophobia until they enter the magnet. Cervical and thoracic spine studies are more likely to produce claustrophobia because the patient enters the magnet head first. Eighty percent of symptomatic patients will experience some sort of anxiety ranging from a slight discomfort to bare tolerance of the study. There is no more important ingredient for successful completion of the examination in an anxious patient than a caring and compassionate technologist who will take the time and effort to "talk" the patient through the study. Mild sedatives, blindfolds, bringing the patient out of the magnet between acquisitions, and having someone accompany the patient during the examination have all been tried with some success. The remaining 20% (or 2% of scheduled patients) will

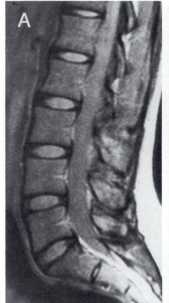
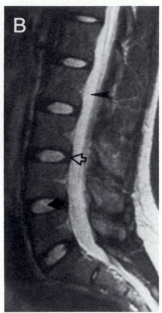

FIG 35–1.
Normal long TR images of the lumbar spine. **A,** proton-density sagittal image of the lumbar spine (spin echo [SE], TR = 2,000 ms, TE = 30 ms, 2 NEX, 5-mm-thick slice, 256 × 192). Flow compensation was used. **B,** T2-weighted sagittal image (SE, TR = 2,000 ms, TE = 80 ms, 2 NEX, 5-mm-thick slice, 256 × 192). Flow compensation was used. Note the nucleus pulposus *(solid arrow),* annulus fibrosus *(open arrow)* and CSF *(arrowhead).*

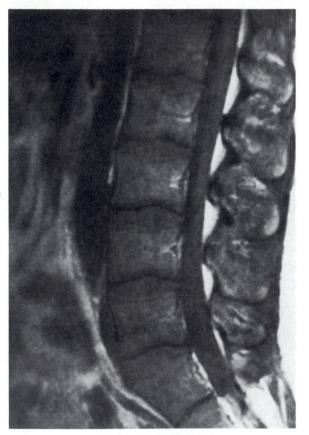

FIG 35–2.
Normal short TR images of the lumbar spine. T1-weighted sagittal image of the lumbar spine (SE, TR = 500 ms, TE = 20 ms, 2 NEX, 5-mm-thick slice, 256 × 256). Note the lack of delineation of the annulus, the posterior longitudinal ligament, and the CSF. Also note the lack of delineation of the annulus from the nucleus pulposus. The increased signal in the vertebral body is due to fat in the bone marrow.

not be able to tolerate the examination under any circumstances short of general anesthesia.

Long TR studies yield proton-density (long TR, short echo time [TE]) and T2-weighted (long TR, long TE) images. The proton-density images are also known as balanced images, having characteristics of both T1 and T2 studies (Fig 35–1,A). T2 images are particularly useful for distinguishing various normal and pathologic tissues. TR is usually 2,000 ms or greater, with echos of 30 and 80 ms. Cardiac gating and/or flow compensation is applied to reduce the effect of spinal fluid movement.[4] T2-weighted images distinguish the signal-intense fluid of the nucleus pulposus from the signal-poor fibrous annulus and yield bright signal from the cerebrospinal (CSF) to produce the "myelogram effect" (Fig 35–1,B).

Pulse sequences using short TR and short TE produce T1-weighted images (Fig 35–2). These are quick studies and are useful for localization. If a high-resolution matrix is employed, images with exquisite anatomic detail can be obtained, especially when thin sections (5 mm or less) are acquired. Since the posterior longitudinal ligament, dura, and CSF all exhibit low signal on T1-weighted images, separation of the interfaces can be difficult. There is virtually no differentiation between the annulus and nucleus pulposus with these sequences. T1-weighted images are very useful for examining fat, static blood, colloid, or melanin, which are all signal intense on T1-weighted images.

Examinations are usually carried out in the orthogonal planes, i.e., coronal, sagittal, and transverse. By simply changing the manner in which data are collected rather than repositioning the patient, oblique planes may be studied.[5] This is very useful in acquiring data through the planes of the intervertebral disks, and recent software improvements permit multiplanar, multiangle acquisitions (Fig 35–3).[6] Complex planes may also be used and are particularly helpful in studying patients with scoliosis (Fig 35–4,A–D).

Although a direct acquisition may be obtained in virtually any desired plane, multiplanar studies may also be accomplished by three-dimensional examination of a block of tissue obtained in a single acquisition.[7] The block may then be studied in any desired plane without the image degradation that is usually seen with CT reformatting. Three-dimensional imaging also permits the use of thin sections (1 to 2 mm) without interslice gaps and with an increased SNR.

Spin-echo imaging subjects the protons of interest to a 90-degree pulse followed by a 180-degree pulse to refocus the dephasing protons. To acquire gradient refocused images, initial flip angles (θ) less than 90 degrees are employed. This is then followed by a gradient pulse.[8] The smaller the initial flip angle, the more T2 weighted is the sequence. The proper combination of flip angle and gradient pulse timing will produce T1-weighted, proton-density, or T2-weighted images in less time than standard spin-echo sequences and result in excellent studies of the CSF, spinal cord, and nucleus pulposus (Fig 35–5). The images incur some contrast loss, and very low flip angles result in significant signal loss.

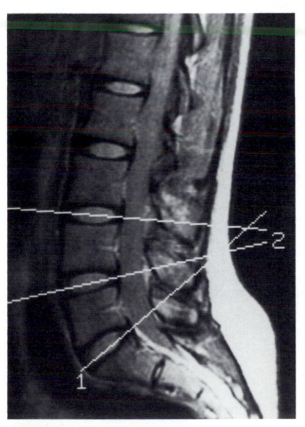

FIG 35–3.
A sagittal image of the lumbar spine demonstrates slice location annotation for a multiangle, multiplanar, axial acquisition.

ANATOMIC CONSIDERATIONS

Suffice it to say that any anatomy visible on CT images of the spine can also be identified on MRI

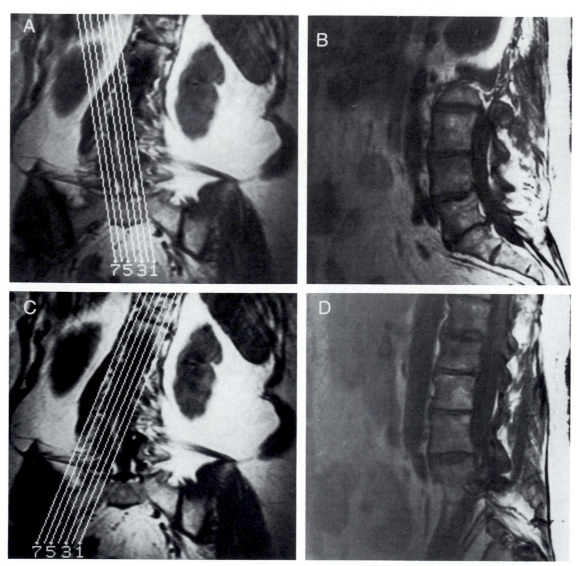

FIG 35–4.
By using a coronal T1-weighted image as a localizer, nonorthogonal planes may be utilized to straighten the scoliosis for full-column imaging in the sagittal plane. **A,** localization for a sagittal full-column image of the lower lumbar spine demonstrated in **B. C,** localization for the upper lumbar spine in **D.**

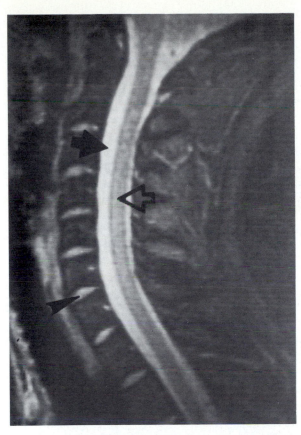

FIG 35–5.
Gradient-refocused sagittal cervical spine image (TR = 400 ms, TE = 20 ms, flip angle = 12 degrees, 4 NEX, 3-mm-thick slice, 256 × 192). Note the CSF *(solid arrow)*, spinal cord *(open arrow)*, and nucleus pulposus *(arrowhead)*.

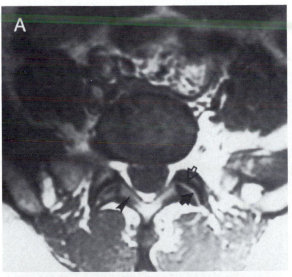

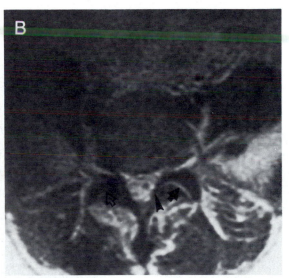

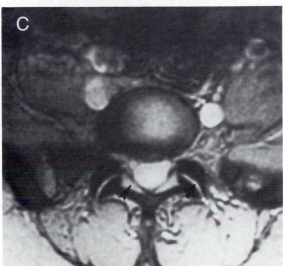

FIG 35–6.
Normal axial images of the lumbar spine. **A,** T1-weighted axial image of the lower lumbar spine (SE, TR = 500 ms, TE = 20 ms, 4 NEX, 4-mm-thick slice, 256 × 192). Note the moderate signal from the articular cartilage *(solid arrow)*, signal void from the cortical bone *(open arrow)*, and moderate signal from the ligamentum flavum *(arrowhead)*. **B,** T2-weighted axial lumbar image (SE, TR = 1,800 ms, TE = 80 ms, 2 NEX, 4-mm-thick slice, 256 × 192). Note the moderate signal from the cartilage of the facet joint on the left *(solid arrow)*. Incidental note of the facet arthropathy on the right should be made *(open arrow)*. The ligamentum flavum is poorly delineated *(arrowhead)*. **C,** gradient-refocused, T2-weighted, axial lumbar image (TR = 350 ms, TE = 18 ms, flip angle = 25 degrees, 4 NEX, 4-mm-thick slice, 256 × 192). Note the increased signal intensity from the articular cartilage *(solid arrow)* and the increased signal intensity from the ligamentum flavum *(arrowhead)* as compared with the T1- and T2-weighted SE axial images.

studies. This is also true of osseous structures, but it must be remembered that MRI and CT demonstrate different bony components. CT yields exquisite detail of cortical bone and the trabecular structure of the vertebral bodies, while MRI demonstrates these structures by their signal void. The bone marrow, because of its fat content, is not well demonstrated on CT but can be critically evaluated on MRI, especially with T1-weighted images (see Fig 35–2).[9] The articular cartilage of facet joints is clearly visible on T1 and proton-density images which produce a moderately bright signal. The cartilage is signal intense on T2-weighted images.[10] Gradient refocused T2-weighted images give better delineation of the cartilage of facet joints than do spin-echo T2-weighted images. Unlike CT, which requires bone and soft-tissue windows to fully evaluate the spinal structures, MRI's extended contrast range permits visualization of both components in a single image (Fig 35–6,A–C).

THE CERVICAL SPINE

Technical Considerations

Studies of the cervical spine are invariably performed with surface coils. A 5-in. circular coil placed posterior to the neck yields a good SNR and

produces high-quality images. More recently, an anterior coil fashioned after the Philadelphia Collar (Wener L. and Schenk J., unpublished data) (Medrad Corp, Pittsburgh) has been designed and produces improved images of the neck, both of the cervical spine and the cervical soft tissues such as the larynx and thyroid (Fig 35–7).

The coronal images are used primarily for localization and are normally obtained with a crude matrix (256×128). The slices are 5 mm thick, are spaced 2.5 mm apart, and have 1 NEX and a 24-cm field of view (FOV).

Using the coronal images, a T1-weighted sagittal series is obtained. Seven 3-mm-thick locations separated by 1.5 mm are planned so that the center slice images the midline of the neural canal. This series will image from foramen to foramen, usually including the vertebral artery within the foramina transversaria. The T1-weighted sequence is obtained at a TR/TE of 500/20, 2 NEX, 24-cm FOV, and a 256×192 matrix. The most useful sagittal sequence is a proton-density and T2-weighted study, which may be obtained with spin-echo or gradient-refocused pulses. Identical locations are programmed to coincide with the T1-weighted acquisition. To reduce flow artifacts induced by CSF motion, cardiac gating and flow compensation are applied during spin-echo acquisitions. TR is dependent on the heart rate but is minimally 2,000

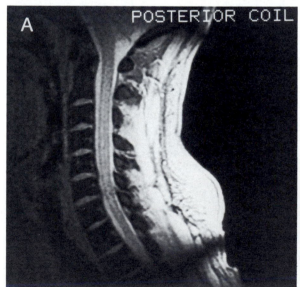
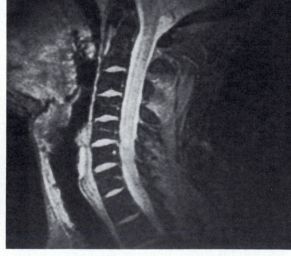

FIG 35–7.
Gradient-refocused images of the cervical spine. **A,** sagittal proton-density image with a posteriorly placed surface coil (TR = 400 ms, TE = 20 ms, flip angle = 12 degrees, 4 NEX, 3-mm-thick slice, 256 × 192). **B,** sagittal proton-density image with an anterior sur- face coil (TR = 400 ms, TE = 20 ms, flip angle = 12 degrees, 4 NEX, 3-mm-thick slice, 256 × 192). Note the improved image quality of the anterior neck structures as well as the improved imaging of the disks and cervical vertebrae with the anterior surface coil.

ms. Two echos of 30 and 80 ms are employed to produce a proton-density image and a heavily weighted T2-weighted image. The matrix is 256 × 192 with a 24-cm FOV and 1 NEX.

Sagittal images obtained with gradient refocusing can be acquired in as short a time as 5 minutes, and cardiac gating is not required. The images are similar to their spin-echo counterparts, but certain differences must be appreciated. The gradient-refocused, proton-density images are a bit more useful than are spin-echo, proton-density images because there is better separation of cord from CSF.

The disk is imaged as signal intense and can be easily identified distinct from bone, which images with a low signal. With gradient-refocused sequences magnetic susceptibility differences are accentuated, and regions with markedly differing signals must be evaluated with caution to avoid exaggerating the size of lesions. Overall, the short imaging time and the high-quality images available with this technique make it the sequence of choice in many institutions. The imaging parameters are TR = 350, TE = 10/20, θ = 12 degrees, 24-cm FOV, 4 NEX, and a 256 × 192 matrix.

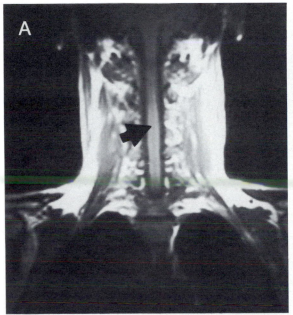

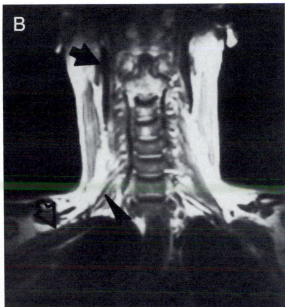

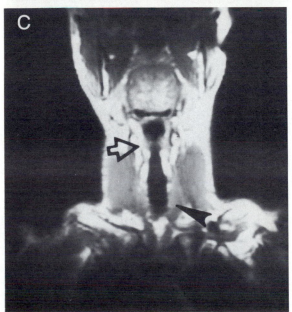

FIG 35–8.
Coronal T1-weighted images of the cervical spine (SE, TR = 500 ms, TE = 20 ms, 2 NEX, 5-mm-thick slice, 256 × 192). **A,** note the cord *(arrow)* and some exiting nerve roots. **B,** the lower cervical roots *(arrowhead)* are descending to form the brachial plexus *(open arrow)*. The carotid bifurcation is demonstrated *(solid arrow)*. **C,** the thyroid gland *(arrowhead)* is noted, as is the larynx *(arrow)*.

Axial images are obtained by using gradient-refocused, T2-weighted sequences. T1-weighted sequences are acquired if necessary. T1-weighted sequences are most helpful postoperatively because metal artifact is less prominent than on gradient-refocused images. The parameters for gradient-refocused images are similar to those used in the sagittal acquisitions. The images are obtained by using oblique planes passing through the planes of the disk and neural foramina. A minimum of three slices are obtained at pathologic levels.

Because the exit zone is oriented at a 45-degree angle to the neural canal, oblique imaging is required for cross-sectional study of the neural foramina. This acquisition is not a part of the routine study but is used in cases of obscure unilateral radiculopathy. Gated spin-echo T2-weighted studies and/or T1-weighted images are acquired by using the same sequences described for the respective sagittal acquisitions.

Normal Anatomy

The spinal cord can be visualized on the coronal images over varying distances depending on the degree of lordosis (Fig 35–8). The exiting roots are imaged and can be traced to the brachial plexus. The major vessels of the aortic arch and neck are identified by their flow void. The supraclavicular area and thyroid gland are also visualized.

A T1-weighted sagittal sequence (500/20) will demonstrate the vertebral bodies and the entire intervertebral disk. The cervical cord is clearly seen because of its moderate signal intensity surrounded by the low-intensity CSF. Because the neural foramina are obliquely oriented to the neural canal, they are not ideally visualized in this plane. The posterior cervical tissues as well as the pharynx, larynx, and thyroid can be evaluated (Fig 35–9).

T2-weighted sagittal images, whether obtained by spin-echo or gradient-refocused sequences, produce an image that has the appearance of a lateral cervical myelogram. Unlike myelography, MRI visualizes the spinal cord directly, surrounded by the signal-intense CSF. On spin-echo acquisitions, the nuclei of the intervertebral disks are variably intense, and the criteria for degenerative disk disease, so reliable in the lumbar spine, are less obvi-

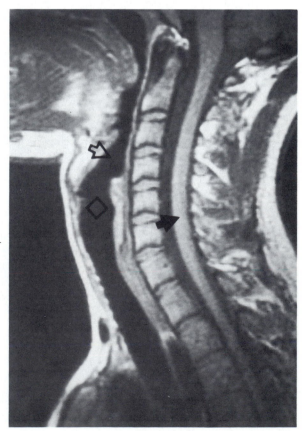

FIG 35–9.
Sagittal T1-weighted image of the cervical spine (SE, TR = 500 ms, TE = 20 ms, 2 NEX, 3-mm-thick slice, 256 × 192). Note the cervical cord *(solid arrow)*. There is signal void in the pharynx *(open arrow)* and larynx *(diamond)*. Again note the loss of delineation of the annulus, the posterior longitudinal ligament, and the CSF.

ous in the cervical region. Also the low signal of the annulus fibrosus, the posterior longitudinal ligament, and the dura is indistinguishable, thus making evaluation of the disk-CSF interface imprecise (Fig 35–10). Gradient-refocused studies are particularly useful in distinguishing the high signal of disk from the low signal of bone. The ligament-dura complex is seen as a thin black line between the white signal of the disk and the white signal of the CSF (Fig 35–11).

On T2-weighted axial studies obtained by gradient-refocused sequences, the bone has low signal, while the disk images with a high signal (Fig 35–12). These sequences are very useful in evaluating the bone-CSF interface. The signal-intense CSF clearly outlines the lower-signal spinal cord white matter and dentate ligaments. The cord central gray matter is discernible as signal intense, and the CSF outlines the exiting root sleeves within the neural foramina (Fig 35–13). T1-

weighted axial images are particularly useful to study spinal cord, bone, and paraspinal abnormalities.

The venous structures are best visualized on the gradient-recalled, T2-weighted axial images. They are signal intense and can be separated from the intense CSF by the signal-poor dura (Fig 35–14). The size and number of these structures in the cervical canal is impressive and should not be confused with vascular abnormalities.[11]

THE THORACIC SPINE

Technical Considerations

Imaging the thoracic spine has problems similar to but more complex than examinations of the cervical spine. This section of the vertebral column is affected by the transverse pulsation of the heart and the respiratory movement of the lungs in

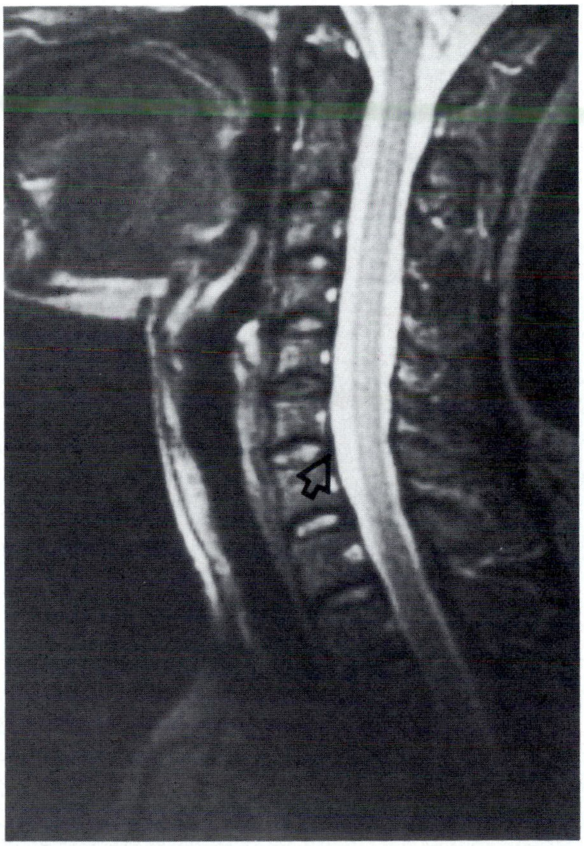

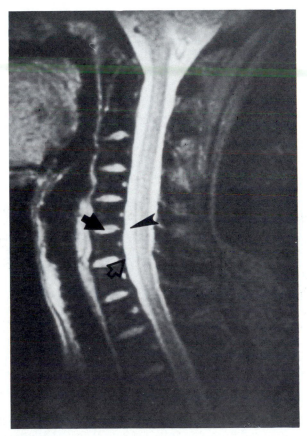

FIG 35–10.
Sagittal, T2-weighted, cardiac-gated image of the cervical spine (SE, TR = 2400 ms, TE = 80 ms, 1 NEX, 3-mm-thick slice, 256 × 192). Flow compensation was also used. Note the decreased signal from the confluence of the annulus fibrosis, the posterior longitudinal ligament, and the dura *(arrow)*.

FIG 35–11.
Sagittal, T2-weighted, gradient-refocused image of the cervical spine (TR = 400 ms, TE = 20 ms, flip angle = 12 degrees, 4 NEX, 3-mm-thick slice, 256 × 192). Note the signal-intense disk *(solid arrow)* and signal-intense CSF *(arrowhead)* sandwiching the posterior longitudinal ligament and dura *(open arrow)*.

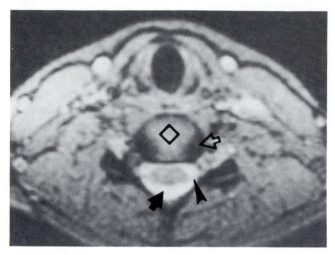

FIG 35–12.
Gradient-refocused, T2-weighted axial image of the cervical spine (TR = 400 ms, TE = 18 ms, flip angle = 12 degrees, 4 NEX, 3-mm-thick slice, 256 × 192). Note the increased signal from the disk *(diamond)*, the signal void from the cortical bone *(open arrow)*, and the dentate ligaments laterally *(arrowhead)*. The signal-intense CSF *(solid arrow)* outlines the spinal cord and dentate ligaments.

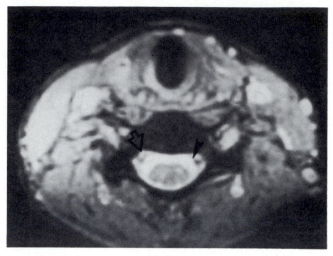

FIG 35–14.
Gradient-refocused, T2-weighted axial image of the cervical spine (TR = 350 ms, TE = 18 ms, flip angle = 12 degrees, 4 NEX, 3-mm-thick slice, 256 × 192). Note the signal-intense epidural veins *(arrow)*. The dura *(arrowhead)* is of low signal intensity, while the vein demonstrates increased signal from the slow venous flow.

addition to the vertical pulsatile movement of the blood and the CSF through the thorax. Sequences must therefore be designed to curtail motion artifacts in perpendicular planes in order to obtain high-quality images of the thoracic spine.

If the phase-encoding direction is anterior to posterior, then swapping the frequency and phase-encoding directions can change the cardiac and respiratory artifacts to an inferosuperior direction, which places them anterior to the vertebral column. Since the phase-encoding direction is then running along the vertical axis of the body, there is more tissue than available field of view, which results in "phase wrap." This phenomenon can be suppressed by software. Flow artifacts may also be greatly reduced by several methods. Saturation or "killer" pulses may be used to supress flow-related enhancement perpendicular to the imaging plane. Cardiac gating and flow compensation (gradient

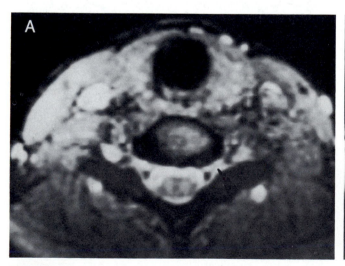

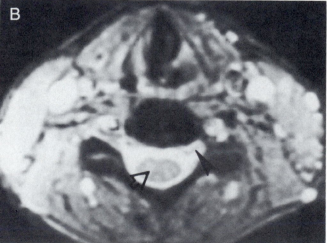

FIG 35–13.
Gradient-refocused, T2-weighted axial images of the cervical spine (TR = 350 ms, TE = 18 ms, flip angle = 12 degrees, 4 NEX, 3-mm-thick slice, 256 × 192). **A,** note the exiting nerve roots *(arrowhead)* in the neural foramen on the left. **B,** the signal-intense central gray matter *(arrow)* is surrounded by low-signal white matter. Note the exiting root *(arrowhead)* on the left course under the pedicle and into the neural foramen.

moment nulling) can also be employed. The principle of flow compensation is to balance phase shifts for both stationary and moving spins. Respiratory gating or compensation is usually not required.

A large-field sagittal image is first obtained by using the body coil and must include the odontoid process. This permits identification of the various thoracic vertebral levels. A T1-weighted coronal localizing study is acquired that yields five 5-mm-thick sections, each separated by 2.5 mm. These images demonstrate the thoracic cord and the paraspinal tissues.

By using the technique of swapping phase and frequency with phase wrap suppression, a series of proton-density and T2-weighted sagittal locations (usually seven) are acquired that extend from foramen to foramen with the center slice in the midline of the neural canal. All images in the thoracic region are 3 mm thick with an interslice gap of 1.5 mm. A 32-cm FOV with two excitations and a high-resolution matrix (256 × 256 or 256 × 192) is used. The TR is minimally 2,000 ms, with two echos of

30 and 80 ms. Signal is received by a large rectangular surface coil placed beneath the patient and centered on the thoracic spine. These may be obtained with spin-echo sequences similar to those used in the cervical spine, i.e., cardiac gated acquisitions with flow compensation, or with gradient-refocused techniques. A T1-weighted study may also be obtained to visualize the spinal cord.

Axial images are obtained at pathologic levels by using T1-weighted images and T2-weighted gradient-refocused images.

Normal Anatomy

The coronal view, depending on the degree of kyphosis, demonstrates varying lengths of the spinal cord. The vertebral bodies, paraspinal tissues, and portions of the aorta are well visualized (Fig 35–15).

The proton-density and T2-weighted spin-echo sagittal studies are the most revealing: they demonstrate the anteriorly positioned spinal cord surrounded by CSF and the conus medullaris. The

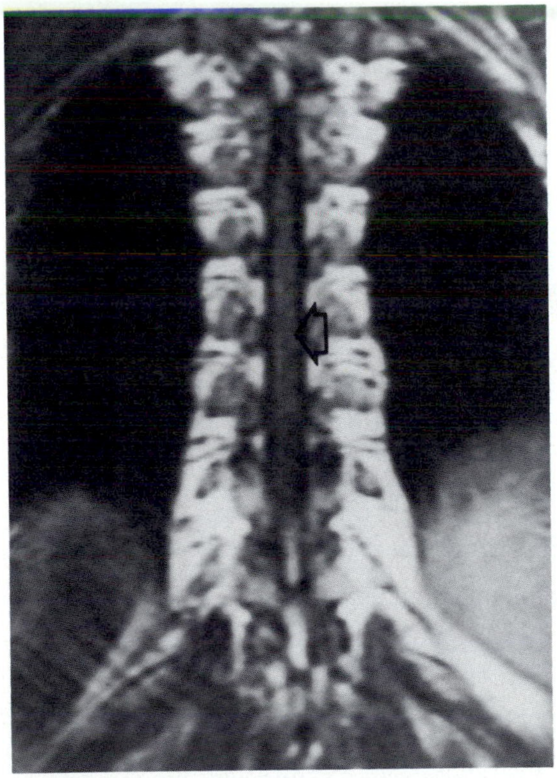

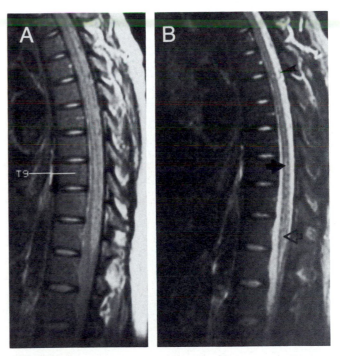

FIG 35–15.
Coronal T1-weighted image through the thoracic spine (SE, TR = 400 ms, TE = 20 ms, 2 NEX, 5-mm-thick slice, 256 × 128). Note the cord *(arrow)* surrounded by low-signal CSF and the paraspinal structures.

FIG 35–16.
Proton-density **(A)** and T2-weighted **(B)** cardiac-gated sagittal images of the thoracic spine (SE, TR = 2,400 ms, TE = 30/80 ms, 2 NEX, 3-mm-thick slice, 256 × 192). Frequency- and phase-encoding directions were swapped to reduce cardiac pulsation artifacts anteriorly and displace them away from the spine. Flow compensation was used. The cord *(closed arrow)* and the conus *(open arrow)* are surrounded by CSF. The venous channels *(arrowhead)* are noted dorsally.

neural foramina have migrated from their 45-degree orientation in the cervical region to a more parallel position relative to the transverse plane of the spine and are well seen in the sagittal plane. The exiting roots, surrounded by fat, can be identified in the inferior portion of the foramina. Extensive vascular channels, usually posterior, are visualized on gated and nongated examinations and should not be confused with vascular malformations (Fig 35–16).

The hydrated nucleus of the normal intervertebral disk is routinely appreciated, and this structure should remain within the disk space. The relationship of the nucleus to the CSF of the anterior subarachnoid space can be assessed.

Attention should be paid to the vertebral bodies that contain yellow marrow. The fatty nature of the marrow yields a high signal on T1-weighted images, but this fades with progressive T2 weighting. There are instances of foci of high signal on the proton-density images that fade on T2 weighting. These are presumed to represent intraosseous lipomatous deposits and are of no clinical consequence (Fig 35–17). On other occasions, areas of

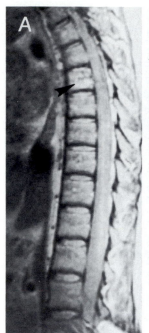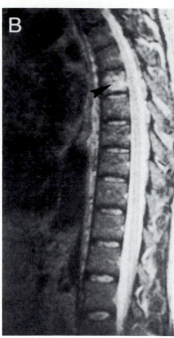

FIG 35–18.
Sagittal proton-density **(A)** and T2-weighted **(B)** cardiac-gated image of the thoracic spine (SE, TR = 2,000 ms, TE = 30/80 ms, 2 NEX, 3-mm-thick slice, 256 × 256). Flow compensation was used. Note the irregular area of increased signal involving the T6 thoracic vertebra *(arrowhead)*. The signal is the same on proton-density and T2-weighted images. This represents a hemangioma.

high signal are seen on both proton-density and T2-weighted studies. These are thought to represent hemangiomas and may be seen occupying portions of or the entire vertebral body. As long as the lesion remains confined to the vertebral body, it, too, is of no clinical moment (Fig 35–18). On the other hand, lesions that have low signal on T1 images and become bright on T2 images should be regarded with suspicion, for this is the imaging pattern of infiltrative processes such as metastatic disease.

THE LUMBAR SPINE

Technical Considerations

Like the other portions of the spine, the lumbar region is best imaged by surface coil. Ideally the study should cover an area from the lower dorsal spine including the conus medullaris to the end of the thecal sac, usually about S2. In most patients, this can be accomplished by using a 24-cm field of view and a rectangular ("license plate") coil. Since the structures are larger in the lower portion of the spine, 5-mm-thick slices are usually adequate in the sagittal plane, although axial stud-

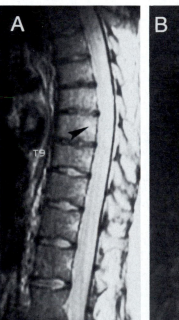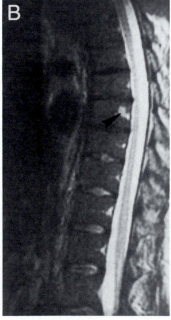

FIG 35–17.
Proton-density **(A)** and T2-weighted **(B)** cardiac-gated sagittal image of the thoracic spine (SE, TR = 2,400 ms, TE = 30/80 ms, 2 NEX, 3-mm-thick slice, 256 × 192). Flow compensation was used. Note the area of fatty deposit *(arrowhead)* in the T8 thoracic vertebra: it demonstrates increased signal on the proton-density image and then fades in intensity on the T2-weighted image. Incidental note of degenerative changes at the T6–7, T7–8, and T8–9 levels should be made. There is slight buckling of the annulus posteriorly at these levels.

ies are normally accomplished with 3- or 4-mm-thick slices. Spinal fluid motion is less of a problem in the caudal sac, but using a flow-compensating sequence will improve the images by reducing CSF motion artifact.

Five localizing images are obtained in the coronal plane by using a TR of 400 ms, TE of 20 ms, 256 × 128 matrix, 1 NEX, and a 32-cm field of view. Phase-wrap suppression is employed, and the study is centered at L3–4.

Using the coronal localizer, proton-density and T2-weighted spin-echo sagittal images are acquired at seven 5-mm sagittal locations with an interslice gap of 1.5 mm, with a TR of 2,000 ms and TEs of 30 and 80 ms. Flow compensation is used. Ideally the initial TE should be 20 ms, but the flow compensation program limits the use of echo delays below 30 ms. The field of view is 24 cm, with a 256 × 192 matrix and 2 NEX. Only spin-echo techniques are used for sagittal imaging in the lumbar region because the gradient-refocused sequences fail to differentiate early degenerative changes from normal disks.

Axial studies are carried out on all pathologic levels. New software permits multislice multiangle acquisitions, and consequently all five lumbar disks can be imaged through the plane of the disk in one series. A minimum of three 3- to 4-mm-thick slices through the disk are obtained that pass through the inferior, middle, and superior compart-ments of the neural foramina. T1-weighted images are obtained with a minimum TR/TE of 500/20, a 256 × 192 matrix, 4 NEX, and a 24-cm field of view, and saturation pulses may be used to reduce flow artifact but are usually not necessary. As stated previously, T2-weighted, gradient-refocused axial images give better detail of the facet joints and cartilage than do T2-weighted, spin-echo axial sequences. For this reason a T2-weighted, gradient-refocused series is obtained by using 350/18 with a θ of 25 degrees, 4 NEX, and a 24-cm field of view.

Oblique imaging may also be used to evaluate the facet joints; this produces images having the same appearance as the familiar "scotty dogs" of the lumbar plain films. These are acquired with T1-weighted sequences oriented perpendicular to the joint of interest.

Oblique imaging is also useful in correcting for scoliosis of the lumbar spine. A correction is applied along the y-axis, which tends to "straighten out" the curvature and permit more accurate sagittal imaging. By using this (straightened out) sagittal image, a second angle may be used to obtain true axial images (see Fig 35–4,A–D).

Normal Anatomy

Coronal T1-weighted images demonstrate the spinal erector musculature on the initial studies.

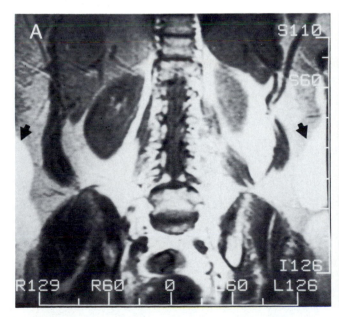
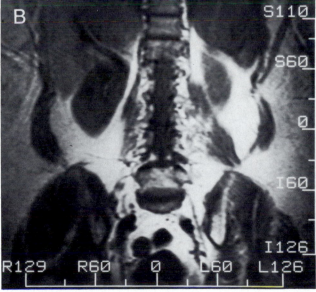

FIG 35–19.
T1-weighted, coronal-localizing images of the lumbar spine (SE, TR = 400 ms, TE = 20 ms, 1 NEX, 5-mm-thick slice, 256 × 128). Flow compensation was used. **A,** without phase wrap. Notice the fold over artifact *(arrow)* on both edges from tissue outside the field of view. **B,** with phase wrap. This artifact is eliminated.

Moving anteriorly, the images visualize the posterior elements, the retrothecal fat pads, the thecal sac and exiting roots and ganglia, and the yellow marrow of the vertebral bodies. The disks can be seen as linear regions of intermediate signal, and hypertrophic changes in the lumbar spine can be appreciated. The kidneys and perirenal areas, the psoas musculature, and the upper structures in the bony pelvis may be evaluated along with portions of the abdominal vascular structures. The liver and spleen are imaged in the upper portion of the abdomen, but care must be taken to avoid calling fold over artifacts pathologic processes. This can be minimized by using phase-wrap suppression (Fig 35–19). By using this suppression the software reduces the number of averages, NEX, by half; however, the SNR remains the same, so there is no loss of image quality.

The sagittal images are the principal diagnostic views yielding essential information on the state of hydration of the intervertebral disk and the size of the thecal sac. Spin-echo proton-density and T2-weighted sequences are the techniques of choice. The fatty marrow of the vertebral bodies outlines these structures on the proton-density images and fades significantly on the T2-weighted images. As previously mentioned, various increased signals can be found in normal vertebrae, most likely representing lipomas or hemangiomas. The anterior internal vertebral plexus (AIVP) can be identified, and the basivertebral vein can be followed as it en-

ters the midportion of the vertebral body. The posterior longitudinal ligament can be seen posterior to the AIVP, attached to the annular fibers at the disk space, and stretched across the posterior concavity of the vertebral body. The posterior longitudinal ligament thins as it extends laterally. The anterior longitudinal ligament can also be identified as a line of low signal characteristic of fibrous structures outlining the anterior aspect of the annulus. The ligament merges imperceptibly with the anterior cortical surface of the vertebral body. The major abdominal vasculature can be identified by the flow void, but this effect is diminished with flow compensation (Fig 35–20).

The normal disk is composed of two elements, the nucleus pulposus, which is composed of a hydrophilic mucopolysaccharide/collagen gel, and the annulus fibrosus, composed of concentric layers of collagen fibers (Sharpey's fibers) that run obliquely between the adjacent vertebral bodies. While some differentiation of these structures is possible on the proton-density images, the true nature of the hydrated nucleus surrounded by the signal-poor annulus is clearly seen on the T2-weighted images (see Fig 35–1,B). The anatomic separation of these elements is not as definite as MRI studies would suggest, but the state of hydration as an indicator of nuclear health and age is obvious on the long TR, long TE studies. This information is virtually absent on T1-weighted images. The nucleus is actually composed of two some-

FIG 35–20.
Proton-density **(A)** and T2-weighted **(B)** sagittal images of the lumbar spine (SE, TR = 2,000 ms, TE = 30/80 ms, 2 NEX, 5-mm-thick slice, 256 × 192). Flow compensation was used. Note the basivertebral vein *(large arrowhead)* enter the vertebral body from the AIVP. Note the signal-poor posterior longitudinal ligament and dura *(open arrow)*, which are inseparable. They are posterior to the AIVP and stretch over the posterior concavity of the vertebral body. The anterior longitudinal ligament *(solid arrow)* is noted as a line of low signal. Note the left renal vein *(small arrowhead)* pass between the aorta and superior mesenteric artery.

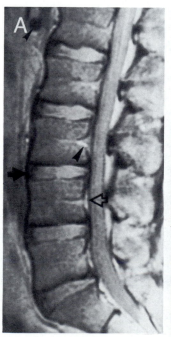
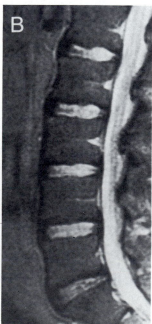

what ameboid cavities stacked on each other and connected by an isthmus that is surrounded by a fibrous annulus. The "cleft" seen on the sagittal images in the center of most of the nuclei is actually the interposition of annular fibers between these two nuclear cavities as seen from the side. The anterior and posterior extremities of the nucleus are bullet shaped, and there is a decrease in signal anteriorly and posteriorly as a result of volume averaging of the nucleus and annulus (Fig 35–21). The thecal sac can be examined as well as the neural structures it contains. The fluid is signal poor on T1-weighted images, and the conus medullaris and roots of the cauda equina are of moderate signal. With progressive T2 weighting, these signals reverse, and the low signal rootlets are outlined by the signal-intense CSF. The various rootlets can be traced to their exit levels with considerable accuracy (Fig 35–22).

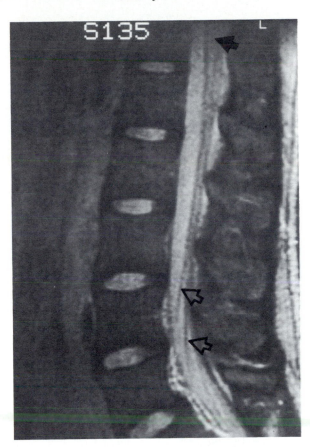

FIG 35–22.
T2-weighted sagittal lumbar image (SE, TR = 2,000 ms, TE = 80 ms, 2 NEX, 5-mm-thick slice, 256 × 192). Flow compensation was used. Note the rootlets *(open arrows)* descend anteriorly from the conus *(closed arrow)* to exit under the pedicles at the appropriate levels.

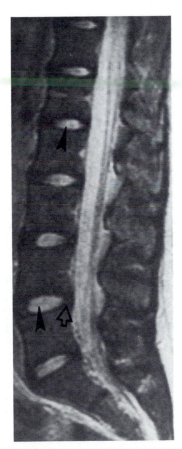

FIG 35–21.
T2-weighted sagittal image of the lumbar spine (SE, TR = 2,000 ms, TE = 80 ms, 2 NEX, 5-mm-thick slice, 256 × 256). Flow compensation was used. Note the fibrous clefts *(arrowheads)* in the various disks as well as a decrease in signal anteriorly and posteriorly secondary to volume averaging of the annulus *(arrow).*

The vertical position of the neural foramina makes the sagittal plane ideal for the evaluation of these structures. The exiting nerve root can be seen as a moderate-signal structure surrounded by perineural fat and accompanied by the sinovertebral artery as it passes beneath the superior margin of the foramen (Fig 35–23). The midportion and the inferior aspect of the foramen are filled with fat and small vessels that can be identified by their flow void. The neural foramen is defined superiorly and inferiorly by the pedicles of the adjacent vertebral bodies. The posterior longitudinal ligament and the annulus form the anterior margin of the lower third of the foramen. The profile of the facet joints and ligamentum flavum can be seen to form the posterior margin of the foramen.[12] The yellow marrow of the articular facets is bounded by the low signal of the cortical bone. The intermediate signal of the articular cartilage of the joint is interposed between the cortical surfaces of the

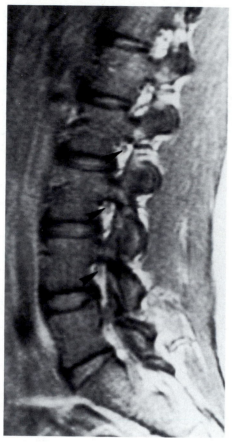

FIG 35–23.
Proton-density sagittal lumbar image through the neural foramen (SE, TR = 2,000 ms, TE = 20 ms, 2 NEX, 5-mm-thick slice, 256 × 256). Flow compensation was used. Note the exiting nerve roots *(arrowheads)* in the upper third of the neural foramina.

superior and inferior facets. Occasionally a fat pad may be seen in the superior aspect of the facet joint (Fig 35–24).

T1-weighted axial images are useful for evaluating the size and contour of the thecal sac. The T1-weighted sequence images the fat in the bone marrow as bright signal and the water in the disk as a lower-signal structure (Fig 35–25,A and B). However, determining slice location as being through the vertebral body or disk based on T1-weighted axial image signal intensity alone is not as reliable as on T2-weighted axial images. This is because of partial-volume artifact and imprecise slice location as well as moderate differences of signal intensity between the disk and vertebral body, particularly in younger people where the red marrow has not been replaced by fat as occurs in osteoporosis. On the T1-weighted axial images the signal-intense epidural fat containing the venous structures can be seen, and the exiting roots and

ganglia are detected within the neural foramina (Fig 35–26,A and B). The retrothecal fat pad is seen along with the ligamentum flavum, to which the anterior recess of the facet joint is attached. Occasionally, a fine line of decreased signal is visible between the articular cartilages of the facet joints, presumably representing a small amount of fluid. The previously described fat pad may be imaged at the superior portion of the facet joint, even projecting into the joint itself. T1-weighted images are excellent for the visualization of paraspinal anatomy, i.e., the psoas muscles and the retroperitoneal structures.

T2-weighted axial images obtained by gradient-refocused sequences image the CSF as high signal and the bone as low signal, thus giving excellent bone-CSF interface differentiation. Nuclear material images with high signal and is surrounded by low-signal annulus fibrosus. This appearance of the disk is opposite that on T1-weighted images, and slice location through the disk is much more apparent on T2 axial images than on T1 axial im-

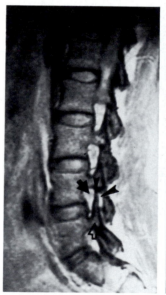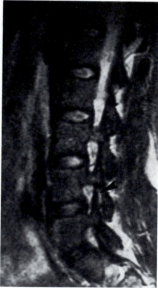

FIG 35–24.
Sagittal proton-density **(A)** and T2-weighted **(B)** off-center images through the facet joints and neural foramina of the lumbar spine (SE, TR = 2,000 ms, TE = 30/80 ms, 2 NEX, 5-mm-thick slice, 256 × 192). Flow compensation was used. On the proton-density image note the nerve root *(solid arrow)* in the upper third of the neural foramen. The fat pad *(large arrowhead)* in the upper portion of the facet joint is demonstrated, and its signal fades on the T2-weighted image. The ligamentum flavum *(small arrowhead)* and the superior articulating facet *(open arrow)* of the lower lumbar vertebra form the posterior aspect of the foramen. The anterior surface is formed by the annulus and posterior longitudinal ligament. Superiorly and inferiorly the pedicles of the adjacent vertebral bodies form the remaining borders.

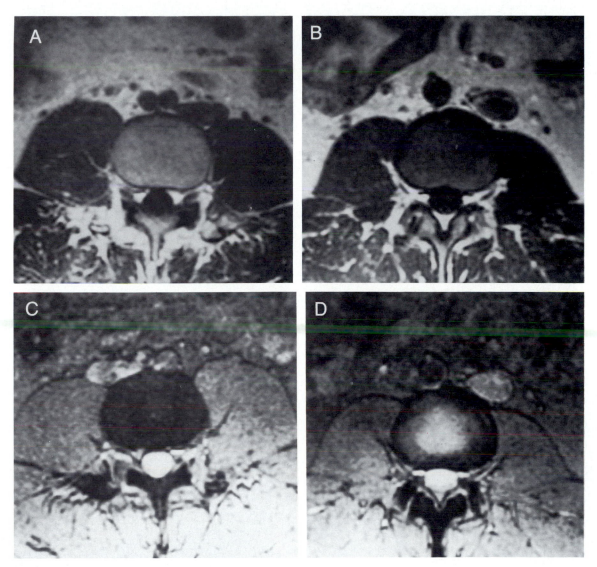

FIG 35–25.

T1-weighted and T2-weighted gradient-refocused axial images through the vertebral body and disk space of a lumbar vertebra. **A** and **B,** SE, TR = 600 ms, TE = 20 ms, 4 NEX, 4-mm-thick slice, 256 × 192. **C** and **D,** TR = 250 ms, TE = 18 ms, flip angle = 25 degrees, 4 NEX, 4-mm-thick slice, 256 × 192. **A,** T1-weighted axial image through a lumbar vertebral body. **B,** through a lumbar disk space. **C,** same location as **A** but is a T2 gradient-refocused image. **D,** same location as **B** but also is a T2-weighted, gradient-re-focused image. Note the increased signal in the fat in the marrow of the vertebral body on the T1-weighted axial image **(A).** The opposite findings are seen in **C,** which is a T2-weighted, gradient-refocused axial image. In **B,** the disk is signal poor as compared with the fat of the marrow on the T1 image. On the T2 axial image **(D),** one sees the signal-intense disk centrally, with the signal decreasing as one goes peripherally to the annulus.

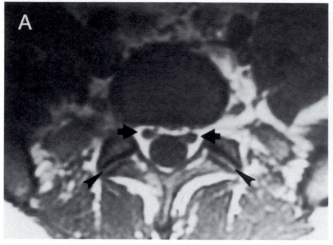

FIG 35–26.
Axial T1-weighted images through the lumbar spine at different levels through the neural foramina (SE, TR = 500 ms, TE = 20 ms, 4 NEX, 4-mm-thick slice, 256 × 192). **A,** through the inferior portion of the neural foramina at L5–S1. Note the descending S1 roots *(arrows)* anterior and lateral to the thecal sac. The articular cartilage *(arrowheads)* of the facet joints is demonstrated and is of moder-ate signal intensity. **B,** through the upper portion of the neural foramina. The dorsal root ganglia *(arrows)* are demonstrated bilaterally. The thecal sac and descending roots as well as the dorsal ganglia are surrounded by signal-intense fat. Multiple small vessels are seen between the thecal sac and the vertebral body. These are of low signal intensity.

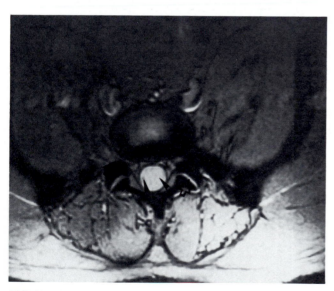

FIG 35–27.
T2-weighted, gradient-refocused axial image through the lumbar spine (TR = 350 ms, TE = 18 ms, flip angle = 25 degrees, 4 NEX, 4-mm-thick slice, 256 × 192). Note the intermediate signal from the rootlets *(arrowheads)* surrounded by signal-intense CSF. Also note the signal-intense articular cartilage of the facet joint *(open arrow)* blend with the ligamentum flavum. Note the exiting nerve root *(solid arrow)* in the neural foramen on the right.

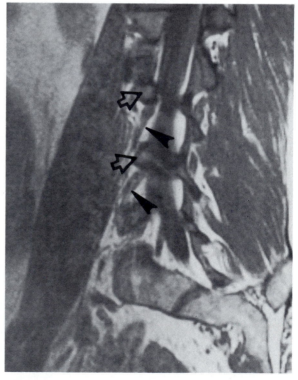

FIG 35–28.
T1-weighted oblique image through the pedicles of the lumbar spine (SE, TR = 600 ms, TE = 20 ms, 4 NEX, 3-mm-thick slice, 256 × 256). Note the nerve roots *(arrowheads)* exit beneath the pedicles *(arrows)*.

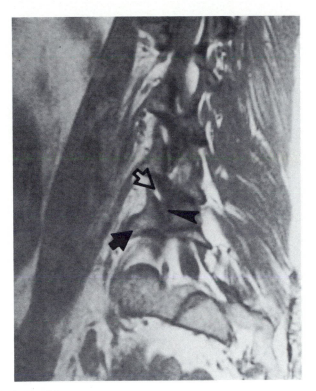

FIG 35–29.
T1-weighted oblique image through the facet joints of the lumbar spine (SE, TR = 600 ms, TE = 20 ms, 4 NEX, 3-mm-thick slice, 256 × 256). Note the moderate signal from the articular cartilage *(arrowhead)*, fat pad *(open arrow)* in the superior aspect of the facet joint, and the "scotty dog" appearance of the articular facets *(solid arrow)*.

ages (see Fig 35–25,C and D). The articular cartilage of the facet joint images brightly. The rootlets are seen as intermediate signal surmounted by the intense signal of the CSF (Fig 35–27).

Oblique images can demonstrate the origin of the nerve root sleeves and the axillary regions with exquisite detail. The roots can be traced through the neural foramina and into the paraspinal area (Fig 35–28). The relationship of the root to the pedicle is well visualized. This projection will also produce the "scotty dog" appearance of the ipsilateral neural arch. The structures of the facet joint described above can be seen with clarity (Fig 35–29).

SUMMARY

MRI studies of the spine have become more popular and more useful as the acquisition tech-niques have improved. Thin slices, high-resolution matrices, reasonable study times, and visualization of the planes of interest have all combined to increase the demand for these examinations. In many hands, the added information without the need for radiation or contrast has made MRI of the spine the first evaluation. The radiologist is obligated to become familiar with the technical and anatomic information necessary to best serve his patients.

REFERENCES

1. Mitchell DG, Burk DL Jr, Vinitski S, The biophysical basis of tissue contrast in extracranial MR imaging. *AJR* 1987; 149:831–837.
2. Axel L: Surface coil magnetic resonance imaging. *J Comput Assist Tomogr* 1984; 8:381–384.
3. Berger PE, Atkinson D, Wilson WJ, et al: High resolution surface coil magnetic imaging of the spine: Normal and pathological anatomy. *Radiographics* 1986; 6:573–601.
4. Rubin JB, Enzmann DR, Wright A: CSF-gated MR imaging of the spine: Theory and clinical implementation. *Radiology* 1987; 163:784–792.
5. Edelman RR, Stark DD, Saini S, et al: Oblique planes of section in MR imaging. *Radiology* 1986; 159:807–810.
6. Reicher MA, Lufkin RB, Smith S, et al: Multiple-angle, variable-interval, nonorthogonal MRI. *AJR* 1986; 147:363–366.
7. Gallimore GW Jr, Harms SE: Selective three dimensional MR imaging of the spine. *J Comput Assist Tomogr* 1987; 11:124–128.
8. Wehrli FW: *Introduction to Fast-Scan Magnetic Resonance.* Milwaukee, General Electric Co, 1986.
9. Wener L, Cohen PAM, Schulof R, et al: Imaging studies of skeletal metastatic problems. Presented at the 72nd RSNA, Chicago, December 1986.
10. Schellinger DR, Wener L, Ragsdale BD, et al: Facet joint disorders and their role in the production of back pains and sciatica. *Radiographics* 1987; 7:923–944.
11. Flannigan BD, Lufkin RB, McGlade C, et al: MR imaging or the cervical spine: Neurovascular anatomy. *AJNR* 1987; 8:27–32.
12. Ho PSP, Yu S, Sether L, et al: Ligamentum flavum: Apperance on sagittal and coronal MR images. *Radiology* 1988; 168:469–471.

36

CT of Degenerative and Nonneoplastic Spine Disorders

Susan S. Kemp, M.D.

Jeffrey M. Rogg, M.D.

Since the publication of the first edition of this work, magnetic resonance imaging (MRI) has evolved as an important imaging modality for evaluation of spinal disorders. However, MRI has not replaced computed tomography (CT) and myelography in the evaluation of radiculopathy.[1] Each modality has specific advantages. Preliminary prospective reports suggest that the complimentary use of MRI and CT may increase diagnostic accuracy[2, 3] and together they may provide a noninvasive alternative to myelography.[2, 3]

High-resolution CT scanners are currently capable of thinner sections than MRI scanners are. CT images provide superior distinction between soft tissue and bone, particularly in the lateral spinal canal and neural foramina.[1-4] MRI provides noninvasive evaluation of the spinal cord and subarachnoid space and produces multiplanar information without the image degradation inherent in CT reformations.

The following discussion will examine the current CT evaluation of intervertebral disk disease, spinal stenosis, and nonneoplastic disorders of the craniocervial junction.

ATLANTOAXIAL DISORDERS

A variety of nonneoplastic disorders may give rise to atlantoaxial instability. In addition to rheumatoid arthritis (RA), these include ankylosing spondylitis (AS),[5] Down syndrome,[6, 7] pharyngeal infection,[5] and os odontoideum. AS may result in odontoid erosion and mild atlantoaxial subluxation that is less severe than in RA.[8] Atlantoaxial instability is much less frequent in AS than RA.[5]

Atlantoaxial subluxation may occur in as many as 20% of patients with Down syndrome.[6, 7] Although the etiology is uncertain, there is speculation that laxity of the transverse ligament is responsible. Alternatively, there may be abnormal development of the odontoid process.[7]

Os odontoideum represents an unfused apical segment of the odontoid process. There is debate as to whether this is congenital[9] or acquired, possibly due to trauma.[10] This abnormality results in instability of the atlantoaxial articulation with the possibility of subluxation and cord compression[11] (Fig 36-1).

CT Findings

Plain films in flexion are necessary to identify atlantoaxial subluxation. Plain films in extension and conventional tomography are useful to further define the bony anatomy and to demonstrate encroachment upon the spinal canal. Noncontrast CT is useful for evaluation of the bony spinal canal and ligamentous anatomy, and provides some information regarding encroachment upon the subarachnoid space.[6] Intrathecal contrast may be necessary to better define cord compression.[7, 12, 13]

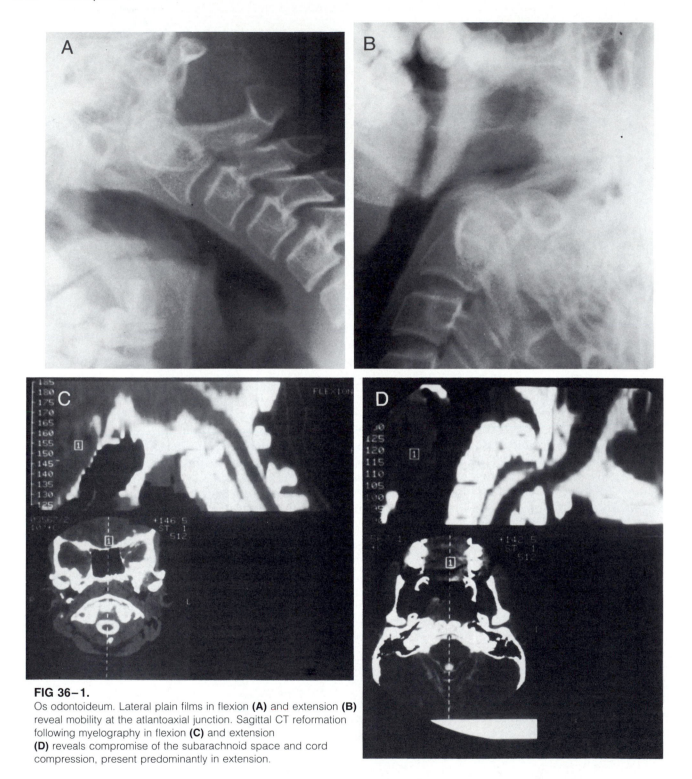

FIG 36–1.
Os odontoideum. Lateral plain films in flexion **(A)** and extension **(B)** reveal mobility at the atlantoaxial junction. Sagittal CT reformation following myelography in flexion **(C)** and extension **(D)** reveals compromise of the subarachnoid space and cord compression, present predominantly in extension.

Axial images and sagittal reformations[12] may be performed in flexion and extension[13] (Fig 36–1,C and D) or neutral positions to provide information regarding mobility. MRI can assess the degree of cord compression without the need for instillation of intrathecal contrast.

CERVICAL SPINE DISORDERS

Rheumatoid Arthritis

The cervical spine is commonly affected in RA.[8, 14] Rheumatoid synovitis results in ligamentous abnormality and eventual rupture, articular cartilage destruction, and bony changes that include osteoporosis, erosion, and cyst formation.[15] These changes cause alignment abnormalities that most frequently involve the craniovertebral and upper cervical levels.[16] Atlantoaxial impaction (also known as vertical subluxation, cranial settling, or pseudobasilar invagination) results from bony erosion of occipitoatlantal and atlantoaxial joints. This may prove fatal as a result of medullary compression by the odontoid[17] or vertebral artery occlusion.[18]

Atlantoaxial subluxation (Figs 36–2 and 36–3) results from damage or disruption of the transverse alar and apical ligaments.[15] The subluxation is usually anterior,[15–17] but lateral subluxation and rare posterior subluxation may occur. The latter can only occur if there is an odontoid abnormality such as massive erosion, fracture, or congenital deformity.[17] Atlantoaxial subluxation may occur early and becomes significantly more common later in the course of RA.[14]

The likelihood of developing neurologic signs appears to be influenced by the following factors: gender (being more prominent in males); degree of subluxation, particularly if it is greater than 9 mm; and the presence of atlantoaxial impaction.[16] Lateral atlantoaxial subluxation may also predispose the patient to the development of neurologic findings.[16] Atlantoaxial impaction developing in the presence of atlantoaxial subluxation may actually reduce the measured C1–2 subluxation in spite of progressive narrowing of the spinal canal and spinal cord compression.[16, 19]

Subaxial subluxation may be identified at mul-

tiple levels early in the disease.[14] Erosive changes are characteristic of the disease, and the absence of osteophytes is a helpful distinction to identify rheumatoid changes.[20] However, discovertebral narrowing and osteophyte formation can occur and may represent superimposed degenerative changes in response to underlying rheumatoid abnormality.[14]

CT Findings

Lateral conventional C-spine radiography is the preferred screening examination.[21] Flexion and extension views are necessary to determine the degree of subluxation.[20, 21] CT, particularly with multiplanar reformation (see Fig 36–2), can demonstrate bony changes and canal encroachment and may add significant information to conventional tomography.[21] Flexion and neutral or extension CT views are helpful in assessing the degree of subluxation.[13, 17] Rotational subluxation may be better assessed by CT than by plain films.[19]

Noncontrast CT at the atlantoaxial junction demonstrates odontoid erosion (Fig 36–2,A), an increase in the preodontoid space (Fig 36–3,A), and thickening of the transverse ligament with decreased density identified between the ligament and the odontoid.[17] Additional CT findings include reduced anteroposterior (AP) diameter of the spinal canal at the atlantoaxial level, subaxial subluxations, coexisting osteophyte formation, and sclerosis.[17] In the case of atlantoaxial impaction, the odontoid process may be demonstrated within the foramen magnum (Fig 36–3,C).[17]

Myelography followed by contrast-enhanced

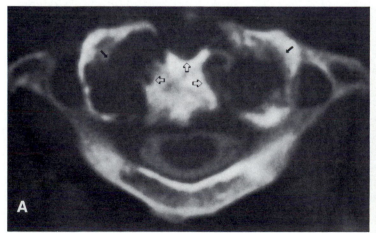

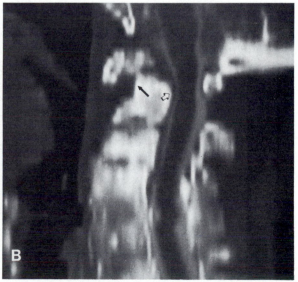

FIG 36–2.
Rheumatoid arthritis with atlantoaxial subluxation. **A,** an axial postmyelogram CT reveals erosive changes of the odontoid *(open arrows)* and atlas *(arrows).* **B,** sagittal reformations better illustrate the degree of subluxation *(arrow),* cord compression, and compromise of the subarachnoid space *(open arrow).*

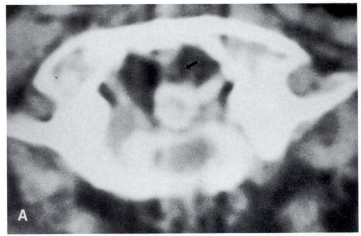

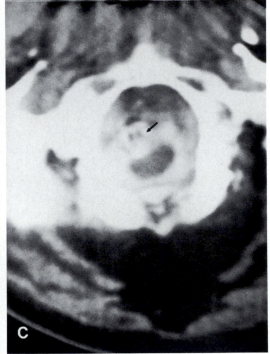

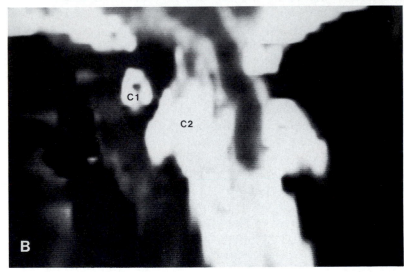

FIG 36–3.
Rheumatoid arthritis with atlantoaxial subluxation and cranial settling. **A,** axial postmyelogram CT. Note the marked prominence of the preodontoid space *(arrow)* and flattening of the cervical cord. **B,** sagittal reformation demonstrates marked subluxation and cord deformity. **C,** cranial settling as evidenced by the presence of the odontoid process within the foramen magnum *(arrow),* which is causing compression at the cervicomedullary junction.

CT is particularly helpful in the assessment of the degree of cord compression if atlantoaxial subluxation is severe (greater than 8 mm) and if there is atlantoaxial impaction.[19] CT with intrathecal contrast demonstrates cord deformity and atrophy better than myelography does alone (Figs 36–2,B and 36–3,B).[19] CT cisternography of the craniocervical junction employs lower contrast doses than myelography does and, with multiplanar reformations, provides an examination that may obviate the need for conventional myelography.[12]

Initial reports of MRI evaluation of the craniocervical junction in RA are promising.[22, 23] MRI may replace myelography due to superior cord visualization and assessment of clinically important features without the need for invasive procedures.[23]

Cervical Disk Herniation

Intervertebral disk herniation in the cervical spine is less frequent than in the lumbar spine. Of cases that come to surgery, the C5–6 level is the most frequently involved, followed by C6–7.[24, 25] C4–5, C3–4, and C7–T1 are involved in decreasing order of frequency and much less frequently than the first two stated levels.[25] A syndrome of acute disk herniation can be distinguished from chronic disk herniation. The former is seen most frequently in younger patients[25] with a history of antecedent trauma.[26] Radiculopathy and/or myelopathy may result from cervical disk herniation. Symptomatology is dependent upon the location and extent of the compression by the soft-tissue mass.

Cervical intervertebral disks are thin, and there is a paucity of epidural fat resulting in limited contrast within the cervical spinal canal. These anatomic features necessitate a tailored approach to CT of the cervical spine that includes thin (1.5 mm) sections with angulation through the intervertebral disks.[27, 28] A bolus injection of intravenous contrast[29–31] enhances the dura and epidural venous plexus and permits delineation of exiting nerve roots. CT examination may be performed following the introduction of intrathecal contrast for myelography.[32-35] This technique permits evaluation of the cord, exiting nerve roots, and surrounding subarachnoid space and outlines any disk protrusions.

A comparison of CT with myelography suggests that the accuracy of CT is equal to[36, 37] or better than myelography[38, 39] for disorders in the cervical spine. CT myelography may add significant additional information regarding characterization of the abnormality, lateralization if the myelogram was indeterminate, demonstration of the abnormalities distal to a block, and cord atrophy and foraminal narrowing not appreciated on myelography.[36, 40] CT with intrathecal contrast is more accurate than myelography is in the identification of central disk herniation[41]; however, investigators make the point that ventral abnormalities and bulging ligamenta flava appear less marked on CT myelography than on plain-film myelography.[36, 37, 42] This has been attributed to accentuation of these abnormalities in

hyperextension, the position required for myelography. Myelography is a practical examination to survey the entire cervical spine. A detailed CT examination directed toward abnormalities identified by myelography or suspected clinically can then be performed.[42]

A comparison of CT and surface-coil MRI in the evaluation of cervical radiculopathy suggests that CT is superior in evaluation of the neural foramina[3] and in distinguishing osteophyte from disk material. However, surface-coil MRI may be more effective in evaluation of the lower cervical interspaces where beam-hardening artifact from the shoulder limits the CT examination.[43, 44] Some authors suggest that MRI, because of its noninvasive nature, should be used as an initial screening examination coupled with plain films. In this scheme, CT with or without intrathecal contrast is reserved for difficult or questionable cases.

CT Findings

A cervical disk herniation on CT appears as a slightly hyperdense soft-tissue mass[31] projecting

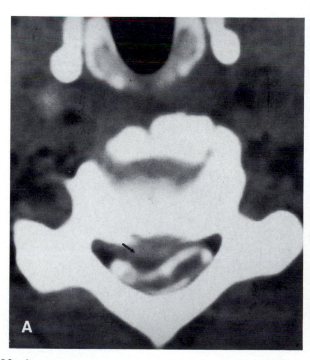
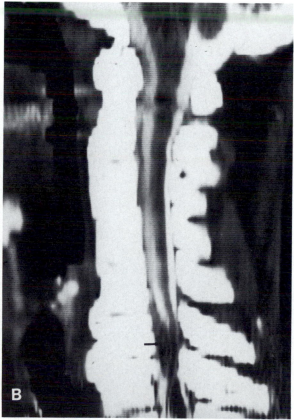

FIG 36-4.
Cervical disk herniation with cord compression. **A,** postmyelogram CT demonstrates disk herniation with marked cord compression *(arrow).* **B,** sagittal reformation also illustrates the degree of cord compression *(arrow).*

centrally, paracentrally, or posterolaterally from the disk space into the spinal canal[45] or neural foramen (Fig 36–4). The disk material is usually identified on several adjacent slices including at the disk level.[46] With intravenous enhancement, the slightly hyperdense disk material appears relatively lucent adjacent to an enhancing marginal blush (Fig 36–5).[30, 31] Free disk fragments may be surrounded by enhancement.[30] Retrocorporeal enhancement is normally not seen caudal to the C2–3 level,[30] and subtle disk herniations may be detected solely by the presence of linear enhancement posterior to the vertebral body without any subjacent lucency.

Compression of the thecal sac and distortion of the cord are better identified in the presence of intrathecal contrast (Fig 36–6).[28] Localized, sharply demarcated distortion of the thecal sac with a moderate- to large-sized extradural soft-tissue mass suggests that the disk has perforated the posterior longitudinal ligament.[47] Cord compression or rotation may be the secondary manifestation of a large herniated disk (Fig 36–7).[36]

There are rare reports of intradural herniation of disk material in the cervical spine. The intradural location of the disk fragment and its relationship to the cord are demonstrable on CT with intrathecal contrast.[48]

A rare condition known as calcification of the intervertebral disk occurs in childhood. This typically occurs in the lower cervical spine and may less frequently occur in the thoracic or lumbar spine.[49] Herniation of disk material may be demonstrated by CT as well as MRI.[50] This disorder typically pursues a benign clinical course with spontaneous resorption of the herniated nuclear material[49] and resolution of symptoms.[50]

Cervical Spinal Stenosis

Spinal stenosis represents narrowing of the spinal canal and may be congenital or acquired.[51] Achondroplasia with progressive stenosis of the canal in the craniocaudal direction is an example of congenital stenosis.[52] Subclinical developmental narrowing of the spinal canal[52] caused by short pedicles and thick laminae[53] may play an important role in the development of acquired spinal stenosis. Patients may become symptomatic only when degenerative changes occur later in life.[52] Spondylosis, Paget's disease,[54] and acromegaly[55] are examples of acquired etiologies for spinal stenosis.

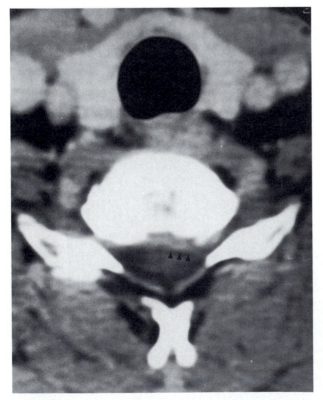

FIG 36–5.
Cervical disk herniation demonstrated with intravenous contrast. Retrocorporeal enhancement *(arrowheads)* delineates the extent of this asymmetrical disk herniation. Retrocorporeal enhancement is not normally observed caudal to C2.

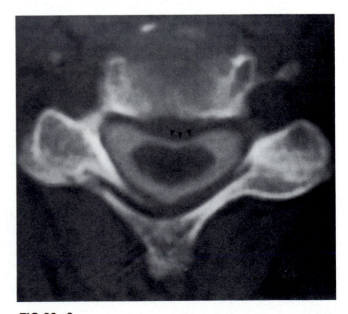

FIG 36–6.
Central cervical disk herniation *(arrowheads)* as seen on postmyelogram CT.

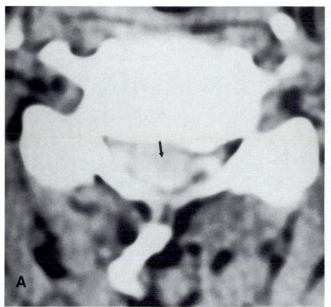 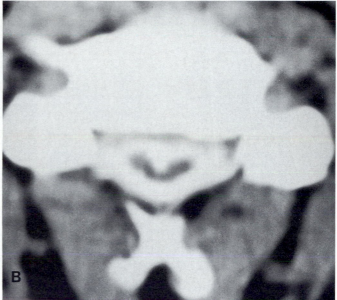

FIG 36–7.
Cervical disk herniation with cord compression. **A,** postmyelogram CT reveals a large disk herniation *(arrow)* causing severe cord compression. **B,** atrophic changes are present in the cord just above the compression.

Cervical spondylosis is a common degenerative disorder causing acquired spinal stenosis, which may result in myelopathy or radiculopathy. However, changes are frequently identified radiographically that do not correlate with symptoms. When symptomatology presents, it is usually of longer duration and more insidious in onset than isolated disk herniation[56, 57] and not necessarily related to an antecedent traumatic event.

The pathogenesis is multifactorial. The nucleus pulposus becomes desiccated with aging, and defects appear in the annulus fibrosus as the disk space narrows. These changes occur most frequently at C5–6, followed by C6–7 and then the other cervical vertebral levels.[58] This permits closer approximation of the uncinate processes and subsequent development of spur formation encroaching upon the intervertebral foramina.[58, 59] Herniation of disk material may occur. Spur formation develops adjacent to the discovertebral junction.[58, 59] Apophyseal joints are not frequently affected in the cervical spine.[58] However, there are rare reports of cervical synovial cysts in association with degenerative facet joint changes.[60]

Productive bony degenerative change can result in nerve root or cord compression. Spondylotic changes superimposed upon a congenitally narrow canal may contribute to the development of myelopathy.[40, 58, 61] Additional factors influencing the development of myelopathy include dynamic forces (i.e., flexion, extension)[40] and compromise of the spinal cord blood supply.[40, 58, 62]

Ossification of spinal ligamentous structures can occur. The most well described entity is ossification of the posterior longitudinal ligament (OPLL). This disorder is more frequently found in the cervical than the thoracic and lumbar spine and can cause radiculomyelopathy.[59, 63] Calcification or ossification may also occur in the ligamenta flava.[64]

CT Findings

Unenhanced CT can demonstrate the extent of bony encroachment upon the spinal canal and neural foramina and can differentiate soft disk herniation from an osteophyte. However, spinal cord compression is best evaluated with intrathecal contrast.[28, 36, 42] Typical findings include spondylotic spurs projecting into the canal and distorting the thecal sac (Figs 36–8 and 36–9). Focal cord flattening and secondary cord rotation can be identified. Spur formation may encroach upon the neural foramina (Fig 36–10). Laterally located spurs may be myelographically occult but easily identified by CT.[36]

OPLL may be differentiated from spur formation by a thin radiolucent zone between the posterior vertebral body margin and the ossified ligament.[28] Contiguity over several levels is also a helpful distinguishing feature.[59]

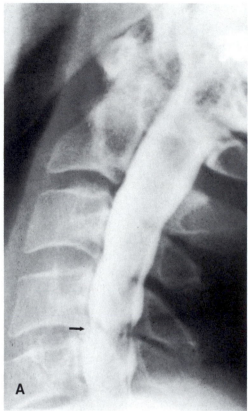

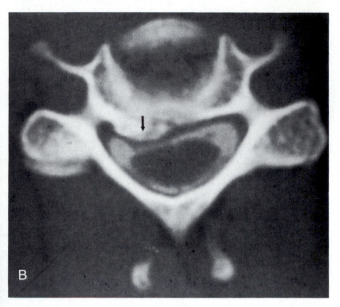

FIG 36–8.
Cervical spondylosis. **A,** a lateral myelographic view reveals a ventral impression from spur formation *(arrow)*. **B,** spur formation is distorting the thecal sac without cord compression.

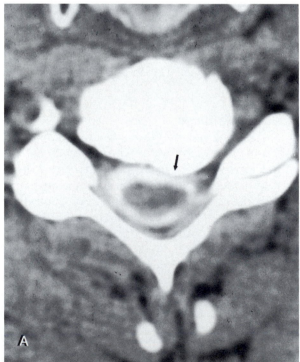

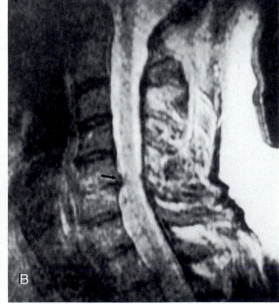

FIG 36–9.
Cervical spur formation effacing the subarachnoid space. **A,** post-myelogram CT demonstrates a spur *(arrow)* without cord compres- sion. **B,** sagittal long–repetition time (TR) MRI illustrates the finding *(arrow)* nonivasively.

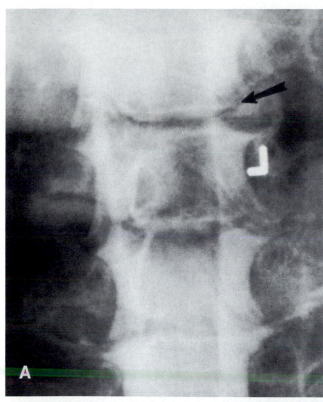

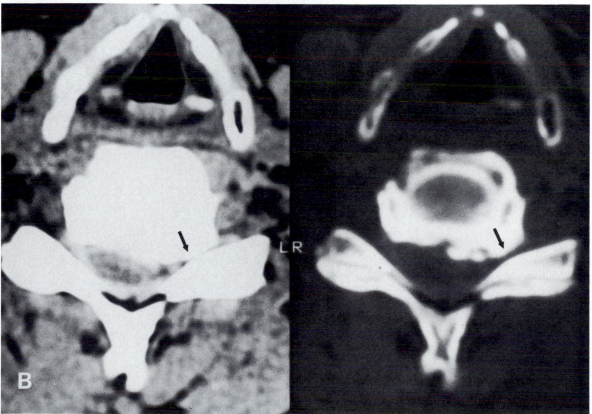

FIG 36–10.
Cervical spondylosis. **A,** an AP myelogram reveals root sleeve cutoff *(arrow).* **B,** postmyelogram CT with a soft-tissue *(left)* and bone *(right)* algorithm. These reveal spur formation compressing and distorting the cord and almost obliterating the left neural foramen *(arrow).*

The AP diameter is the most frequently compromised dimension of the spinal canal in cervical spondylosis.[65] The smallest AP diameter of the cervical spinal canal normally occurs at C3 through C5, with the smallest cross-sectional area at C4 and C7.[65] One group of investigators found that all patients with spondylosis and AP canal diameters less than 10 mm had quadriplegia. However, these authors caution that quantitative data alone will permit underestimation of the extent of the spondylosis.[65]

The normal cervical cord on CT myelography is elliptical in shape and somewhat flattened in appearance at C4 and C5.[66] The anterior and posterior median fissures normally may be difficult to identify. Progressive changes in the appearance of the cord occur with increasing severity of compression (Fig 36–11). The ventral surface of the cord is initially flattened by an osteophyte. This progresses to central infolding and widening of the ventral fissure, which results in a bean-shaped appearance of the cord. The lateral funiculi become tapered and point toward the anterolateral aspects of the canal,[40, 67] possibly due to tension from the dentate ligaments.[67] The anterolateral and posterolateral funiculi of the cord become atrophic. A notchlike deformity of the dorsal surface of the cord may represent dorsal column atrophy.[67]

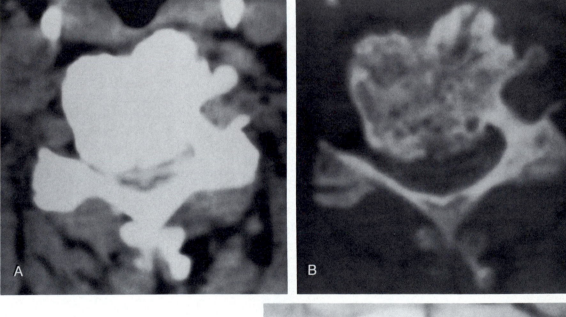

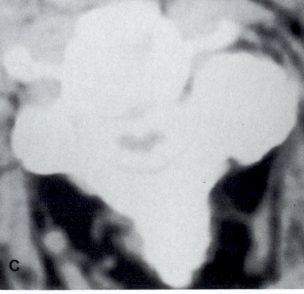

FIG 36–11.
Cervical spondylosis with cord compression and atrophy. Postmyelogram CT with soft-tissue **(A)** and bone windows **(B)** demonstrates severe spondylosis with marked spinal cord compression. One level down **(C)**, the spinal cord is atrophic secondary to the compression and resultant ischemia above.

CT with intrathecal contrast may also provide prognostic information. An approximate 30% reduction in cord cross-sectional area may be necessary to produce long-tract signs.[68] One report suggests that recovery of function is poor after decompression if the cord is markedly atrophic with a relatively capacious subarachnoid space.[36]

Phantom studies suggest that absolute measurement of cord dimensions can be changed by varying the window level and width or the density of contrast. The use of high concentrations of intrathecal contrast and the widest window width that allows a sharp boundary between cord and contrast permit performance of consistent measurements.[69]

THORACIC SPINE DISORDERS

Thoracic Disk Herniation

Intervertebral disk herniation is rare in the thoracic spine[70–74] but, when present, most frequently occurs at caudal levels, below T8.[70, 71] There are reports of involvement at more than one level (Fig 36–12).[71, 72, 75] The incidence is greatest in the fourth to sixth decades of life,[70, 71] with equal[71] to slight male predominance.[70] While trauma may play a role in acute disk herniation, degenerative changes within the disk seem to be more important.[70] The frequent occurrence of disk space calcification within the affected disk may support this view.[71]

Spinal cord dysfunction results from local compression and vascular insufficiency.[72] Back and radicular pain are the most common presenting symptoms, followed by sensory disturbances. Incidental CT detection of asymptomatic calcified thoracic disk herniation has been reported.[76]

A rare pediatric condition, calcification of the intervertebral disk, occurs more frequently in the cervical than thoracic spine.[49] Herniation of the calcified disk may be demonstrable (Fig 36–13). The natural history is typically benign, with spontaneous regression of the displaced disk.[49]

CT Findings

CT is valuable in the diagnosis of thoracic disk herniation.[70, 72, 74] Calcification of the disk protrusion is present on plain films in 55% of cases.[71] CT without intrathecal contrast may demonstrate a cal-

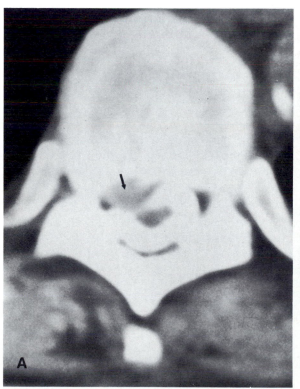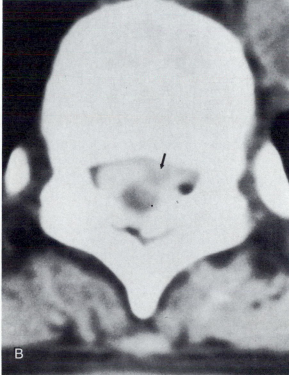

FIG 36–12.
Thoracic disk herniation at two levels. **A,** axial postmyelogram CT reveals paracentral disk herniation *(arrow).* **B,** at a separate level, a second paracentral herniation is identified on the contralateral side *(arrow).*

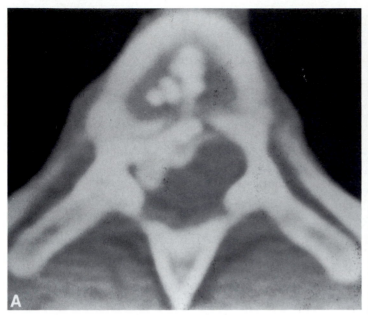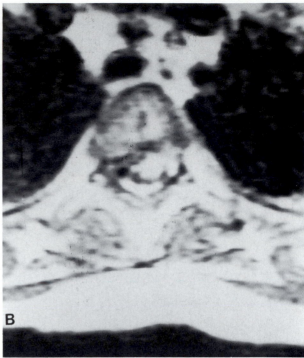

FIG 36–13.
Calcified thoracic disk protrusion in a child. **A,** an axial CT image demonstrates calcification of the intervertebral disk in the midthoracic level with protrusion of calcified disk material into the spinal canal to the right. **B,** axial short-TR (TR = 800 ms, echo time [TE] = 28 ms) MRI reveals spinal canal encroachment by the disk herniation, but calcification of the disk material is poorly demonstrated.

cified mass within the spinal canal (Fig 36–13).[76, 77] The disk herniation is most frequently central or paracentral.[70, 71] However, lateral protrusions can occur.[70, 72] Intrathecal contrast is necessary to outline the configuration of the compressed spinal cord and the disk protrusion (Fig 36–14). It may be difficult to separate a dense, calcified disk from the contrast column. An examination before and after the administration of intrathecal contrast may be complimentary. Abnormalities on plain-film myelography can suggest the appropriate level(s) for CT examination.

Thoracic Spinal Stenosis

The most common cause for acquired spinal stenosis is spondylosis, which is rare in the thoracic region.[78] Degenerative changes in the intervertebral disks occur more frequently in the lumbar and cervical spine than in the thoracic spine.[59] However, apophyseal joint osteoarthritis occurs,[79] as does osteophyte formation, which may compromise the spinal canal.[59]

OPLL and ossification of the ligamentum flavum (OLF) may contribute to spinal stenosis and resulting radiculomyelopathy.[63, 64, 80–82] OPLL is more common in the cervical spine,[59] and a minor-

ity of these patients will have associated thoracic OPLL.[63] Alternatively, when this abnormality occurs in the thoracic spine, it is frequently associated with cervical OPLL,[63] and T4 through T7 are the most frequently affected levels.[59] The abnormalities often involve two or more ligamentous structures.[63]

The clinical significance of these changes may depend upon the presence of congenital bony spinal stenosis. This may be due to focal idiopathic congenitally short pedicles and/or thickened laminae,[83] or it may be related to a more generalized disorder such as achondroplasia and result in spinal stenosis that is progressive caudally.

There are rare reports of epidural lipomatosis resulting in thoracic spinal cord compression.[84–87] This may occur in association with exogenous steroid therapy[84–87] or morbid obesity.[88]

CT Findings

OPLL appears as calcific density that may be separable from the posterior margin of the vertebral body by a radiolucent zone (Fig 36–15).[28, 80] This is distinguishable from a calcified herniated disk by its extension over several levels and identification at a distance from the disk space. The ossification may be laminated in nature.[81] The liga-

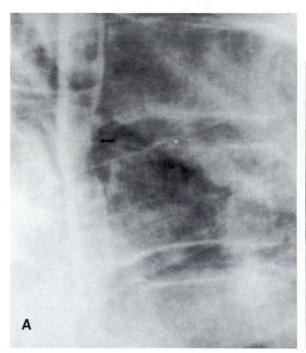

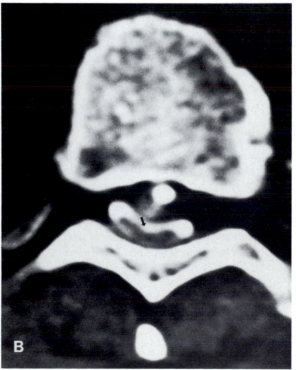

FIG 36–14.
Thoracic disk herniation. **A,** a lateral myelogram reveals ventral extradural impression *(arrow)* at the disk space with cord compres- sion. **B,** postmyelogram CT reveals disk herniation *(arrow)* causing cord compression.

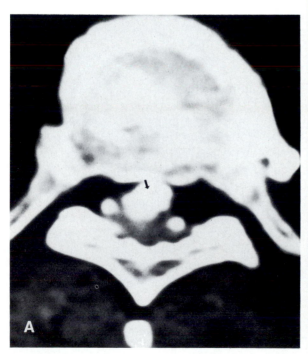

FIG 36–15.
Ossification of the posterior longitudinal ligament in the thoracic spine. **A,** postmyelogram CT reveals dense ventral calcification at the level of the myelographic block *(arrow)*. **B,** just distal to the block, although calcification is less apparent, cord compression is obvious *(arrow)*.

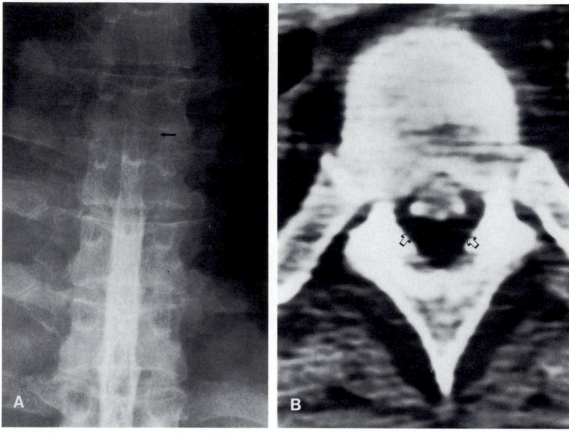

FIG 36–16.
Epidural lipomatosis. **A,** an AP myelogram reveals a complete extradural block in the midthoracic spine *(arrow).* **B,** postmyelogram CT near the level of the block reveals fat within the canal that is compressing the cord *(open arrows).* This abnormality extended over several levels.

mentum flavum is most heavily calcified adjacent to the superior articular process, in the capsular portion of the ligament.[64] Noncontrast CT can illustrate the extent of spinal canal compromise. In multilevel involvement, intrathecal contrast will show effacement of the subarachnoid space[89] and may delineate the clinically important levels by defining the degree of cord compression.

CT evaluation in epidural lipomatosis reveals a density characteristic of fat within the spinal canal (Fig 36–16).[84–88] Spinal cord compression in this condition frequently results from excessive accumulation of fat dorsal to the cord. Intrathecal contrast provides further delineation of the degree of cord compression and outlines focal epidural fatty deposition.

LUMBAR DISK HERNIATION

The clinical lumbar disk syndrome results from a variety of pathologic processes including disk herniation, spondylosis, and congenital spinal stenosis.[90, 91] Disk herniation alone is seen only in a small proportion of patients presenting with sciatica.[90, 92] Disk herniation may be present incidently in as many as 20% of asymptomatic patients[93] and may go on to subsequently produce clinically significant radiculopathy.[94] History alone (both demographic and symptomatic) cannot accurately predict the likelihood of disk herniation on CT.[95] Interestingly, a correct CT interpretation is more likely without a clinical history.[96] Because of the difficulty in determining the significance of positive radiologic findings, a precise correlation of CT findings with the patient's clinical symptoms is necessary to accurately direct a surgical approach.[97]

Disk herniation refers to rupture of the nucleus pulposus through a defect in the annulus fibrosus. The posterior longitudinal ligament is adherent to[98, 99] and serves to reinforce the midline annulus fibrosus, which is thinnest posteriorly.[59, 92] In addition, the nucleus pulposus is normally eccentrically positioned somewhat posteriorly.[59] Therefore, herniation of disk material most frequently occurs posterolaterally[92, 100] and less frequently occurs centrally[101] or laterally (Fig 36–17).[102] Central disk herniation may be subjacent to the posterior longitudinal ligament or may be extruded through or around the posterior longitudinal ligament into the vertebral canal or intervertebral foramen.[103, 104] Free fragments of disk material may migrate superiorly (Fig 36–18), inferiorly (Fig 36–19), or laterally.[103, 104] There is disagreement regarding which direction free disk fragments most frequently migrate.[103–105] However, superiorly extruded fragments may migrate a greater distance[103] and result in compression of the rostral exiting nerve root as well as the traversing nerve root at the level of the herniated disk[102] (Fig 36–20).

Rare instances of intradural herniation of disk material have been reported.[106–108] Speculation regarding pathogenesis suggests that adhesions between the dura, annulus, and/or posterior longitudinal ligament permit intradural disk extrusion.

Follow-up CT studies of disk herniation over time suggest that herniated disks may spontaneously regress.[109, 110]

A bulging annulus fibrosus must be distinguished from disk herniation (Fig 36–21). With advancing age, desiccation of the nucleus pulposus and loss of elasticity of the annulus allows the intervertebral space to diminish in height and permits bulging of the annulus.[111] With severe changes, the incidence and degree of disk displacement are reduced.[59]

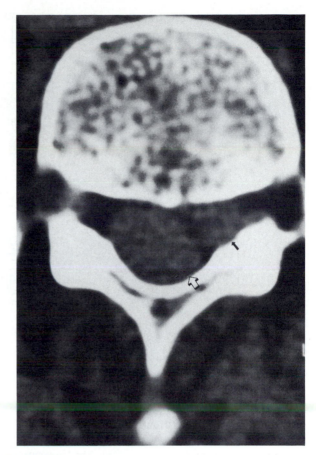

FIG 36–18.
Free disk fragment that has migrated superiorly from the L4–5 disk space. The thecal sac *(open arrow)* is distorted, and the disk fragment *(arrow)* fills the left lateral recess.

Plain CT is accurate in diagnosing disk herniation[112–114] and had been the initial procedure of choice for the evaluation of suspected disk disease until the advent of MRI. The accuracy of noncontrast CT compares favorably[104, 115–119] or may be slightly less accurate[97] than myelography in the diagnosis of disk herniation. CT is particularly helpful at L5–S1 where the ventral epidural space may be patulous,[104, 120–122] in the diagnosis of lateral disk herniation, and in cases of myelographic block related to disk herniation.[117] Myelography provides the advantage of evaluating the conus region and thus revealing a possible occult spinal tumor that might otherwise be missed.[97]

Initial performance of plain CT of the lumbar spine reduces the need for subsequent myelography in the diagnosis of disk disease.[118, 119] In questionable cases, myelography may then be performed,[39] followed by CT myelography in specific locations directed by the plain-film myelogram.[117–119] When compared with myelography, CT with intrathecal contrast provides additional di-

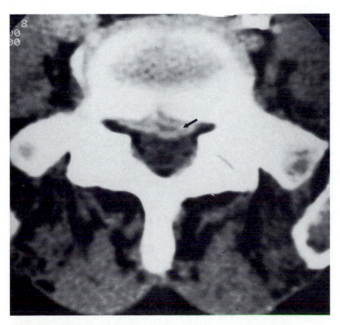

FIG 36–17.
L5–S1 disk herniation *(arrow)* slightly eccentric to the left.

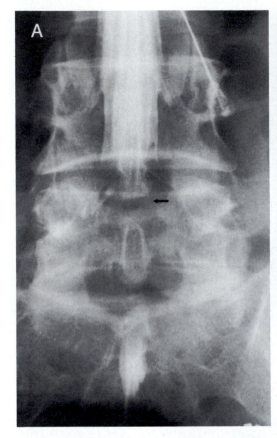

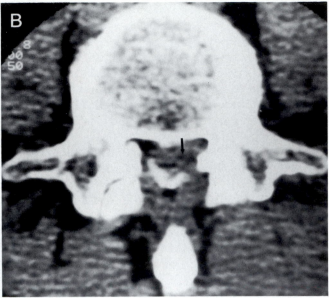

FIG 36–19.
L4–5 disk herniation with inferior migration of a disk fragment. **A,** an AP myelographic film reveals a block to contrast flow at the L4–5 disk space *(arrow).* **B,** postmyelogram CT demonstrates that the inferior migration of disk material *(arrow),* to the L5 vertebral body level, is causing marked distortion of the thecal sac.

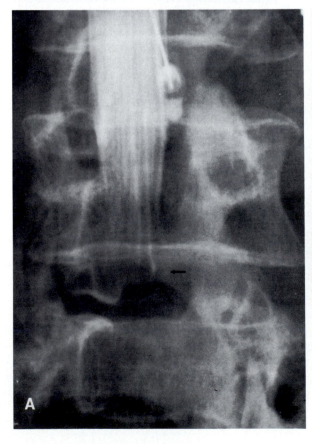

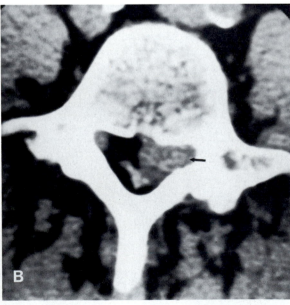

FIG 36–20.
Disk herniation with superior migration of a free fragment. **A,** a myelogram reveals a block at L4–5 *(arrow).* **B,** an axial CT slice at L5 vertebral body levels reveals a disk fragment *(arrow)* in the lateral recess that is compressing the traversing nerve root.

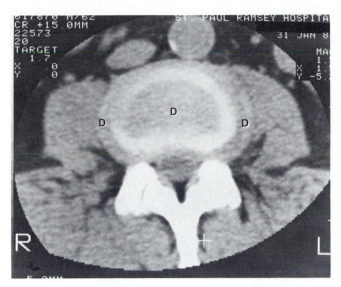

FIG 36–21.
Bulging disk *(D)*. The diffuse appearance is characteristic of degenerative bulging. There is no encroachment on the dural sac and probably no compression of the traversing roots.

agnostically useful information,[122, 124–126] particularly in difficult cases where a distinction between soft-tissue structures within the canal is obscure as in patients with spinal stenosis, conjoined nerve roots, perineural cysts, synovial cysts, and neurofibromas.[117, 120, 127]

The role of MRI in this diagnostic sequence has yet to be determined. However, some authors suggest that MRI may be equivalent to CT and myelography and that CT and MRI can be employed in a complementary fashion, perhaps obviating the need for myelography (Fig 36–22).[2]

Intravenous contrast has been useful in differentiating recurrent disk herniation from fibrous scars in the postoperative patient,[128–132] and intravenous contrast subjectively improves delineation of intraspinal soft tissues.[133] It seems logical that intravenous contrast enhancement might be helpful in distinguishing a ventral epidural venous plexus from disk herniation in difficult cases.

Multiplanar reconstruction usually does not contribute important diagnostic information when axial images are carefully analyzed for disk herniation. However, reformations may provide additional confirmation of an abnormality suspected by axial images (Fig 36–23). Reformation imposes the limitation that slices cannot be angled parallel to the disk space.[134]

CT Findings

Disk herniation on CT most frequently appears as a focal protrusion of the disk margin displacing the epidural fat.[101, 103, 104] The thecal sac may be indented or displaced, and the affected nerve root

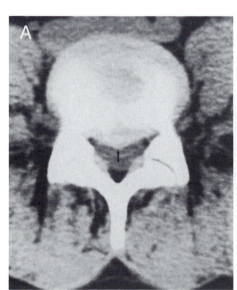

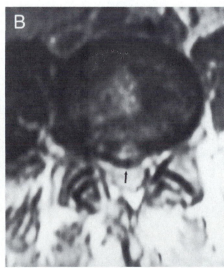

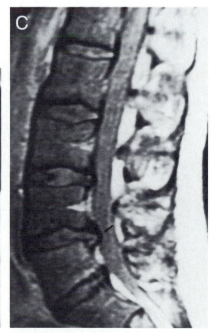

FIG 36–22.
Central L4–5 disk herniation. **A,** CT illustrates central disk herniation with effacement of the thecal sac *(arrow)*. **B,** axial MRI similarly reveals the disk protrusion *(arrow)* and effacement of the thecal sac (TR = 2,500 ms, TE = 30 ms). **C,** sagittal MRI also demonstrates the herniation *(arrow)* (TR = 2,200 ms, TE = 30 ms).

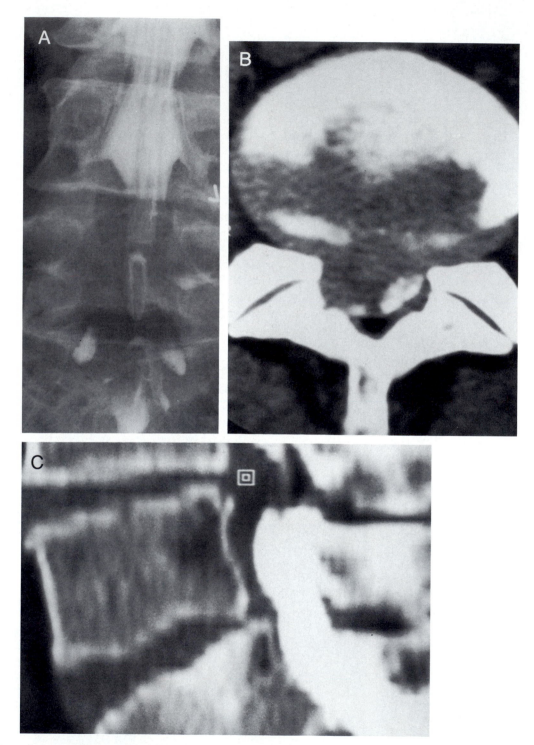

FIG 36–23.
Large L4–5 disk herniation with a free fragment. **A,** an erect mye-lographic view reveals a block to the caudal flow of intrathecal contrast at the L4–5 disk space. **B,** axial CT reveals an enormous fragment markedly compressing the thecal sac and displacing it to the left. **C,** sagittal reformations provide a myelogram-like picture illustrating the large disk herniation.

sheath may be compressed or displaced. Enlargement of the nerve root sheath may be identified superior or inferior to the level of the disk herniation.[104] Calcification[101, 113] (Fig 36–24) or gas (nitrogen)[103, 104, 135] (Fig 36–25) may be identified within the herniated disk. The disk itself is usually hyperdense in comparison to the thecal sac[104] (see Fig 36–17) and nerve root ganglion.[136]

Lateral disk herniation results in the appearance of soft tissue within the neural foramen that displaces the foraminal fat without thecal sac deformity.[102, 127] Disk herniation can also be identified in an extraforaminal location (Fig 36–26).[137, 138] Most extraforaminal disk herniations have an intraforaminal component and frequently occur without coexisting intraspinal disk herniation.[138] Identification depends upon the presence of focal soft tissue of disk density lateral to the neural foramen that may be obliterating perispinal fat and displacing or compressing the exiting nerve root or ganglion.[138] Anterior interverte-

bral disk herniation, although rare, has also been reported.[139]

Extruded intraspinal disk fragments may be contiguous with the originating (parent) disk and, as such, may be difficult to distinguish from a subligamentous herniation by CT.[105] An extruded free fragment that has migrated from the parent interspace appears as a soft-tissue mass that may have irregular margins,[105] displace the thecal sac or root sheath, and distort the epidural fat. The parent disk interspace may have a normal-appearing margin (Fig 36–27).[103, 105] The fragment is usually hyperdense in comparison to the thecal sac but is occasionally isodense.[103] The free fragment that has migrated presents a number of differential diagnostic possibilities to be examined subsequently.

Osseous changes occurring in association with disk herniation include cortical erosion of the adjacent vertebral body, bony sclerosis, and occasional avulsion of the posterior inferior vertebral body

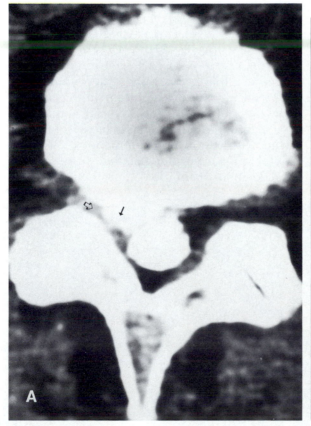

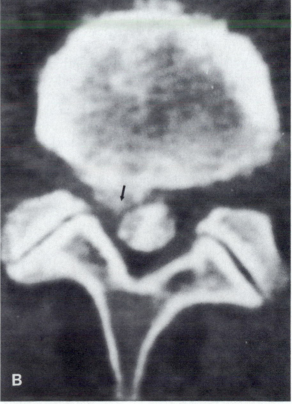

FIG 36–24.
Right lateral calcified disk herniation. **A,** postmyelogram CT reveals a calcified disk protrusion *(arrow)* compressing the thecal sac. Also note the hyperdense disk *(open arrow)* protruding into the neural foramen. **B,** greater window width emphasizes the calcification *(arrow)* and better delineates the thecal sac distortion.

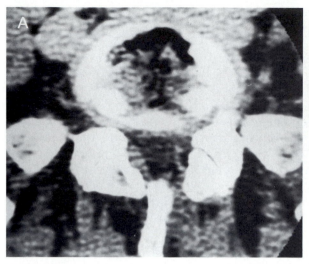
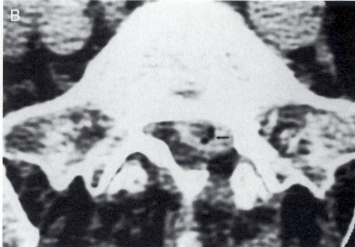

FIG 36–25.
Migration of a free disk fragment containing air. **A,** at the level of the intervertebral disk, a vaccum phenomenon is identified, and only a slight distortion of the posterior disk margin is evident on the left. **B,** 12 mm inferior to **A,** a free disk fragment is identified that contains gas *(arrow)*. There may be some peripheral enhancement. The examination was performed with intravenous contrast.

cortical margin.[140, 141] The latter may be seen on the lateral scout view.

Identification of disk herniation in a stenotic canal may be difficult. In these cases, epidural fat is minimal, and the disk may have an isodense appearance relative to the thecal sac. This may be related to reduced cerebrospinal fluid (CSF) and relatively greater neural tissue in the compressed thecal sac.[104] Alternatively, a massive disk herniation may encompass the entire spinal canal, obliterate fat planes, and compress the thecal sac.[112] Intrathecal contrast may be helpful in identifying the pathology in these cases.

CT distinction between disk herniation and disk bulge depends upon the focality of the protrusion. A bulging disk has a diffusely smooth contour projecting beyond the margins of the vertebral body (see Fig 36–21).[111] Occasionally, the bulge may be asymmetrical.[142] A posterior concavity may be retained, presumably due to reinforcement from an intact posterior longitudinal ligament.[111] Gas may be identifiable within the abnormal disk.[143]

A differential diagnosis of disk herniation includes normal anatomic structures such as an epidural venous plexus; calcified posterior longitudinal ligament or annulus[103]; anatomic variations such

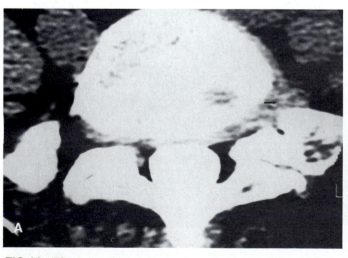
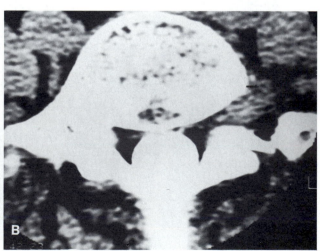

FIG 36–26.
Extraforaminal disk herniation at L5–S1. **A,** disk herniation into the left L5–S1 neural foramen *(arrow)*. **B,** the disk material extends laterally, beyond the neural foramen *(arrow)*.

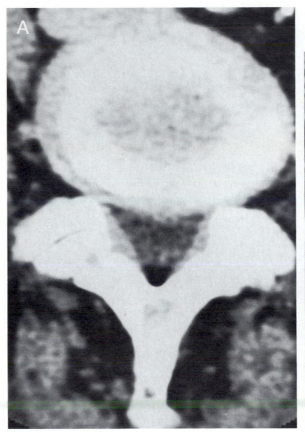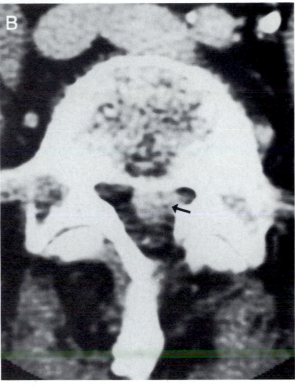

FIG 36–27.
Disk herniation with inferior migration of a free fragment. **A,** a scan through the disk space reveals the convex posterior margin of the intervertebral disk without obvious herniation. **B,** a CT slice inferior to the disk space reveals a large free fragment *(arrow)* markedly distorting the thecal sac.

as conjoined nerve root sleeves[127, 136, 144, 145] and perineural cysts[103, 105]; primary or secondary neoplasms such as neurofibromas,[136, 146] metastasis, or lymphoma[36, 145]; and synovial facet joint cysts.[103, 147, 148] Other processes that obliterate epidural fat including epidural abscess and postoperative scarring may also be difficult to distinguish from disk herniation.[101] Intravenous contrast may aid in identification of the basivertebral venous plexus, which is seen behind the vertebral body and is frequently associated with a small cap of bone.[103]

A conjoined root sleeve represents a common anatomic variation in 5% of all lumbar myelograms[149] and is most frequently identified at L5–S1.[103, 127] CT findings include widening of the adjacent bony lateral recess and a density of the conjoined root sleeve that is similar to the thecal sac. The roots may separate and exit through different foramina, or they may exit by the same foramen (Fig 36–28). Similarly, the density of a perineural cyst or dilated nerve root sheath will approximate

the density of the thecal sac. Confirmation with intrathecal contrast may be necessary in difficult cases (Fig 36–29).

A neurofibroma may have the appearance of an entirely extradural mass, and it may not be detectable by myelography[146] and needs to be distinguished from lateral disk herniation. CT findings include a soft-tissue mass with smooth margins identified in the neural foramen with a density similar to the thecal sac (but less than disk material) and that may enhance with intravenous contrast.[105, 136] Associated erosion of the adjacent bone may be identified.[105, 136]

Primary or metastatic neoplasms may arise in or destroy adjacent bone and may infiltrate paraspinal musculature. A history of primary or metastatic carcinoma may be helpful in these cases.[136] Tumor may enhance with intravenous contrast. Myelography and CT with intrathecal contrast should be helpful if tumor is suspected.

Facet joint synovial cysts are low-attenuation

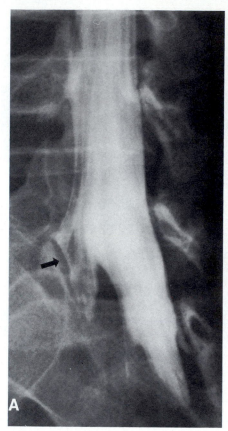

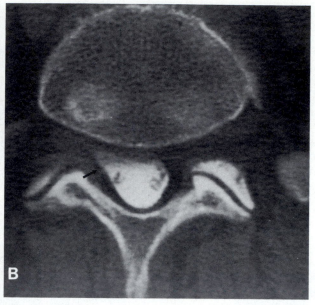

FIG 36–28.
Conjoined root sheath. **A,** a myelogram reveals a conjoined root sheath *(arrow).* The nerve roots are exiting through their respective foramina. **B,** axial postmyelogram CT reveals the asymmetrical thecal sac *(arrow).*

masses projecting into the posterolateral portion of the spinal canal (Fig 36–30).[103] They arise adjacent to degenerated facet joints and characteristically occur at the L4–5 level.[148] Calcification is frequently identified in the cyst wall.[103, 147, 148] Percutaneous injection of contrast into the facet joint may opacify the cysts and confirm the diagnosis.[147, 148]

Lumbar Spinal Stenosis

Spinal stenosis represents narrowing of the spinal canal and may result in spinal cord/cauda equina compression or isolated nerve root entrapment. Lumbar spinal stenosis may be a more common cause of back pain and sciatica than disk herniation is.[92, 150] Both soft-tissue and bony changes contribute to the compromise of the spinal canal (Table 36–1). Spondylosis and Paget's disease represent acquired etiologies for spinal stenosis. Achondroplasia is an example of congenital spinal stenosis. The development of spondylosis in a spinal canal that is already congenitally subclinically compromised may result in symptomatic spinal stenosis.[52]

TABLE 36–1.

Classification of Lumbar Spinal Stenosis*

I. Congenital-developmental stenosis
   A. Idiopathic
   B. Achondroplastic
II. Acquired stenosis
   A. Degenerative stenosis
      1. Central portion of canal
      2. Peripheral portion of canal and nerve canals
      3. Degenerative spondylolisthesis
   B. Combined stenosis: Any possible combination of developmental stenosis, degenerative stenosis, and HNP†
   C. Spondylolisthetic stenosis
   D. Postoperative stenosis
      1. Postlaminectomy
      2. Postfusion
      3. Postchemonucleolysis
   E. Post-traumatic stenosis (late changes)
   F. Miscellaneous
      1. Paget's disease
      2. Fluorosis

* From Arnoldi CC, Brodsky AE, Cauchoix J, et al: *Lumbar Spinal Stenosis and Nerve Root Entrapment Syndromes: Clinical Orthopaedics and Related Research,* no. 115. Philadelphia, JB Lippincott, 1976, pp 4–5. Used by permission.
† HNP = herniated nucleus pulposus.

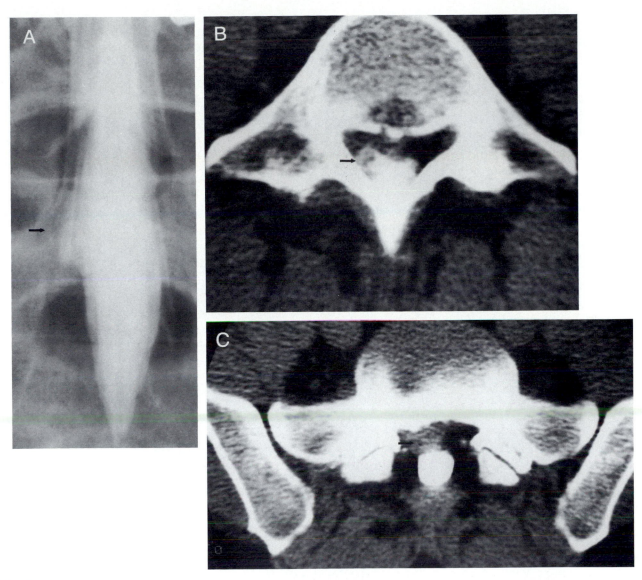

FIG 36–29.
Disk herniation below a conjoined root sleeve. **A,** myelography reveals conjoined L5–S1 root sleeves on the right *(arrow),* and no abnormal impression was identified upon the thecal sac. **B,** post-myelogram CT demonstrates the conjoined root sheath *(arrow)* as it approaches the foramen in the lateral recess at L5. **C,** herniated disk fragment identified inferior to the nerve root sheath *(arrow).*

Acquired spondylotic stenosis represents a degenerative process predominantly involving the facet joints and intervertebral disk. The changes take place over time as a result of repeated minor trauma. Rotational injury results in circumferential annular tears. This in combination with desiccation of the nucleus pulposus results in a loss of disk height, may contribute to a bulging annulus, and causes the formation of osteophytes.[59, 151] Progressive degenerative changes in the facet joints lead to osteophyte formation and joint instability.[15]

Stenosis may be central, lateral, or a combination of both. Central stenosis refers to compromise of the bony spinal canal bounded by the pedicles laterally; facet joints, laminae, and spinous processes posteriorly; and the intervertebral disk anteriorly.

Lateral stenosis is a term encompassing lateral recess (subarticular) stenosis and foraminal stenosis. Lateral recess or subarticular stenosis refers to the entrapment of the traversing nerve root as it obliquely descends and approaches the pedicle in the lateral recess. The lateral recess is bounded posteriorly by the superior articular facet, laterally by the pedicle, and anteriorly by the posterior surface of the vertebral body (Fig 36–31). Neural fo-

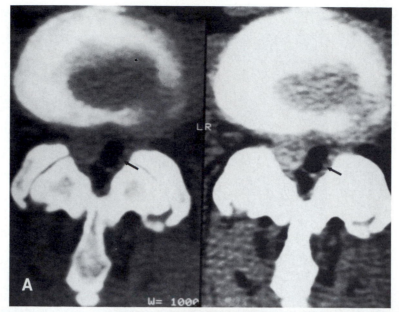

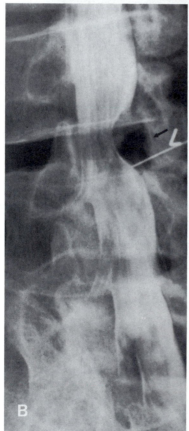

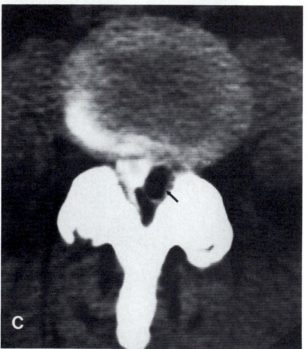

FIG 36–30.
Gas-containing synovial cyst. **A,** plain CT at bone *(left)* and soft-tissue *(right)* windows reveals a gas-containing mass *(arrow)* in the posterolateral spinal canal, adjacent to the narrowed left facet joint. **B,** a myelogram reveals an extradural impression upon the thecal sac *(arrow)*. Gas density in the cyst can be identified. **C,** CT following a myelogram better illustrates the distortion of the thecal sac *(arrow)*.

raminal stenosis involves the exiting nerve as it passes under the pedicle in the upper portion of the intervertebral foramen.

The inclination of the articular processes favors a slight posterior and inferior subluxation (or retrolisthesis) of the upper vertebral body (Fig 36–32).[152–154] With these changes, the superior articular facet of the inferior vertebral body is positioned closer to the disk space and vertebral body, and this narrows the lateral recess and neural fora-

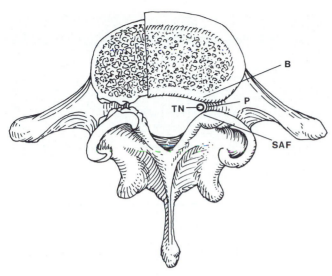

FIG 36–31.
The lateral recess. Note the normal left side and lateral recess stenosis on the right. The boundaries of the lateral recess are the vertebral body *(B)*, upper border of the pedicle *(P)*, and base of the superior articulating facet *(SAF)* *(TN = traversing nerve).*

men.[150] This focal stenosis is augmented by the formation of osteophytes on the medial edge and anterior surface of the superior articular process of the inferior vertebral body and/or the inferior articular process of the superior vertebral body.[150, 155] The lateral recess is narrowest at the rostral border of the corresponding pedicle. Therefore, spur formation of the superior articular facet at the same level is also likely to cause nerve root compression in the lateral recess.[156, 157]

Additional factors contributing to lumbar spinal stenosis include degeneration of the ligamenta flava[158] and posterior longitudinal ligament that is characterized by a loss of elasticity, calcification, and even ossification (Fig 36–33).[59] Ligamentous changes alone may result in significant symptomatic spinal stenosis.

Usually, the degenerative process results in a loss of epidural fat, but stenosis caused by excess epidural fat as a result of steroid treatment or marked obesity has been reported.[88, 159]

CT Appearance

The spinal canal is somewhat oval in shape at the L1 level and becomes more triangular in shape caudally at L5 to S1.[160] A bulging annulus, prominent ligamenta flava, and osteophytes projecting from the vertebral body compromise the canal centrally most at the disk level, thus accounting for the "hourglass" appearance of the thecal sac seen at myelography. This corresponds to a trefoil shape of

the stenotic spinal canal on axial CT images (Fig 36–34).

A scheme to quantify the size of the bony central canal has been proposed[161]; however, this does not account for the soft-tissue contribution to compression of the cauda equina, which may be significant.

There may be considerable compression of the thecal sac, and epidural fat may be reduced in the stenotic spinal canal.[153] An absence of this natural contrast may make the thecal sac difficult to distinguish from surrounding tissues without intrathecal contrast. However, a lumbar puncture for installation of contrast may be technically difficult in these patients.

Facet joint osteophyte formation can contribute to both central and lateral stenosis. Additional changes that may be observed in the facet joints include spur formation, subchondral sclerosis, and

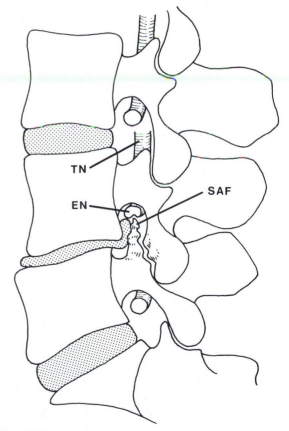

FIG 36–32.
Changes producing foraminal (lateral) stenosis. With loss of the disk space, the superior articulating facet *(SAF)* moves superiorly toward the upper neural foramen to compress the exiting nerve. Posterior spondylolisthesis of the body above and osteophytes on the SAF cause further narrowing *(TN = traversing nerve; EN = exiting nerve in upper neural foramen).*

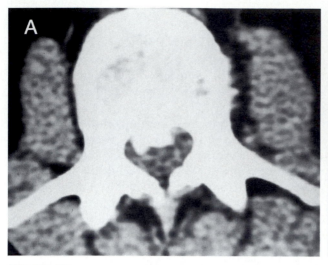
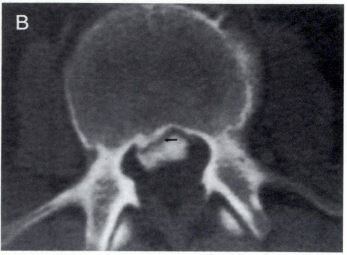

FIG 36–33.
Ossification of the posterior longitudinal ligament in the lumbar spine demonstrated with soft-tissue **(A)** and bone **(B)** windows. Note that this can be differentiated from calcified disk material by the presence of a cleft *(arrow)* between the area of calcification and the vertebral body. Also, this is seen at the midvertebral body level. There is substantial compromise of the spinal canal due to the ossified ligament.

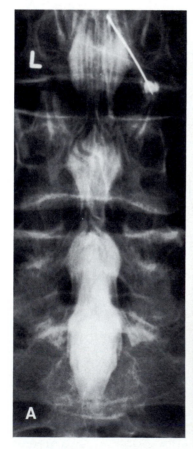
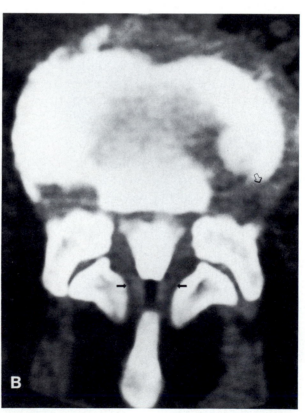

FIG 36–34.
Lumbar spinal stenosis. **A,** a myelogram reveals narrowing of the thecal sac at the disk space levels. Note the tortuosity of the nerve roots between the areas of compression. **B,** a bulging annulus *(open arrow)* and prominence of the ligamentum flavum *(arrows)* contribute to the compression of the thecal sac. The scan was performed without gantry angulation.

vaccum phenomenon (Fig 36–35).[162] Pagetic modeling with expansion of the vertebral body, facets, and laminae can cause symptomatic spinal stenosis (Fig 36–36).[54]

Lateral recess stenosis frequently results from spur formation of the superior articular facet.[156, 157] CT is of great utility in assessment of the lateral recess (Fig 36–37). AP measurements of the lateral recess of 3 mm or less strongly suggest stenosis.[150, 156, 157] However, interobserver variation may make such measurements unreliable.[163] The changes appear to occur most frequently at L4–5.[154–156] Myelography alone is inadequate for detecting compression in the lateral recess and neural foramen.[153, 157] This is principally because the nerve root sheath terminates at or near the dorsal root ganglion.[102]

Osteophytes projecting from the facet joints,[152, 153, 155, 164] subluxation (particularly anterior spondylolisthesis with an intact posterior arch),[164] and disk herniation with superior migration all may compress the nerve root within the neural foramen, thus accounting for the radiculopathy. These processes result in obliteration of the perineural fat in the neural foramen.[152] It is important to evaluate the superior aspect of the neural foramen just inferior to the pedicle on axial images to assess significant nerve root compression (Fig 36–38). In order to adequately evaluate suspected lateral stenosis, axial images must be taken from the pedicles of one vertebral level to the pedicles of the next. Scanning exclusively through the intervertbral disk space may result in overlooking symptomatically significant disease. Sagittal reformations may be particularly helpful in evaluation of the neural foramina.[153]

A normal variation, the foraminal spur, is a bony projection extending into the neural foramen from either the pars interarticularis or pedicle.[165] It is generally located dorsal to the nerve root and is thought to represent ossification of the ligamentum flavum at its point of insertion.[165] Sagittal reformation may be helpful in confirming the presence of this anomaly.

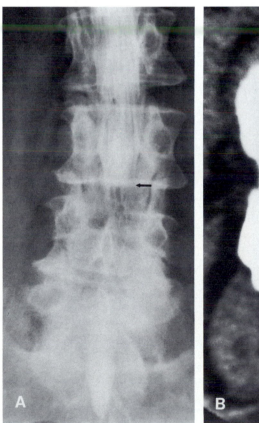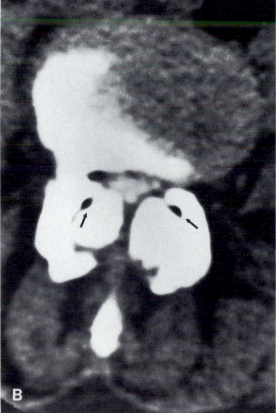

FIG 36–35.

Spinal stenosis. **A,** an AP myelogram reveals a partial block to the caudal flow of contrast at L3–4 *(arrow).* **B,** postmyelogram CT demonstrates marked compression of the thecal sac. Note the vacuum phenomenon in facet joints bilaterally *(arrows).*

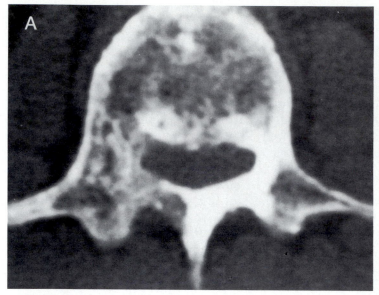

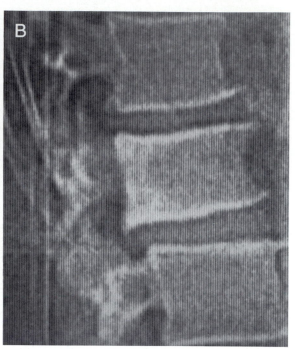

FIG 36–36.
Paget's disease of the lumbar spine. **A,** note the mottled sclerotic changes in the verebral body. The spinal canal at this level is compromised in the AP dimension. **B,** a lateral scout view reveals a thickened cortex characteristic of Paget's disease.

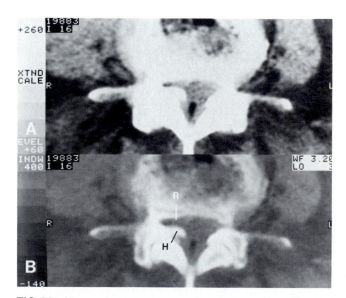

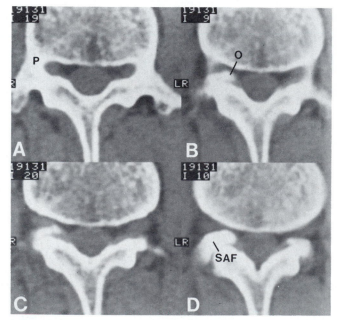

FIG 36–38.
Foraminal (lateral) stenosis. **A,** level of the pedicle *(P)*. **B** and **C,** a few millimeters below at the upper foramen where the exiting nerve passes. The osteophyte *(O)* from the superior articulating facet *(SAF)* produces definite narrowing on the right. The left foramen is normal. **D,** lower foramen, which normally has a small sagittal diameter. Note the large *SAF* on the right. The normal left side would appear narrowed if evaluated at this level.

FIG 36–37.
Lateral recess stenosis. **A,** soft-tissue setting. **B,** bone setting. The lateral recess *(R)* is deep transversely and narrow sagittally because of a hypertrophied superior articulating facet *(H)*. This patient also has central stenosis, which tends to push the nerve laterally into the narrowed recess.

Spondylolysis and Spondylolisthesis

Spondylolysis refers to a defect in the pars interarticularis and may be associated with spondylolisthesis, that is, anterior subluxation of the affected vertebral body. The pars defect is thought to represent an acquired traumatic lesion[166] and is usually bilateral.[166–169] Changes of spondylolysis and/or spondylolisthesis are present in about 4% of all lumbar spine examinations.[167] Pars defects may be associated with congenital anomalies including spina bifida, hypoplastic facets, and anomalous laminae.[166, 168]

Spondylolisthesis can be classified into the fol-lowing types according to etiology[170]: (1) type I—dysplastic, involving the upper sacrum or neural arch of L5; (2) type II—isthmic, representing a defect in the pars interarticularis, which may result from fracture or elongation of the pars; (3) type III—degenerative (spondylotic) spondylolisthesis resulting from degenerative changes in the facet joints and disk with joint instability and subluxation; (4) type IV—traumatic, due to fractures other than in the pars (Fig 36–39); (5) type V—pathologic etiologies resulting from a generalized spine disorder such as Paget's disease; and (6) iatrogenic, from extensive laminectomy and facetectomy.[166] Isthmic (spondylolytic) and degenerative

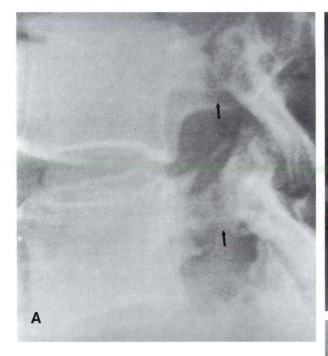
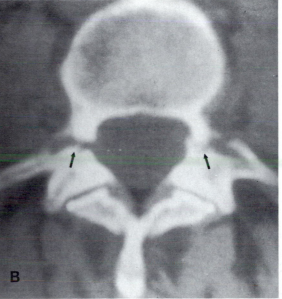
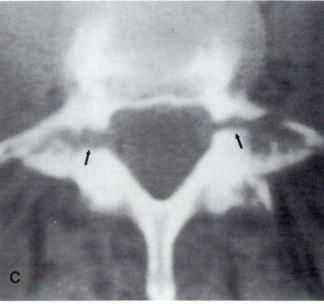

FIG 36–39.
Bilateral lumbar pedicle fractures at multiple levels. **A,** a lateral plain film reveals pedicle fractures *(arrows)*. These unusual defects could result in type IV (traumatic) spondylolisthesis. **B** and **C,** axial CT reveals bilateral defects in pedicles *(arrows)* at multiple levels.

(spondylotic) are the most common types of spondylolisthesis.[167, 169]

Spondylolytic spondylolisthesis occurs most frequently in young males at L5–S1[167, 169] and may result in varying degrees of severity of spondylolisthesis.[169] Spondylotic (degenerative) spondylolisthesis most frequently occurs in older females at L4–5[167, 169] and commonly results in a minor degree of subluxation.[169]

CT Findings

Axial CT findings of spondylolysis consist of a defect in the pars interarticularis that is usually bilateral and best seen at[171] or slightly cephalad to the pedicles (Fig 36–40).[167] Identification of a complete cortical ring outlining the spinal canal on one slice at a given vertebral level above the neural foramina excludes spondylolysis.[167, 171] The pars defect usually has jagged irregular margins with frequent sclerosis of the pars or adjacent lamina.[167, 168] Fragmentation of the lamina adjacent to the defect may be seen.[172] AP elongation of the canal may be present.[167, 168] Differentiation between

the facet joint and a pars defect is based on location (Fig 36–41): the former is seen on slices at the level of the neural foramina, not the pedicles; smooth cortical margins are present in facet joints; and notches may be present adjacent to facet joints where the joint capsules attach.[168]

Identification of the pars interarticularis defect may be easier with CT sagittal reformation, and better evaluation of the neural foramina is also possible (Fig 36–42).[166, 168, 169] Coronal CT reformations may demonstrate free bony fragments.[166] To optimally perform reformations, gantry angulation parallel to the disk space cannot be performed, and thinner sections (3 mm or less) are preferable. The location of the pars defect at the level of the pedicles emphasizes the need to scan through the pedicles and not the disk space exclusively in patients with suspected spondylolysis. Spondylolysis can be identified on the lateral localizing image in many cases.[168] Sagittal MRI can demonstrate the spondylolytic defect in the fatty marrow of the pars.[173]

Findings of spondylolisthesis in the axial plane

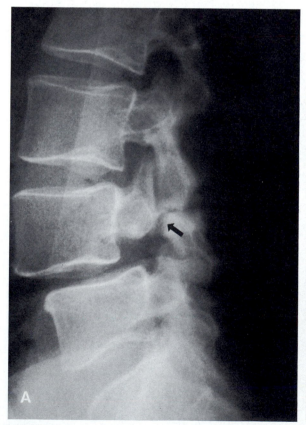

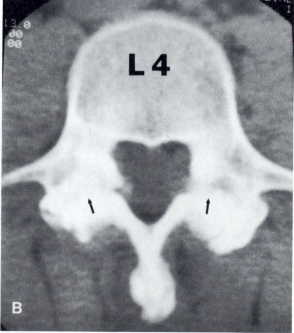

FIG 36–40.
Spondylolysis with spondylolisthesis. **A,** a lateral plain film reveals pars interarticularis defects *(arrow)* and anterior displacement of L4 on L5. **B,** axial CT reveals an elongated canal resulting from spondylolisthesis. Pars defects are indicated *(arrows).*

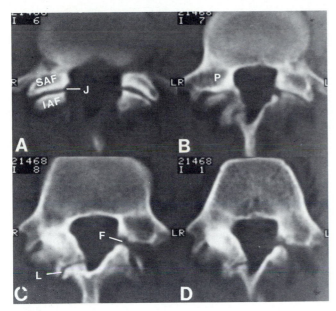

FIG 36–41.
Spondylolysis of L5. **A,** facet joint *(J)* *(SAF* = superior articular facet; *IAF* = inferior articular facet). **B,** a few millimeters below **A,** lower part of the facet joints *(P* = pedicle of L5). **C,** classic lysis or fracture *(F)* of the pars interarticularis on the left and an unusual fracture or lysis of the lamina *(L)* on the right. **D,** the lower aspect of the fractures are seen. Careful attention to the sequence of anatomy is necessary in order not to confuse the lysis with the facet joints.

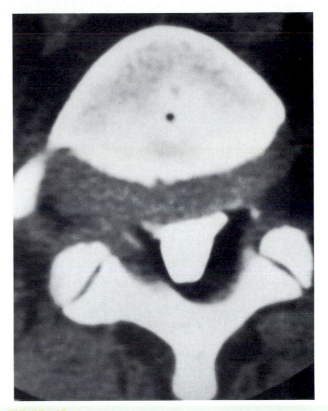

FIG 36–43.
Pseudobulging disk in spondylolisthesis.

include the pseudobulging disk (Fig 36–43), which represents the annulus extending from the posterior edge of the anteriorly displaced vertebral body to the posterior edge of the lower vertebral body. An axial slice through the disk space reveals disk material posterior to the superior vertebral body, and this reflects the anterior position of the superior vertebral body rather than the posterior protrusion of the disk. The pseudobulging disk has an indistinct margin and great transverse breadth and appears to extend laterally into the neural foramina.[167] Fibrocartilage buildup contributes to this.[167, 169] A vacuum phenomenon within the facet joint may accompany spondylotic spondylolisthe-

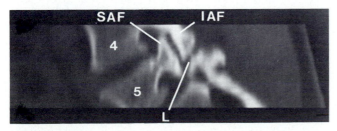

FIG 36–42.
Reformatted image showing spondylolysis of the pars of L5 (*4* and *5* = lumbar vertebrae; *SAF* = the superior articulating facet of L5; *IAF* = inferior articulating facet of L4; *L* = lysis of the L5 pars).

sis.[174] There is a decreased AP diameter of the canal beginning at the level of the disk space and extending caudally. Portions of several vertebral levels may be identified on a single slice due to the exaggerated lordosis accompanying severe spondylolisthesis. The lateral scout view or sagittal reformations should confirm a spondylolisthesis suspected on the axial images.[166]

Abnormalities associated with spondylolysis and/or spondylolisthesis include nerve root canal stenosis and fibrocartilaginous soft tissue adjacent to the pars defect, which may compromise the spinal canal.[166, 169] Spinal stenosis is seen predominantly in patients with spondylotic spondylolisthesis. This is related to a degenerative change[169] that is responsible for instability and to the presence of an intact neural arch.[175]

Disk herniation is uncommon in association with spondylolysis or spondylolisthesis. It most frequently occurs at the level above a spondylolytic spondylolisthesis[166] and at the same level as a spondylotic spondylolisthesis. The CT interpretation of disk herniation in the presence of spondylolisthesis[169] must be cautiously made, and sagittal reformations are necessary for confident diagnosis.[166, 169]

REFERENCES

1. Haughton VM: MR imaging of the spine. *Radiology* 1988; 166:297–301.
2. Modic MT, Masaryk TJ, Boumphrey F, et al: Lumbar herniated disk disease and canal stenosis: Prospective evaluation by surface coil MR, CT, and myelography. *AJNR* 1986; 7:709–717.
3. Modic MT, Masaryk TJ, Mulopulos GP, et al: Cervical radiculopathy: Prospective evaluation with surface coil MR imaging, CT with metrizamide, and metrizamide myelography. *Radiology* 1986; 161:753–759.
4. Modic MT, Pavlicek W, Weinstein MA, et al: Magnetic resonance imaging of intervertebral disk disease. *Radiology* 1984; 152:103–111.
5. Sharp J, Purser DW: Spontaneous atlantoaxial dislocation in ankylosing spondylitis and rheumatoid arthritis. *Ann Rheum Dis* 1961; 20:47–74.
6. Miller GOR, Grace MGA, Lampard R: Computed tomography of the upper cervical spine in Down syndrome. *J Comput Assist Tomogr* 1986; 10:589–592.
7. Hungerford GD, Akkaraju V, Rawe SE, et al: Atlanto-occipital and atlantoaxial dislocations with spinal cord compression in Down syndrome: A case report and review of the literature. *Br J Radiol* 1981; 54:758–761.
8. Bland JH: Rheumatoid arthritis of the cervical spine. *J Rheumatol* 1974; 1:319–342.
9. Wollin DG: The os odontoideum. *J Bone Joint Surg [Am]* 1963; 45:1459–1471.
10. Fielding JW, Griffin PP, et al: Os odontoideum: An acquired lesion. *J Bone Joint Surg [Am]* 1974; 56:187–190.
11. Minderhoud JM, Broakman R, Penning L: Os odontoideum: clinical, radiologic and therapeutic aspects. *J Neurol Sci* 1968; 8:521–544.
12. LaMasters DL, Watanabe TJ, Chambers EF, et al: Multiplanar metrizamide-enhanced CT imaging of the foramen magnum. *AJNR* 1982; 3:485–494.
13. Osborne D, Triolo P, Dubois P, et al: Assessment of craniocervical junction and atlanto-axial relation using metrizamide-enhanced CT in flexion and extension. *AJNR* 1983; 4:843–845.
14. Wolf BK, O'Keeffe D, Mitchell DM, et al: Rheumatoid arthritis of the cervical spine: Early and progressive radiographic features. *Radiology* 1987; 165:145–148.
15. Lipson SJ: Rheumatoid arthritis of the cervical spine. *Clin Orthop* 1984; 182:143–149.
16. Weissman BNW, Aliabadi P, Weinfeld MS, et al: Prognostic features of atlanto-axial subluxation in rheumatoid arthritis patients. *Radiology* 1982; 144:745–751.
17. Castor WR, Miller JDR, Russell AS, et al: Computed tomography of the craniocervical junction in rheumatoid arthritis. *J Comput Assist Tomogr* 1983; 7:31–36.
18. El-Khoury GY, Wener MH, Menezes AH, et al: Cranial settling in rheumatoid arthritis. *Radiology* 1980; 37:637–642.
19. Laasonen EM, Kankaanpaa U, Paukku P, et al: Computed tomographic myelography (CTM) in atlanto-axial rheumatoid arthritis. *Neuroradiology* 1985; 27:119–122.
20. Park WM, O'Neill M, McCall IW: The radiology of rheumatoid involvement of the cervical spine. *Skeletal Radiol* 1979; 4:1–7.
21. Braunstein EM, Weissman BN, Seltzer SE, et al: Computed tomography and conventional radiographics of the craniocervical region in rheumatoid arthritis: A comparison. *Arthritis Rheum* 1984; 27:26–31.
22. Aisen AM, Martel W, Ellis JH, et al: Cervical spine involvement in RA: MR imaging. *Radiology* 1987; 165:159–163.
23. Bundschuh C, Modic MT, Kearney F, et al: Rheumatoid arthritis of the cervical spine: Surface-coil MR imaging. *AJNR* 1988; 9:565–571.
24. Simeone FA, Rothman RH: Cervical disc disease, in Rothman RH, Simeone FA (ed): *The Spine*, ed 2. Philadelphia, WB Saunders Co, 1982, p 497.
25. Lunsford LD, Bissonette DJ, Janetta PJ: Anterior surgery for cervical disc disease. Part I: Treatment of lateral cervical disc herniation in 253 cases. *J Neurosurg* 1980; 53:1–11.
26. Shapiro R: The herniated intervertebral disk, in Shapiro R (ed): *Myelography*, ed 4. Chicago: Year Book Medical Publishers, Inc, 1984, p 475.
27. Orrison WW, Johansen JG, Eldevik OP, et al: Optimal computed-tomographic techniques for cervical spine imaging. *Radiology* 1982; 144:180–182.
28. Scotti G, Scialfa G, Pieralli S, et al: Myelopathy and radiculopathy due to cervical spondylosis: Myelographic-CT correlations. *AJNR* 1983; 4:601–603.
29. Heinz ER, Yeates A, Burger P, et al: Opacification of epidural venous plexus and dura in evaluation of cervical nerve roots: CT technique. *AJNR* 1984; 5:621–624.
30. Russell EJ, D'Angelo CM, Zimmerman RD, et al: Cervical disk herniation: CT demonstration after contrast enhancement. *Radiology* 1984; 152:703–712.
31. Baleriaux D, Noterman J, Ticket L: Recognition of cervical soft disk herniation by contrast-enhanced CT. *AJNR* 1983; 4:607–608.
32. DiChiro G, Schellinger D: Computed tomography of spinal cord after lumbar intrathecal introduction of metrizamide (computer-assisted myelography). *Radiology* 1976; 120:101–104.
33. Coin CG, Chen Y-S, Keranen V, et al: Computer

assisted myelography in disk disease. *J Comput Assist Tomogr* 1977; 1:398–404.

34. Arii H, Takahashi M, Tamakawa Y, et al: Metrizamide spinal computed tomography following myelography. *Comput Tomogr* 1980; 4:117–125.

35. Dublin AB, McGahan JP, Reid MH, et al: The value of computed tomographic metrizamide myelography in the neuroradiological evaluation of the spine. *Radiology* 1983; 146:79–86.

36. Badami JP, Norman D, Barbara NM, et al: Metrizamide CT myelography in cervical myelopathy and radiculopathy: Correlation with conventional myelography and surgical findings. *AJR* 1985; 144:675–680.

37. Sobel DF, Barkovich AJ, Munderloh SH: Metrizamide myelography and postmyelographic computed tomography: Comparative adequacy in the cervical spine. *AJNR* 1984; 5:385–390.

38. Landman JA, Hoffman JC, Braun IF, et al: Value of computed tomographic myelography in the recognition of cervical herniated disk. *AJNR* 1984; 5:391–394.

39. Daniels DL, Grogan JP, Johansen JG, et al: Cervical radiculopathy: Computed tomography and myelography compared. *Radiology* 1984; 151:109–113.

40. Yu YL, Stevens JM, Kendall B, et al: Cord shape and measurements in cervical spondylotic myelopathy and radiculopathy. *AJNR* 1983; 4:839–842.

41. Nakagawa H, Okumura T, Sugiyama T, et al: Discrepancy between metrizamide CT and myelography in diagnosis of cervical disk protrusions. *AJNR* 1983; 4:604–606.

42. Yu YL, du Boulay GH, Stevens JM, et al: Computed tomography in cervical spondylotic myelography and radiculopathy: Visualization of structures, myelographic comparison, cord measurements and clinical utility. *Neuroradiology* 1986; 28:221–236.

43. Brown BM, Schwartz RH, Frank E, et al: Preoperative evaluation of cervical radiculopathy and myelography by surface-coil MR imaging. *AJNR* 1988; 9:859–866.

44. Karnaze MG, Gado MH, Sartor KJ, et al: Comparison of MR and CT myelography in imaging the cervical and thoracic spine. *AJNR* 1987; 8:983–989.

45. Coin CG, Coin JT: Computed tomography of cervical disk disease: Technical considerations with representative case reports. *J Comput Assist Tomogr* 1981; 5:275–280.

46. Miyasaka K, Isu T, Iwasaki Y, et al: High resolution computed tomography in the diagnosis of cervical disc disease. *Neuroradiology* 1983; 24:253–257.

47. Isu T, Iwasaki Y, Miyasaka K, et al: A reappraisal of the diagnosis in cervical disc disease: The posterior longitudinal ligament perforated or not. *Neuroradiology* 1986; 28:215–220.

48. Eisenberg RA, Brener AM, Northup HM: Intradural herniated cervical disk: A case report and review of the literature. *AJNR* 1986; 7:492–497.

49. Mainzer F: Herniation of the nucleus pulposus. *Radiology* 1973; 107:167–170.

50. McGregor JC, Butler P: Disc calcification in childhood: Computed tomographic and magnetic resonance imaging appearance. *Br J Radiology* 1986; 59:180–182.

51. Arnoldi CC, Brodsky AE, Chauchoix J, et al: Lumbar spinal stenosis and nerve root entrapment syndromes: A definition and classification. *Clin Orthop* 1975; 115:4–5.

52. Roberson GH, Llewellyn HJ, Taveras JM: The narrow lumbar spinal canal syndrome. *Radiology* 1973; 107:89–97.

53. Verbiest H: Pathomorphologic aspects of developmental lumbar stenosis. *Orthop Clin North Am* 1975; 6:177–196.

54. Zlatkin MB, Lordar PH, Hadjipavlou AG, Levine JJ: Paget disease of the spine: CT with clinical correlation. *Radiology* 1986; 160:155–159.

55. Gelman MI: Cauda equina compression in acromegaly. *Radiology* 1974; 112:357–360.

56. Lunsford LD, Bissonette DJ, Zoreb DS: Anterior surgery for cervical disc disease. Part 2: Treatment of cervical spondylotic myelopathy in 32 cases. *J Neurosurg* 1980; 53:12–19.

57. Simeone FA, Rothman RH: Cervical disc disease, in Rothman RH, Simeone FA (eds): *The Spine*, ed 2. Philadelphia, WB Saunders Co, 1982, p 453.

58. Payne EE, Spillane JD: The cervical spine. An anatomicopathological study of 70 specimens (using a special technique) with particular reference to the problem of cervical spondylosis. *Brain* 1957; 80:571–591.

59. Resnick D: Degenerative diseases of the vertebral column. *Radiology* 1985; 156:3–14.

60. Patel SC, Sanders WP: Synovial cyst of the cervical spine: Case report and review of the literature. *AJNR* 1988; 9:602–603.

61. Epstein JA, Carras R, Hyman RA, et al: Cervical myelopathy caused by developmental stenosis of the spinal canal. *J Neurosurg* 1979; 51:362–367.

62. Ehni G: Stenosis and cervical myelopathy (letter). *J Neurosurg* 1980; 52:290.

63. Miyasaka K, Kaneda K, Ito T, et al: Ossification of spinal ligaments causing thoracic radiculomyelopathy. *Radiology* 1982; 143:463–468.

64. Miyasaka K, Kaneda K, Sato S, et al: Myelopathy due to ossification or calcification of the ligamentum flavum: Radiologic and histologic evaluations. *AJNR* 1983; 4:629–632.

65. Stanley JH, Schabel SI, Frey GD, et al: Quantitative analysis of the cervical spinal canal by com-

puted tomography. *Neuroradiology* 1979; 18:57–62.

66. Thijssen HOM, Keyser A, Horstink MWM, et al: Morphology of the cervical spinal cord on computed myelography. *Neuroradiology* 1979; 18:57–62.

67. Mawad ME, Hilal SK, Fetell MR, et al: Patterns of spinal cord atrophy by metrizamide CT. *AJNR* 1983; 4:611–613.

68. Penning L, Wilmink JT, Van Woerden HH, et al: CT myelographic findings in degenerative disorders of the cervical spine: Clinical significance. *AJR* 1986; 146:793–801.

69. Rosenbloom S, Cohen WA, Marshall C, et al: Imaging factors influencing spine and cord measurements by CT: A phantom study. *AJNR* 1983; 4:646–649.

70. Arce CA, Dohrmann GJ: Thoracic disc herniation. *Surg Neurol* 1985; 23:356–361.

71. McAllister VL, Sage MR: The radiology of thoracic disc protrusion. *Clin Radiol* 1976; 27:291–299.

72. Bhole R, Gilmer RE: Two-level thoracic disc herniation. *Clin Orthop* 1984; 190:129–131.

73. Michowiz SD, Rappaport HZ, Shaked I, et al: Thoracic disc herniation associated with papilledema. *J Neurosurg* 1984; 61:1132–1134.

74. Hochman MS, Pena C, Ramirez R: Calcified herniated thoracic disc diagnosed by computerized tomography. *J Neurosurg* 1980; 52:722–723.

75. Alvarez O, Rogue CT, Pampati M: Multilevel thoracic disc herniations: CT and MR studies. *J Comput Assist Tomogr* 1988; 12:649–652.

76. Ryan RW, Latty JF, Kozic Z: Asymptomatic calcified herniated thoracic discs: CT recognition. *AJNR* 1988; 9:363–366.

77. VanDuym FCVA, Van Wiechan PJ: Herniation of calcified nucleus pulposis in the thoracic spine. *J Comput Assist Tomogr* 1983; 7:1122–1123.

78. Shapiro R: The narrow spinal canal, in Shapiro R (ed): *Myelography*, ed 4. Chicago, Year Book Medical Publishers, Inc, 1984, p 501.

79. Jaspan T, Holland IM, Punt JA: Thoracic spinal canal stenosis. *Neuroradiology* 1987; 29:217.

80. Ono M, Russell WJ, Kudo S, et al: Ossification of the thoracic posterior longitudinal ligament in a field population. *Radiology* 1982; 143:469–474.

81. Murakami J, Russell WJ, Hayabuchi N, et al: Computed tomography of posterior longitudinal ligament ossification: Its appearance and diagnostic value with special reference to thoracic lesions. *J Comput Assist Tomogr* 1982; 6:41–50.

82. Williams DM, Gabrielsen TO, Latack JT: Ossification in the caudal attachments of the ligamentum flavum. *Radiology* 1982; 145:693–697.

83. Govani AF: Developmental stenosis of a thoracic vertebra resulting in narrowing of the spinal canal. *AJR* 1971; 112:401–404.

84. Jungreis CA, Cohen WA: Spinal cord compression induced by steroid therapy: CT findings. *J Comput Assist Tomogr* 1987; 11:245–247.

85. Pennisi AK, Meisler WJ, Dira TS: Case report. Lymphomatosis meningitis and steroid-induced epidural lipomatosis: CT evaluation. *J Comput Assist Tomogr* 1985; 9:595–598.

86. Quint DJ, Boulos RS, Sanders WP, et al: Epidural lipomatosis. *Radiology* 1988; 169:485–495.

87. Buthiau D, Rette JC, Ducerveau MN, et al. Steroid-induced spinal epidural lipomatosis: CT survey. *J Comput Assist Tomogr* 1988; 12:501–503.

88. Badami JP, Hinck VC: Symptomatic deposition of epidural fat in morbidly obese women. *AJNR* 1982; 3:664–665.

89. Gellad F, Rao KCVG, Joseph PM, et al: Morphology and dimensions of the thoracic cord by computer-assisted metrizamide myelography. *AJNR* 1983; 4:614–617.

90. Paine KWE, Huang PWH: Lumbar disc syndrome. *J Neurosurg* 1972; 37:75–82.

91. Rothman RH, Simeone FA, Bernini PM: Lumbar disc disease, in Rothman RH, Simeone FA (eds): *The Spine*, ed 2. Philadelphia, WB Saunders Co, 1982, p 521.

92. Carrera GF, Williams AL, Haughton VM: Computed tomography in sciatica. *Radiology* 1980; 137:433–437.

93. Wiesel SW, Tsourmas N, Feffer HL, et al: A study of computer assisted tomography. 1. The incidence of positive CAT scans in an asymptomatic group of patients. *Spine* 1984; 9:549–551.

94. Wilberger JE, Pang D: Syndrome of the incidental herniated lumbar disc. *J Neurosurg* 1983; 59:137–141.

95. Giles DJ, Thomas RJ, Osborn AG, et al: Lumbar spine: Pretest predictability of CT findings. *Radiology* 1984; 150:719–722.

96. Eldevik OP, Dugstad G, Orrison WW, et al: The effect of clinical bias on the interpretation of myelography and spinal computed tomography. *Radiology* 1982; 145:85–89.

97. Bell GR, Rothman RH, Booth RE, et al: A study of computer-assisted tomography. II. Comparison of metrizamide myelography and computed tomography in the diagnosis of herniated lumbar disc and spinal stenosis. *Spine* 1984; 9:552–556.

98. Haughton VM, Syversten A, Williams AL: Soft-tissue anatomy within the spinal canal as seen on computed tomography. *Radiology* 1980; 134:649–655.

99. Haughton VM, Williams AL: CT anatomy of the spine: *CRC Crit Rev Diagn Imaging* 1981; 13:173–192.

100. Rothman RH, Simeone FA, Bernini PM: Lumbar disc disease, in Rothman RH, Simeone FA (eds):

The Spine, ed 2. Philadelphia, WB Saunders Co, 1982, p 521.

101. Williams AL, Haughton VM, Syversten A: Computed tomography in the diagnosis of herniated nucleus pulposus. *Radiology* 1980; 135:95–99.
102. Williams AL, Haughton VM, Daniels DL, et al: CT recognition of lateral lumbar disk herniation. *AJR* 1982; 139:345–347.
103. Dillon WP, Kaseff LG, Knackstedt VE, et al: Computed tomography and differential diagnosis of extruded lumbar disc. *J Comput Assist Tomogr* 1982; 6:874–887.
104. Fries JW, Abodeely DA, Vijungco JG, et al: Computed tomography of herniated and extruded nucleus pulposus. *J Comput Assist Tomogr* 1982; 6:874–887.
105. Williams AL, Haughton VM, Daniels DL, et al: Differential CT diagnosis of extruded nucleus pulposus. *Radiology* 1983; 148:141–148.
106. Graves VB, Finney HL, Mailarder J: Intradural lumbar disk herniation. *AJNR* 1986; 7:495–497.
107. Barbera J, Gonzalez-Darder JG, Garcia-Vazquez FG: Intraradicular herniated lumbar disc. *J Neurosurg* 1984; 60:858–860.
108. Kaiser MC, Sandt G, Roilgen A, et al: Intradural disk herniation with CT appearance of gas collection. *AJNR* 1985; 6:117–118.
109. Guinto FC, Hashim H, Stumer M: CT demonstration of disk regression after conservative therapy. *AJNR* 1984; 6:632–633.
110. Teplick JG, Haskin ME: Spontaneous regression of herniated nucleus pulposus. *AJNR* 1985; 6:331–335.
111. Williams AL, Haughton VM, Meyer GA: Computed tomographic appearance of the bulging annulus. *Radiology* 1982; 142:403–408.
112. Firooznia H, Benjamin V, Kricheff II, et al: CT of lumbar spine disk herniation: Correlation with surgical findings. *AJNR* 1984; 5:91–96.
113. Rovira M, Romero F, Ibarra B, et al: Prolapsed lumbar disk: Value of CT in diagnosis. *AJNR* 1983; 4:593–594.
114. Gulati A, Weinstein R, Studdard E: CT scan of the spine for herniated discs. *Neuroradiology* 1981; 22:57–60.
115. Haughton VM, Eldevik OP, Magnaes B, et al: A prospective comparison of computed tomography and myelography in the diagnosis of herniated lumbar disks. *Radiology* 1982; 142:103–110.
116. Bosacco SJ, Berman AT, Garbarino JL, et al: A comparison of CT scanning and myelography in the diagnosis of lumbar disc herniation. *Clin Orthop* 1984; 190:124–128.
117. Dublin AB, McGahan JP, Reid MH: The value of computed tomographic metrizamide myelography in the neuroradiological evaluation of the spine. *Radiology* 1983; 146:79–86.

118. Raskin SP, Keating JW: Recognition of lumbar disk disease: Comparison of myelography and computed tomography. *AJNR* 1982; 3:215–221.
119. Schipper J, Karduan JWPF, Braakman R, et al: Lumbar disk herniation: Diagnosis with CT or myelography? *Radiology* 1987; 165:227–231.
120. Anand AK, Lee BCP: Plain and metrizamide CT of lumbar disk disease: Comparison with myelography. *AJNR* 1982; 3:567–571.
121. Meyer GA, Haughton VM, Williams AL: Diagnosis of lumbar disk with computed tomography. *N Engl J Med* 1979; 301:1166–1167.
122. Barrow DL, Wood JH, Hoffman JC: Clinical indications for computer-assisted myelography. *Neurosurg* 1983; 12:47–57.
123. Moufarrij NA, Hardy RW, Weinstein MA: Computed tomographic, myelographic and operative findings in patients with suspected herniated lumbar discs. *Neurosurg* 1983; 12:184–188.
124. DiChiro G, Schellinger D: Computed tomography of spinal cord after lumbar intrathecal introduction of metrizamide (computer-assisted myelography). *Radiology* 1976; 120:101–104.
125. Coin CG, Chan Y, Keranen V, et al: Computer-assisted myelography in disc disease. *J Comput Assist Tomogr* 1977; 1:398–404.
126. Arii H, Takahashi M, Tamakawa Y, et al: Metrizamide spinal computed tomography following myelography. *Comput Tomogr* 1980; 4:117–125.
127. Teplick JG, Teplick SK, Goodman L, et al: Pitfalls and unusual findings in computed tomography of the lumbar spine. *J Comput Assist Tomogr* 1982; 6:888–893.
128. Schubiger O, Valavanis A: CT differentiation between recurrent disk herniation and postoperative scar formation: The value of contrast enhancement. *Neuroradiology* 1982; 22:251–254.
129. Teplick JG, Haskin ME: Intravenous contrast-enhanced CT of the postoperative lumbar spine: Improved identification of recurrent disk herniation, scar, arachnoiditis, and diskitis. *AJR* 1984; 143:845–855.
130. Braun IF, Hoffman JC, Davis PC, et al: Contrast enhancement in CT differentiation between recurrent disk herniation and postoperative scar: Prospective study. *AJNR* 1985; 6:607–612.
131. Yang PJ, Seeger JF, Dzioba RB, et al: High-dose IV contrast in CT scanning of the postoperative lumbar spine. *AJNR* 1986; 7:703–707.
132. Weiss T, Treisch J, Kazner E, et al: CT of the postoperative lumbar spine: The value of intravenous contrast. *Neuroradiology* 1986; 28:241–245.
133. Wilmink JT, Roukema JG, VandenBurg W: Effects of IV contrast administration on intraspinal and paraspinal soft tissues: A CT study 2. Visual assessment. *AJNR* 1988; 9:191–193.

134. Rosenthal DI, Stauffer AE, David KR, et al: Evaluation of multiplanar reconstruction in CT recognition of lumbar disk disease. *AJNR* 1984; 5:307–314.

135. Yetkin Z, Chintapalli K, Daniels DL, et al: Gas in spinal articulations. *Neuroradiology* 1986; 28:150–153.

136. Gado M, Patel J, Hodges FJ: Lateral disk herniation into the lumbar intervertebral foramen: Differential diagnosis. *AJNR* 1983; 4:598–600.

137. Novetsky GJ, Berlin L, Epstein AJ, et al. The extraforaminal herniated disk: Detection by computed tomography. *AJNR* 1982; 3:653–655.

138. Osborne AG, Hood RS, Sherry RG, et al: CT/MR spectrum of far lateral and anterior lumbosacral disk herniations. *AJNR* 1988; 9:775–778.

139. Johansen JG: Demonstration of anterior intervertebral disc herniation by CT. *Neuroradiology* 1987; 29:214.

140. Vadala G, Dore R, Garbagna P: Unusual osseous changes in lumbar herniated disks: CT features. *J Comput Assist Tomogr* 1985; 9:1045–1049.

141. Kaiser MC, Capesius P, Viega-Pires JA, et al: A sign of lumbar disk herniation recognizable on lateral CT generated digital radiograms. *J Comput Assist Tomogr* 1984; 8:1066–1071.

142. Kieffer SA, Sherry RG, Wellenstein DE, et al: Bulging lumbar intervertebral disk: Myelographic differentiation from herniated disk with nerve root compression. *AJR* 1982; 138:709–716.

143. Resnick D, Niwayama G, Guerra G, et al: Spiral vacuum phenomena: Anatomical study and review. *Radiology* 1981; 139:341–348.

144. Hoddick WK, Helms CA: Bony spinal cord changes that differentiate conjoined nerve roots and differentiation from a herniated nucleus pulposus. *Radiology* 1985; 154:119–120.

145. Helms CA, Dorwart RH, Gray M: The CT appearance of conjoined nerve roots and differentiation from a herniated nucleus pulposus. *Radiology* 1982; 144:803–807.

146. Yang WC, Zappulla R, Malis L: Neurolemmoma in lumbar intervertebral foramen. *J Comput Assist Tomogr* 1981; 5:904–906.

147. Casselman ES: Radiologic recognition of symptomatic spinal synovial cysts. *AJNR* 1985; 6:971–973.

148. Hemminghytt S, Daniels DL, Williams AL, et al: Intraspinal synovial cysts: Natural history and diagnosis by CT. *Radiology* 1982; 145:375–376.

149. Meyer GD: Computed tomographic myelography in degenerative disc disease and spinal stenosis, in Latchaw RE (ed): *Computed Tomography of the Head, Neck, and Spine*, ed 1. Chicago, Year Book Medical Publishers, Inc, 1985, p 621.

150. Kirkaldy-Willis WH, Wedge JH, Yong-Hing K, et al: Lumbar spinal nerve root entrapment. *Clin Orthop* 1982; 169:171–178.

151. Kirkaldy-Willis WH, Wedge JH, Yong-Hing K, et al: Pathology and pathogenesis of lumbar spondylosis and stenosis. *Spine* 1978; 3:319–328.

152. Risius B, Modic MT, Hardy RW, et al: Sector computed tomographic spine scanning in the diagnosis of lumbar nerve root entrapment. *Radiology* 1982; 143:109–114.

153. McAfee PC, Ullrich CG, Yuan HA, et al: Computed tomography in degenerative spinal stenosis. *Clin Orthop* 1981; 161:221–234.

154. Epstein JA, Epstein BS, Rosenthal AD, et al: Sciatica caused by nerve root entrapment in the lateral recess: The superior facet syndrome. *J Neurosurg* 1972; 36:584–589.

155. Reynolds AF, Weinstein PR, Wachter RD: Lumbar monoradiculopathy due to unilateral facet hypertrophy. *Neurosurg* 1982; 10:480–486.

156. Ciric I, Mikhael MA, Tarkington JA, et al: The lateral recess syndrome: A variant of spinal stenosis. *J Neurosurg* 1980; 53:433–443.

157. Mikhael MA, Ciric I, Tarkington JA, et al: Neuroradiologic evaluation of the lateral recess syndrome. *Radiology* 1981; 140:97–107.

158. Randall BC, Muraki AS, Osborn RE, et al: Epidural lipomatosis with lumbar radiculopathy: CT appearance. *J Comput Assist Tomogr* 1986; 10:1039–1041.

159. Stollman A, Pinto R, Benjamin V, et al: Radiologic imaging of symptomatic ligamentum flavum thickening with and without ossification. *AJNR* 1987; 8:991–994.

160. Matozzi F, Moreau JJ, Jiddane M, et al: Correlative anatomic and CT study of the lumbar lateral recess. *AJNR* 1983; 4:650–652.

161. Ullrich CG, Binet EF, Sanecki MG, et al: Quantitative assessment of the lumbar spinal cord by computed tomography. *Radiology* 1980; 134:137–143.

162. Carrera GF, Haughton VM, Syversten A, et al: Computed tomography of the lumbar facet joints. *Radiology* 1980; 134:145–148.

163. Beers GJ, Carter AP, Leiter BE, et al: Interobserver discrepancies in distance measurements from lumbar spine CT scans. *AJNR* 1984; 5:787–790.

164. Epstein JA, Epstein BS, Lavine LS, et al: Lumbar nerve root compression at the intervertebral foramina caused by arthritis of the posterior facets. *J Neurosurg* 1973; 39:362–369.

165. Helms CA, Sims R: Foraminal spurs: A normal variant in the lumbar spine. *Radiology* 1986; 160:153–154.

166. Rothman SLG, Glenn WV: CT multiplanar reconstruction in 253 cases of lumbar spondylolysis. *AJNR* 1984; 5:81–90.

167. Teplick JG, Laffey PA, Berman A, et al: Diagnosis and evaluation of spondylolisthesis and/or spondylolysis on axial CT. *AJNR* 1986; 7:479–491.

168. Grogan JP, Hemminghytt S, Williams AL, et al: Spondylolysis studied with computed tomography. *Radiology* 1982; 145:737–742.

169. Elster AD, Jensen KM: Computed tomography of spondylolisthesis: Patterns of associated pathology. *J Comput Assist Tomogr* 1985; 9:867–874.

170. Wiltse LL, Newman PH, NacNeb I: Classification of spondylolysis and spondylolisthesis. *Clin Orthop* 1976; 117:23–29.

171. Langston JW, Gavant ML: "Incomplete ring" sign: A single method for CT detection of spondylolysis. *J Comput Assist Tomogr* 1985; 9:728–729.

172. Amato M, Totty WG, Gilula LA: Spondylolysis of the lumbar spine: Demonstration of defects and laminal fragmentation. *Radiology* 1984; 153:627–629.

173. Johnson DW, Farnum GN, Latchaw RE, et al: MR imaging of the pars interarticularis in patients with spondylolisthesis. *AJNR* 1988; 9:1215–1220.

174. Lefkowitz DM, Quencer RM: Vacuum facet phenomenon: A computed tomographic sign of degenerative spondylolisthesis. *Radiology* 1982; 144:562.

175. Newman PH: The etiology of spondylolisthesis. *J Bone Joint Surg [Br]* 1963; 45:39–59.

37

Magnetic Resonance Imaging of Degenerative Diseases of the Spine

Louis Wener, M.D.

Stanley M. Perl, M.D.

GENERAL CONSIDERATIONS

Since humans began to walk erect, the spine has become a source of various ailments producing symptoms ranging from mild discomfort to incapacitation with gross neurologic abnormality. Because of the frequency and severity of these ailments, physicians have been trying to image the spinal column and its contents in an effort to establish the causal factors of spinal disease and, it is hoped, prescribe the appropriate therapy. Magnetic resonance imaging (MRI), with its expanded soft-tissue contrast, multiplanar capability, and noninvasive nature, has added another dimension to this effort.

Plain-film study of the spine left much to be desired, for the neurologic tissues were not imaged. Air myelography was introduced in 1919 by Dandy,[1] and iodized oil studies began in 1922 with the use of Lipiodol.[2] Myelography continued to be the mainstay of spinal canal examinations until the advent of computed tomography (CT), which proved more efficacious for the diagnosis of lumbar disk abnormalities.[3] The computerized techniques are preferred in the lumbar region because they afford direct visualization of the spinal structures and neural elements rather than depending on indirect evidence of abnormalities by their effect on a column of opaque material. A combination technique using contrast-enhanced CT studies may still be the study of choice in the cervical spine.[4, 5]

MRI was quickly recognized as an excellent imaging modality in the study of the spine but was hampered by poor resolution caused by thick slices and a poor signal-to-noise ratio (SNR) in body-coil images.[6, 7] Although carefully performed CT remains an excellent modality for spinal studies,[8] the advent of thinner slices and surface-coil development has catapulted MRI studies of the spine to the forefront of spinal examinations.

As mentioned previously, spinal studies require a good SNR in thin slices for clear spatial resolution and should be performed with surface coils adapted to the region of interest. Anatomy is best studied with T1-weighted images. T2-weighted acquisitions yield physiologic information about the disk and "opacify" the thecal space and its contents. The patient should be made as comfortable as possible to minimize motion artifacts and adjunctive measures such as gating, flow compensation, phase wrap suppression, and saturation pulses to reduce flow artifacts are employed as necessary to produce sharp images. The slice thickness should be 5 mm or less depending on the section of spine being imaged.

CERVICAL SPONDYLOSIS

Ehni[9] describes a motion segment as two contiguous vertebrae and their supporting structures that permit movement and ensure unrestricted passage of the neural elements and their nutrient vessels. He refers to cervical arthrosis as "degenerative disease of the cervical joints with all the neurological consequences." Whether the initial lesion begins with degeneration of the intervertebral disk and progresses to overproduction of bone resulting in osteophytes and arthritis of the Luschka and diarthrodial joints or whether this represents several different degenerative processes remains a matter of debate.[10] In any event, there is a decrease in protoglycan of the hyaline cartilage that results in a loss and ulceration of the articular surface; this is followed by proliferation of new bone about the joints that produces osteophytosis.

The relationship between the pathologic findings of cervical spine degeneration (spondylosis) and clinical symptomatology is vague and has been extensively studied.[11, 12] By the beginning of the fifth decade, there seems to be a decreasing correlation between anatomic findings and clinical manifestations. By the seventh decade, clinical symptoms and anatomic changes correlate in only one of four patients. This condition becomes symptomatic when the bony overgrowth compresses the exiting nerve roots within the neural foramina or the spinal cord within the neural canal (Fig 37–1). Anterior subarachnoid space impingement in a congenitally narrow canal, especially in combination with hypertrophy of the ligamentum flavum posteriorly, may cause stenosis of the neural canal.

CT has been very useful in delineating the new bone production and, when used with intrathecal contrast, is an excellent examination of cervical pain syndromes secondary to osteoarthritis.[13] The development of gradient-refocused MRI sequences has added a new dimension to the study of this condition, requires no injections, and appears to be useful in differentiating an osteophyte from herniation of nuclear material.

DEGENERATIVE DISK DISEASE

Since the historic treatise of Mixter and Barr[14] established the relationship between the intervertebral disk and sciatica, the majority of diagnostic emphasis has been placed on examining the state of the disk. The ability of MRI to differentiate between the annulus and nucleus gives a greater in-

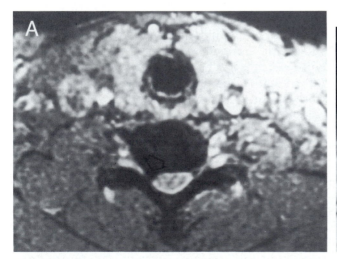
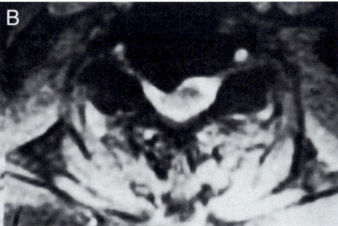

FIG 37–1.
Cervical spondylosis. **A,** T2-weighted gradient-refocused axial image through the neural foramina at the cervical level (TR = 500 ms, TE = 20 ms, flip angle = 18 degrees, number of excitations [NEX] = 4, 3-mm-thick slice, 256 × 192 matrix) demonstrates a spur *(open arrow)* originating from the right uncovertebral joint and compromising the medial aspect of the neural foramen and conse-quently the exiting root at this level. **B,** In a different patient, a T2-weighted gradient-refocused axial image through the neural foramina at the C5–6 level demonstrates a very large posterior vertebral body and uncinate spur compressing the right side of the spinal cord and narrowing the right neural foramen. (**B,** Courtesy of Richard E. Latchaw, M.D., Englewood, Colo.)

sight into the role of the disk components in various back syndromes.

To comprehend the significance of the imaging characteristics of the intervertebral disk, one should study carefully the work of Arthur Naylor,[15] whose presentation on the characteristics of the degenerating disk can be used to explain the imaging parameters seen on magnetic resonance studies. The intervertebral disk is composed of two elements, the nucleus pulposus, which is made up of a hydrophilic mucopolysaccharide/collagen system, and the annulus fibrosus, which is formed by concentric layers of collagen fibers (Sharpey's fibers) that run obliquely between the adjacent vertebral bodies. The consistency of the nucleus is that of a gel because of the hydrophilic nature of the mucopolysaccharide. The collagen serves as the connective tissue. The human disk has a blood supply until the age of 8 years, after which it rapidly loses its direct vascular connections. The water content of the nucleus is highest in the newborn, gradually decreasing with age, especially after the fifth decade. In the adult, the vertebral body end plate has numerous perforations through which liquids diffuse between the vertebral body, bone marrow, and the hydrophilic mucopolysaccharide/collagen gel of the nucleus.

Naylor believes the following to be the course of events in the formation of a degenerated, herniated nucleus pulposus. A disturbance, etiology yet unknown, in the balance of mucopolysaccharide synthesis/depolymerization occurs in favor of depolymerization, which transiently increases the fluid content of the disk and thus increases intradiscal pressure. Simultaneously there is reduction in the mucopolysaccharide content of the disk and fibrillation and percipitation of the collagen. Annular fibers reorient themselves to accommodate the increased volume of the nucleus. The water then diffuses out through the pores in the end plates, the volume of the nucleus is therefore less, the annular fibers reorient themselves again, and a new equilibrium within the nucleus is achieved. However, with less hydrophilic mucopolysaccharide in the nucleus, there is less water-binding capacity of the nucleus. As this process is repeated, a desiccated, degenerated nucleus occurs. The function of the gel-like nucleus is to transmit forces evenly to the annulus. Once the gel is partially dehydrated, it is unable to distribute force evenly to the annulus, and this results in excessive stress conveyed to focal areas of the annulus that results in annular tears and nuclear herniation. This the-ory may explain the phenomenon reported by Teplick and Haskin[16] of the "disappearing herniated disk." With varying intradiscal pressure and subsequent changes in orientation of the annular fibers, herniations of nuclear material may protrude through an annular tear and then be retracted back into the nucleus.

As expected, magnetic resonance images the normal nucleus as signal poor on T1-weighted sequences and signal intense on T2-weighted sequences because of the water content of the normal nucleus. The well-hydrated, diffusely bulging disk that one frequently sees on MRI could be explained by Naylor's initial stage of degeneration with increased water content of the nucleus and reorientation of the annular fibers to accommodate the increased volume of the nucleus. This progressive degenerative process is manifested on MRI as an irregularity of the "oyster-shaped" nucleus, particularly in the region of the cleft. The normal

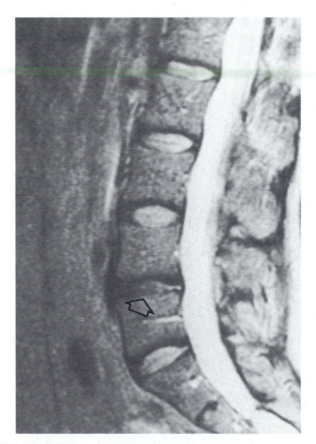

FIG 37–2.
Degenerative disk disease seen on a sagittal T2-weighted lumbar image (spin-echo [SE], TR = 2,000 ms, TE = 80 ms, 2 NEX, 5-mm-thick slice, 256 × 192). Flow compensation was used. Note the decreased signal from the L4–5 disk space secondary to degeneration and desiccation of the nucleus pulposus.

bullet-shaped posterior extremity of the nucleus begins to flatten and may assume a fishtail configuration. These morphologic changes are accompanied by a continuum of low to absent signal from the nucleus on T2-weighted images (Fig 37–2) and coincide with the changes Naylor describes. The absent signal of a degenerated disk on T2-weighted images was one of the initial observations with MRI of the spine.[17] When the disk space is narrowed, there may be some buckling of the annulus that, by occupying space, can cause symptoms identical to a herniated nucleus pulposus (Fig 37–3,A and B).

This process occurs normally with aging but may be accelerated by trauma, surgery, or other unusual stresses. Advancing age results in fissuring of the annulus. Trauma can also produce tears in the annular fibers. The external lamellae can heal, but the internal rings will not. If Naylor's theory is valid, a situation in which the increase in intradiscal tension is combined with the weakness of the annulus may permit herniation of the nucleus pulposus through an annular rent. When this occurs, the herniation consists of a hyperhydrated nucleus that is no longer in contact with the vertebral body

end plates and thus may be excluded from the fluid-exchange mechanism. This may explain the usual MRI finding of a herniated nucleus pulposus that is signal intense on T2-weighted images and a degenerated nuclear remnant within the disk space imaging with a low or absent signal. Extruded fragments, although separated from the parent disk, also seem to retain the hyperhydrated state and image with high signal on T2-weighted images (Fig 37–4).[18]

The disruption or stretching of the annular fibers alone may be a source of back pain. It is now well accepted that compression of the roots by the herniated nuclear material frequently presents as a radiculopathy. It is important to remember, however, that herniated nuclei can be silent and critical clinical correlation is required for an accurate assessment of back syndromes. The degeneration of the nucleus with a consequent loss of disk space height may also impose stresses on the posterior elements of the "motion segment"[19] that result in various low back syndromes mimicking radiculopathy.

As the nucleus degenerates and the disk begins to bulge, it will usually distend posteriorly be-

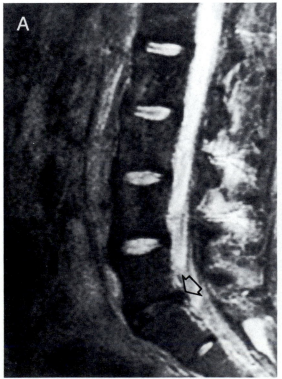

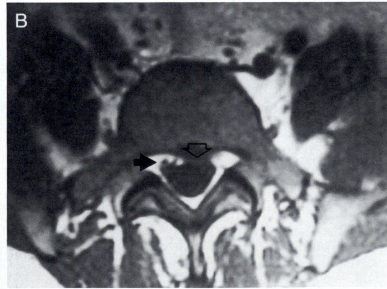

FIG 37–3.
Degeneration of the L5–S1 disk with buckling of the annulus posteriorly that is compromising the S1 root on the left. **A,** a T2-weighted, spin-echo sagittal image through the lumbar spine. **B,** a T1-weighted axial image through the lumbar spine at the same level. **A:** SE, TR = 2,000 ms, TE = 20 ms, 2 NEX, 4-mm-thick slice, 256 × 192. Flow compensation was used. **B:** SE, TR = 600 ms, TE = 20 ms, 4 NEX, 4-mm-thick slice, 256 × 192. This patient presented with an S1 radiculopathy on the left. Note the degeneration of the L5–S1 disk with loss of signal from the disk and the annulus *(open arrow)* buckled posteriorly. In **B,** one may see the annulus *(open arrow)* compromise the S1 root on the left. The S1 root on the right *(closed arrow)* appears to be surrounded by signal-intense fat.

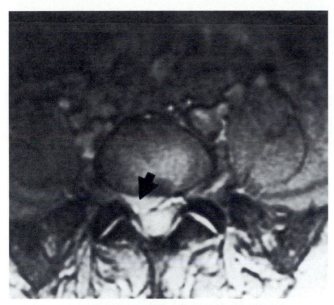

FIG 37–4.
Hyperhydrated extruded disk fragment seen on a gradient-refocused T2-weighted axial image through the lumbar disk space (TR = 350 ms, TE = 18 ms, flip angle = 25 degrees, 4 NEX, 4-mm-thick slice, 256 × 192). A hyperhydrated extruded fragment of nuclear material *(arrow)* is demonstrated. The descending and exiting roots on the right are probably compromised by this fragment.

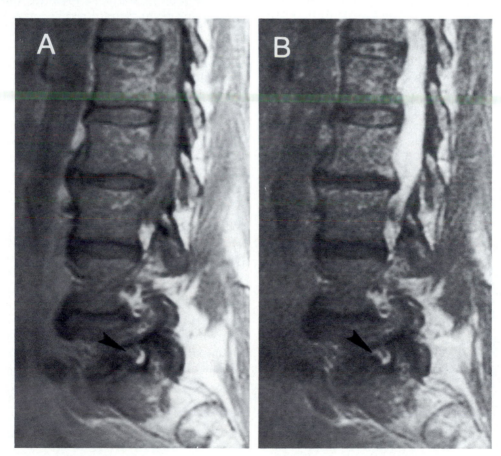

FIG 37–5.
An extruded fragment of nuclear material is demonstrated in the neural foramen of the lumbar spine. Off-center sagittal proton-density **(A)** and T2-weighted image **(B)** are shown (SE, TR = 2,000 ms, TE = 30/80 ms, 2 NEX, 5-mm-thick slice, 256 × 192). Note the extruded fragment *(arrowheads)* in the neural foramen. The exiting nerve root is displaced posteriorly and is not well seen on the proton-density image because it blends with the decreased signal of the annulus and posterior longitudinal ligament. On the T2-weighted image **(B)**, the nerve root appears to be displaced and flattened from its anterior surface.

cause of the relative weakness of the posterior longitudinal ligament. This will push the posterior longitudinal ligament backward, and the resultant mass may cause back pain and radiculopathy by direct compression of the neural elements. It may, however, bulge anteriorly and displace the anterior longitudinal ligament forward. This latter condition is less common because of the strength of the anterior longitudinal ligament and is not associated with radiculopathy. The annular distension could conceivably result in back pain.

The posterolateral protrusion of the disk encroaches on the inferior portion of the neural foramen, which is usually occupied by fat and exiting vessels. The intermediate signal of the exiting nerve can be seen in the superior third of the foramen, above the protruding disk (Fig 37–5,A and B). MRI studies of the spine are performed with the patient in the supine position. However, one should consider that the vertical stress of the erect position may compress the foramen and bring the nerve into contact with the bulging disk, thereby resulting in radicular symptoms.

Naylor's work is oriented to the lumbar region, but the changes he described can also be seen in the thoracic spine. The technical requirements of MRI studies in this area are critical and require surface-coil imaging, thin sections, and motion suppression to achieve reliable results.[20]

The state of hydration of the cervical interver-tebral disk nucleus is quite variable and is not a reliable index of degeneration. The separation of annulus and nucleus is not as dramatic as in the lumbar region, and the volume of the nucleus is approximately 0.5 cc or 20% to 25% of that of the lumbar nuclei (Rollins S., unpublished data). Extrusion of the entire nucleus would be expected to produce a sphere 7 mm in diameter. The degenerative mechanism seems to be similar to that described in the lumbar area since the "soft disk" herniation is seen as a knuckle of increased signal on T2-weighted images. This is true whether the images are acquired by spin-echo or gradient-refocused sequences (Figs 37–6 and 37–7).

MOTION SEGMENT DISORDERS

The motion segment includes the facet joints, which are gliding diarthrodial joints with lax capsules richly innervated with pain fibers.[19] In addition to direct compression of neural elements by various pathologic states of the facet joint, pain may also be initiated by irritation of the nerve fibers of the capsule. This latter situation can produce referred pain indistinguishable from radicular pain but will be relieved by intra-articular injection of anesthetics and steroids. Critical assessment and identification of the site of the clinical abnormality is essential to proper and efficacious treatment planning.

Facet anatomy is well visualized on MRI studies. The dense cortical bone is seen as a line of signal void, while the articular cartilage images with an intermediate signal on spin-echo, proton-density images and becomes signal intense on T2-weighted images. Occasionally a thin line of decreased signal is seen between the cartilages of the facets and represents a small amount of fluid in the joint space. The contiguity of the cartilage and the ligamentum flavum is well demonstrated, and the extensions of the joint spaces into the posterior recess can also be visualized (Fig 37–8,A and B). The exiting nerve roots are readily seen, particularly on oblique images, and the relationship of these structures to the facet joint can be assessed (Figs 37–9 and 37–10).

Arthropathy can be demonstrated as a decrease in articular cartilage within the facet joint space. This is manifested by MRI as a reduced or irregular intense cartilage signal on T2-weighted images (Fig 37–11).

In the pathologic state, the overgrowth of bone

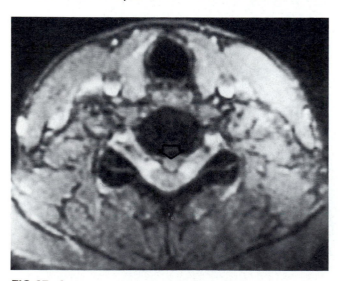

FIG 37–6.
Extruded cervical disk seen in a T2-weighted gradient-refocused axial image of the cervical spine through the level of the neural foramina (TR = 350 ms, TE = 18 ms, flip angle = 12 degrees, 4 NEX, 3-mm-thick slice, 256 × 192). The extruded fragment *(arrow)* is signal intense. The dura is signal poor and is displaced posteriorly by the fragment.

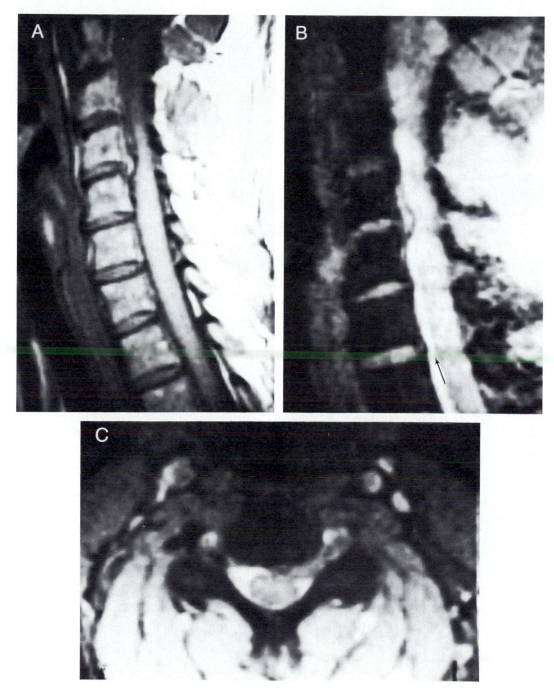

FIG 37–7.
Herniated nucleus pulposus at C4–5. Sagittal T1-weighted **(A)** and T2-weighted gradient-refocused **(B)** sequences demonstrate the large disk protrusion at the C4–5 level with elevation of the posterior longitudinal ligament. An axial **(C)** gradient-refocused image demonstrates the large disk fragment extending into the left lateral recess and occupying all of the left neural foramen. (Courtesy of Richard E. Latchaw, M.D., Englewood, Colo.)

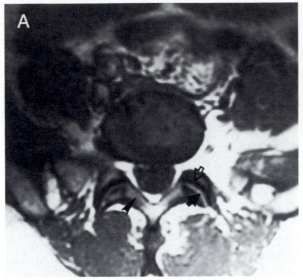

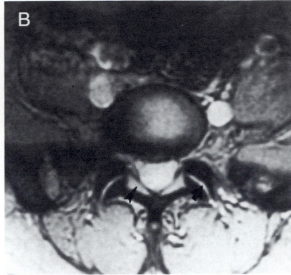

FIG 37–8.
Facet anatomy. **A,** T1-weighted axial lumbar image. **B,** T2-weighted gradient-refocused axial lumbar image (**A:** SE, TR = 600 ms, TE = 20 ms, 4 NEX, 3-mm-thick slice, 256 × 192; **B:** TR = 350 ms, TE = 18 ms, flip angle = 25 degrees, 4 NEX, 4-mm-thick slice, 256 × 192). In **A,** a T1-weighted axial image, note the signal-poor cortical bone of the facet joint *(open arrow)* and the moderate sig-

nal-intense cartilage of the facet joint *(closed arrow)*. Note the ligamentum flavum *(arrowhead)* join the anterior portion of the cartilage of the facet joint. In **B,** a T2-weighted gradient-refocused axial image, the articular cartilage *(arrow)* is a brighter in signal than on the T1-weighted image. The ligamentum flavum *(arrowhead)* is also better delineated than on the T1-weighted image.

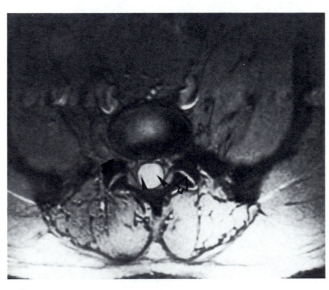

FIG 37–9.
Nerve root anatomy seen in a T2-weighted gradient-refocused axial image through the lumbar spine, (TR = 350 ms, TE = 18 ms, flip angle = 25 degrees, 4 NEX, 4-mm-thick slice, 256 × 192). Note the intermediate signal from the rootlets *(arrowheads)* surrounded by signal-intense cerebrospinal fluid. Also note the signal-intense articular cartilage of the facet joint *(open arrow)* blend with the ligamentum flavum. Note the exiting nerve root *(solid arrow)* in the neural foramen on the right.

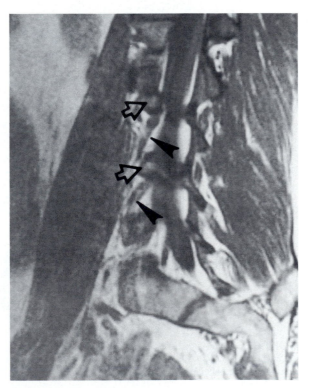

FIG 37–10.
Nerve root anatomy seen in a T1-weighted oblique image through the pedicles of the lumbar spine (SE, TR = 600 ms, TE = 20 ms, 4 NEX, 3-mm-thick slice, 256 × 256). Note the nerve roots *(arrowheads)* exit beneath the pedicles *(arrows)*.

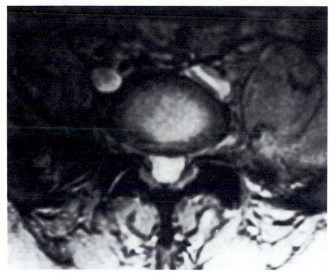

FIG 37–11.
Unilateral facet arthropathy seen in a T2-weighted gradient-refocused axial lumbar image (TR = 350 ms, TE = 18 ms, flip angle = 25 degrees, 4 NEX, 3-mm-thick slice, 256 × 192). Note the lack of signal from the articular cartilage of the facet joint on the left. Bony overgrowth is also noted on the left.

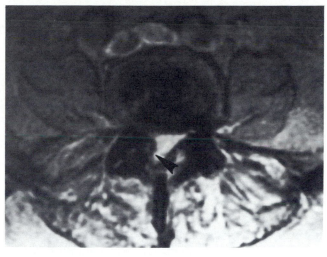

FIG 37–12.
Facet hypertrophy causing lateral stenosis on the right with subsequent compromise of the exiting root and thecal sac in a T2-weighted gradient-refocused axial image of the lumbar spine through the neural foramina (TR = 400 ms, TE = 18 ms, flip angle = 30 degrees, 4 NEX, 4-mm-thick slice, 256 × 192). Bilateral facet overgrowth is noted to compromise the neural foramina bilaterally. There is a diffusely bulging annulus. A small synovial cyst *(arrowhead)* along the medial aspect of the facet joint on the right further compromises the canal.

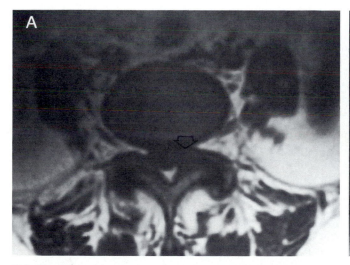

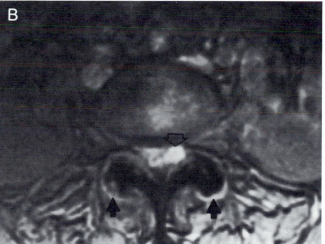

FIG 37–13.
Axial T1-weighted **(A)** and gradient-refocused T2-weighted **(B)** images through the L4–5 disk space demonstrate a synovial cyst compromising the medial aspect of the neural foramen on the left **(A:** SE, TR = 600 ms, TE = 20 ms, 4 NEX, 3-mm-thick slice, 256 × 192; **B:** TR = 350 ms, TE = 18 ms, flip angle = 25 degrees, 4 NEX, 4-mm-thick slice, 256 × 256). The patient presented with an L5 radiculopathy on the left. Note the synovial cyst *(open arrow)* image as water. It is signal poor on the T1-weighted image and signal intense on the T2-weighted image. This cyst is medial to the facet joint on the left, which demonstrates marked degenerative changes, as well as the one on the right. There is an effusion *(closed arrows)* surrounding both facet joints.

from the articular processes in response to an instability syndrome can be appreciated on MRI studies as an irregular increase in the amount of signal null. This may be seen to compromise the exiting roots within the neural foramen (Fig 37–12). Lateral stenosis can also be seen as a result of central hypertrophy of the superior articular facet. The overproduction of bone around defects that is associated with spondylolisthesis is not as clearly defined as with CT studies, but the disk abnormalities are more apparent.

As the facet joints undergo degeneration, synovial cysts or ganglion cysts may occur (Fig 37–13,A and B). These cysts form by a small herniation of synovium through the facet joint capsule and ligamentum flavum. If the communication with the joint persists, this cyst usually resolves over a period of weeks. However, if this communication is obstructed, a ganglion cyst forms. Over a period of time pressure necrosis converts the cyst into a non–synovial-lined cyst with mucoid content.[21] These cysts may cause mass effect and compromise surrounding neurologic structures.

Facet fractures can also be identified on MRI although CT scans reveal this abnormality more graphically.

SUMMARY

The technical improvements in MRI have resulted in a quantum leap in the study of back pain syndromes. It can be effectively used for the diagnosis of degenerative disk disease and can also add valuable information in the study of various bone degenerative states.

Acknowledgments

A special acknowledgment is extended to Alicia Miller, R.T., and Betsy Stine, without whose assistance, perseverance, and attention to detail the completion of this work would not have been possible.

REFERENCES

1. Dandy WC: Roentgenography of the brain after the injection of air into the spinal canal. *Ann Surg* 1919; 70:397.
2. Shapiro R: *Myelography.* Chicago, Year Book Medical Publishers, Inc, 1962.
3. Raskin SP, Keating JW: Recognition of lumbar disc disease: Comparison of myelography and computed tomography. *AJR* 1982; 139:349–355.
4. Orrison WW, Johansen JG, Eldevik OP, et al: Optimal computed tomographic techniques for cervical spine imaging. *Radiology* 1982; 144:180–182.
5. Dublin AB, McGahan JP, Reid MH: The value of computed tomographic metrizamide myelography in the neuroradiological evaluation of the spine. *Radiology* 1983; 146:79–86.
6. Han JS, Kaufman B, El Yousef SJ, et al: NMR imaging of the spine. *AJR* 1983; 141:1137–1145.
7. Norman D, Milis CM, Brant-Zawadzki M, et al: Magnetic resonance imaging of the spinal cord and canal: Potentials and limitations. *AJR* 1983; 141:1147–1152.
8. Modic MT, Masaryk T, Boumphrey F, et al: Lumbar herniated disk disease and canal stenosis: Prospective evaluation by surface coil MR, CT, and myelography. *AJNR* 1986; 7:709–717.
9. Ehni G: *Cervical Arthrosis.* Chicago, Year Book Medical Publishers, Inc, 1984.
10. Bland JH: *Disorders of the Cervical Spine.* Philadelphia, WB Saunders Co, 1987.
11. Friedenberg ZB, Miller WT: Degenerative disc disease of the cervical spine. *J Bone Joint Surg [Am]* 1963; 45:1171–1178.
12. McRae DL: The significance of abnormalities of the cervical spine. *AJR* 1960; 84:3–25.
13. Modic MT, Masaryk TJ, Mulopulos GP, et al: Cervical radiculopathy: Prospective evaluation with surface coil MR imaging, CT with metrizamide and metrizamide myelography. *Radiology* 1986; 161:753–759.
14. Mixter WJ, Barr JS: Rupture of the intervertebral disc with involvement of the spinal canal. *N Engl J Med* 1934; 211:210.
15. Naylor A: The biophysical and biochemical aspects of intervertebral disc herniation and degeneration. *Ann R Coll Surg Engl* 1962; 31:91–114.
16. Teplick JG, Haskin ME: Spontaneous regression of herniated nucleus pulposus. *AJR* 1985; 145:371–375.
17. Modic MT, Pavlicek MS, Weinstein MA, et al: Magnetic resonance imaging of intervertebral disc disease: Clinical and pulse sequence considerations. *Radiology* 1984; 152:103–111.
18. Masaryk TJ, Ross JS, Modic MT, et al: High-resolution MR imaging of sequestered lumbar intervertebral discs. Presented at the 72nd Scientific Assembly and Annual Meeting of the Radiological

Society of North America, Chicago, November 30–December 5, 1986.

19. Schellinger DR, Wener L, Ragsdale BD, et al: Facet joint disorders and their role in the production of back pains and sciatica. *Radiogaphics* 1987; 7:923–944.

20. Ross JS, Perez-Reyes N, Masaryk TJ, et al: Thoracic disc herniation: MR imaging. *Radiology* 1987; 165:511–515.

21. Mani JR: Pitfalls in the computed tomographic diagnosis of herniated disks, in Genant HK (ed): *Spine Update 1984*. Radiology Research and Education Foundation, 1983, pp 79–95.

38

Imaging of the Postoperative Lumbar Spine

Joachim F. Seeger, M.D.

Each year, over 200,000 laminectomies and other back operations are performed in the United States. Up to 30% of these patients are either unimproved or have recurrent symptoms after surgery.[1] Unsuccessful operations have often been the result of faulty patient selection or surgery inappropriate for the offending lesion.[2] Other relatively common causes of unsatisfactory long-term results include inadequate decompression of spinal or foraminal stenosis, residual or recurrent disk herniation, epidural fibrosis, and adhesive arachnoiditis. Less common causes include fusion complications (pseudarthrosis, osseous hypertrophy, bone plug migration), wrong-level surgery, mechanical instability, nerve injuries, and missed diagnoses.

Computed tomography (CT) has had a profound impact on both the pre- and postoperative evaluation of the spine and is currently the most utilized study for assessing postoperative alterations.[3] The development of low-osmolality water-soluble contrast media has made myelography and CT/myelography much safer and less frightening for the patient than in the past and allows for detailed assessment of the contents of the subarachnoid sac not available with plain CT scanning.[4] The more recent, still incompletely tapped resource of magnetic resonance (MR) imaging promises to provide even more information on the postoperative spine than either CT or myelography, especially concerning subtle soft tissue abnormalities such as postoperative hematomas, infections, fibrosis, and sequestered disk fragments.[5]

In order to help provide the best possible care for the postoperative patient, the diagnostic radiol-ogist must become thoroughly familiar with the appropriate applications of the different imaging modalities, and with the imaging appearances of the various back operations, postoperative problems, and complications. The radiologist should develop an understanding of the clinical manifestations of different back problems, such as mechanical back pain, spinal stenosis, and individual nerve root compression syndromes. This requires a close working relationship with the referring surgeon, so that the most appropriate and informative study or studies are obtained for a given clinical situation. Periodic trips to the operating room by the radiologist are also advantageous to develop a first-hand correlation with the imaging findings.

It is the purpose of this chapter to acquaint the radiologist with some of the advantages and disadvantages of the different imaging studies, the various types of spinal operations, the postoperative problems that may occur, and the radiologic assessment of specific problems.

SURGICAL PROCEDURES INVOLVING THE LUMBAR SPINE

There are many different decompressive and stabilizing procedures involving the lumbar spine which vary between the subspecialties of orthopedics and neurosurgery, between individual surgeons, and between institutions.[6, 7] Each has its vocal supporters and detractors. The heated arguments surrounding the merits and disadvantages of the different operations can make for entertaining reading but are beyond the scope of this chapter.[2, 8–10] Only the more commonly encountered procedures will be discussed.

The surgical procedure most difficult to recognize radiologically is the microsurgical diskectomy. In its smallest form, this may only involve an interlaminar fenestration of the ligamentum flavum followed by microscopic diskectomy. Focal absence of the ligamentum flavum may be the one clue on a CT or MR scan that surgery has been performed. Because little epidural fat is removed, there generally is very little postoperative epidural fibrosis.

A more extensive microsurgical procedure is the laminotomy and diskectomy, which usually involves resection of the inferior portion of the superior lamina and the underlying ligamentum flavum (Fig 38–1). For greater caudal exposure the superior margin of the lower lamina may also be removed, and, if lateral exposure is required, the medial portion of the facet joint may also be resected. When done carefully, with little removal of epidural fat, this operation also produces relatively little epidural fibrosis.

Conventional, or nonmicrosurgical diskectomy generally involves resection of the lamina which overlies the disk herniation—a so-called hemilaminectomy. If greater lateral exposure is required, a medial or partial facetectomy may be performed in conjunction with the hemilaminectomy (Fig 38–2). For more medial exposure, a bilateral or complete laminectomy may be performed.

A foraminotomy involves a laminectomy followed by surgical enlargement of the neural foramen and usually requires resection of the anterior surface of the adjacent superior articular facet or the posterolateral surface of the vertebral body or both (Fig 38–3).

The most extensive commonly encountered surgical procedure is the multilevel bilateral laminectomy, facetectomy, and foraminotomy for treatment of spinal canal and foraminal stenoses. This produces a potentially unstable segment of the spine and thus is frequently performed in association with spinal fusion, especially in younger, more active patients. There are many different types of spinal fusions or arthrodeses. Posteromedial fusion, in which small matchstick-sized fragments of cancellous bone are laid over decorticated spinous processes and laminae with additional bone chips packed into denuded facet joints, was performed quite commonly in the past (Fig 38–4). This procedure has currently fallen into disfavor because of a high rate of pseudarthrosis as well as iatrogenic postfusion spinal stenosis. However, posteromedial fusion is still encoun-

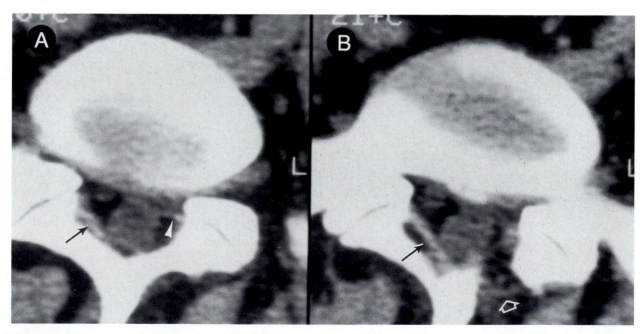

FIG 38–1.
Two contiguous CT slices (**A** and **B**) show there has been a left laminotomy of L5 (**B,** *open arrow).* Note the ligamentum flavum on the right and its absence on the left *(arrows).* There is only a mini-mal epidural scar on the left (**A,** *arrowhead)* secondary to the left microdiskectomy.

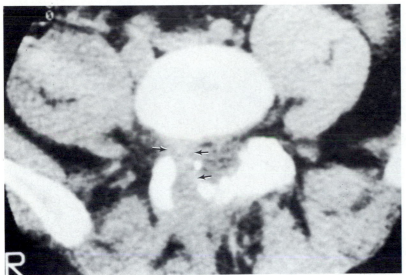

FIG 38–2.
A right hemilaminectomy and partial facetectomy have resulted in significant epidural scar *(arrows)* within the right spinal canal and neural foramen.

tered quite frequently by the radiologist because many patients return years after fusion with symptoms of spinal stenosis.

The intertransverse or posterolateral fusion (PLF) is currently the most frequently performed arthrodesis. This procedure is usually done to treat mechanical low back pain disorders producing intractable and disabling pain, often in association with complete laminectomy and facetectomy. Autologous strips of iliac bone are placed between the denuded posterior margins of the laminae bilaterally. Most of the fusions are carried down to the sacrum to provide complete immobilization of the lower lumbar spine (Fig 38–5). However, some surgeons may elect to perform only a so-called floating fusion between two affected lumbar vertebrae. Occasionally the fusions are reinforced with metallic distraction-fixation devices, such as Knodt rods.[9] The posterolateral arthrodeses have a fairly high rate of fusion, generally recorded as 90% with single-level and 80% with two-level fusion.[9]

The anterior lumbar interbody fusion (ALIF) involves placing wedges of bone, usually from an iliac donor site, into an intervertebral disk space via a transperitoneal or retroperitoneal approach. This procedure is rarely done today because of a high rate of pseudarthrosis and frequent operative complications. More common is the posterior lumbar interbody fusion (PLIF) in which bone plugs are placed from behind into the intervertebral disk space following laminectomy and diskectomy to provide both stability and maintenance of height of the disk space and lateral foramina (Fig 38–6). Although this is a compressive-type fusion, there still

is a fairly high incidence (15%–30%) of pseudarthrosis.

Degenerative scoliosis, when it is unstable and progressive, is occasionally treated with Harrington rod distraction.[11] This can be particularly effective in relieving associated neural foraminal stenosis without the necessity of laminectomy and foraminotomy (Fig 38–7).

Nearly all patients that have undergone laminectomies and diskectomies will demonstrate variable degrees of postoperative epidural fibrosis at the site of surgery. Surgeons often place a small fat graft at the site of hemilaminectomy or a large fat graft in an area of extensive laminectomy in order to fill the dead space and promote hemostasis and thus prevent significant postoperative fibrosis.[12] A large full-thickness fat graft when scanned acutely may present as a mass and distort the subarachnoid sac. However, with time, the fat graft usually decreases in volume and the subarachnoid sac returns to a more normal configuration or may even dilate (Fig 38–3,B).

IMAGING STUDIES

Plain Film Radiographs

Although plain films are generally considered only adjuncts to the more sophisticated cross-sectional imaging techniques, they may play an important role in evaluation of certain postoperative conditions. The anteroposterior (AP) and lateral views are quick and relatively inexpensive means of screening the entire lumbosacral spine and may occasionally reveal abnormalities that could be

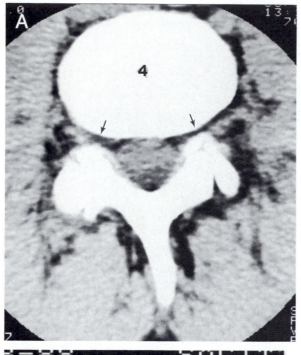

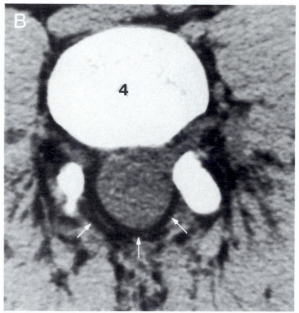

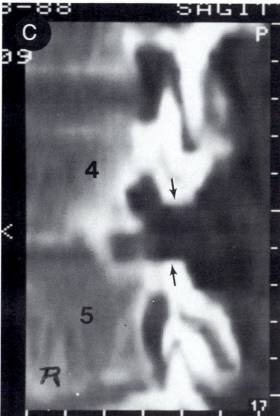

FIG 38–3.
Surgery for foraminal stenosis. **A,** a preoperative CT scan
shows bilateral foraminal stenoses *(arrows),* worse on the
left, mostly due to facet hypertrophy and associated
capsular calcification. **B,** a postoperative scan at the same
level shows a complete laminectomy, bilateral facetectomies,
and foraminotomies. An extensive fat graft *(arrows)* placed
around the sac has prevented epidural scar formation. Note
compensatory dilatation of the sac reflecting the
laminectomy. **C,** a parasagittal multiplanar reconstruction
clearly shows the partial resections of the inferior L4 and
superior L5 facets *(arrows)* to produce the foraminotomy.

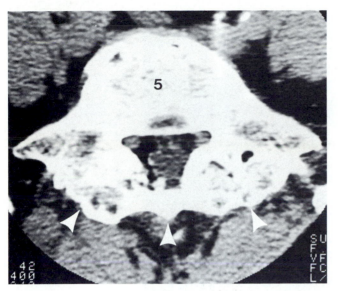

FIG 38–4.
A posteromedial fusion *(arrowheads)* has resulted in complete ankylosis of the facet joints and a solid union between L5 and S1.

overlooked at CT or magnetic resonance imaging (MRI), such as early ankylosing spondylitis, spondylolysis without spondylolisthesis, and lesions of the upper lumbar spine or lower sacrum and pelvis not included on the routine CT scan.

They also provide a quick assessment of the extent, level, and type of previous surgery by demonstrating the laminectomy defect, fusion masses, and other postoperative changes, including metallic fixation devices. Routine oblique views of the postoperative lumbar spine are generally unnecessary, unless there is a strong suspicion of spondylolysis.

In patients presenting with mechanical low back pain, plain films with flexion and extension and perhaps lateral bending views may be especially useful in demonstrating postoperative spinal instability or failure of fusion not appreciated on the more static CT or MR images.

Myelography

For over 30 years, and up until the mid-1970s, iophendylate (Pantopaque), a nonwater-soluble oily iodinated fatty ester, was the myelographic contrast agent of choice in the United States. Unfortunately, iophendylate alone or in combination with surgery produced arachnoiditis in over 25% of cases and it has been incriminated as one of the causes of the so-called failed back surgery syndrome.[13] Although no longer used, residual

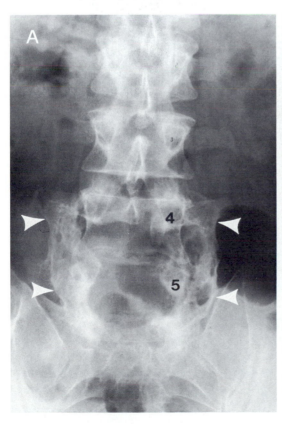

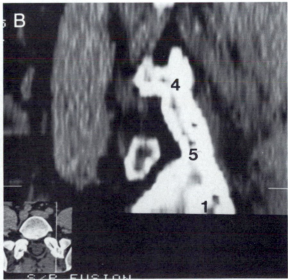

FIG 38–5.
A, an AP radiograph reveals a partial L4 and complete L5 and S1 laminectomies, facetectomies and bilateral lateral fusions *(arrows)* from the transverse processes of L4 to the sacrum. **B,** a parasagittal reformatted CT image through the left fusion mass confirms solid bony union from L4 to the sacrum.

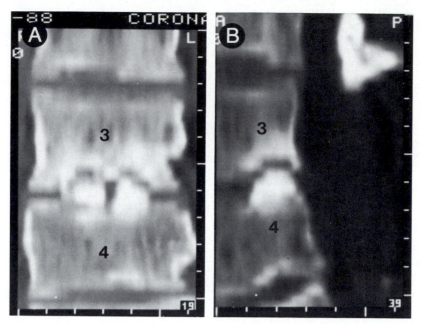

FIG 38–6.
Coronal **(A)** and sagittal **(B)** MPRs of a posterior lumbar interbody fusion show two dowels of iliac bone inserted into the L3–4 inter- space. Note the lucency and adjacent sclerosis along the superior margins of the dowels consistent with nonunion.

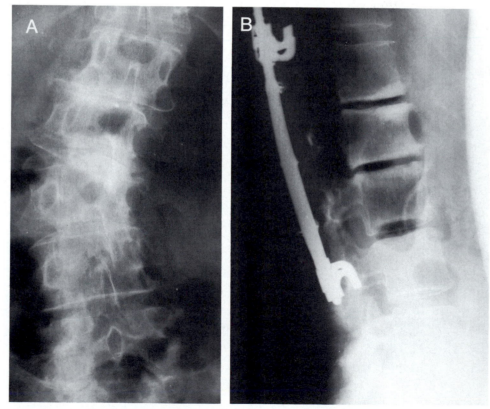

FIG 38–7.
A 67-year-old woman underwent Harrington rod placement be- tween T12 and L4 to correct a progressive degenerative scoliosis of the lumbar spine. **(A)** a preoperative AP film and **(B)** a postop- erative lateral film show excellent correction of the scoliosis.

iophendylate is frequently seen during evaluation of the postoperative spine.

Iophendylate was replaced in the mid-1970s by metrizamide (Amipaque), a water-soluble, nonviscous absorbable contrast medium which provided much better visualization of the subarachnoid sac and lumbar nerve roots but produced a fairly high incidence of toxic side effects, including severe headaches, nausea and vomiting, and frequent pain during injection of a subarachnoid sac plagued by prior arachnoiditis. Metrizamide itself, however, did not contribute to the arachnoiditis.

During the past several years, new nonionic low-osmolality contrast agents such as iohexol (Omnipaque) and iopamidol (Isovue) have completely replaced metrizamide. These media have all of the advantages of metrizamide as well as a low incidence of toxic side effects.

Despite these advancements, myelography in the postoperative spine is still limited to showing defects involving the subarachnoid sac and its contents and often produces negative results with far-lateral disk herniations and foraminal stenoses. When the sac is congenitally short or small, it is not possible to visualize pathologic changes at the lumbosacral junction. Myelography is not very helpful in differentiating postoperative fibrosis from recurrent disk herniation. On the other hand, because of excellent spatial resolution, myelography is still the most sensitive study for visualizing individual nerve roots and for demonstrating mild or even moderate arachnoiditis. When combined with lateral flexion-extension views, myelography provides an excellent dynamic assessment of spinal stenosis caused by postoperative instability, information which may be overlooked with static CT or MRI studies, which are performed with the patient in a supine and slightly flexed position. Myelography can also be performed in patients with Harrington or other rods, which usually produce excessive artifacts on CT or MRI. Myelography is often used in conjunction with CT scanning (CT myelography) to utilize the best features of both studies.

Computed Tomography

The development of spinal CT scanning in the late 1970s and early 1980s truly revolutionized the radiologic assessment of the postoperative spine. The axial cross-sectional images provide information on the spinal canal and neural foramina not available on plain films or myelography. Before CT, many patients with radiculopathy underwent inadequate or misdirected surgery on the basis of a myelographic defect, such as a presumed bulging or herniated disk, when the true cause of symptoms was an unrecognized foraminal or perhaps a subarticular recess stenosis.[14] Additional advantages of CT scanning over myelography are more reliable differentiation between bulging and herniated disks and identification of far-lateral or intraforaminal disk herniations that produce no myelographic defects.[15]

CT scanning can also demonstrate postoperative soft tissue changes, such as ligamentous hypertrophy, facet capsular laxity and subluxation, and epidural fibrosis. CT provides elegant definition of postoperative bony changes, including laminectomies, facetectomies, foraminotomies, and fusions. Pseudarthrosis can frequently be demonstrated with CT, particularly with multiplanar reformation through the fusion mass.

Postoperative spinal CT also has certain advantages over MRI, including superior definition of bone detail, and the ability to scan the spine quite successfully in the presence of postoperative wires or sutures which may produce significant magnetic susceptibility artifacts on the MR scan.

CT scanning also has some disadvantages in comparison with myelography or MRI. Because axial scanning is usually limited to preselected levels, tandem lesions or more distant lesions, such as at the conus medullaris, may be overlooked. This is generally not a problem in the postoperative spine, particularly when there is good clinical correlation. As opposed to MRI or myelography, plain CT scanning generally cannot clearly define intrathecal abnormalities, such as arachnoiditis or even a tumor within the subarachnoid sac. CT scanning may also occasionally miss an isodense extruded or sequestrated disk fragment which may be very obvious on the myelogram or CT myelogram.

Magnetic Resonance Imaging

High-resolution surface-coil MR imaging of the spine is rapidly becoming as accurate as CT scanning for diagnosing herniated nucleus pulposus (HNP) and spinal canal stenosis. Preliminary experience with the intravenous paramagnetic contrast agent gadolinium diethylenetriamine pentaacetic acid (DTPA) suggests MRI is even better than intravenously enhanced CT in the differentiation of disk vs. scar. The excellent signal-to-noise ratio achieved with the high-field-strength magnets makes MRI quite competitive with myelography and CT myelography for demonstrating the individual lumbar nerve roots within the subarachnoid sac.

The greatest advantage of MRI of the postoperative spine is its ability to combine some of the best features of CT scanning and myelography, in that it is noninvasive, is sensitive to lateral disk disease and lateral canal and foraminal stenosis, and can image the entire lumbosacral spine, including the conus medullaris, at one sitting.

The disadvantages of MRI in comparison with CT in the postoperative spine are its insensitivity to partly calcified or ossified lesions and its decreased sensitivity in demonstrating pseudarthrosis and facet joint changes. However, it is very likely that some of these disadvantages will have already been overcome at the time of publication of this chapter.

POSTOPERATIVE SPINAL PROBLEMS

Postoperative spinal problems can generally be categorized as immediate or delayed. Considerations in patients who have undergone decompres-

sive spinal surgery with little or no relief or a worsening of symptoms in the early postoperative period include epidural hematoma; recurrent disk herniation; failure to identify and remove a sequestered disk fragment; inadequate decompression of central, lateral, or foraminal stenosis; a completely missed diagnosis, such as a tumor of the conus medullaris or sacrum or a disk at another level; and infection such as diskitis or epidural abscess. Considerations with delayed postoperative spinal problems include recurrent disk herniation at the same or at a different level, epidural fibrosis, development of foraminal or lateral recess stenosis, mechanical instability and associated progressive degenerative changes, fusion overgrowth, arachnoiditis, and a migrating bone plug.

Most of these postoperative problems can be diagnosed quite accurately with one or more of the various radiologic imaging procedures, particularly high-resolution CT scanning or MRI.

RADIOLOGIC ASSESSMENT OF SPECIFIC PROBLEMS

Epidural Scar vs. Herniated Disk

Distinguishing recurrent HNP from postoperative scar formation is often impossible clinically,

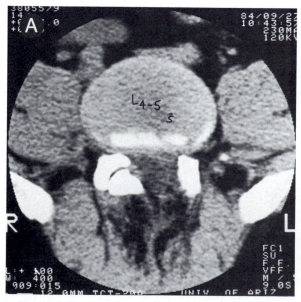 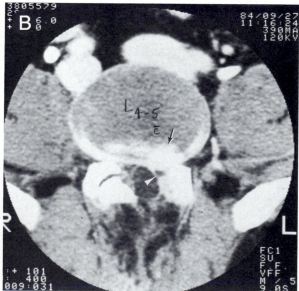

FIG 38–8.
Recurrent left radiculopathy 2 years following laminectomy and left L4–5 diskectomy. **A,** an unenhanced CT scan shows soft tissue within the spinal canal on the left, slightly less dense than the disk, and producing no obvious compression of the sac. Epidural fibrosis should be favored, but a small associated herniated nucleus pulposus cannot be excluded. **B,** the enhanced study at the same level shows intense soft tissue enhancement, mostly on the left, clearly highlighting the low-density subarachnoid sac and also surrounding the descending left L5 nerve root *(arrowhead)*. The diskectomy site itself also enhances *(arrow)*, reflecting infiltration by scar. There is no recurrent disk herniation.

and yet such differentiation is very important for patient management, since reoperation of scar generally leads to a poor surgical result, as opposed to removal of a reherniated disk.[16, 17] Myelography alone is unreliable in discriminating between disk herniation and epidural fibrosis, and conventional CT scanning is only moderately reliable, having a reported accuracy of only 43% to 60%.[18, 19] Typi-

cally, epidural scar is more diffuse, irregular, and less dense than herniated disk on plain CT, and tends to contour around and retract rather than compress the neural sac. In this situation, scar is relatively easy to diagnose with plain CT (see Fig 38–2). However, scar in the anterior and anterolateral epidural space may occasionally present as a mass with a density and configuration similar to a

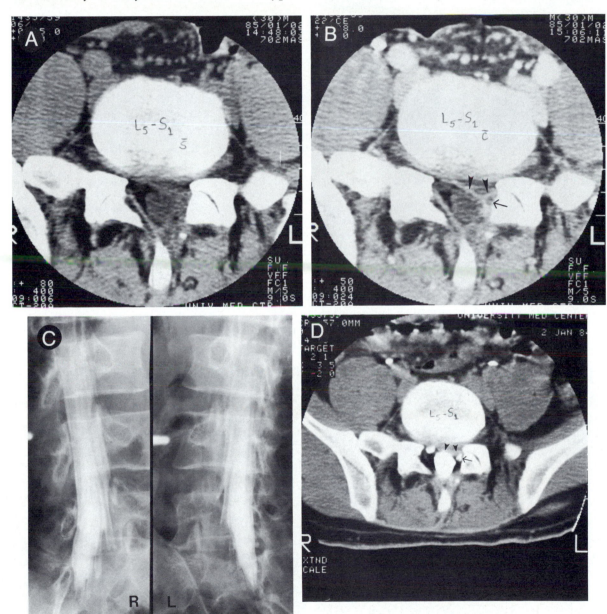

FIG 38–9.
Recurrent left-sided S1 radiculopathy 1 year after a left laminectomy and L5–S1 diskectomy. **A,** the unenhanced CT scan shows absence of the left ligamentum flavum and considerable fibrosis along the left lateral margin of the sac. The posterior disk margin and left S1 nerve are not clearly defined. **B,** following intravenous enhancement, a moderate recurrent herniated nucleus pulposus covered by a thin layer of enhancing scar becomes apparent *(ar-* *rowheads),* producing posterior displacement of the left S1 nerve *(arrow),* which is also surrounded by enhancing perineural fibrosis. **C,** a subsequent myelogram shows compression of the left S1 nerve compared to its mate on the right *(arrows)* and a follow-up CT myelogram **(D)** provides excellent correlation with the enhanced CT scan **(B).**

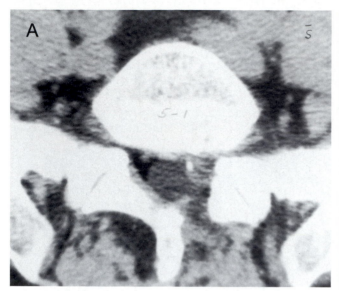 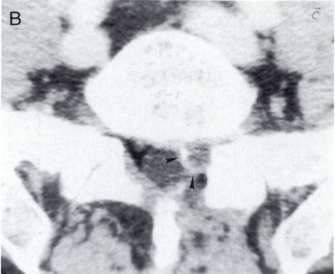

FIG 38–10.
Recurrent left S1 radiculopathy 9 months after left L5–S1 diskectomy. **A,** an unenhanced CT scan just rostral to the posterior disk margin shows a soft tissue mass with a fleck of calcium along its medial margin within the anterior left spinal canal. The sac is displaced slightly toward the right. Recurrent disk herniation should be favored. **B,** an enhanced scan clearly shows the large nonenhancing extruded disk fragment wrapped in enhancing epidural scar *(arrowheads).*

recurrent disk herniation, or a combination of disk herniation and scarring may occur. In such cases neither myelography nor plain CT scanning will prove helpful.

On the other hand, CT scanning with intravenous contrast enhancement has been reported by several investigators to be effective in distinguishing recurrent disk herniation from epidural scar.[3, 18–23] This is because epidural fibrosis almost always enhances uniformly whereas with disk herniation enhancement is usually limited to a thin band at the peripheral margin of the disk. For optimum success, such a study requires meticulous attention to technique, including the use of thin,

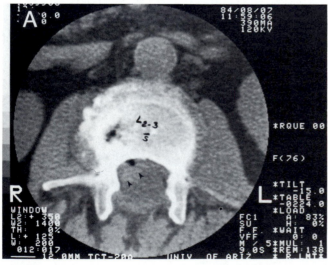 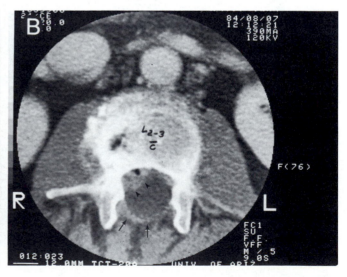

FIG 38–11.
A 76-year-old woman developed right quadriceps weakness 4 years following decompressive surgery from L2 to L5 for spinal stenosis. **A,** an unenhanced CT scan reveals a very subtle soft tissue density *(arrowheads)* containing a small gas bubble in the right anterior spinal canal. **B,** the enhanced scan shows definite enhancement of the soft tissue mass *(arrowheads)* similar in density to the enhancing scar contouring the posterior margin of the sac *(arrows).* Although it is unusual for a herniated disk to enhance, the focal mass effect and the associated gas bubble favored a herniated nucleus pulposus. At surgery, a large disk fragment infiltrated by scar tissue was removed.

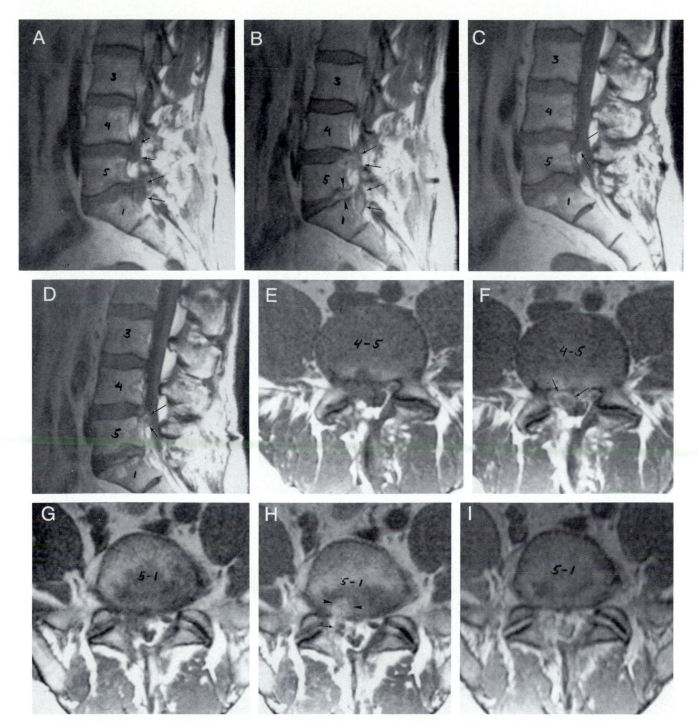

FIG 38–12.
Recurrent right buttock and leg pain 2 years following right laminectomies at L4–5 and L5–S1. **A,** an unenhanced T1-weighted parasagittal MR scan just to the right of the midline shows soft tissue isointense to the disks at both L4–5 and L5–S1 *(arrows).* **B,** these soft tissues enhance following gadolinium-DTPA *(arrows)* reflecting epidural fibrosis. Note enhancing granulation tissue within the original L5–S1 diskectomy site *(arrowheads).* **C,** an unenhanced midline MR scan shows a more discrete focus of soft tissue *(arrows)* just caudal to the bulging L4–5 annulus. **D,** the enhanced scan shows this to be a nonenhancing extruded disk fragment wrapped in enhancing fibrosis *(arrows).* **E,** Unenhanced and **F,** enhanced axial MR scans at L4–5. The disk fragment and surrounding scar **F,** *(arrows)* are clearly shown on the enhanced study. **G,** the T1-weighted unenhanced scan at L5–S1 shows soft tissue in the canal on the right which could be scar, a herniated nucleus pulposus, or both. **H,** the enhanced study clearly reveals this to be enhancing epidural fibrosis surrounding and not displacing the right S1 nerve *(arrow).* Note disk enhancement at the prior surgical site *(arrowheads).* **I,** an unenhanced balanced image (long TR, short TE) also suggests scar, which typically becomes hyperintense to disk on balanced and T2-weighted scans. However, the T1-weighted scans without and with contrast greatly increase the confidence level.

contiguous, or slightly overlapping slices (3–5-mm-thick), pre- and postenhancement scans through precisely the same levels and with the same gantry angulation, and, for the enhanced study, rapid administration of 70 to 80 g of iodine, starting the scan sequence when half the contrast medium has been injected. The patient must also remain motionless between the two studies. The accuracy of enhanced lumbosacral CT scanning in diagnosing recurrent disk herniation has been reported to range from 65% to 100%.[18, 19, 21] Admittedly, the data in most comparison studies are skewed, since surgery is generally not performed on those patients in whom the enhanced CT scan is interpreted as epidural fibrosis. In our own series, there has been excellent correlation between enhanced CT scanning and surgical findings in 18 of 21 cases (86%) (Figs 38–8 through 38–11).

Recently, at least two studies have shown good correlation between unenhanced MR scanning and surgical results in 79% and 86% of postoperative levels respectively,[24, 25] thus comparing very favorably with intravenous contrast–enhanced CT scanning. The obvious advantage of MRI is that the patient is subjected to neither ionizing radiation nor to a large iodine bolus, with the associated risk of a severe contrast reaction.

Even more recently, enhanced MRI using gadopentatate dimeglumine (gadolinium DTPA) has further advanced the differentiation of postoperative scar and recurrent disk.[26] The discomfort and

risk of intravenous gadolinium is negligible when compared to intravenous iodine salts. T1-weighted scans are obtained before and immediately after injection of the contrast medium, since scar tissue enhances intensely and immediately whereas disk material does not. However, disk may enhance 30 to 60 minutes later, though not to the same degree as scar.[27] Our usual protocol is to obtain unenhanced T1-weighted (short TR, short TE) spin-echo sagittal and axial scans and T2-weighted gradient-echo sagittal scans, repeating the T1-weighted sagittal and axial scans after intravenous contrast enhancement. The intense enhancement generally allows for easy discrimination between scar and the subarachnoid sac, nerve roots and adjacent disk margin, or disk fragment, which is often not possible on the unenhanced study. Occasionally, the enhancing scar may obscure very small disk fragments, or the size of the disk may be underestimated. It is also noteworthy that enhancement of the parent disk or the site of disk curettage may occur in up to 30% of cases, presumably secondary to infiltration by scar. The normal epidural venous plexus and the dorsal root ganglia also show enhancement with gadolinium and should not be mistaken for scar.

A prospective study of 30 patients with so-called failed back surgery syndrome conducted at Case Western Reserve showed accurate differentiation between scar and recurrent disk in all 19 reoperated cases.[26] MRI has now become the study

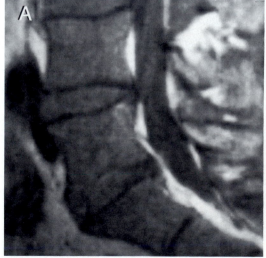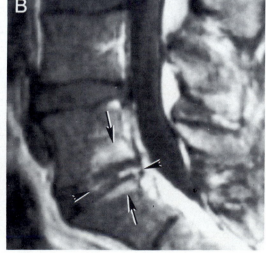

FIG 38–13.
Recurrent low back pain 2 years after L5–S1 diskectomy. Comparison of the T1-weighted unenhanced **(A)** and enhanced **(B)** MR scans shows enhancement of the site of disk curettage (**B,** *arrowheads*) and enhancement of reactive vascular infiltration of the adjacent marrow (**B,** *arrows*), findings often seen after disk surgery. Similar disk and adjacent marrow enhancement can occasionally occur even without surgery when there is acute disk degeneration.

TABLE 38-1.
MRI and CT Criteria of Postoperative Scar vs. Herniated Nucleus Pulposus

Lesion	Morphology	Mass Effect	CT Unenhanced	CT Enhanced	MRI Unenhanced T1-Weighted	MRI Enhanced T1-Weighted	MRI Unenhanced T2-Weighted
Epidural fibrosis	Often linear; extends above and below disk; conforms to epidural space; tends to retract sac	Occasional	Tends to be less dense than disk (50–80 HU)	Enhances; becomes denser than disk	Hypo- or isointense to disk	Enhances; becomes hyperintense to disk	Usually hyperintense to disk; posterior scar more variable
Herniated disk	Contiguous with disk	Yes	Same density as parent disk (80–120 HU)	No enhancement; may be covered by enhancing scar	Hypo- or isointense to disk	No or delayed enhancement; may be covered by enhancing scar	Hypo-, iso-, or hyperintense to disk
Free fragment	Usually well-circumscribed; near, but not contiguous with disk	Yes	Same density as disk; slightly denser than sac	Same density as disk; may be "wrapped" in enhancing scar	Hypo- or isointense to disk	Hypo- or isointense to disk; may be "wrapped" in enhancing scar	Usually hyperintense; may be surrounded by hypointense band

of choice in discriminating between fibrosis and disk herniation (Figs 38–12 and 38–13).

Table 38–1 provides a comparison of CT and MRI in differentiating epidural fibrosis from recurrent disk herniation.

Arachnoiditis

Although there are many possible etiologies, adhesive arachnoiditis of the lumbar spine is most commonly due to prior iodophendylate myelography and surgery.[13, 28] Arachnoiditis is often associated with chronic low back pain and variable neurologic deficits.[29] It is important to demonstrate the presence of arachnoiditis in the patient with failed back surgery, since this may explain the patient's symptoms and the surgeon is reluctant to operate when there is arachnoiditis.

In early or mild cases, adhesions occur in the nerve root sleeves, leading to blunting and rounding of the sleeves. This finding is best demonstrated with myelography and is generally of no clinical significance. With progression, the descending nerve roots may adhere to the subarachnoid sac and are then no longer visible within the sac on the myelogram. The roots of the cauda equina may also adhere to one another and become matted. These latter findings are clearly defined by myelography and CT myelography but

can also be seen with MRI (Figs 38–14 and 38–15).[30] Although clumping of nerves can be seen on T1-weighted scans, the diagnosis is usually facilitated on T2-weighted scans because of the high contrast between the high signal intensity of cerebrovascular fluid (CSF) and the low signal of the nerves. With more severe arachnoiditis, it may be difficult to determine where the spinal cord ends and the cauda equina begins because the clumped nerves are the same size and produce the same signal intensity as the conus medullaris. With further progression, the entire thecal sac can become so thickened and constricted as to produce a complete block at myelography. Occasionally, this myelographic finding may be difficult to differentiate from tumor, particularly CSF seeding. MRI may also be confusing in such cases. A CT myelogram obtained several hours after the myelogram usually allows seepage of some contrast medium through the site and will often clarify the intrathecal pathology, also demonstrating adhesions above and below the site of the myelographic block.

Rarely, calcification or ossification may occur within the arachnoidal adhesions (arachnoiditis ossificans).[31] This is readily demonstrated on CT scans but is usually not apparent with MRI (Fig 38–16). Preliminary experience with enhanced MRI has shown only mild enhancement of adhesive arachnoiditis.[5]

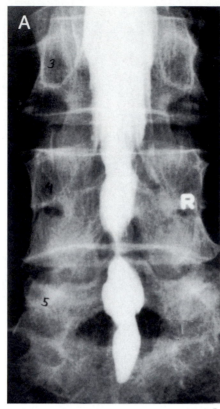
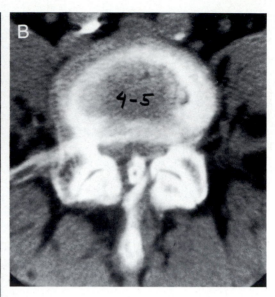

FIG 38–14.
A 41-year-old woman with severe back and leg pain 4 years after L4–5 laminotomy and diskectomy. **A,** an AP film at myelography shows severe stenosis at L4–5. Irregular narrowing of the sac above and below this level, nonvisualization of the lower nerve root sleeves, and an "empty" appearance to the sac are consistent with adhesive arachnoiditis. **B,** an axial CT scan through L4–5 shows posterior bulging of the disk and bony and ligamentous hypertrophy but also confirms the presence of arachnoiditis. Only one nerve *(arrow)* is visualized within the sac.

Infection

Postsurgical infections after diskectomy are uncommon, and are usually confined to the disk space.[32] It is very rare for such diskitis to extend into the epidural space or paravertebral soft tissues. Clinically, the patient is usually asymptomatic for the first few days or weeks after surgery, but then returns with severe back pain at the surgical site, generally without radiculopathy. Fever and leukocytosis may be absent, but the sedimentation rate is always elevated.[33, 34] Needle biopsy of the disk usually yields a negative culture, especially if there is no pus to be aspirated. Recently, automated aspiration biopsy with the nucleotome (Surgical Dynamics, Inc., San Leandro, Calif.) has been advocated as an effective means of obtaining an accurate histologic and bacteriologic diagnosis.[35]

Plain radiographs are the simplest and most cost-effective way of showing the characteristic findings of progressive disk space narrowing and irregular destruction of the adjacent end plates but these changes generally do not occur in the first 2 to 8 weeks.[36] If there is clinical suspicion of diskitis and the plain films are negative, or if there is a question of an associated paravertebral or epidural component, or compression of the cauda equina, MRI is the study of choice. Because of its great soft tissue sensitivity, MRI will detect changes in the disk and adjacent end plates and bone marrow when the plain films or bone scans are still negative.[37] The sagittal scans in particular are best for showing abnormalities and for ruling out extraosseous extension. Axial CT through the disk is also quite sensitive in showing early destruction of the bony end plates and for evaluating the paraspinous soft tissues (Fig 38–17).

The clinical treatment usually involves immobilization. With bacteriologic diagnosis, the patient can be placed on effective antibiotics for more rapid recovery. Rarely, an epidural abscess may occur after disk surgery (Fig 38–18).

Hematoma and Pseudomeningocele

A postoperative hematoma is generally epidural and presents with neurologic deficit in the im-

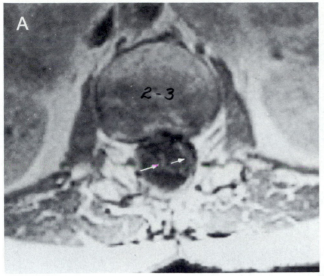

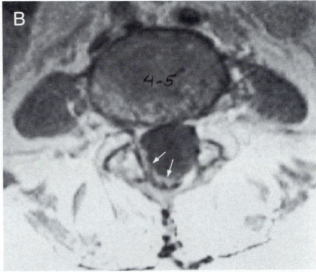

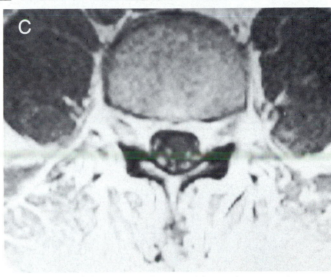

FIG 38–15.
A 60-year-old woman who underwent prior L2–S1 laminectomies and fusions. **A,** T1-weighted axial MR scan through L2–3 shows mild nerve root adhesions *(arrows).* **B,** a similar scan through L4–5 shows more severe adhesions of nerves to the periphery of the sac *(arrows).* **C,** a normal scan of another patient for comparison.

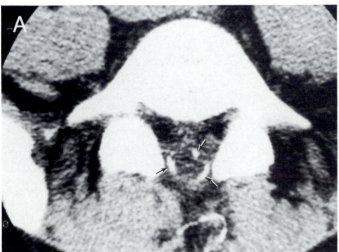

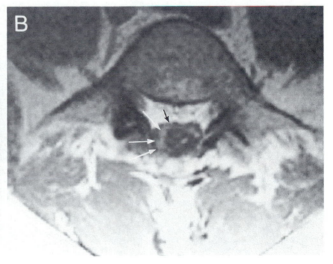

FIG 38–16.
A, an unenhanced CT scan shows calcification along the margins of the subarachnoid sac *(arrows)* in this 36-year-old man who had prior L5–S1 laminectomy. **B,** a T1-weighted MRI at the same level does not demonstrate the calcification but shows the thickened sac with adherent nerve roots *(arrows).*

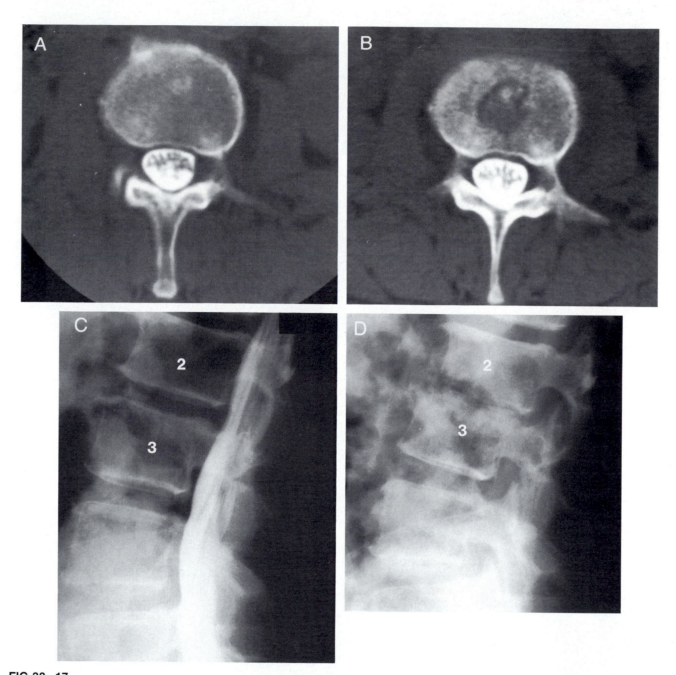

FIG 38–17.

A 65-year-old man underwent a left L2–3 diskectomy for a far-lateral disk herniation. **A,** a preoperative CT myelogram at the level of the inferior end plate of L2 is unremarkable. **B,** a repeat scan done 4 weeks later, after the patient had developed severe pain at the operative site, showed early resorption of the end plate. **C,** the myelogram at that time showed no bony change. **D,** 4 weeks later, end-plate destruction was obvious at L2–3. *Facing page,* the T1-weighted **(E)** and T2-weighted **(F)** MR scans showed obvious involvement of the disk and adjacent marrow, with no associated epidural extension.

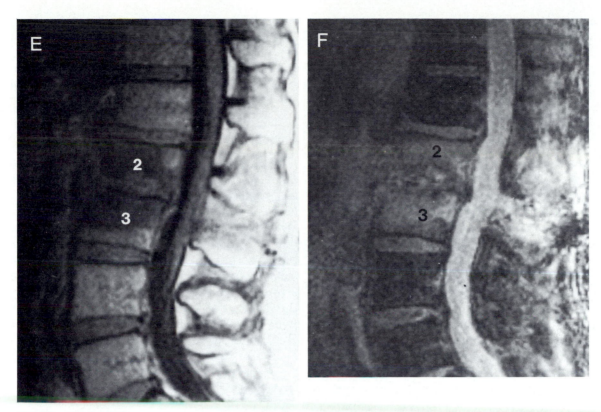

FIG 38–17   (cont.).

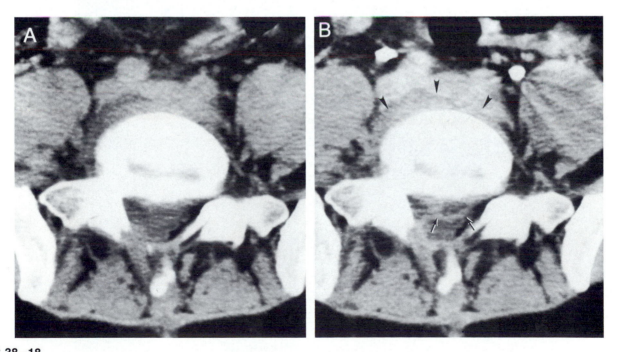

FIG 38–18.

A 35-year-old male developed recurrent back pain and radiculopathy 10 days after surgery. Unenhanced **(A)** and enhanced **(B)** CT scans through L5–S1 show an anterior epidural mass with marginal enhancement (B, *arrows*) which looks very much like a recurrent disk herniation. However, the low density of the mass and the associated paraspinous soft tissue fullness (B, *arrowheads*) should raise the suspicion of inflammatory disease. An epidural abscess was treated by surgical drainage.

mediate postoperative period. Myelography may be extremely difficult and confusing because of compression and obliteration of the sac by the hematoma (Fig 38–19). Because it is noninvasive and sensitive to soft tissue abnormalities, MRI is probably now the first study of choice. Sagittal MRI is particularly useful because it provides rapid assessment of the complete rostrocaudal extent of the lesion.

A pseudomeningocele is usually caused by a small dural tear at the time of surgery which either allows progressive herniation of the arachnoid membrane through the rent[38] or produces a CSF leak into the soft tissues which eventually develops a fibrous capsule.[39] As opposed to a hematoma, a pseudomeningocele usually does not produce symptoms until weeks or months after the surgery.

The lesion is readily demonstrated by CT or MRI as a well-circumscribed mass posterior to the thecal sac that is of CSF density or signal intensity. Of course, if the cyst contains blood or xanthochromic fluid, the signal intensity will be different.

The actual rent usually cannot be defined with either study but may be shown at myelography and especially with follow-up CT myelography (Fig 38–20). If there is any question that the cyst represents an abscess, a percutaneous aspiration can easily be performed.

Spinal Stenosis

Stenosis of the spinal canal can be developmental, acquired, or both, and can involve the central canal, the lateral recesses, the neural foramina, or a combination of the above. The role of spinal stenosis in failed back surgery is often difficult to define. Was the stenosis overlooked at the time of initial surgery? Did it develop as a cause of the surgery, or did it occur much later due to progressive spondylosis? There is little doubt that prior to the advent of CT scanning, many diskectomies were performed on the basis of myelographic defects which were in fact secondary to bony and ligamentous hypertrophy, with or without associated

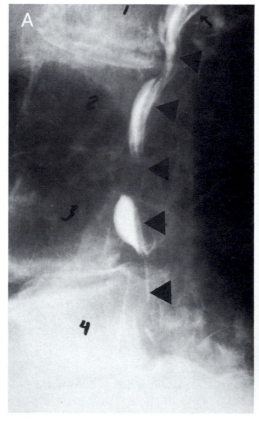 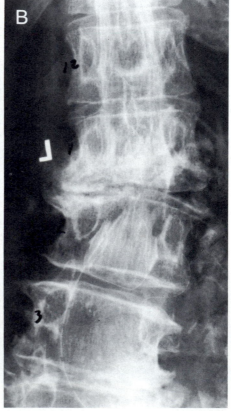

FIG 38–19.
Twelve hours after L2–5 laminectomy for spinal stenosis, this 72-year-old woman developed lower extremity paralysis. **A,** AP and lateral views **(B)** of an emergency myelogram via C1–2 puncture reveal a large, mostly dorsal mass narrowing the sac (**A,** *arrowheads*) from L1–2 to a virtually complete block at L4. An epidural hematoma was evacuated.

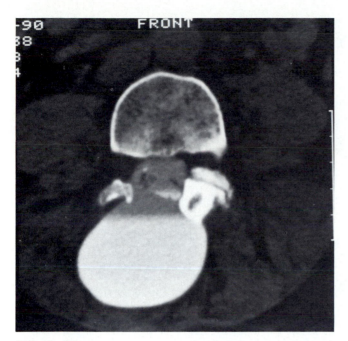

FIG 38–20.
A CT myelogram of a patient who had undergone laminectomy 5 years earlier demonstrates leakage of CSF and contrast medium through a right-sided arachnoid rent into a large pseudomeningocele.

bulging or herniation of the disk. Since the neural foramina could not be assessed with myelography, many central canal decompressions were performed without treating associated neural foraminal or lateral recess stenosis. Even an appropriate

diskectomy may lead to subsequent foraminal stenosis as a result of progressive settling of the disk space and consequent rostral migration of the superior articular facet into the neural foramen. Some investigators have suggested that lateral or foraminal stenosis continues to be the most common cause of the failed back surgery syndrome.[1, 14]

Interruption of the posterior joints and ligaments without stabilization may lead to excessive mobility, hypertrophic degenerative changes, and a subsequent mechanical stenosis. Another commonly encountered problem is spinal stenosis immediately above or below a successful spinal fusion that is due to increased stress and mobility of the unfused segment, and which leads to bony and soft tissue hypertrophy (Fig 38–21).

Fusion Complications

Of the estimated 10,000 spinal fusions performed annually, approximately 30% to 40% experience recurrent or persistent pain. Identifying the specific cause of the pain is often difficult, but fusion arthrodesis has been incriminated as one of the causes. Assessment of structural integrity of the fusion mass can often be done successfully with plain films (Fig 38–22). If there is uncertainty, thin-section CT scanning using sagittal and coronal reformations is the next procedure of choice (Fig 38–23). MRI is of only limited value in the detec-

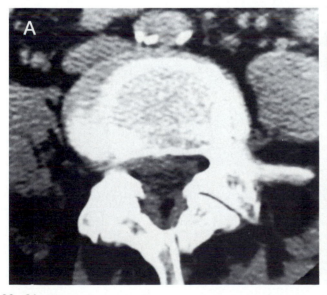
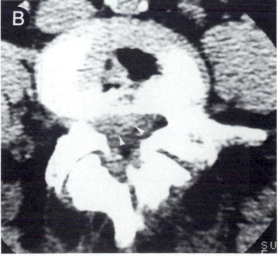

FIG 38–21.
A preoperative **(A)** and a 9-months postoperative **(B)** scan through the L4–5 disk of the same patient shown in Figure 38–7 show interval development of disk degeneration and gas, progressive facet joint hypertrophy, and a moderate, right-sided posterior disk herniation (**B,** *arrowheads*) reflecting the added stresses at L4–5 caused by the more rostral fusion.

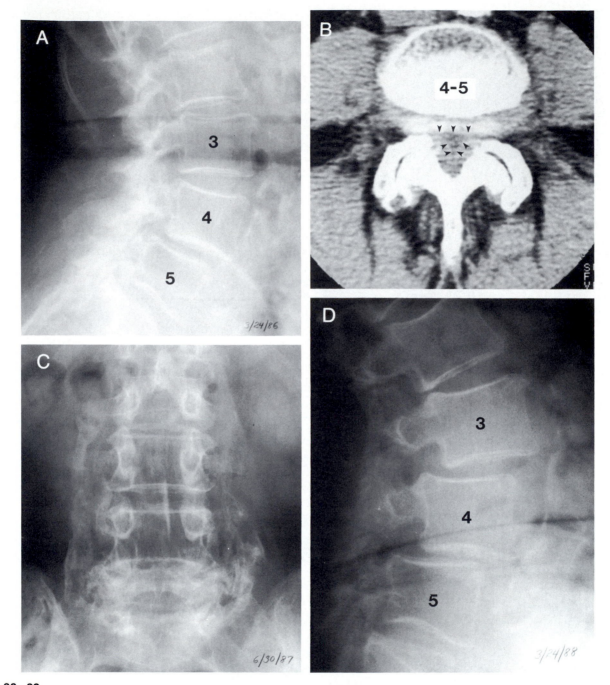

FIG 38–22.

A preoperative lateral spine film **(A)** and an axial CT scan **(B)** shown severe spinal canal stenosis at L4–5 (**B**, *arrowheads*) due to degenerative spondylolisthesis and ligamentous hypertrophy in this 75-year-old woman. **C,** a postoperative film shows overly gen-

erous laminectomies and facetectomies from L2–L4 and a lateral fusion from L2–S1. **D,** a lateral film obtained 9 months later shows progressive spondylolisthesis at L4–5 and a new listhesis at L3–4 reflecting fusion failure.

tion of pseudarthrosis, due to the low T1 and T2 signal of fusion mass.

Even more important is functional assessment of the fusion. Plain films utilizing lateral flexion-extension views are best in this regard and may detect motion even when the fusion appears structur-

ally intact. Motion and distractive forces are necessary for gas to occur in the disk or in the facet joints. The plain film demonstration of intradiskal gas is thus another sign of functional instability. CT is even more sensitive than plain films in detecting gas within the disk or facet joints at the

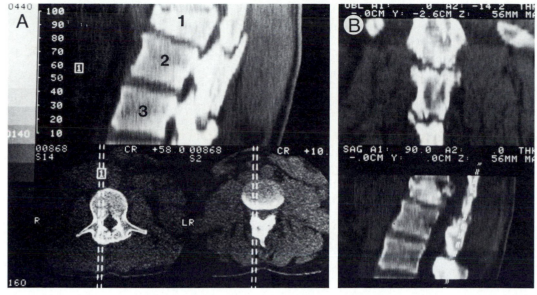

FIG 38–23.

A 30-year-old man with persistent pain 2 years after posterior T12–L3 fusion for a compression fracture of L1. The stability of the fusion could not be assessed with plain films. Sagittal **(A)** and coronal **(B)** reformatted CT images clearly show pseudarthroses of the fusion mass at L1–2 and L2–3.

level of fusion. MRI may also be of value in functional assessment of a fusion. Reactive hyperemia and scar within the marrow adjacent to a disk strongly suggests biomechanical stress from motion and will produce decreased T1 and increased T2 signal intensity. On the other hand, a successful fusion will relieve such stress and the bone marrow will often undergo fatty conversion, resulting in a high T1 signal and a low signal on a T2-weighted image.

Planar bone scintigraphy and especially single photon emission tomography (SPECT) are especially sensitive in detecting pseudarthrosis.[40] Precise localization of the defect allows the surgeon to re-fuse without having to take down the entire fusion.

Other fusion complications include osseous hypertrophy resulting in spinal stenosis and bone plug migration causing cauda equina or local nerve root impingement.

SUMMARY

Whether to rely on CT scanning or MRI in evaluation of the postoperative spine has not yet been completely resolved. To some extent, this issue is influenced by the available equipment. The new, fast CT scanners (less than 1 or 2 seconds per slice) can produce a study of the lumbosacral spine from L3 to S1 in less than 10 minutes. If needed, additional intravenously enhanced scans can be obtained in 5 or 10 minutes. Use of nonionic iodinated contrast agents makes the study very safe but also adds significantly to the cost. In addition to providing reliable discrimination between scar and recurrent disk in over 80% of cases, CT currently has certain advantages over MRI, including speed, cost, availability, better definition of associated postoperative or degenerative bony changes, the ability to reliably differentiate disk from bony spur, a slightly better signal-to-noise ratio and spatial resolution, the ability to perform contiguous or overlapping slices, and no significant problems with claustrophobia. CT can also show disk calcification and inspissated or adherent iophendylate which might otherwise be overlooked with MRI. The advantages of speed and spatial resolution are more apparent when comparing CT to low-field-strength magnets.

On the other hand, surface-coil MRI has the advantage of demonstrating a larger area than is usually covered with routine CT, including the conus medullaris and lower thoracic spinal cord, and has the additional advantage of multidimensional imaging capability. Every disk can be enhanced and visualized simultaneously with sagittal MRI, whereas usually only two or three disk levels are optimally enhanced with axial CT. Sagittal scans are often more sensitive than axial scans in demonstrating subtle disk protrusions and can also show polypoid disk herniations and free disk fragments that might be very difficult to appreciate on axial views. Enhanced MRI appears to be more specific than enhanced CT in discriminating between recurrent disk and scar.

From a practical perspective, routine CT scanning, using contrast enhancement when necessary, does very well in differentiating reherniated disk from scar in the postoperative spine. Further study with MRI or CT myelography is only infrequently necessary. It should also be remembered that most postoperative back failures are not due to disk herniation or scar but rather to persistent spinal canal or neural foraminal stenosis. Axial CT performs very well in this regard and may still have some advantages over MRI. Occasional patients will require additional CT or CT myelography after either conventional CT or MRI to clarify associated bony vs. ligamentous abnormalities and to clearly define individual nerve roots.

REFERENCES

1. Heithoff KB, Burton CV: CT evaluation of the failed back surgery syndrome. *Orthop Clin North Am* 1985; 16:417–444.
2. Fager CA: Lumbar microdiscectomy: A contrary opinion. *Clin Neurosurg* 1986; 33:419–456.
3. Teplick JG, Haskin ME: Review: Computed tomography of the postoperative lumbar spine. *AJR* 1983; 141:865–884.
4. Voelker JL, Mealey J Jr, Eskridge JM, et al: Metrizamide-enhanced computed tomography as an adjunct to metrizamide myelography in the evaluation of lumbar disc herniation and spondylosis. *Neurosurgery* 1987; 20:379–384.
5. Ross JS: Magnetic resonance imaging of the postoperative spine. *Top Magn Reson Imaging* 1988; 1:39–52.
6. Mall JC, Kaiser JA: The usual appearance of the postoperative lumbar spine. *RadioGraphics* 1987; 7:245–269.
7. Fraser RD, Hall DJ: Surgical and interventional procedures for low back pain and sciatica. *Curr Imaging* 1989; 1:225–230.
8. Maroon JC, Abla AA: Microlumbar discectomy. *Clin Neurosurg* 1986; 33:407–417.
9. Sypert GW: Low back pain disorders: Lumbar fusion? *Clin Neurosurg* 1986; 33:457–483.
10. Feffer HC, Wiesel SW, Cuckler JM, et al: Degenerative spondylolisthesis: To fuse or not to fuse. *Spine* 1985; 10:287–289.
11. Swank S, Lonstein JE, Moe JH, et al: Surgical treatment of adult scoliosis. A review of two hundred and twenty-two cases. *J Bone Joint Surg [Am]* 1981; 63:268–287.
12. Kiviluoto O: Use of free fat transplants to prevent epidural scar formation. *Acta Orthop Scand [Suppl]* 1976; 164:3–75.
13. Burton CV: Lumbosacral arachnoiditis. *Spine* 1978; 3:24–30.
14. Burton CV, Kirkaldy-Willis WH, Yong HK, et al: Causes of failure of surgery on the lumbar spine. *Clin Orthop* 1981; 157:191–199.
15. Nelson MJ, Gold LH: CT evaluation of intervertebral foramina lesions with normal or nondiagnostic myelograms. Report of ten cases. *Comput Radiol* 1983; 7:155–160.
16. Finnegan WJ, Fenlin JM, Marvel JP, et al: Results of surgical intervention in the symptomatic multiply-operated back patient. *J Bone Joint Surg [Am]* 1979; 61:1077–1082.
17. Law JD, Lehman RAW, Kirsch WM: Reoperation after lumbar intervertebral disk surgery. *J Neurosurg* 1978; 48:259–263.
18. Braun IF, Hoffman JC Jr, Davis PC, et al: Contrast enhancement in CT differentiation between recurrent disk herniation and postoperative scar: Prospective study. *AJNR* 1985; 6:607–612.
19. Firooznia H, Kricheff II, Rafii M, et al: Lumbar spine after surgery: Examination with intravenous contrast enhanced CT. *Radiology* 1987; 163:221–226.
20. Schubiger O, Valavanis A: CT differentiation between recurrent disc herniation and postoperative scar formation: The value of contrast enhancement. *Neuroradiology* 1982; 22:251–254.
21. Teplick JG, Haskin ME: Intravenous contrast-enhanced CT of the postoperative lumbar spine: improved identification of recurrent disk herniation, scar, arachnoiditis, and diskitis. *AJNR* 1984; 5:373–383.
22. Weiss T, Treisch J, Kazner E, et al: CT of the postoperative lumbar spine: The value of intravenous contrast. *Neuroradiology* 1986; 28:241–245.
23. Yang PJ, Seeger JF, Dzioba RB, et al: High-dose IV contrast in CT scanning of the postoperative lumbar spine. *AJNR* 1986; 7:703–708.
24. Bundschuh CV, Modic MT, Ross JS, et al: Epidural fibrosis and recurrent disk herniation in the lumbar spine: MR imaging assessment. *AJNR* 1988; 9:169–178.
25. Sotiropoulos S, Chafetz NI, Lang P, et al: Differentiation between postoperative scar and recurrent disk herniation: Prospective comparison of MR, CT, and contrast-enhanced CT. *AJNR* 1989; 10:639–643.
26. Hueftle M, Modic MT, Ross JS, et al: Lumbar spine: Postoperative MR imaging with Gd-DTPA. *Radiology* 1988; 167:817–824.
27. Ross JS, Delamarter R, Hueftle MG, et al: Gadolinium-DTPA–enhanced MR imaging of the

postoperative lumbar spine: Time course and mechanism of enhancement. *AJNR* 1989; 10:37–46.

28. Simmons JD, Newton TH: Arachnoiditis, in Newton TH, Potts DG (eds): *Computed Tomography of the Spine and Spinal Cord.* San Anselmo, Calif, Clavadel Press, 1983, pp 223–229.

29. Shaw MOM, Russel JA, Grossart KW: The changing pattern of spinal arachnoiditis. *J Neurol Neurosurg Psychiatry* 1978; 41:97–107.

30. Ross JS, Masaryk TJ, Modic MT, et al: MR imaging of lumbar arachnoiditis. *AJNR* 1987; 8:885–892.

31. Naikin L: Arachnoiditis ossificans. Report of a case. *Spine* 1978; 3:83–86.

32. Dall BE, Rowe DE, Odette WG, et al: Postoperative discitis—diagnosis and management. *Clin Orthop* 1987; 224:138–146.

33. Taylor TKF, Grainger WD: Disc space infection as a complication of disc surgery. *J Bone Joint Surg [Am]* 1973; 55:435–438.

34. El-Gindi S, Aref S, Andrew J: Infection of intervertebral discs after operation. *J Bone Joint Surg [Am]* 1976; 58:114–116.

35. Onik G, Shang Y, Maroon JC: Automated percutaneous biopsy in postoperative diskitis: A new method. *AJNR* 1990; 11:391–393.

36. Ross PM, Fleming JL: Vertebral body osteomyelitis: Spectrum and natural history: A retrospective analysis of 37 cases. *Clin Orthop* 1976; 118:190–198.

37. Unger E, Moldofsky P, Gatenby R, et al: Diagnosis of osteomyelitis by MR imaging. *AJR* 1988; 150:605–610.

38. Teplick JG, Peyster RG, Teplick S, et al: CT identification of post laminectomy pseudomeningocele. *AJNR* 1983; 4:179–182.

39. Patronas NJ, Jafer J, Brown F: Pseudomeningoceles diagnosed by metrizamide myelography and computerized tomography. *Surg Neurol* 1981; 16:188–191.

40. Slizofski WJ, Collier BD, Flatley TJ, et al: Painful pseudoarthrosis following lumbar spinal fusion: detection by combined SPECT and planar bone scintigraphy. *Skeletal Radiol* 1987; 16:136–141.

39

Tumors and Infections of the Spine and Spinal Cord

Charles A. Jungreis, M.D.

William E. Rothfus, M.D.

Richard E. Latchaw, M.D.

Computed tomography (CT) and magnetic resonance imaging (MRI) of the spine have gained great popularity due to their ability to provide a tremendous amount of information with minimal if any discomfort and danger to the patient. Scanning allows precise evaluation of bone destruction, associated paraspinal masses, and the degree of cord and/or nerve root compression (Fig 39–1). Nevertheless, different diseases may have similar appearances, and despite the most sophisticated examinations, differentiating infection from neoplastic disease may still be difficult. In this chapter we will generally not attempt to advocate CT vs. MRI as the method of examination since many factors will determine which examination is used for a particular patient. Often both examinations will be required, depending on the clinical situation.

TECHNIQUES OF EXAMINATION

Plain CT may be all that is needed for the evaluation of a single focus of bone destruction such as a bony metastasis, a primary neoplasm of bone, or a disk space infection with destruction of the adjacent vertebrae. High-resolution scanners afford good definition of both the epidural spread of such neoplastic and infectious processes and the paraspinal component as well. Since acquiring axial images through the entire spine is not practical, zeroing in on an area of interest is essential. Thus, a good clinical examination, plain films, or radionuclide scans become very important. Our routine CT scans of the spine consist of contiguous 3- or 5-mm-thick sections through the area of interest, depending on the size and extent of the expected pathology. Soft-tissue and/or bone algorithms might be performed, depending on the clinically suspected lesion. Better definition may be afforded by thinner cuts, and thinner cuts also provide better reformatted sagittal and coronal images if these are desired. Reformatted images are particularly useful in evaluating structures such as vertebral end plates that lie in the axial plane. Five-millimeter cuts spaced every 3 mm also give excellent reformatted images. Scanning is performed with either 0-degree angulation of the gantry or with angulation parallel to the disk space. For example, our usual examination of a patient suspected of having degenerative disk disease consists of 3-mm-thick contiguous slices that angle parallel to each disk space and cover the region from the pedicle above the disk to the pedicle below. We do not routinely employ reformatted images.

Intravenously enhanced CT scans may provide additional information over nonenhanced CT. Mainly, the dura can frequently be enhanced adequately enough to clearly define the margins of the thecal sac. In addition, many disease processes en-

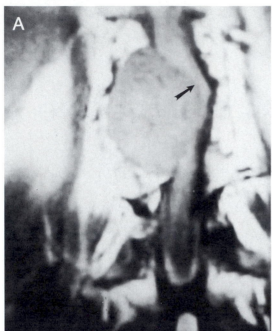
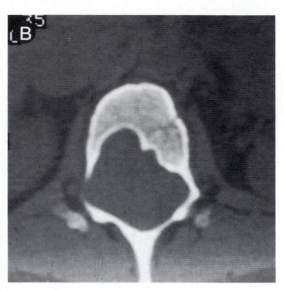

FIG 39–1.
Neurofibroma. **A,** coronal MRI (T1 weighted) shows a large mass centered at the L2 level and displacing the conus medullaris *(arrow)*. **B,** axial CT through L2 shows the tremendous remodeling of the vertebra without actual bone destruction. The cortex is very well demonstrated and is intact.

hance, again providing additional information. For instance, inflammatory tissue tends to enhance, and the epidural extent may be more easily demonstrated with enhanced CT. Certain primary bone tumors like hemangiomas and plasmacytomas tend to enhance markedly, a characteristic that can help define their extent.

CT performed following the administration of intrathecal contrast (myelography) often affords spectacular anatomy with clear definition of the thecal sac and of the neural elements contained within. Currently, CT follows virtually every myelogram that is performed with rare exceptions, with the myelogram used as a localizing process to direct us to regions of interest for CT studies.

Delayed CT scanning following myelography with water-soluble contrast agents has been advocated as a method to demonstrate areas of fluid collections within the cord.[1] The "imbibition" of contrast into syringohydromyelia/tumor cysts has been demonstrated.[2] However, appropriate delay after the initial scan is arguable due to the variations in rates of contrast uptake and dissipation in various lesions. In the past, delayed scans of 6, 12, and 24 hours have been performed to look for cystic areas within the cord. However, this technique of demonstrating cysts has been not only inconsistent but also misleading. Imbibition may occur in injured cord that has no cyst and cause a false-positive re-

sult. Conversely, false-negative results or equivocal results are common. With the advent of MRI and ultrasound, this technique has lost some popularity but occasionally can be helpful.

In general there are two great advantages of MRI over CT in evaluating the spine. The first is that because MRI has great sensitivity to soft-tissue contrast, the spinal cord is seen with excellent definition. Both the external margins and internal structure of the cord are superbly demonstrated with MRI. The other advantage of MRI over CT is in determining appropriate regions of interest since sagittal (and coronal) images of large areas of the spine can be covered relatively easily with MRI. Subsequent high-resolution examinations may then be directed to a region of interest. Surface coils are very useful for this purpose. In practice the use of surface coils is routine. The surface-coil size is determined by the size of the area to be examined. Most manufacturers provide multiple shapes and sizes from which to choose.

For example, our current adult lumbar examination begins with a sagittal series that includes the entire lumbar spine. When using an appropriately sized surface coil (5 by 11 in.) on which the patient rests, images in all three planes can be obtained with little effort and only several minutes of additional time for each set of images. Our slice thickness is generally 5 mm in both sagittal and axial planes. Depending on the size of the area of interest as determined on the initial sagittal series, spacing between axial slices can be chosen and can be minimal (1 mm or less). Images based on T1 contrast, spin-density contrast, or T2 contrast information can be obtained with the same patient position and coil position. While short repetition time (TR) images (T1 contrast or T1-weighted images) are generally quicker to obtain than long TR images (T2 contrast or T2-weighted images), either or both might be required in any particular case, depending on the suspected pathology and relative contrast between tissues. Partial flip angle images may also be obtained with most equipment using the same coil and may provide useful information. In addition, the use of the intravenously administered paramagnetic contrast agent gadolinium—diethylenetriamine pentaacetic acid (DTPA) can greatly increase the tissue contrast between areas that enhance and areas that do not. This type of enhancement is analogous to enhancement on CT following iodinated contrast administration, but MRI appears to be more sensitive to small amounts of contrast than does CT. Contrast-enhanced MRI holds great promise in the evaluation of tumors of the spine and spinal cord. Finally, our routine examinations include software able to help compensate for flow (FLOWCOMP, GE Medical Systems, Milwaukee) and cardiac gating, techniques that help decrease motion artifacts.

TUMORS OF BONE

Hemangioma

Hemangioma represents the most common neoplasm of the bony spine and occurs in almost 11% of autopsy specimens.[3] It occurs most often in the lower thoracic and upper lumbar segments (Fig 39–2).[4] It is a benign lesion, although it may attain considerable size. Hemangioma consist of abnormal vascular channels in a fatty matrix. The usual vertebral trabeculae appear decreased in number, with the remaining trabeculae appearing thickened. The vast majority of hemangiomas are confined to the vertebral body, often involving only a portion of the vertebral body. However, it may spread along the contiguous bony structures to involve the posterior elements. It may break through the cortex to extend into the epidural and/or paraspinal spaces. Epidural extension may produce significant cord compression (Fig 39–3). Usually, an hemangioma is demonstrated as an in-

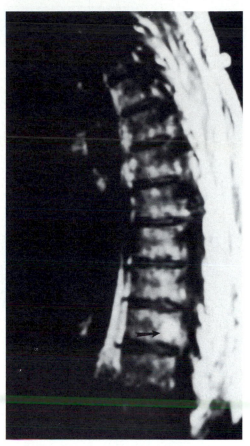

FIG 39–2.
Hemangioma. A sagittal T1-weighted image shows a small lower thoracic hemangioma *(arrow)* with the characteristic high signal on this sequence.

cidental finding on an examination performed for other reasons. The object in identifying a hemangioma is to avoid an erroneous diagnosis of malignant or infectious look-alikes. In those patients with signs of cord compression, evaluation becomes aimed at the usual parameters, like epidural extent and osseous integrity.

A stippled appearance on axial CT is typical. That is, the remaining trabeculae appear as dense nodules in a background of fat (Fig 39–4). Nevertheless, plasmacytoma and lymphoma can give an almost identical appearance on CT. Paget's disease may be confused with hemangioma but is usually distinguished by cortical thickening and overall enlargement of the vertebra. Enhancement of a hemangioma with intravenous contrast may be dramatic, although the degree of enhancement is usually less than expected for the presumed degree of vascularity.

The MRI appearance reflects the various components of a hemangioma in a relatively unique

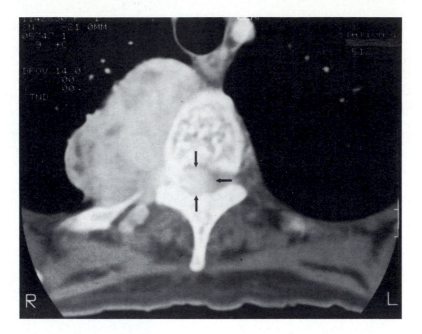

FIG 39–3.
Hemangioma. Contrast CT through the thoracic spine demonstrates a large paraspinal mass that extends into the spinal canal as well *(arrows)*. Also notice the thickened trabecular pattern in the vertebral body. The spinal canal has been severely compromised by the intraspinal extent of this mass. (Courtesy of Ronald Miller, M.D., Omaha.)

pattern. The fat provides a high signal on the T1-weighted images (Fig 39–5), while the cellular (watery) components probably provide the typical high signal seen on the T2-weighted images. Blood flow and/or thrombosis of vascular channels appears to contribute little to this pattern. The region of increased signal may be mottled rather than homogeneous. If extraosseous extension is present, that portion may differ in signal characteristics from the intraosseous portion.[3]

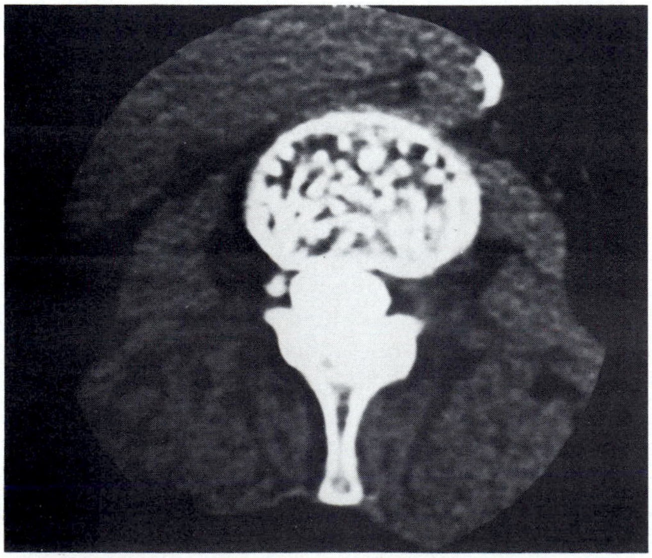

Osteochondroma

Osteochondroma is an unusual tumor of the spine, but when it occurs, it most commonly involves the spinous process (Fig 39–6). The CT characteristics are similar to those on plain films and include a margin of cortical bone surrounding an inner, less dense component of chondroid tissue that may or may not be calcified.

Osteoid Osteoma and Osteoblastoma (Giant Osteoid Osteoma)

The classic location of an osteoid osteoma is the pedicle of a thoracic or upper lumbar vertebra. Occasionally other portions of the neural arch are affected. The usual patient is a young male presenting with back pain that is worse at night and relieved with aspirin. Plain films and CT demonstrate a sclerotic focus of bone usually no bigger than 1 to 2 cm. Either plain-film tomography[5] or appropriate CT windows may demonstrate a small radiolucent nidus of only several millimeters in diameter that lies centrally within the sclerotic area.

Histologically osteoblastoma is very similar to osteoid osteoma. However, osteoblastoma is gener-

FIG 39–4.
Vertebral hemangioma. CT demonstrates the typical stippled appearance in the body.

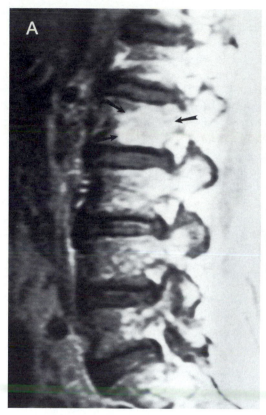

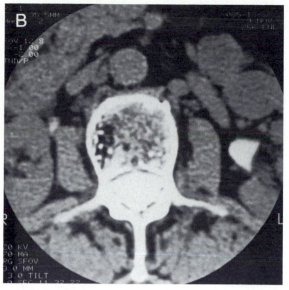

FIG 39–5.
Hemangioma of L2. **A,** sagittal T1-weighted MRI shows a hemangioma *(arrows)* in the body of L2. **B,** axial CT shows that only a portion of the vertebral body is affected; the stippled trabeculae are apparent in the background matrix of fat.

ally larger and is characterized by a diffuse lytic expansion of a portion of the neural arch with cortical thinning. There is a predilection for occurring in the cervical spine. Intraspinal and paraspinal extension by a soft-tissue mass may be present and may compress the spinal cord and/or nerve roots.

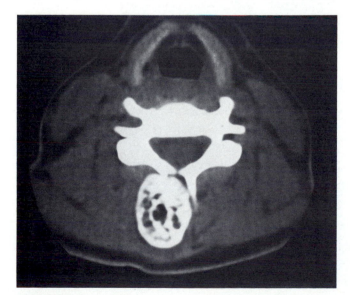

FIG 39–6.
Osteochondroma of the cervical spine. Axial CT demonstrates the pedunculated mass protruding from the spinous process.

Radiographically, "aneurysmal" changes in the bone may be present and make differentiation from an aneurysmal bone cyst difficult. In fact, pathologically the two entities may be found contiguously, which supports the school that contends that aneurysmal bone cyst is a "secondary" lesion.[6] Some controversy does exist pathologically with respect to the actual categorization of osteoblastoma, aneurysmal bone cyst, and giant-cell tumor.

Aneurysmal Bone Cyst

An aneurysmal bone cyst (ABC) is comprised of large blood-filled cavities and is not usually considered a true neoplasm. Its etiology is uncertain, but it is seen frequently in areas of previous trauma and in areas of bone harboring a concurrent osteoblastoma or giant-cell tumor.[6] One patient developed an ABC during pregnancy at a site of fibrous dysplasia.[7] Thus it has sometimes been considered a "secondary" lesion. The hallmark of an ABC is tremendous expansion of a bone with marked thinning of the cortex. While any bone in the body may be involved, one fifth of ABCs involve the spine, particularly the posterior elements. The differential diagnosis includes osteoblastoma, giant-cell tumor, and malignant round-cell tumors (Ewing's sarcoma, plasmacytoma). Due to the expansion of the bone, the neural elements including the cord can be compressed. The symptoms may include local pain and swelling as well as neurologic deficits related to the neural compression.

Imaging will demonstrate a multiloculated expansive process that appears to originate within the bone but may extend intraspinally and paraspinally. The origin usually appears in the posterior elements but an ABC may extend into the vertebral body. Intravenous contrast CT may demonstrate enhancement.

Angiography and embolization may be of value preoperatively. This lesion is histologically benign and therefore theoretically curable.

Giant-Cell Tumor

The majority of giant-cell tumors are histologically benign, but it may progress to malignancy. Giant-cell tumor generally involves the sacrum,

with a presentation in other portions of the spine being distinctly uncommon.[8] In contrast to the thin but relatively well-defined cortical expansion of an ABC, the giant-cell tumor typically has poorly defined margins in an expansive area, and actual bone destruction at the margins may be apparent. Giant-cell tumor is rare before the age of 20 years, whereas ABC commonly occur before the age of 20 years. Giant-cell tumor generally involves the sacrum, and ABC generally does not.[8]

Surgical resection may be curative, although local recurrence and/or progression to malignancy may occur, just as in other locations in the body. Imaging is important in the evaluation of both the paraspinal and intraspinal extent.

Chordoma

The chordoma arises from notochordal cell rests within a disk space, thereby providing the mechanism to spread into contiguous vertebral bodies. In this sense, it may mimic disk space in-

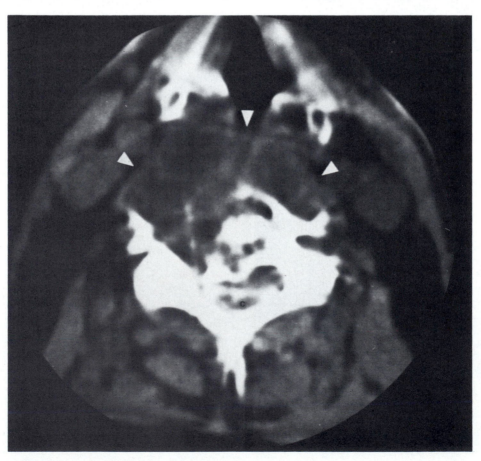

FIG 39–7.
Chordoma. This irregular mass has destroyed much of the right side of this cervical vertebral body and spread into the prevertebral space *(arrowheads)*. There is flattening of the cord *(c)*, which is outlined by water-soluble contrast that had been instilled intrathecally prior to scanning (CT/myelography).

fection. The most common locations for chordoma are the sphenoid bone and clivus, with the sacrum the next most common. Chordomas may occur anywhere along the rest of the spine, but such involvement accounts for fewer than 15% of cases.

Chordoma is characterized by a poorly marginated destructive mass often with large dense calcifications within it (Fig 39–7).[9]

Paget's Disease

Paget's disease is not a form of neoplasia but is considered here because of differential diagnosis. Paget's disease classically has three phases, including an initial lytic phase, a second phase characterized by mixed osteolytic and osteoblastic components, and a tertiary diffuse osteoblastic phase. When a vertebral segment is involved, the hallmark is one of enlargement of the bone with thickening of the cortex and prominence of the trabecular pattern (Fig 39–8). There may be sufficient enlargement of a vertebral body and neural arch to produce compression of the spinal cord and/or nerve roots, although this is uncommon.

Metastatic Tumor

Metastases are the most common malignancy of the spine. While a single focus may be the reason for evaluation, multiple foci are often evident, even on the initial scan. Metastases may be lytic, blastic, or a combination of both. The most common osteolytic metastases are from carcinoma of the breast, lung, and kidney. Multiple myeloma/plasmacytoma may also appear as an osteolytic lesion and be indistinguishable from an osteolytic metastasis of any origin. The most common osteoblastic metastases are from carcinoma of the prostate gland (Fig 39–9) in males and from carcinoma of the breast in females.

Axial CT with or without intravenous contrast can be helpful in evaluation of a focus of disease, particularly with respect to the intraspinal and paraspinal extension. However, since obtaining axial images of the entire spine is not usually practical, the region of interest must usually be determined either clinically, with plain films, by radionuclide scanning, or in conjunction with myelography. CT performed with intrathecal contrast (CT myelography) is a superb method to demonstrate the anatomy (Fig 39–10). An advantage of MRI is the ease with which sagittal sections of the entire spine can be obtained and then used to focus on regions of interest for higher-resolution study.[10]

Replacement of the normal marrow within a vertebral body, cortical destruction, and intraspinal and paraspinal extension is common. By CT, the normal fine trabecular pattern will be absent, being replaced by a soft-tissue mass. MRI (Figs 39–11 and 39–12) will demonstrate replacement

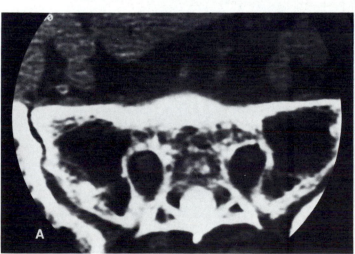

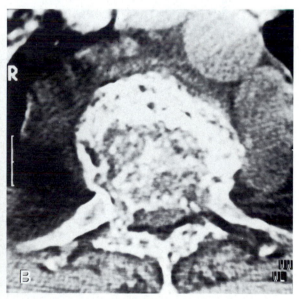

FIG 39–8.
Paget's disease. **A,** CT of the sacrum shows thickening of the cortex and a more lucent trabecular pattern in the body of the sacrum. **B,** a different patient shows involvement of the body and posterior elements with abnormal soft tissues compromising the spinal canal and extending into the paraspinal and the prevertebral spaces.

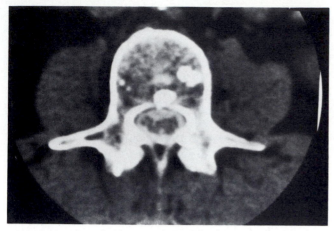

FIG 39–9.
Prostatic carcinoma. Multiple well-defined blastic metastasis dot the medullary cavity of the vertebral body.

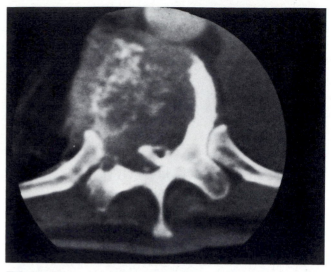

FIG 39–10.
Lung carcinoma metastatic to the thoracic spine. Not only has this metastasis destroyed much of the body of the vertebra, but it also extends into the spinal canal and is narrowing the subarachnoid space (outlined with water-soluble contrast).

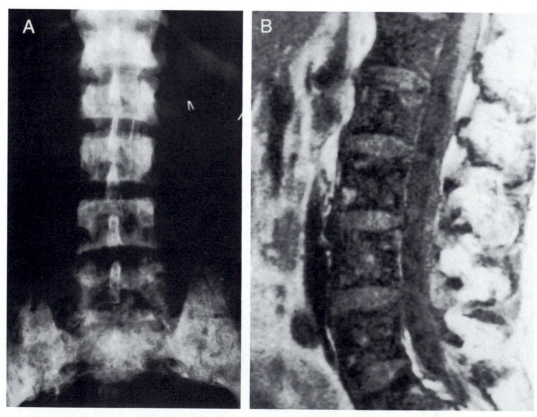

FIG 39–11.
Prostatic carcinoma. **A,** a plain film of the lumbosacral spine demonstrates extensive blastic changes. **B,** sagittal T1-weighted MRI demonstrates complete replacement of the normal marrow in all of the visualized vertebra.

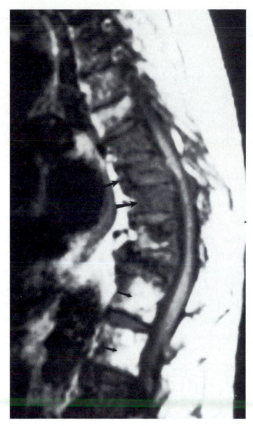

FIG 39–12.
Diffuse thoracic metastasis. Sagittal T1-weighted MRI shows that the marrow has been replaced by tumor in many of the midthoracic vertebra as evidenced by the loss of the "fatty" signal expected in normal marrow (*large arrows* = metastasis; *small arrows* = normal marrow)

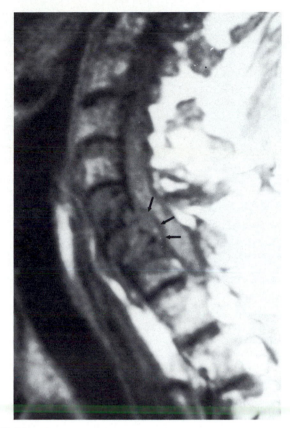

FIG 39–13.
Cervical metastasis. A sagittal T1-weighted image shows that multiple vertebrae are affected and epidural extension *(arrows)* compresses the spinal cord.

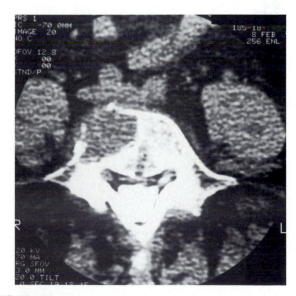

FIG 39–14.
Metastasis to L5. CT/myelography was performed. The plain films were unremarkable. However, CT demonstrates the defect in the body of the vertebrae with relative sparing of the pedicles and posterior elements. Notice the cortical disruption on the right anterolateral aspect of the body.

of the normal "fatty" marrow by tissues of signal characteristics differing from marrow. Typically, a metastasis will have lower signal than marrow on a T1-weighted image and higher signal on a T2-weighted image. Such signal changes, however, are not specific for metastatic disease. One report has utilized ratios of relaxation times in an attempt to be more specific, although the reliability of that method still needs further confirmation.[11] Mass extending beyond the confines of the expected cortex indicates bone destruction (Fig 39–13).

With both CT and MRI, one appreciates a tendency for the vertebral body to be involved more extensively and earlier than the posterior elements (Fig 39–14). The classic "absent pedicle" seen on plain films and for many years taken as an early radiographic sign of metastases often represents a later phase of bone destruction when the process has extended into the pedicle from the vertebral body.

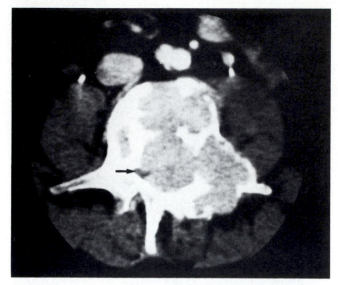

FIG 39–15.
Plasmacytoma. Following intravenous contrast administration, the expansile lesion enhances homogeneously. The tumor fills most of the spinal canal, and only a very compromised portion of the thecal sac can still be identified *(arrow)*.

Plasmacytoma and Multiple Myeloma

Neoplasia involving plasma cells results in plasmacytoma in the isolated form and multiple myeloma in the diffuse form. Many patients presenting with a solitary plasmacytoma will eventually develop multiple myeloma. A solitary plasmacytoma is characterized by diffuse expansion of a vertebral body or neural arch, and contrast enhancement may be prominent (Fig 39–15). Multiple myeloma may appear as a diffuse abnormal marrow.

INTRASPINAL TUMORS

Introduction

Intraspinal tumors traditionally have been divided into the following three categories, depending upon their location: epidural, intradural-extramedullary, and intramedullary neoplasms. This classification allows for specific differential diagnoses because certain tumors characteristically occur in each of the three locations. The "classic" myelographic appearance for each of these categories can be extended to explain the appearance on CT and MRI (Fig 39–16). For example, on myelography epidural tumors produce contralateral displacement of the entire thecal sac and intrathecal contents, with obtuse margins characterizing the filling defect. Sagittal MRI will appear similar

to a lateral myelographic film. When a complete epidural block is present on myelography, there is a horizontal limitation to the contrast column that represents the level of compression. The interface at the level of the block may have a characteristic "paint brush" appearance in the cauda equina, which is due to the presence of contrast material around nerve roots that are compressed in a diffuse manner through the relatively thick dura.

In contrast, intradural-extramedullary tumors are sharply marginated masses that by their presence separate the cord and dura on the ipsilateral side and displace the spinal cord in a contralateral direction. Thus the subarachnoid space on the same side as the mass just above and below the mass is enlarged. The subarachnoid space on the opposite side is diminished as the displaced cord is pushed against the opposite dura. Axial images will reflect these variations in the size of the subarachnoid space (Fig 39–17). The sharp margination typical of intradural-extramedullary tumors is due to the close approximation between the contrast material and the mass, the two often being separated only by a thin layer of arachnoid. The difference in appearance between epidural and intradural masses, therefore, to a large degree is a function of the relationship of mass to dura. Intramedullary neoplasms, on the other hand, are characterized by diffuse enlargement of the spinal cord that produces a "cigar" shape. In a single AP or lateral view on myelography such an appearance can be simulated by compression of the cord by an extramedullary mass. It is therefore essential on myelography to obtain at least two perpendicular views to demonstrate into which category the lesion falls. CT and MRI both can demonstrate axial anatomy and therefore are excellent methods of demonstrating into which category a lesion will fall. Furthermore, both CT and MRI can demonstrate adjacent bone involvement and paraspinal extension.

Epidural Neoplasms

Primary and Metastatic Disease

The great majority of epidural neoplasms are secondary to tumors of the vertebra that have extended into the epidural space (Fig 39–18). The primary tumors of bone have been discussed above. But even more common than primary bone tumors are metastatic tumors to the vertebrae. Vertebral metastases have also been discussed above, but their appearance will be reemphasized. The

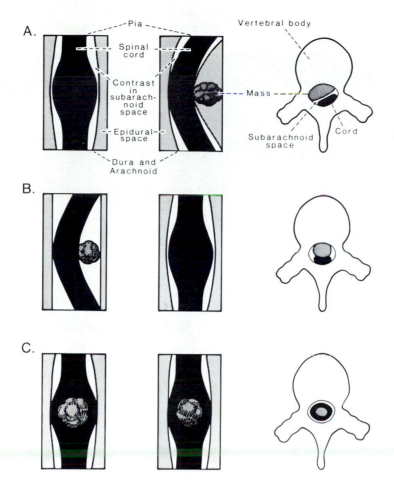

FIG 39-16.
Spinal tumors. The three common locations for spinal tumors are depicted schematically. On the left is the myelographic appearance in anteroposterior (AP) and lateral projections. On the right is the correlative axial appearance that will be seen with either MRI or CT. **A,** extradural mass. **B,** intradural-extramedullary mass. **C,** intramedullary mass.

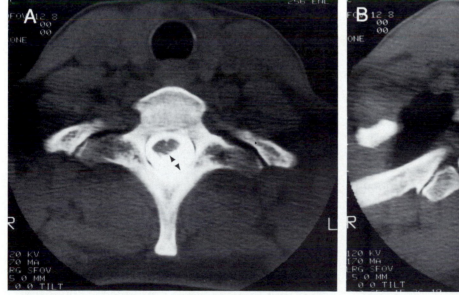
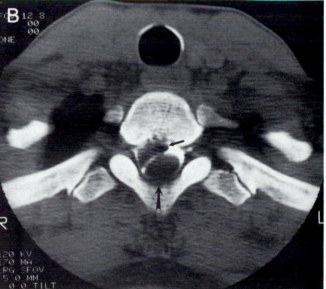

FIG 39-17.
Intradural extramedullary neurofibroma: two adjacent sections from a CT/myelogram. **A,** the section just above the mass demonstrates a widened subarachnoid space *(arrowheads)* on the side with the tumor. **B,** the section through the mass *(large arrow)* shows compression of the spinal cord *(small arrow)*. Notice the smooth margin that the tumor makes with the contrast material.

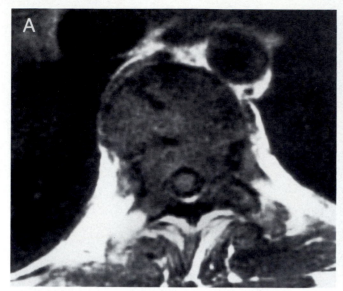
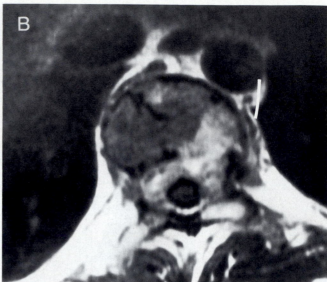
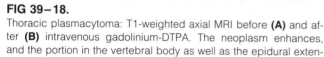

FIG 39–18.
Thoracic plasmacytoma: T1-weighted axial MRI before **(A)** and after **(B)** intravenous gadolinium-DTPA. The neoplasm enhances, and the portion in the vertebral body as well as the epidural exten- sion is delineated. (From Sze G, Krol G, Zimmerman R, et al: *Radiology* 1988; 167:217–223. Used by permission.)

bodies of the vertebrae rather than the pedicles and lamina are most frequently involved, and therefore epidural extension most frequently begins in the anterior spinal canal. This is only a trend, and epidural extension from any direction can and does occur (see Figs 39–10 and 39–13). Metastasis directly to the epidural space without vertebral involvement is usually via the epidural venous plexus from neoplasms of the pelvis (i.e., prostate and ovarian carcinoma). While this form of epidural metastasis via the venous plexus does occur, such a pattern of disease spread is less common than is extension from the vertebrae. Hence, metastatic epidural disease is usually associated with and secondary to vertebral metastases.

Both CT and MRI can readily demonstrate the bone changes from metastases to the spine. Similarly, epidural as well as paraspinal extent can be evaluated with both modalities. As stated previously, localizing a region of interest is very helpful prior to scanning. Plain films, clinical suspicions, or myelography may be utilized prior to CT. MRI generally has the advantage that an image with a large field of view in the sagittal plane is easily obtained as the initial sequence and can be used to focus the rest of the examination.

Lymphoma

Lymphoma frequently involves the vertebrae but may present in the epidural soft tissues with-

out discernible bone involvement.[12] When bone is affected, marginal erosion may be secondary to chronicity of the lymphomatous masses, or there may be frank bone destruction. In contrast to the usual appearance of metastatic disease, lymphoma often has a longer segment of involvement, often circumferential around the thecal sac (Fig 39–19). Epidural soft tissue replacing the epidural fat and compressing the thecal sac is the appearance on imaging studies. Associated areas of lymphomatous involvement such as in the retroperitoneum can usually be evaluated during imaging of the spine and may aid in making a diagnosis.

Neoplasms Involving Neural Foramina

Extradural Schwannoma and Neurofibroma.— The terms *schwannoma, neurofibroma,* and *neurilemoma* in our context are synonymous. Neurofibromas usually originate in the intradural extramedullary space along nerve roots. Extension into the extradural space as well as growth through the neural foramen into the paraspinal tissues is common and is a relatively unique pattern of growth. Occasionally, these neural tumors may be strictly extradural and/or extraspinal in location (Fig 39–20). A neurofibroma may be well circumscribed or plexiform in nature with poor margination and insinuate itself into surrounding tissues. Size can range from several millimeters to many centimeters. Multiplicity is common. Often, associ-

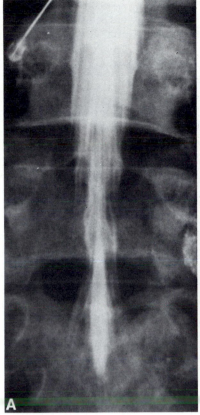
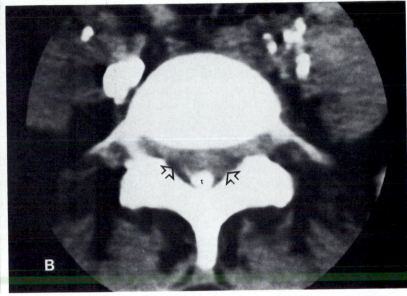

FIG 39–19.
Lymphoma. **A,** a myelogram demonstrates a long extradural defect that concentrically constricts the thecal sac at the L4 level. **B,** CT shows the lymphomatous tissue *(arrows)* in the epidural space. The normal epidural fat has been displaced.

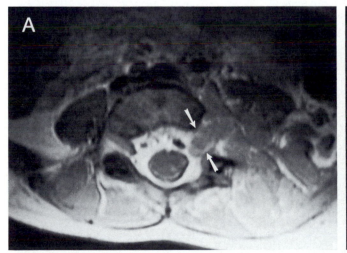
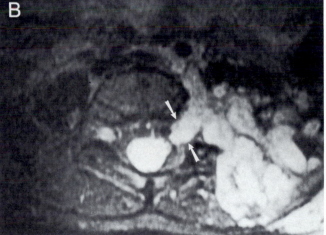

FIG 39–20.
Plexiform neurofibroma. **A,** axial MRI (T1 weighted). **B,** axial MRI (T2 weighted). Notice the multilobulated mass in the left paraspinal region that displaces the left psoas muscle anteriorly and extends through an enlarged intervertebral foramen *(arrows)* into the spinal canal. There may be a small neurofibroma in the right intervertebral foramen as well.

ated bone changes are apparent including abnormally formed vertebral bodies, a wide intervertebral foramen, and angular kyphosis (Fig 39–21). The vertebral anomalies may occur at sites remote from the neurofibroma.

A small extradural neurofibroma may be impossible to differentiate from other small neoplasms. Associated bone changes or the lack thereof may help. Difficulty in differentiating a small neurofibroma from disk material (i.e., herniation) or even from a root cyst can occur. On intravenously enhanced CT, a neurofibroma typically enhances homogeneously, unlike disk material (Fig 39–22). A root cyst can be identified as containing cerebrospinal fluid (CSF) with intrathecal contrast or with MRI.

Neuroblastoma.—Neuroblastoma and ganglioneuroma may originate not only in the adrenal medulla but also in the paraspinal sympathetic chain. These tumors frequently grow in a "dumbbell" fashion through a neural foramen to produce an intraspinal epidural mass.[13] Compression of the spinal cord may be the presenting symptom in such children.[14] A neuroblastoma actually originating within the spinal canal, however, is rare.[14] Bone metastases from neuroblastoma are common and are not restricted to the spine.

Imaging generally shows a paraspinal mass, commonly with punctate calcifications, that may extend into the epidural space. Patient age (the peak incidence is in children less than 3 years old) and associated bone destruction are helpful data to be correlated with the imaging studies in coming to a diagnosis.

Epidural Lipomatosis
Deposition of adipose tissue in the epidural space, while not truly neoplastic and usually benign, may on rare occasions become symptomatic. In patients with long-standing high corticosteroid levels of either exogenous or endogenous etiology, a manifestation of the classic centripetal fat deposition of the cushingoid patient may be abnormal

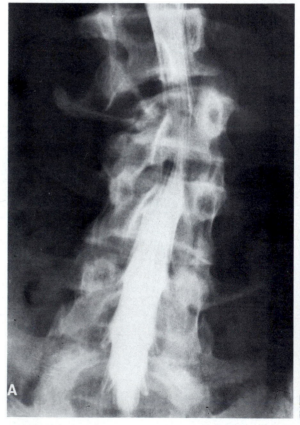

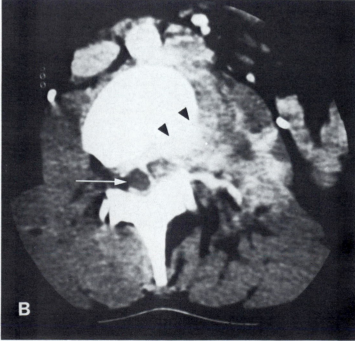

FIG 39–21.
Plexiform neurofibroma. **A,** an angular scoliosis is present, and the thecal sac is narrowed by an extradural mass at the same level. **B,** CT following intravenous contrast shows the irregularly enhancing mass that is wrapping around the thecal sac *(arrow).* The neural foramen *(arrowheads)* is widened, and the mass infiltrates the psoas muscle.

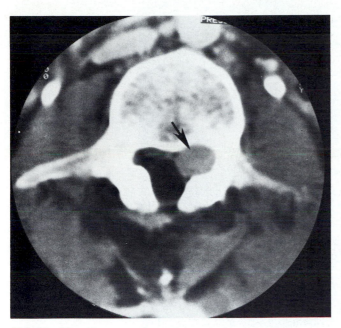

FIG 39–22.
Small neurofibroma. Intravenously enhanced CT at L2 demonstrates a well-circumscribed, homogeneously enhancing schwannoma *(arrow)* involving the left side of the spinal canal. The tumor produces local deformity of the lateral recess and slightly displaces the thecal sac, the margins of which are slightly thickened by scar tissue from previous surgery.

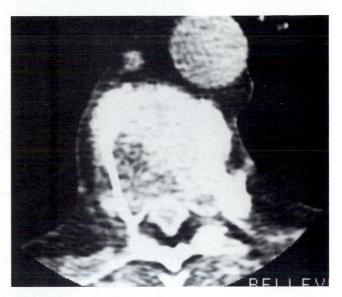

FIG 39–23.
Epidural lipomatosis. CT/myelography demonstrates abundant epidural fat in the posterior spinal canal that is flattening the posterolateral thecal sac.

epidural collections of fat sufficient to cause actual cord compression.[15–19] These same patients are also at risk of steroid-induced osteopenia with resultant vertebral compression fractures and cord compression. Either mechanism alone or in some combination may occur. CT/myelography has been useful in the evaluation of such patients by demonstrating the epidural fat, osseous integrity, and cord compression (Fig 39–23). MRI might provide an alternative means of evaluation.[20]

Intradural Extramedullary Lesions

The major differential diagnosis of intradural extramedullary masses is between neurofibroma/schwannoma and meningioma, with metastatic tumor being a distant third. Nonneoplastic cysts are rarer still.

Neurofibroma/Schwannoma

Intradural neurofibroma (or schwannoma) may exist alone or be associated with epidural and paraspinal extension via an enlarged vertebral foramen (Fig 39–24). On the side of the cord with the tumor, the subarachnoid space is widened above and below the tumor as the cord is pushed away from the dura. On the opposite side, as expected, the cord and dura are apposed, and the subarachnoid space is diminished. CT with intrathecal contrast (CT/myelography) usually demonstrates this anatomy exquisitely (see Fig 39–17). MRI is also effective in demonstrating this anatomy (Fig 39–25). Both examinations are excellent methods of evaluating paraspinal extent.

By either CT/myelography or MRI, a neurofibroma usually has sharply defined smooth borders with imaging characteristics of soft tissue in contrast to the surrounding CSF. Since multiplicity is common, one should closely observe other nerve roots for additional small neurofibromas.

Meningioma

Meningioma accounts for approximately 40% of all spinal tumors. It is far more common in women than in men and generally occurs in the thoracic spine. The appearance is frequently indistinguishable from a neurofibroma. However, meningioma tends to be located in the posterior portion of the spinal canal, while neurofibroma tends to be placed anterolaterally along exiting roots. Also, meningioma calcifies in either a psammomatous or globular pattern more commonly than neurofibroma does (Fig 39–26). Finally, while a dumbbell meningioma extending through a neural foramen does occur, such an appearance is unusual and far more characteristic of a neurofibroma.

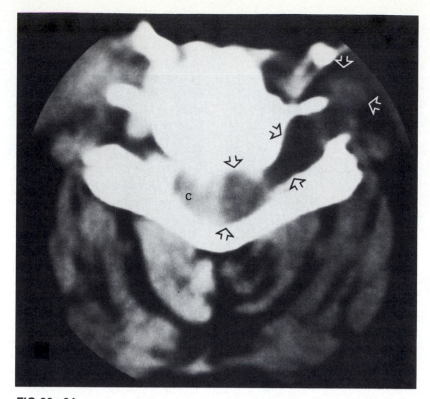

FIG 39–24.
"Dumbbell" neurofibroma. CT/myelography demonstrates the tumor *(arrows)*, which
is both intraspinal and extraspinal in location. The cord *(c)* is displaced to the opposite side.

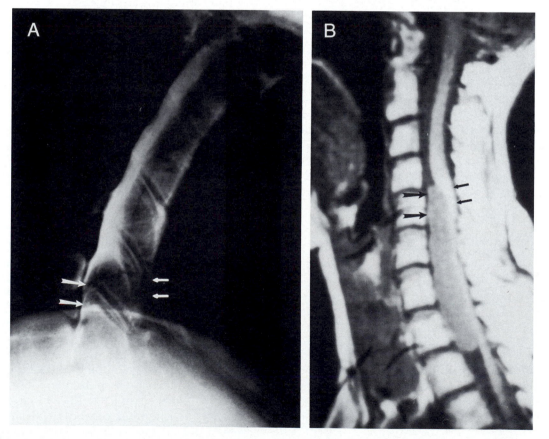

FIG 39–25.
Cervical neurofibroma. The typical appearance of an intradural extramedullary mass is apparent. **A,** a lateral view of a myelogram
shows that the cord *(small arrows)* is displaced posteriorly by the
anteriorly located mass *(large arrows)*. **B,** sagittal T1-weighted MRI
correlates well with the myelogram. Notice on both images that the
subarachnoid space is widened just above and below the mass.
The interface of the mass with the subarachnoid space is rounded
with acute angles at the margins *(small arrows = cord; large arrows = mass)*.

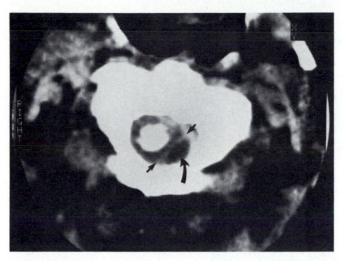

FIG 39–26.
Meningioma. CT/myelography demonstrates a large calcified meningioma that occupies most of the spinal canal. A thin rim of contrast *(small arrows)* separates the meningioma from the cord *(curved arrow).*

Lipomas

An intradural lipoma is usually an associated finding in congenital malformations and will be addressed in that section. Occasionally, it occurs as an isolated lesion that may or may not be symptomatic (Fig 39–27).

Metastases

"Drop mets" or "dropped metastases" actually represent metastatic implants in the subarachnoid space from dissemination of a primary tumor through the CSF spaces. The most common primary tumor that tends to spread in this fashion is medulloblastoma.[21] Ependymoma, pineal teratoma, and glioblastoma multiforme are also known to metastasize via CSF pathways (Fig 39–28). Such seeding may occur along the outer aspect of the spinal cord, along nerve roots, or even in the axillary pouch of a nerve root. Spread to the intradural space is unusual for hematogenous dissemination of primary tumors not of central nervous system origin, but occasionally this does occur. One report documented leukemic infiltrates (chloromas) that had formed in multiple root sheaths with an appearance indistinguishable from multiple small neurofibromas (Fig 39–29).[22]

The characteristics of "drop mets" are not usually specific but are usually interpreted in a clinical context that aids in the diagnosis. For example, children with medulloblastoma routinely require evaluation for subarachnoid metastases with either

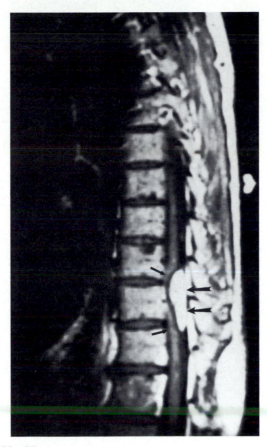

FIG 39–27.
Subdural lipoma. Sagittal T1-weighted MRI demonstrates the lipoma *(large arrows)* that is compressing the spinal cord *(small arrows).*

MRI or CT/myelography. A nodule or filling defect in such a clinical context is strong evidence for "drop mets." Perhaps the most difficult aspect of imaging in this context is to exclude early or small metastases. Of course the larger the mass, the more easily visualized by any imaging modality.

Cysts

Neurenteric Cyst.—The neurenteric cyst is a congenital anomaly in which there is a connection between the gut or lung, the spinal column, and frequently the intraspinal contents as well. The fistulous connection may be patent or atretic and is lined with respiratory or gastrointestinal epithelium. The abnormal connection passes through a vertebral body and produces an anomalous bony structure that may be as subtle as a small midline cleft in the posterior aspect of the vertebral body.[23] When the fistulous connection is patent, development of a chemical meningitis may produce symptoms. If the intraspinal component compresses the

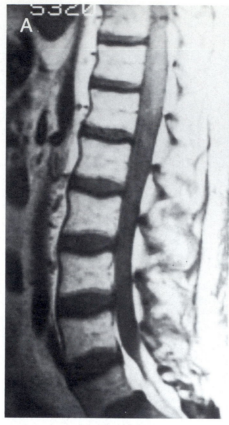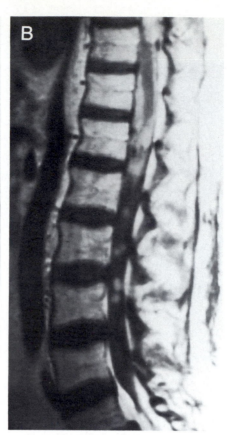

FIG 39–28.
"Drop mets": T1-weighted sagittal MRI before **(A)** and after **(B)** intravenous gadolinium-DTPA. Numerous metastatic nodules enhance within the subarachnoid space in this patient with cerebral glioblastoma. (From Sze G, Abramson A, Krol G, et al: *AJNR* 1988; 9:153–163. Used by permission.)

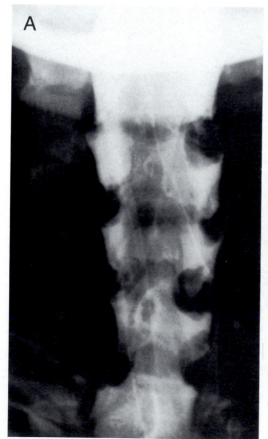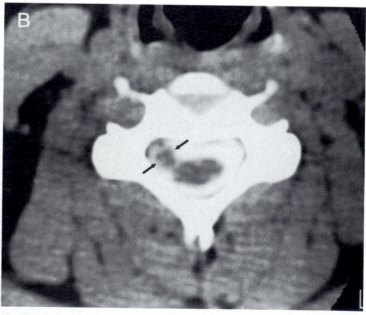

FIG 39–29.
Leukemic infiltrate (chloromas): CT/myelography. **A,** an AP film shows filling defects at the level of each exiting route. The appearance is indistinguishable from multiple small neurofibromas. **B,** CT shows the filling defect *(arrows)* in the right lateral recess.

spinal cord, clinical evidence of cord compression may be apparent.

The intraspinal cyst is usually intradural and extramedullary in position but may be firmly adherent to the pia so that it appears to be intimately related to the spinal cord (Fig 39–30). Appreciation of an associated anomalous vertebral body is helpful in arriving at the correct diagnosis.

Arachnoid Cyst.—An arachnoid cyst of the spine is similar to an intracranial arachnoid cyst in that it may be congenital in origin, may develop due to adhesions from infection or trauma, and if large enough, may produce compression of the central nervous system (spinal cord). A large cyst may smoothly erode the bone and cause bone deformity.[24] The congenital variety is most common in the lumbosacral spine. This root cyst ("Tarlov cyst") may appear on bone films or noncontrast CT as areas of bone remodeling that requires differentiation from a slow-growing tumor (Fig 39–31). Occasionally, an arachnoid cyst may herniate through

a dorsal defect into the extraspinal space or may be present in both compartments. Nevertheless, the cyst usually communicates with the subarachnoid space through a narrow neck, although that neck may be very narrow and cause a relative block to the flow of CSF in and out of the arachnoid cyst.

Because of the variability with which an arachnoid cyst communicate with the subarachnoid space, a spectrum of imaging appearances may occur. On CT myelography, for instance, early scans may demonstrate poor contrast uptake or no contrast accumulation within the cyst, although the cyst may be of CSF density. Delayed scans may demonstrate subsequent accumulation of contrast within the cyst as the normal subarachnoid space is cleared of contrast.

MRI may demonstrate a CSF collection. However, MRI may demonstrate a fluid collection that differs from the rest of the CSF in signal due to the possible difference in protein content within a poorly irrigated cyst or due to a difference in CSF flow as compared with the rest of the subarachnoid

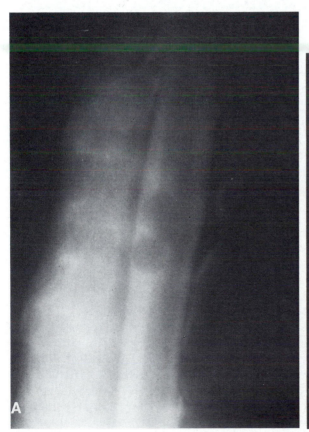
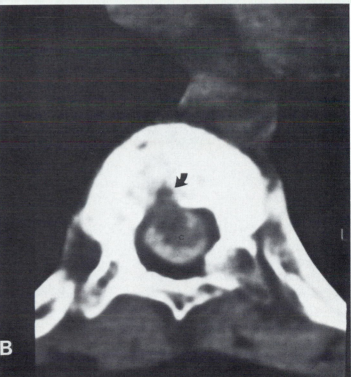

FIG 39–30.
Neurenteric cyst. **A,** film from a myelogram demonstrates a bilobed intradural extramedullary mass displacing the cord. **B,** CT following the myelogram shows the mass abutting the cord (c) and extending into a defect in the posterior vertebral body *(arrow)*, a finding characteristic of a neurenteric cyst.

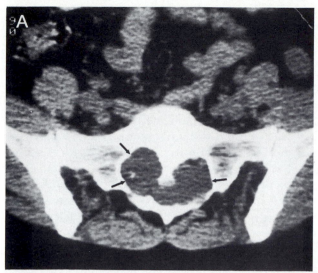

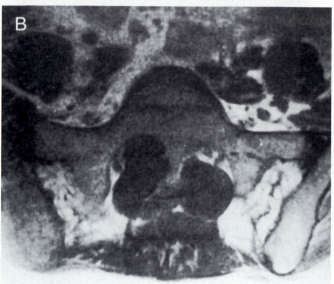

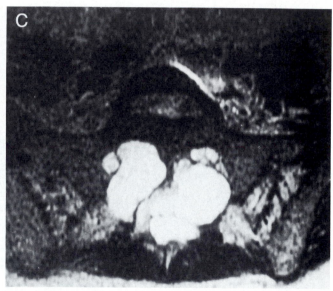

FIG 39–31.
Root cysts (Tarlov cysts). **A,** noncontrast CT shows a soft-tissue mass *(arrows)* that has smoothly eroded the sacrum. The differential diagnosis includes slow-growing neoplasms like neurofibromas. **B,** T1-weighted MRI at the same level. **C,** T2-weighted MRI at the same level. Signal characteristics are those of CSF. Multiple cysts are present, in this case ranging in size up to several centimeters in diameter.

space. Signal differences due to physiologic motion, of course, would not be as apparent on cardiac-gated MRI.

Both CT and MRI can demonstrate associated spinal cord compression (Fig 39–32). In cases of arachnoid cyst secondary to leptomeningeal irritation, a multicompartmental cyst or multiple cysts may be present, each with its own slightly different characteristics.

Arachnoid Adhesions

Arachnoid adhesions (arachnoiditis) is the development of fibrous septa within the subarachnoid space. The neural elements can be displaced, compressed, and retracted and lead to severe pain. Intrathecal contrast may not flow freely and may even be blocked. In the cauda equina the roots are typically plastered to the periphery of the sac and give an amorphous appearance to the contrast that remains centrally (Fig 39–33). Causes include previous infection, trauma, and previous surgery.

Dural Vascular Malformation

A radiculomeningeal vascular malformation is a small vascular malformation or small arteriovenous shunt in the dura that has a relatively slow flow but drain intradurally to spinal cord veins. It is usually in the lower thoracic or upper lumbar spine of middle-aged men who present with signs of myelopathy including lower extremity weakness and pain and with urinary difficulties. While this arteriovenous malformation (AVM) is not actually within the spinal cord, the venous drainage from the cord is altered, and venous hypertension may

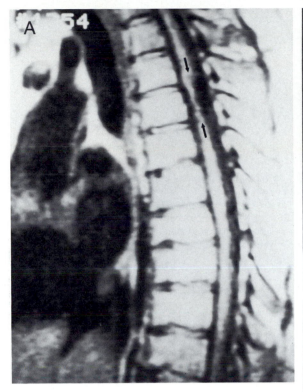

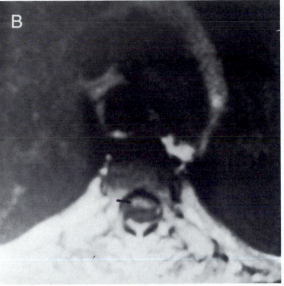

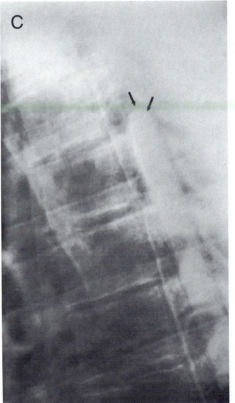

FIG 39–32.
Arachnoid cyst. **A,** sagittal T1-weighted MRI. The spinal cord is compressed *(arrows)* by a cyst that lies posterior to the cord. **B,** an axial T1-weighted image at the level of the lesion shows that the spinal cord *(arrow)* is flattened. **C,** a lateral view from a myelogram shows contrast in a blind-ending pouch *(arrows)* posterior in the canal.

cause cord ischemia with consequent symptoms. The nidus of the malformation requires angiography to be demonstrated. However, the large draining veins within the subarachnoid space can be easily identified with myelography or MRI.[25] The serpentine filling defects on myelography will demonstrate evidence of flow on MRI. Furthermore, MRI may show evidence of associated cord edema or ischemia as areas of decreased signal on T1-weighted images and increased signal on T2-weighted images.

Intramedullary Expansions

The differential diagnosis of an intramedullary expansion includes the two common gliomas, as-

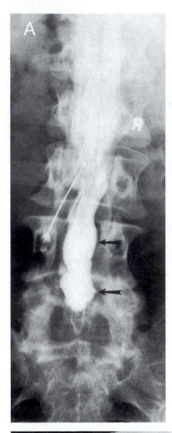

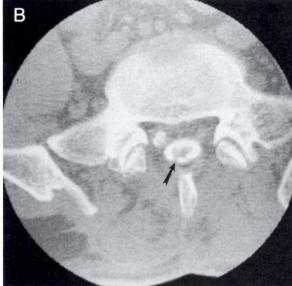

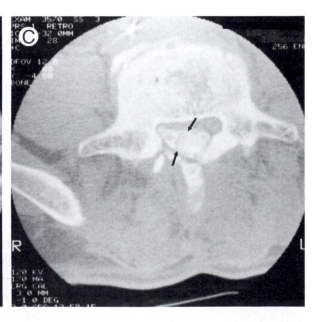

FIG 39–33.
Arachnoiditis. **A,** a myelogram demonstrates abnormal configuration of the distal thecal sac. The contrast at the L4 and L5 levels *(arrows)* is amorphous, and the contrast column ends prematurely at the top of L5. Numerous septations are also apparent. **B,** a CT section shows abnormal clumping of the roots in the center of the thecal sac with a small attachment posteriorly *(arrow).* **C,** an adjacent CT section shows curvilinear septations *(arrows)* that represent fibrous septa and/or clumped nerve roots.

trocytoma and ependymoma; hemangioblastoma; AVM; syringohydromyelia; multiple sclerosis and other forms of myelitis; and rarely metastatic neoplasm. Myelographically, these intramedullary processes cause cord expansion with narrowing of the surrounding subarachnoid space by the enlarged cord. Abnormally enlarged associated blood

vessels can be identified on myelography. Usually the length of the expansion can also be identified on a myelogram. However, the internal characteristics of the lesion are generally not elucidated with myelography. Both CT and MRI, however, frequently afford such evaluation. The advantage therefore of CT and MRI in evaluating an intramedullary expansion is the ability to see the internal characteristics of the lesion.

CT with intravenous contrast enhancement may demonstrate areas of enhancement within a lesion. CT with intrathecal water-soluble contrast (CT/myelography) may demonstrate areas within an enlargement that absorb the water-soluble contrast, a characteristic originally thought to indicate areas of cyst formation that we now know can also occur in any areas of abnormal cord, i.e., solid portions of tumors, areas of myelitis, areas of gliosis, and myelomalacia (Figs 39–34 and 39–35). MRI is probably the most helpful examination in demonstrating the internal signal characteristics and therefore the components of an intramedullary expansion.

Ultrasound has also been utilized to demonstrate solid vs. cystic components of an expansion.[26] The difficulty with ultrasound, of course, is access since the ultrasound must be performed at the time of surgery (intraoperatively) or through a prior laminectomy. When such access is available, however, good definition of cystic and solid components can be accomplished.

An intramedullary expansion can range in length from barely detectable to involvement of the entire spinal cord. The size or length of the lesion generally is not helpful in distinguishing the histology. For example, a cystic astrocytoma may involve nearly the entire spinal cord. Likewise, syringomyelia can involve the entire spinal cord. The required therapy, however, for these two abnormalities is quite different. Therefore, most of the imaging efforts will be aimed at analyzing the internal structure of the lesion.

Intramedullary Glioma

Astrocytoma is the most common intramedullary neoplasm involving the spinal cord, followed in frequency by ependymoma. Ependymoma has a predilection for the lower spinal cord, conus medullaris, and filum terminale.[27] Differentiation of tumors from each other is usually not possible with the following exception. An ependymoma that involves the filum terminale and conus tends to grow exophytically and therefore may appear to be an intradural-extramedullary mass (Fig 39–36).

If the expansion of the cord is great enough, routine myelography may demonstrate a block to the flow of contrast. Nevertheless, CT may demonstrate intrathecal contrast that has passed the myelographic block. Differences in the CSF space above and below the block are reflected by MRI where, particularly if no cardiac gating is utilized on long TR/long echo time (TE) images (T2-weighted images), the nonflowing CSF below a block can appear increased in signal as compared with the CSF above the level of a block.

An important concept regarding intramedullary neoplasms is that they may have large cystic components. Such characteristics are very important since the surgical management will be quite different, depending on the particular makeup of a tumor. For instance, a 2-cm astrocytoma at C5 may have a large associated cyst that extends inferiorly to T5. Surgical resection of this enlargement need only be directed to the solid 2-cm mass at C5. The entire cyst does not need removal, only decompression. In contrast, a large syrinx generally is not resected but merely drained at the caudal end.

Cysts associated with tumors fall into three

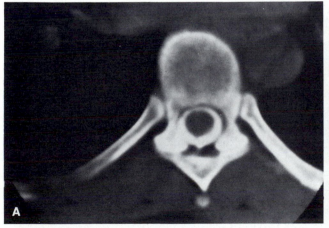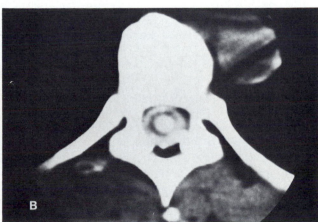

FIG 39–34.
Thoracic syringomyelia. **A,** the cord is diffusely expanded in this CT performed immediately after myelography. **B,** delayed scan shows dense accumulation of contrast within the cyst.

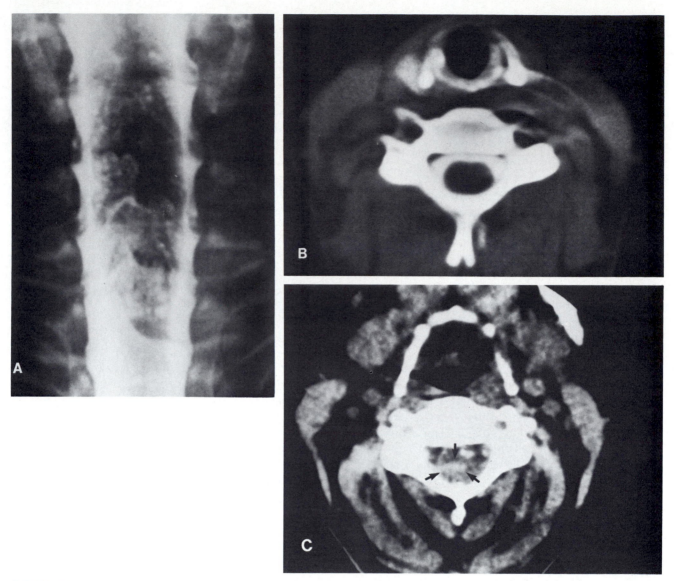

FIG 39–35.
Cervical astrocytoma. **A,** myelography shows a diffusely expanded spinal cord over several cervical segments. **B,** CT following myelography confirms cord enlargement. **C,** a scan performed 24 hours later demonstrates accumulation of contrast *(arrows)* within the tumor. Several other scattered densities in the spinal canal represent residual contrast (iophendylate) from a previous myelogram.

categories: proximal, distal, and intratumoral. The proximal cyst is cephalad to the solid portion of the neoplasm. The distal cyst is caudal to the solid component of the neoplasm. An intratumoral cyst is a cystic area within the solid portion, usually representing a necrotic area. More than one type of cyst may be present in any case.[28]

Thus, great pains must be taken to analyze the intramedullary expansion with respect to the solid vs. cystic components. CT with intrathecal water-soluble contrast has been utilized since a cystic area often imbibes the contrast on delayed images preferentially with respect to solid components. However, we have not found this to be a reliable method for demonstrating cystic areas within the cord since contrast may be imbibed into areas of cord damage such as from trauma or inflammation (Fig 39–37). Furthermore, water-soluble contrast usually permeates a normal spinal cord to some degree and increases the difficulty in interpretation of delayed scans.

In this regard, MRI appears very promising[29] but may still be misleading at times.[30] On T1-weighted images the solid tumor is usually rela-

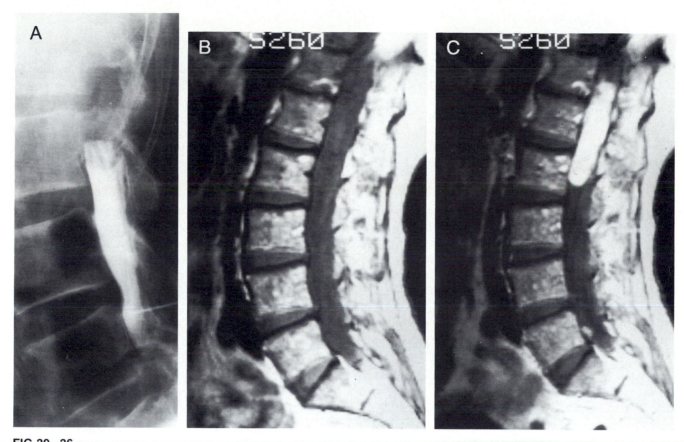

FIG 39—36.
Ependymoma of the conus medullaris and filum terminale. **A,** lumbar myelogram showing a block of contrast by the inferior margin of the tumor. The interface is indistinguishable from that formed by an intradural extramedullary mass. **B,** T1-weighted sagittal MRI appears normal. **C,** T1-weighted sagittal MRI after administration of intravenous gadolinium-DTPA demonstrates tumor. (From Sze G, Abramson A, Krol G, et al: *AJNR* 1988; 9:153—163. Used by permission.)

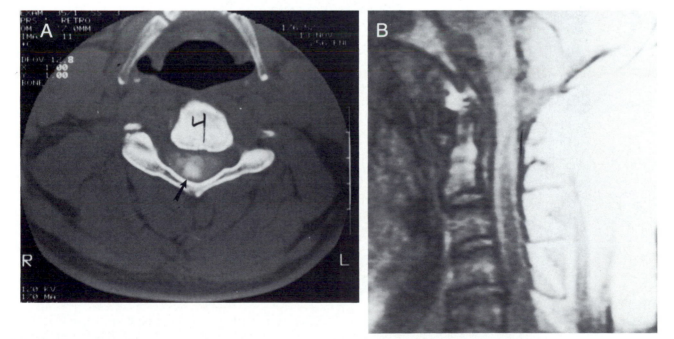

FIG 39—37.
Post-traumatic gliosis. **A,** delayed CT following myelography shows contrast accumulation *(arrow)* within the cord. **B,** sagittal T1-weighted MR shows abnormally decreased signal throughout most of the cervical cord in this patient who sustained a C5 fracture with spinal cord injury several months earlier. At surgery no cord cysts could be found. The cord was diffusely gliotic.

tively isosignal but may be slightly increased or decreased in signal when compared with normal cord. The morphology of the expansion is usually well seen on the T1-weighted images. Gadolinium-enhanced images might also help identify the solid portion (Fig 39–38). On T2-weighted images the tumor is usually hyperintense to normal cord. If present, the associated cysts usually are considerably decreased in signal on T1-weighted images and increased in signal on T2-weighted images. In fact, the signal from the solid and cystic components may be very similar on the T2-weighted images and require evaluation of the T1-weighted images to see the difference (Fig 39–39). Also, due to the protein content of a tumor-associated cyst, which is usually between 2 and 4 gm/100 cc,[31] the signal from a tumor cyst will be slightly greater than CSF on the T1-weighted images.[28] This feature usually allows differentiation of a tumor-associated cyst from syringohydromyelia, which typically contains "pure CSF." At times, despite complete evaluations, the distinction between the tumor cyst (with a high protein content) and the solid component of the tumor will simply not be clear (Fig 39–40). Furthermore, syringohydromyelia that for some reason (previous surgery, hemorrhage) has an elevated protein concentration will not be distinguishable from a tumor-associated cyst. In practice, the neuroradiologist will be asked to demonstrate the site of greatest expansion and then to provide the extent of solid vs. cystic components. Surgical exploration will begin at the site of maximal enlargement and the presumed solid portion. The solid component will either undergo

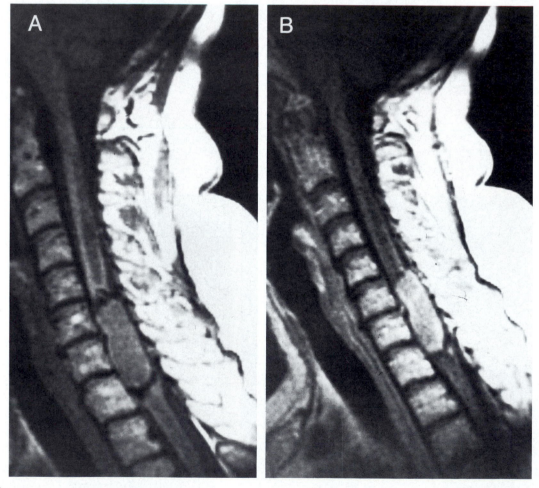

FIG 39–38.
Cervical astrocytoma: sagittal T1-weighted MRI before **(A)** and after **(B)** the intravenous administration of Gd-DTPA. The solid tumor enhances. Proximal and distal cysts in the cord are present. The cysts are slightly higher in signal than CSF is but do not enhance. They were reactive in nature rather than neoplastic at surgery. (From Sze G: *Radiol Clin North Am* 1988; 26:1009–1024. Used by permission.)

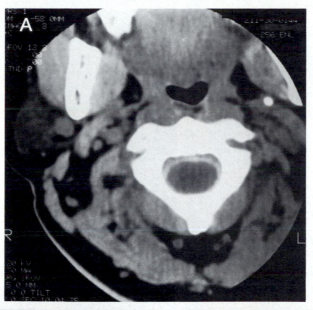

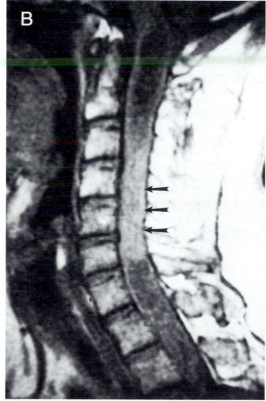

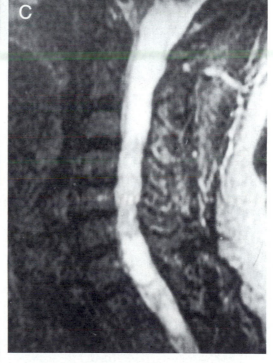

FIG 39–39.
Cervical ependymoma. **A,** postmyelogram CT shows a diffusely expanded spinal cord. **B,** sagittal T1-weighted MRI demonstrates the solid portion of the tumor *(arrows)* extending from C4 to C6 with both proximal and distal intramedullary cysts. **C,** T2-weighted sagittal MRI. Notice that the cysts are higher in signal than the solid portion of the tumor is.

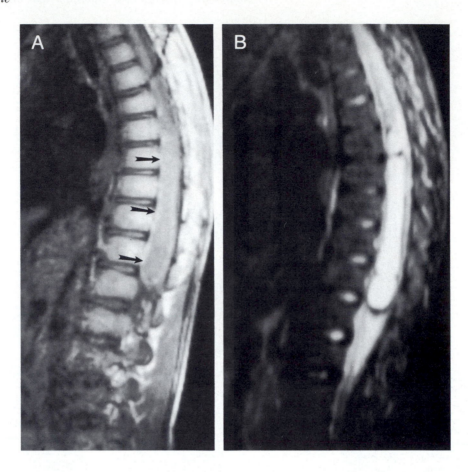

FIG 39–40.
Thoracic astrocytoma. **A,** a sagittal T1-weighted image shows a diffusely expanded distal cord *(arrows)* that is abnormally decreased in signal on this sequence. **B,** a T2-weighted image shows abnormally increased signal in the cord. At surgery, no cysts were demonstrated. The expansion was from solid tumor and involved the entire lower thoracic cord.

biopsy or be excised. Exploration cephalad and caudad will proceed, often aided by intraoperative ultrasound, until the solid component is removed and only the cystic component remains. Postoperatively, the morphology and signal characteristics of the spinal cord can be distorted, and a recurrent tumor can be difficult to detect. Serial scans may be useful in this regard.

Hemangioblastoma

Hemangioblastoma of the spinal cord may occur as an isolated lesion. However, often they are multiple, and approximately one third are associated with the von Hippel–Lindau syndrome. The von Hippel–Lindau syndrome consists of spinal and cerebellar hemangioblastomas, retinal angiomas, pancreatic and renal cysts, and occasionally hypernephromas. A hemangioblastoma is characterized by a very vascular nodule frequently with a large accompanying cyst.

Myelography may demonstrate a diffuse intramedullary expansion representing the combination of solid tumor and cyst. A preoperative diagnosis of hemangioblastoma in such a case may not be possible. Enlargement of spinal cord vasculature, however, may suggest the appropriate diagnosis. In such a case, CT scanning following a bolus of intravenous contrast material may show the nodular portion of the expansion (Fig 39–41). Spinal cord angiography is definitive. A patient with a spinal cord hemangioblastoma in general should have appropriate imaging studies of the entire CNS as well as of the kidneys.

MRI may be very useful to demonstrate the cystic component of a hemangioblastoma and may also identify the abnormal vessels in the spinal canal. Due to the vascularity of the nodular component, a gadolinium-enhanced scan appears to be the most sensitive means by which one is able to identify this tumor.

Arteriovenous Malformation

AVM of the spinal cord may diffusely expand the cord. Abnormally large numbers and sizes of

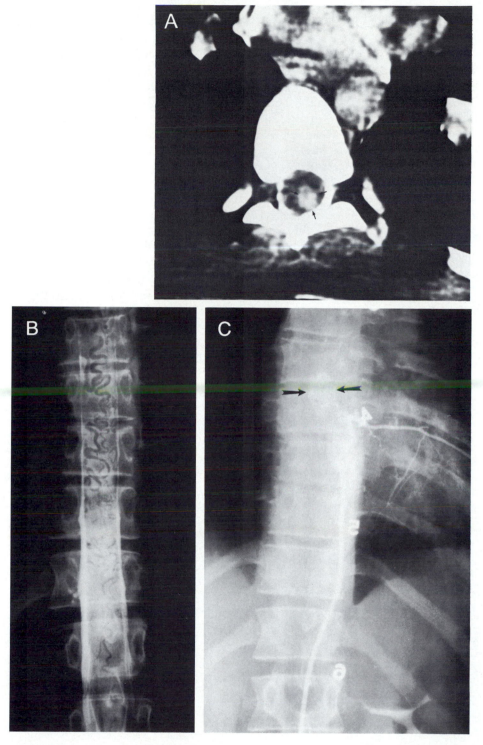

FIG 39–41.

Hemangioblastoma. **A,** thoracic CT following intravenous contrast demonstrates a dense enhancing nodule *(arrows).* The remainder of the expanded cord (surrounded by intrathecal contrast) is lucent and represents cyst. **B,** the myelogram demonstrates a dif- fusely expanded cord with numerous serpentine filling defects indicative of the large vessels associated with this tumor. **C,** a spinal angiogram demonstrates the tumor nodule *(arrows).*

vessels are the hallmark, and may be demonstrated as serpentine filling defects in the CSF by myelography. MRI has the ability to obtain images that may show the course of the abnormal vessels with their expected signal void (Fig 39–42). Angiography is definitive.

Large spinal vessels are not pathognomonic of a cord AVM. Occasionally, an AVM of the spinal dura occur with large draining veins in the subarachnoid space (see above, "Dural Vascular Malformation"). Enlarged and numerous vessels may also be seen with hemangioblastoma and in cases where a highly compressive lesion of any etiology has caused compromise of the normal spinal drainage with secondary vascular distension. In cases of high-grade degenerative spinal stenosis the nerve roots in the cauda equina may become redundant and give a serpentine appearance that mimics the appearance of an abnormal tangle of vessels.

Syringohydromyelia

Syringomyelia refers to cystic degeneration within the spinal cord. Hydromyelia refers to cystic dilatation of the central canal of the spinal cord.

Controversy exists regarding the origins of these two lesions. In practice, however, differentiation is usually impossible and frequently unnecessary. Important is the general association of Chiari malformations with hydromyelia and the association of cord tumors with cysts of the cord. Thus, a cystic expansion of the cord should alert one to the possibility of a Chiari malformation with its frequently associated hydrocephalus or to the possibility of an associated intramedullary neoplasm.

By CT, syringohydromyelia appears as an area of low attenuation that may absorb intrathecal contrast on delayed CT scans. Delayed scanning is usually performed between 6 and 24 hours. Since the absorption of contrast is not consistent, several scans might be required over that time interval to identify imbibition of contrast into cystic areas (Fig 39–43).

MRI can usually demonstrate a cystic cavity in the spinal cord on a single examination (Fig 39–44). The cord is usually but not always expanded. The cavity often extends over many segments and may appear septated or "beaded."[32] The signal from the cavity should be that of CSF with

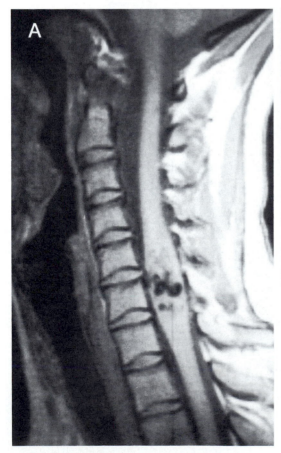

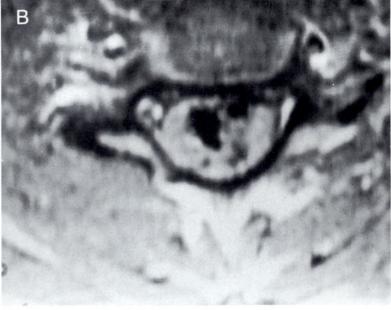

FIG 39–42.
Cervical AVM. **A,** a sagittal T1-weighted image demonstrates fusiform expansion of the lower cervical cord in which are numerous areas of signal void indicative of fast flow in the abnormal vessels. **B,** an axial image at the level of the malformation demonstrates the diffusely expanded cord that almost entirely fills the spinal canal. Again demonstrated are areas of signal void within the abnormal vessels.

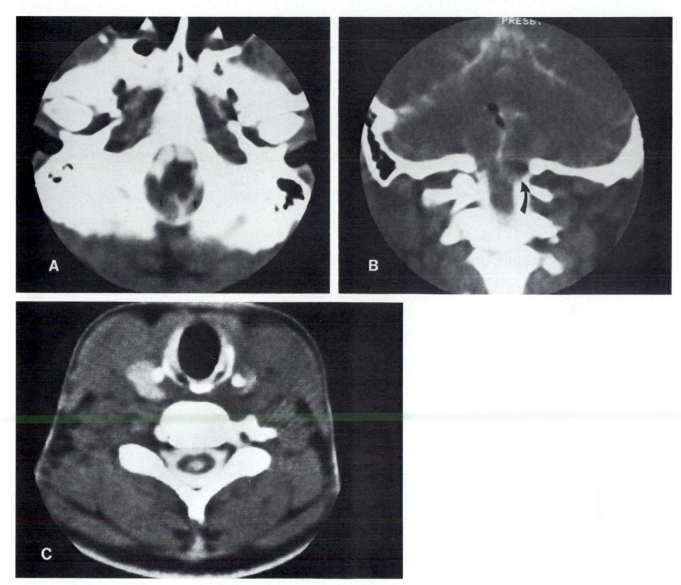

FIG 39–43.
Hydromyelia and Chiari malformation. **A,** axial CT following a myelogram at the foramen magnum shows caudally placed tonsils *(t)*. **B,** a coronal section delineates the caudal bulge of the tonsil *(ar-* *row)* below the foramen magnum. **C,** A well-defined central collection of contrast accumulates within the cervical cavity on a delayed scan.

low signal on T1-weighted images and high signal on T2-weighted images. A "flow void" or loss of expected signal intensity may occur if free communication of the cavity exists with the subarachnoid space. Yet this is not specific for syringohydromyelia since it has also been seen in tumor-associated cysts.[32] Cardiac-gated images might minimize this type of signal loss. At the interface with cord parenchyma gliotic changes may occur and may be evident on MRI as isosignal or areas of only slightly decreased signal on T1-weighted images and as areas of increased signal on T2-weighted images.

Usually the difficulty is in differentiating a true syrinx or hydromyelia from a cyst associated with a tumor. Generally tumor-associated cysts have a protein content higher than the CSF of a true syrinx, and therefore the signal from tumor-associated cysts on some sequences will vary from CSF.[28, 31] Thus, if a cystic dilatation consistently has the signal characteristics of nonflowing CSF on multiple MRI sequences and therefore cannot be differentiated from CSF, the diagnosis of syringohydromyelia is more likely than the diagnosis of a cyst associated with a tumor. Also, with either CT or MRI, if an associated malformation such as a Chiari mal-

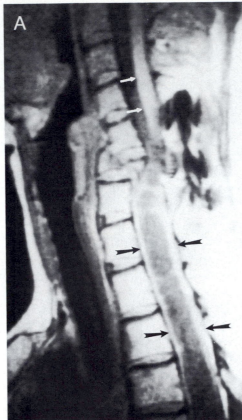

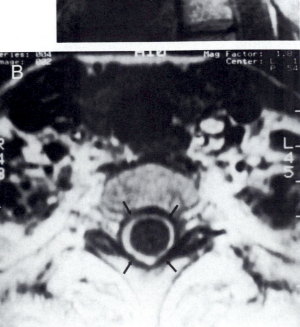

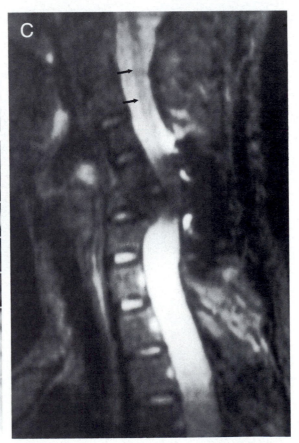

FIG 39–44.
Post-traumatic syrinx. **A,** a sagittal T1-weighted image shows the fracture/dislocation at C5–6. Areas of signal void in the posterior soft tissues are related to wires placed during surgery. Above the level of trauma, the cord *(small arrows)* has a normal configuration and signal. Below the level of trauma, the cord is markedly expanded *(large arrows)* and is abnormally decreased in signal. Several septations are also apparent. **B,** axial T1-weighted MRI through the lower cervical spine shows the centrally located cyst within the cord and the expanded cord *(arrows)*. **C,** T2-weighted sagittal MRI demonstrates that the cystic portion increases dramatically in signal while the relatively normal cord above the level of the injury *(arrows)* remains less in signal than the surrounding CSF. Also notice that the metallic artifact degrades the images more on this long TR image than on the short TR images (as expected).

formation is demonstrated, this would favor the diagnosis of syringohydromyelia rather than a tumor-associated cyst.

Occasionally, myelomalacia following trauma can be difficult to distinguish from a small nontrau-

matic cyst by any method (see Fig 39–37). CT/myelography may demonstrate a slight enlargement of the cord that may imbibe contrast on delayed scans. MRI may demonstrate abnormal signal within the cord. However, if multiple MRI sequences are performed, the signal will not be consistent with CSF unless actual large areas of cavitation have developed.

Multiple Sclerosis

An intramedullary expansion indistinguishable from a neoplasm can occur during the acute phase of multiple sclerosis when it involves the spinal cord. Imaging of the brain may be helpful when the diagnosis of demyelinating disease is suspected since usually cerebral plaques are also present (Fig 39–45).

Metastases

Hematogenous metastases to the spinal cord parenchyma are quite rare. Breast carcinoma and lung carcinoma occasionally metastasize to the spinal cord by the hematogenous route. However,

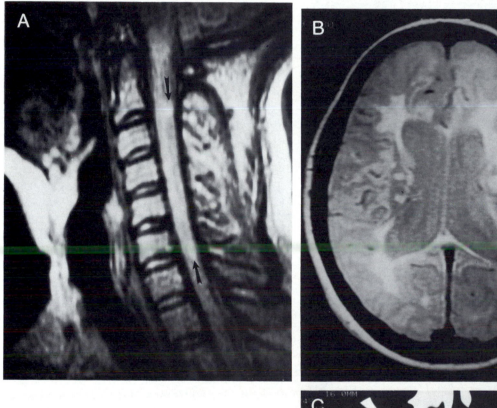

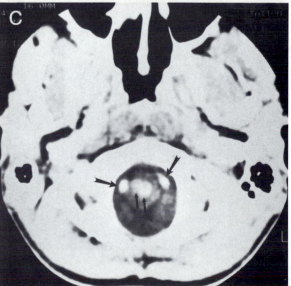

FIG 39–45.
Multiple sclerosis. **A,** a sagittal T1-weighted image shows several areas in the cervical cord that are abnormally increased in signal *(arrows)*. **B,** a head scan (long TR, short TE image) shows the diffusely abnormal periventricular signal in this patient with multiple sclerosis. Isolated abnormalities in the cord can occur in this disease but are more commonly associated with intracranial disease. **C,** intravenous enhanced CT at the cervicomedullary junction in a different patient demonstrates an enhancing plaque *(small arrows)* within the parenchyma. Notice the adjacent vertebral arteries *(large arrows)*.

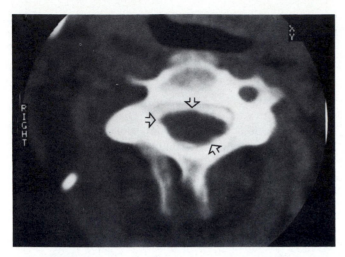

FIG 39–46.
Metastatic medulloblastoma. CT/myelography of the cervical cord shows an intramedullary expansion as well as nodular excrescences along the cord surface (arrows). The expanded cord is from direct extension from the posterior fossa tumor. The surface nodularity may actually represent associated subarachnoid metastasis.

most intramedullary metastases are direct extensions of posterior fossa neoplasms, like a medulloblastoma (Fig 39–46).[33]

Hematomyelia

Cord expansion may be secondary to intraparenchymal hemorrhage following trauma. We

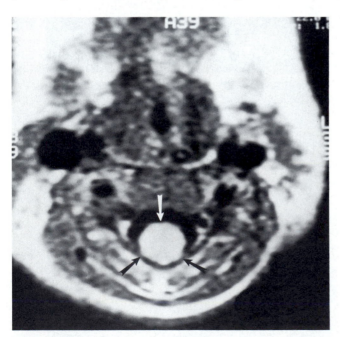

FIG 39–47.
Hematomyelia. Axial T1-weighted MRI through the cervical cord defines a swollen cord of high signal (arrows) following trauma.

have not observed a "surgically drainable" clot under these circumstances but rather a diffusely swollen, hemorrhagic cord. The signal on MRI will vary with the age of the hemorrhage (Fig 39–47).

SPINAL INFECTION

Spinal infection, whether it relates to the bone of the vertebral column or its enclosed soft tissues, is usually diagnosed by clinical findings—backache, muscle spasm, fever, elevated sedimentation rate, elevated white blood count. Imaging techniques are important in localizing and demonstrating the extent of the infection. Vertebral involvement, epidural involvement, and paraspinal extension are demonstrated with either CT or MRI and are characterized by bone destruction, obliteration of the normal epidural and paraspinal fat and tissue planes, narrowing of the disk space, and an inflammatory mass or actual abscess. As emphasized previously, CT is not a screening tool and is best utilized in conjunction with conventional radiographs, radionuclide scans, or a myelogram. MRI has the advantage of easily obtaining sagittal images of long sections of the spine. Axial images with either CT or MRI frequently are the most helpful in evaluating the extent of disease, particularly with respect to the spinal cord.

Disk-Related Infection

So-called disk space infection represent the most common type of spinal infection. There are three basic syndromes of disk space infection, only two of which actually originate from the disk. A complicating factor in considering these syndromes is the fact that infectious agents have not been isolated in all instances. Even with newer methodology for isolating anaerobic bacteria and fungi, a specific etiologic agent is not always found.

The first syndrome is that of vertebral osteomyelitis (also called infectious spondylitis). Primarily a disease of adults, it may be pyogenic or nonpyogenic, acute or chronic.[34-36] Osteomyelitis is believed to be a result of hematogenous seeding of infection into the subchondral region of the vertebral body. Although spread through Batson's plexus of paravertebral veins provides a means of explaining the association of infectious spondylitis with pelvic infection and instrumentation,[37] arterial seeding is more plausible as a mode of spread in the spondylitis associated with distant infections of the skin, indwelling catheters, periodontal disease, and pulmonary disease.[38-41] Bacteria lodge and grow in the low-flow subchondral vascular arcades and cause destruction of the vertebral body, especially along the end plate. The disk is only secondarily involved, while the subjacent vertebral body is infected by contiguous infection or through small collateral channels.[34] Narrowing of the disk space with destructive changes of both adjacent end plates is strong evidence for disk space infection. In contrast, neoplastic disease tends to be on one side or the other of a disk space and tends not to involve the disk space. *Staphylococcus aureus* is the most common infecting organism; however, a wide variety of anaerobic and aerobic organisms have been isolated.

The second syndrome is postoperative disk space infection, which includes any exposure of the disk to the outside environment, including lumbar puncture, myelography, discography, chemonucleolysis, lumbar sympathectomy, epidural anesthesia, or laminectomy.[42-46] The infective agent is introduced directly into the disk and spreads through the avascular disk and subsequently into the contiguous subchondral bone. Clinically there is usually a lag of several weeks between the time of surgery and the development of symptoms or radiographic findings. Again, *Staphylococcus* species are the most common offending agents.[46]

The third syndrome is childhood discitis. This is an inflammatory but not necessarily infectious condition of the spine that causes a wide spectrum of symptoms, including leg or back pain, tenderness, or toxemia. Although the symptoms and radiographic changes suggest a pyogenic etiology, only 30% to 40% of patients are found to have positive cultures, and antibiotics do not necessarily alter the course of the disease; there is a wide spectrum of virulence.[47-51] The presumed cause is hematogenous spread of bacteria or virus to the disk. (The disk is vascularized for the first three decades, after which vascularity regresses.[52]) Secondary involvement of the adjacent vertebral end plates (osteomyelitis) leads to bony weakening and herniation of the disk into the vertebral body.

The conventional radiographic hallmark of these syndromes is irregularity of the vertebral end plates with narrowing of the intervening disk space. However, there can be considerable lag between the onset of symptoms and the plain-film radiographic demonstration of disease. Therefore,

the normal plain film may not exclude osteomyelitis.[34, 36, 40] Radionuclide bone scans are very sensitive to early osteomyelitis. High-resolution CT, being more sensitive than plain films to bony destruction, helps improve early detection (Fig 39–48).[51, 53, 54] MRI is also much more sensitive to early disease than plain films are.

Early changes within the bone as depicted by CT may show small areas of rarefaction in the subchondral bone. The cortex may demonstrate small areas of irregularity or small areas of absence, which eventually may coalesce into large areas of destruction.[51, 55] Reformatted images may help to see the end plate changes. Epidural and paraspinal extension is well demonstrated with CT (Figs 39–49 and 39–50). Intravenous contrast may enhance the dura to better define the limits of the dura vs. the infection in the epidural space. In addition, the inflammatory tissues may enhance. Involvement of two adjacent end plates across a disk space is strong evidence for infection vs. tumor since tumor tends to involve only one side of the disk space.[55]

By MRI, the signal within the marrow of the involved vertebrae becomes abnormal in a pattern suggesting that the marrow fat is replaced by tissues having a more "watery" content. That is, the signal will be decreased on the short TR, short TE (T1-weighted) images and increased on the long TR, long TE (T2-weighted) images in contrast to

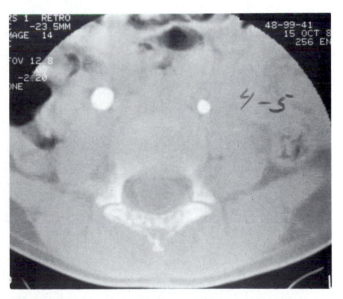

FIG 39–48.
Fungal osteomyelitis. Axial CT at the lumbar (L4–5) level shows partially destroyed posterior elements with a permeative pattern secondary to *Aspergillus* infection in this child.

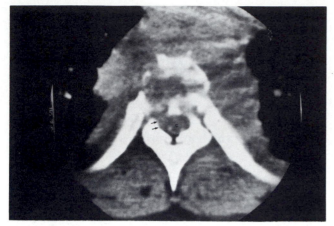

FIG 39–49.
Vertebral osteomyelitis. CT demonstrates that much of the vertebral body is destroyed. Large paravertebral abscesses are present bilaterally. Epidural extension *(arrows)* is apparent and displaces the slightly opacified thecal sac and spinal cord *(c)*.

the usual marrow signal. Sagittal images easily demonstrate the narrowed disk space. The disk will have signal characteristics that follow those of the involved adjacent bone.[56, 57] Such a signal pattern in a disk is different than the signal pattern from a disk that is decreased in height due to de-

generation. While both infection and degeneration can cause decreased disk height, infection tends to have high signal on T2-weighted images, and degeneration usually has low signal on T2-weighted images. The axial images, as with CT, are helpful at delineating epidural and paraspinal extension (Fig 39–51).

Advanced osteomyelitis may result in a weakened vertebral body that may fragment and collapse.[55, 58] The cortical margins of the body tend to fracture outward, which gives an expanded appearance to the vertebra. The infected disk may blend on both CT and MRI with the tissues of the eroded end plates, especially when disk space narrowing is severe. The inflammatory mass and/or bone fragments may displace and compress the thecal sac. The confines of the thecal sac, therefore, are important to define by whatever method is chosen.

In the chronic or healing phase of infectious spondylitis, new bone formation occurs at the margins of the vertebral bodies and may cause fusion between vertebral bodies.

The changes secondary to postoperative infectious discitis may be difficult to distinguish from benign changes that may occur as a normal response to disk surgery. Occasionally, the noninfec-

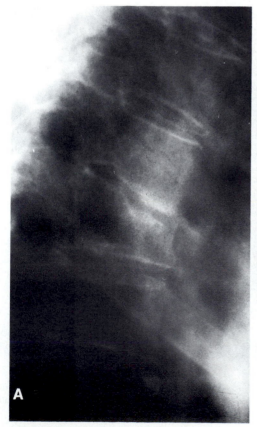

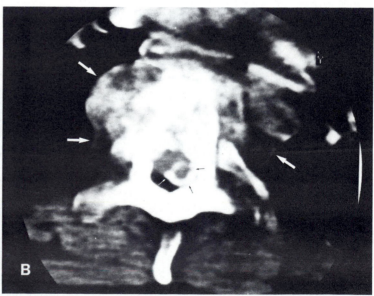

FIG 39–50.
Tuberculous spondylitis. **A,** a lateral plane film demonstrates destruction of the anterosuperior margin of a midthoracic vertebral body. **B,** CT/myelography demonstrates the accompanying paraspinal abscess *(large arrows)* and the epidural extension displacing the opacified thecal sac *(small arrows)*.

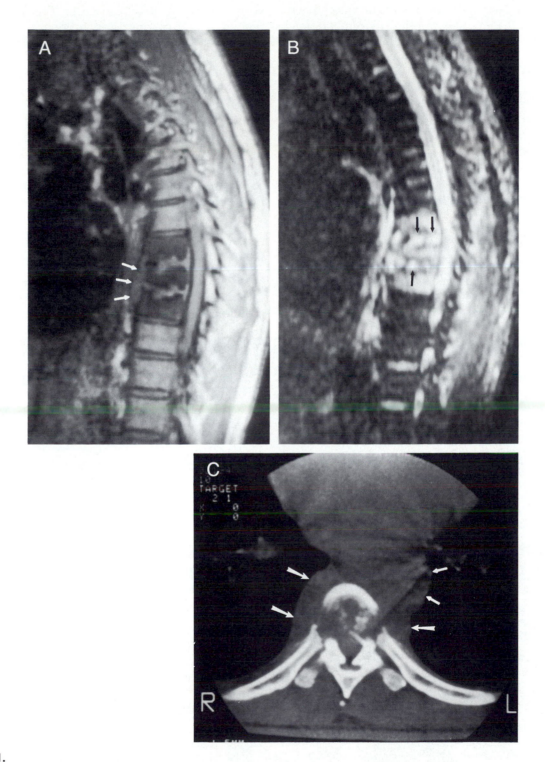

FIG 39–51.
Vertebral osteomyelitis/discitis. **A,** Sagittal T1-weighted MRI shows two abnormal disk spaces between three abnormal vertebral bodies. Notice the anterior paravertebral extension *(arrows).* **B,** T2-weighted MRI shows the increased signal in the disk spaces *(ar-* *rows)* as well as in the infected vertebral bodies. **C,** axial CT shows bone destruction and paraspinal extension *(large arrows)* that includes the aorta *(small arrows).*

tious postoperative changes result in disk space collapse and adjacent subchondral margin rarefaction, presumably as a result of ischemia analogous to osteitis pubis.[59] However, involvement is limited to those areas and does not extend significantly into the epidural or paravertebral regions as it does in infection. Extensive involvement should alert one to the possibility of active infection.

Imaging studies cannot reliably predict the specific agent causing the spondylitis or discitis. However, certain characteristics suggest nonpyogenic agents like tuberculosis or fungi. Tuberculous spondylitis tends to involve the anterior third of the vertebral body, is slowly progressive, and relatively preserves the disk space.[60–63] Involvement of the posterior elements is more characteristic of tuberculous than pyogenic osteomyelitis. Defects of the anterior aspects of several vertebral bodies (subligamentous spread), especially when associated with a paravertebral (psoas) abscess, is very suggestive of tuberculosis (Fig 39–52).[61] Although both pyogenic and tuberculous infections may have paraspinal abscesses, tuberculous abscesses have a greater tendency for calcification, thick enhancing rims, and extensive spread.[60]

Fungal infection can be indistinguishable from pyogenic or tuberculous infection. When multiple well-defined vertebral body and posterior element lytic lesions are seen without disk space involvement, a diagnosis of coccidioidal or cryptococcal spondylitis may be suggested.[63, 64]

Definitive diagnosis of the organism usually requires biopsy. Biopsies may be guided by either CT or MRI (Fig 39–53).

Other Spinal Infections

Extraosseous epidural abscess may arise from direct hematogenous seeding or from extension of a paravertebral (psoas) abscess through the neural

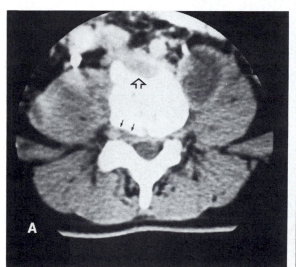
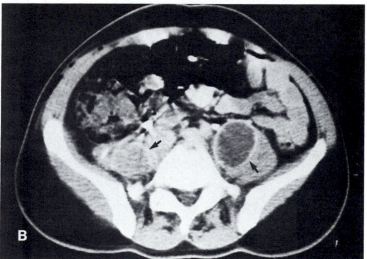
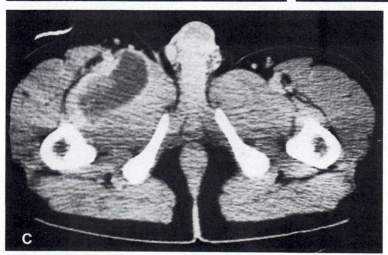

FIG 39–52.
Tuberculous spondylitis. **A,** CT shows a focal area of destruction of the anterior vertebral body *(large arrow)* and epidural abscess in the right neural foramen *(small arrows).* Bilateral psoas abscesses are also present. **B,** at a lower level the bilateral psoas abscesses *(arrows)* can still be seen. **C,** the right psoas abscess has tracked into the leg.

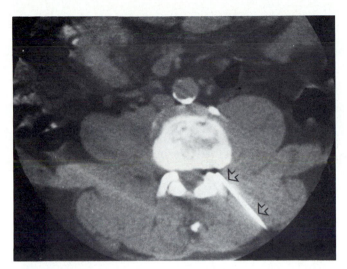

FIG 39–53.
CT-guided biopsy. The biopsy needle *(arrows)* has been directed through the paravertebral muscles to obtain a specimen near the posterior aspect of the disk.

foramen.[52] The imaging appearance is similar to an epidural abscess associated with disk-related infection, except neither the disk nor the adjacent vertebrae are involved. Differentiation from epidural metastases may be difficult. Both CT and MRI can demonstrate the compression of the thecal sac. Most extraosseous extradural abscesses are pyogenic, but a few cases of tuberculous abscess have been reported.[65]

Empyema of the subdural space is rarely encountered. It is not associated with osteomyelitis but results from metastatic seeding (usually *S aureus*) from distant infected sources.[66] Myelographically it presents as single or multiple defects simulating epidural masses or arachnoid adhesions.

An intramedullary abscess similarly is rare. Myelographically, it is indistinguishable from other intramedullary lesions and cause fairly focal cord widening. The thoracic cord is most commonly affected.[67] The CT and MRI features have not been described, but one might expect enhancement with intravenous contrast in the area of low density on CT and abnormal signal on MRI (low signal on T1- and high signal on T2-weighted images). Myelitis of uncertain etiology but presumably viral without clear abscess formation also occurs. Focal cord widening can be demonstrated with either CT or MRI, and abnormal signal on MRI may simulate the pattern seen in multiple sclerosis or a neoplasm.

Finally, neurosarcoid has been reported to occur within the spinal cord.[68] A fusiform swelling of the cord with increased signal on T2-weighted images describes the MRI characteristics. While nonspecific, they do allow differentiation from syringo-hydromyelia, AVM, and lipoma.

Acknowledgment

Many thanks go to Ms. Kelly Morris and to Mrs. Betsy Cervone for their preparation of this manuscript.

REFERENCES

1. Aubin ML, Vignaud J, Jardin C, et al: Computed tomography in 75 clinical cases of syringomyelia. *AJNR* 1981; 2:199–204.
2. Pinto RS, Kricheff II, Epstein F, et al: A practical approach to the neuroradiologic investigation of spinal cord cysts. Presented at the 21st Annual Meeting of the American Society of Neuroradiology, San Francisco, June 5–9, 1983.
3. Ross JS, Masaryk TJ, Modic MT, et al: Vertebral hemangiomas: MR imaging. *Radiology* 1987; 165:165–169.
4. Schmorl G, Junghanns H, Beseman EF (trans-ed): *The Human Spine in Health and Disease*, ed 2. New York, Grune & Stratton, 1971.
5. Freiberger RH: Osteoid osteoma of the spine: A cause of backache and scoliosis in children and young adults. *Radiology* 1960; 75:232–235.
6. Levy WM, Miller AS, Bonakarpour A, et al: Aneurysmal bone cyst secondary to other osseous lesions: A report of 57 cases. *Am J Clin Pathol* 1975; 63:1–8.
7. Mintz MC, Dalinka MK, Schmidt R: Aneurysmal bone cyst arising in fibrous dysphasia during pregnancy. *Radiology* 1987; 165:549–550.
8. Dahlin DC: *Bone Tumors: General Aspects and Data on 6,221 Cases*, ed 3. Springfield, Ill, Charles C Thomas, Publishers, 1978.
9. Firooznia H, Pinto RS, Lin JP, et al: Chordoma: Radiologic evaluation of 20 cases. *AJR* 1976; 127:805–979.
10. Smoker WRK, Godersky JC, Knutzon RK, et al: The role of MR imaging in evaluating metastatic spinal disease. *AJNR* 1987; 8:901–908.
11. Sugimura K, Yamasaki K, Kitagaki H, et al: Bone marrow diseases of the spine: Differentiation with T1 and T2 relaxation times in MR imaging. *Radiology* 1987; 165:541–544.
12. Epstein BS: *The Spine*, ed 4. Philadelphia, Lea & Febiger, 1976.
13. Fagan CJ, Swischuk LE: Dumbbell neuroblastoma or ganglioneuroma of the spinal canal. *AJR* 1974; 120:453–460.

14. Latchaw RE, L'Heureux PR, Young G, et al: Neuroblastoma presenting a central nervous system disease. *AJNR* 1982; 3:623–630.

15. Lee M, Lekias J, Gubboy SS, et al: Spinal cord compression by extradural fat after renal transplantation. *Med J Aust* 1975; 1:201–203.

16. Butcher DL, Sahn SA: Epidural lipomatosis: A complication of corticosteroid therapy. *Ann Intern Med* 1979; 90:60.

17. Lipson SJ, Naheedy MH, Kaplan MM, et al: Spinal stenosis caused by epidural lipomatosis in Cushing's syndrome. *N Engl J Med* 1980; 302:36.

18. Chapman PH, Martuza RL, Poletti CE, et al: Symptomatic spinal epidural lipomatosis associated with Cushing's syndrome. *Neurosurgery* 1981; 8:724–727.

19. Randall BC, Muraki AS, Osborn RE, et al: Epidural lipomatosis with lumbar radiculopathy: CT appearance. *J Comput Assist Tomogr* 1986; 10:1039–1041.

20. Jungreis CA, Cohen WA: Spinal cord compression induced by steroid therapy: CT findings. *J Comput Assist Tomogr* 1987; 11:245–247.

21. Polmeteer FE, Kernohan JW: Meningeal gliomatosis: A study of forty-two cases. *Arch Neurol Psychiatry* 1947; 57:593–616.

22. Eelkema E, Johnson DW, Latchaw RE: Multiple spinal granulocytic sarcomas simulating neurofibromatosis: A case report and review. *AJNR* 1989; 10:542–544.

23. Bently JFR, Smith JR: Developmental posterior enteric remnants and spinal malformations: The split notochord syndrome. *Arch Dis Child* 1960; 35:76–86.

24. Kendall BE, Valentine AR, Keis B: Spinal arachnoid cysts: Clinical and radiological correlation with prognosis. *Neuroradiology* 1982; 22:225–234.

25. Masaryk TJ, Ross JS, Modic MT, et al: Radiculomenigeal vascular malformations of the spine: MR imaging. *Radiology* 1987; 164:845–849.

26. Raghavendra BN, Epstein FJ, McCleary L. Intramedullary spinal cord tumors in children: Localization by intraoperative sonography. *AJNR* 1984; 5:395–397.

27. Haft H, Ransohoff J, Carter S: Spinal cord tumors in children. *Pediatrics* 1959; 23:1152–1159.

28. Jungreis CA, Chandra R, Kricheff II, et al: In vitro magnetic resonance properties of CNS neoplasms and cysts. *Invest Radiol* 1988; 23:12–16.

29. Scotti G, Scialfa G, Colombo N, et al: Magnetic resonance diagnosis of intramedullary tumors of the spinal cord. *Neuroradiology* 1987; 29:130–135.

30. Goy AMC, Pinto RS, Raghavendra, BN, et al: Intramedullary spinal cord tumors: MR imaging, with emphasis on associated cysts. *Radiology* 1986; 161:387–390.

31. Gardner WJ, Collis JS Jr, Lewis LA: Cystic brain tumors and the blood-brain barrier. *Arch Neurol* 1963; 8:291–298.

32. Sherman JL, Barkovich AJ, Citrin CM: The MR appearance of syringomyelia: New observations. *AJNR* 1986; 7:985–995.

33. Deutsch M, Reigel DH: The value of myelography in the management of childhood medulloblastoma. *Cancer* 1980; 45:2194–2197.

34. Stauffer RN: Pyogenic vertebral osteomyelitis. *Orthop Clin North Am* 1975; 6:1015–1027.

35. Bonfiglio M, Lange TA, Kim YM: Pyogenic vertebral osteomyelitis: Disc space infections. *Clin Orthop* 1973; 96:234–247.

36. Digby JM, Kersley JB: Pyogenic non-tuberculous spinal infection: An analysis of thirty cases. *J Bone Joint Surg [Br]* 1979; 61:47–55.

37. Batson OV: The function of the vertebral veins and their role in the spread of metastases. *Ann Surg* 1940; 112:138–149.

38. Wiley AM, Trueta J: The vascular anatomy of the spine and its relationship to pyogenic vertebral osteomyelitis. *J Bone Joint Surg [Am]* 1959; 41:796–809.

39. Sapico FL, Montgomerie JZ: Vertebral osteomyelitis in intravenous drug abusers: Report of three cases and review of the literature. *Rev Infect Dis* 1980; 2:196–206.

40. Musher DM, Thorsteinsson SB, Minuth, JN, et al: Vertebral osteomyelitis: Still a diagnostic pitfall. *Arch Intern Med* 1976; 136:105–110.

41. Waldvogel FA, Vasey H: Osteomyelitis: The past decade. *N Engl J Med* 1980; 303:360–370.

42. Baker AS, Ojemann RG, Morton MD, et al: Spinal epidural abscess. *N Engl J Med* 1975; 293:463–468.

43. Stern WE, Crandall PH: Inflammatory intervertebral disc disease as a complication of the operative treatment of lumbar herniations. *J Neurosurg* 1959; 16:261–276.

44. Pilgaard S: Discitis (closed space infection) following removal of lumbar intervertebral disc. *J Bone Joint Surg [Am]* 1969; 51:713–716.

45. Lindholm TS, Pylkkanen P: Discitis following removal of intervertebral disc. *Spine* 1982; 7:618–622.

46. Rawlings CE, Wilkins RH, Gallis HA, et al: Postoperative intervertebral disc space infection. *Neurosurgery* 1983; 13:371–375.

47. Smith RF, Taylor TK: Inflammatory lesions of intervertebral discs in children. *J Bone Joint Surg [Am]* 1967; 49:1508–1520.

48. Pritchard AE, Thompson WAL: Acute pyogenic infections of the spine in children. *J Bone Joint Surg [Br]* 1960; 42:86–89.

49. Menelaus MB: Discitis: An inflammation affecting the intervertebral discs in children. *J Bone Joint Surg [Br]* 1964; 46:16–23.

50. Grunebaum M, Horodniceanu CH, Mukamel M, et al: The imaging diagnosis of nonpyogenic discitis in children. *Pediatr Radiol* 1982; 12:133–137.

51. Sartoris DJ, Moskowitz PS, Kaufman RA, et al:

Childhood discitis: Computed tomographic findings. *Radiology* 1983; 149:701–707.

52. Conventry MB, Ghormley RK, Kernohan JW: The intervertebral disc: Its microscopic anatomy and pathology. I. Anatomy, development, and pathology. *J Bone Joint Surg [Am]* 1945; 27:105–112.

53. Golumbu C, Firooznia H, Rafii M: CT of osteomyelitis of the spine. *AJNR* 1983; 4:1207–1211.

54. Larde D, Mathiew D, Frija J, et al: Vertebral osteomyelitis: Disc hypodensity on CT. *AJNR* 1982; 139:963–967.

55. Price AC, Allen JH, Eggers FM, et al: Intervertebral disc space infection: CT changes. *Radiology* 1983; 149:725–729.

56. Angtuaco EJ, McConnell JR, Chadduck WM, et al: MR imaging of spinal epidural sepsis. *AJNR* 1987; 8:879–883.

57. Modic MT, Feiglin DH, Piraino DW, et al: Vertebral osteomyelitis: Assessment using MR. *Radiology* 1985; 157:157–166.

58. Hermann G, Mendelson DS, Cohen BA, et al: Role of computed tomography in the diagnosis of infectious spondylitis. *J Comput Assist Tomogr* 1983; 7:961–968.

59. Lowman RM, Robinson F: Progressive vertebral interspace changes following lumbar disc surgery. *AJR* 1966; 97:664–671.

60. Whelan MA, Naidich DP, Post JD, et al: Computed tomography of spinal tuberculosis. *J Comput Assist Tomogr* 1983; 7:25–30.

61. Chapman M, Murray RD, Stoker DJ: Tuberculosis of the bones and joints. *Semin Roentgenol* 1979; 14:266–282.

62. Allen EH, Cosgrove D, Millard FJC: The radiological changes in infections of the spine and their diagnostic value. *Clin Radiol* 1978; 29:31–40.

63. Goldman AB, Freiberger RH: Localized infectious and neuropathic diseases. *Semin Roentgenol* 1979; 14:19–31.

64. McGahan JP, Graves DS, Palmer PES: Coccidioidal spondylitis: Usual and unusual radiographic manifestations. *Radiology* 1980; 136:5–9.

65. Chin D, Barrow D, Edis R, et al: Extraosseous extradural tuberculous granuloma of the spine. *Surg Neurol* 1983; 19:428–430.

66. Fraser RAR, Ratzan K, Wolpert SM, et al: Spinal subdural empyema. *Arch Neurol* 1973; 28:235–238.

67. Brant-Zawadzki M: Infections, in Newton TH, Potts DG (eds): *Computed Tomography of the Spine and Spinal Column.* San Anselmo, Calif, Clavadel Press, 1983, pp 205–221.

68. Kelly RB, Mahoney PD, Cawley KM: MR demonstration of spinal cord sarcoidosis: Report of a case. *AJNR* 1988; 9:197–199.

40

Spinal Trauma

Richard H. Daffner, M.D.

William E. Rothfus, M.D.

Computerized medical imaging has been one of the greatest breakthroughs in the history of medicine. The development of computed tomography (CT) in the early 1970s enabled radiologists to obtain cross-sectional images through areas of the body that were hitherto unseen by noninvasive methods. As computers became more sophisticated and CT scanners were improved, there was a concomitant increase in the amount of diagnostic information that could be obtained from this examination. The principles of computerized imaging derived from CT were applied in the 1980s to information gathered by magnetic resonance imaging (MRI), and thus a whole new field of diagnostic radiology was born. While initial work on comparison of CT and MRI was being done, it became apparent that MRI had many advantages over CT, namely the ability to image in any plane (sagittal, coronal, oblique, as well as transverse) and that certain anatomic structures or abnormalities could be enhanced by manipulating scanning parameters.

Early in the development of both of these imaging methods evidence showed that each could be extremely useful for the evaluation of patients with vertebral trauma.[3, 4, 11, 17, 19, 22, 27, 29-32] This chapter will discuss the use of CT and MRI in the evaluation of patients with vertebral trauma. The methods and techniques described are those that the authors are currently using at Allegheny General Hospital, Pittsburgh. The Trauma Center at Allegheny General Hospital sees approximately 200 patients with vertebral injuries each year. These patients provide the basis for our experience.

COMPUTED TOMOGRAPHY

The CT examination is relatively easy to perform on the patient with vertebral trauma. All that is required from the patient's standpoint is that he lie in a supine position and not move. Before an examination is begun it is necessary that all life support functions be properly monitored. Our CT rooms are equipped with ceiling- and wall-mounted oxygen, vacuum, and electrical outlets. A closed-circuit television camera monitors the patient in the gantry. The electrocardiogram monitor is placed in a position where it may be seen from the control booth. In an acutely injured patient, it may be necessary to pharmacologically induce immobility to obtain an adequate study.

In our institution, the standard procedure for evaluating patients with suspected vertebral injuries by CT begins by determining the levels for examination from plain films as well as from the CT scout view. We cannot overemphasize the value of plain films for the assessment of vertebral injuries. A complete set of plain films should be obtained before each examination. From these films and from the CT scout views it is then possible to determine the levels of examination.[7]

The type of scout view will depend upon the

area being studied. In the cervical region, if an injury is at C5 or above, a lateral scout view is obtained; from C6 through T8, it is performed in the anteroposterior (AP) position. In the lumbar region, the scout view may be either AP or lateral. This procedure will allow accurate identification of all levels in the study. A full-size view is included with and without level annotation from the final study.

Once the levels of examination have been determined, we image from one complete vertebral level above the area of suspected injury to one complete vertebral level below. All sections are obtained at 4- to 5-mm intervals without overlap. It is not necessary to use intravenous contrast enhancement. Filming is performed by utilizing both bone and soft-tissue windows. For bone we prefer a window of 1,500 Hounsfield units (HU) with a level of 150 HU.

The CT examination for patients with vertebral injury has a number of major advantages over conventional tomography. The foremost of these is the ease with which the examination may be performed. In addition, CT provides an additional

plane of examination, and this in turn results in an abundance of information regarding the injury (Figs 40–1 and 40–2). CT provides additional information on the extent of injury that has been already diagnosed on plain radiographs (Figs 40–3 and 40–4).[15] More importantly, CT can demonstrate additional fractures that were either not seen on plain films or totally unsuspected (Figs 40–5 and 40–6).[32] These injuries usually involve the laminae, pedicles, or articular pillars. Of primary concern to the attending neurosurgeon as well as to the patient's prognosis is the ability of CT to easily demonstrate the presence and degree of vertebral canal encroachment (Figs 40–7 and 40–8). In the same regard, fractures that would involve the structures making up the intervertebral foramina and involve peripheral nerve can also be demonstrated (Fig 40–9). CT is also useful in assessing patients with locked or perched facets.[13, 27, 35] In these instances, the images of both facets are clearly demonstrated (Fig 40–10).[21] In this way, CT is useful in augmenting a plain-film diagnosis.[1, 7, 11, 13, 21, 25, 30]

Sagittal and coronal reconstruction may be per-

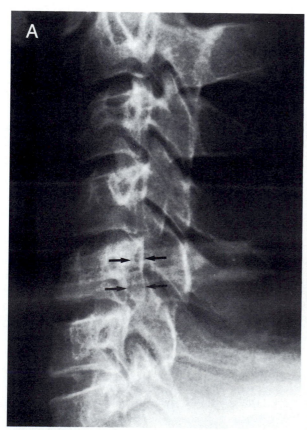

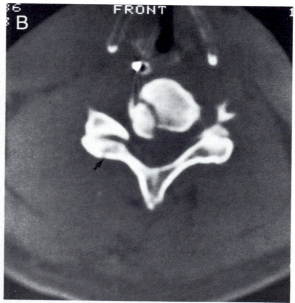

FIG 40–1.
C5 burst fracture. **A,** a lateral radiograph shows posterior displacement of a portion of the body of C5 that results in duplication of the posterior vertebral body line *(arrows)*. **B,** a CT scan shows the vertical fracture through the body of C5 on the right side. Note the posteriorly displaced fragment that accounts for the duplicate posterior vertebral body line images on the plain film. In addition, there is a fracture through the articular pillar on the right side *(arrow)*. (From Daffner RH: *Imaging of Vertebral Trauma.* Aspen Publishers, Inc, 1988. Used by permission.)

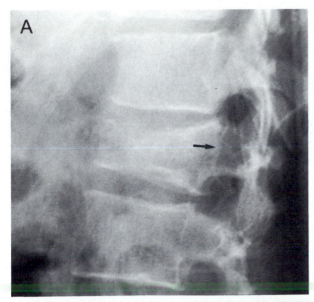

FIG 40–2.
Lumbar burst fracture. **A,** a lateral radiograph shows compression of the body of L1 with retropulsion of bone fragments into the vertebral canal *(arrow)*. **B,** a CT scan shows multiple fractures in the body of L1. Note the compromise of the vertebral canal by retropulsed bone fragment *(arrows)*. **C,** sagittal reconstruction through the region clearly shows the displaced bone fragment *(arrow)*. The ability to perform multiplanar reconstruction is a definite advantage of CT.

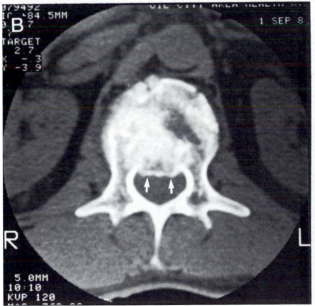

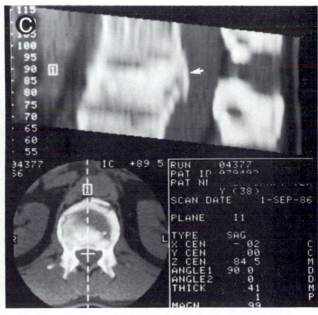

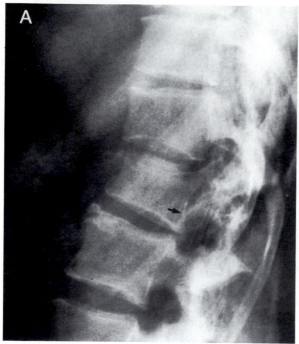

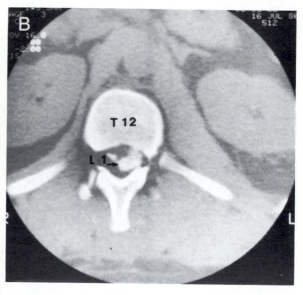

FIG 40–3.
Use of CT to provide additional information. **A,** a lateral radiograph shows a burst fracture of L1. The posterior vertebral body line of L1 is visible inferiorly *(arrow).* The upper portion of that line is missing. **B,** a CT scan made at the T12 level shows intracanalicular bone fragments from L1 *(arrow).* (From Daffner RH: *Imaging of Vertebral Trauma.* Aspen System Publishers, Inc, 1988. Used by permission.)

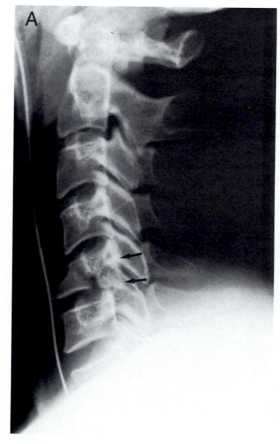

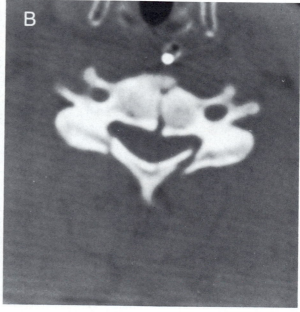

FIG 40–4.
Cervical burst fracture–subluxation. **A,** a lateral radiograph shows a burst fracture of C5 with retrolisthesis of the posterior portions of C5 *(arrows)* and the vertebrae above. **B,** a CT scan shows, in addition to the body fracture, that there are bilateral laminar fractures as well. These were not detected on plain films.

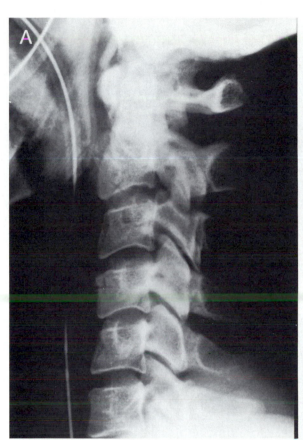
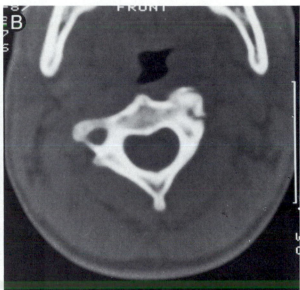
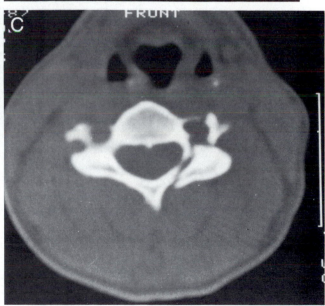

FIG 40–5.
Occult cervical fractures. **A,** a lateral radiograph shows a normal cervical column. **B,** a CT scan of the inferior aspect of C2 shows a fracture involving the lower body of C2 and the transverse foramen on the left. **C,** a section through C3 shows fractures through the lamina and transverse foramen on the left.

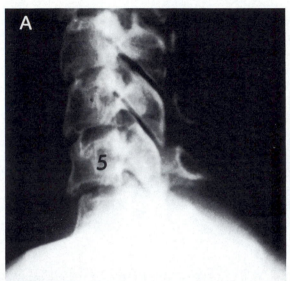

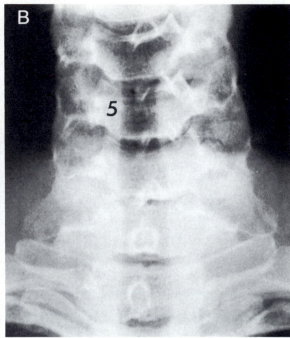

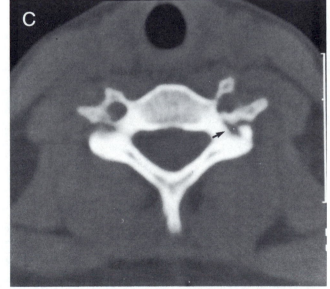

FIG 40–6.
Unilateral facet lock. **A,** a lateral radiograph shows
anterolisthesis of C5 on C6. **B,** a frontal radiograph shows
the spinal processes of C5 and above rotated to the left.
C, a CT scan shows an occult fracture of the C5 pillar on
the left side *(arrow)*.

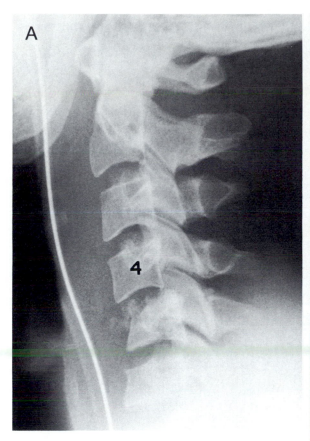

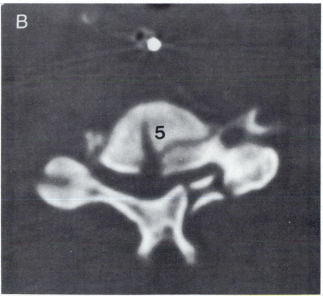

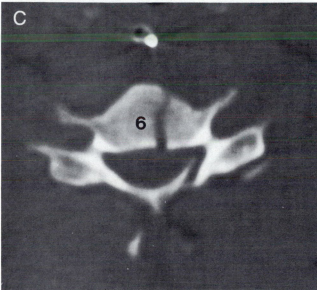

FIG 40–7.
Canal encroachment. **A,** a lateral radiograph shows a comminuted fracture of C5 with anterolisthesis of C4 on C5. **B,** a CT scan through C5 shows the marked degree of canal encroachment as a result of the dislocation. **C,** a section through C6 shows occult fractures in that vertebra. (From Daffner RH: *Imaging of Vertebral Trauma.* Aspen Publishers, Inc, 1988. Used by permission.)

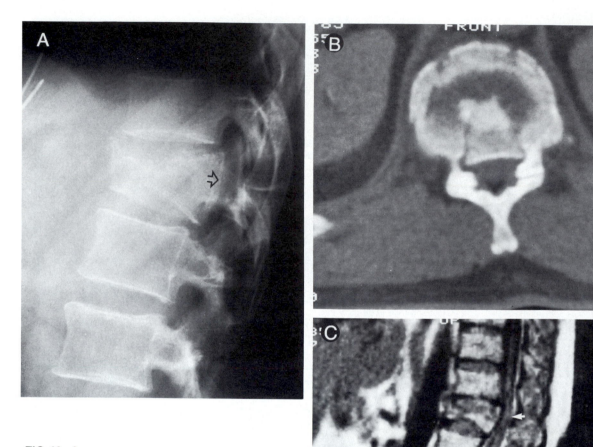

FIG 40–8.
Burst fracture of T12. **A,** a lateral radiograph shows typical
findings of a burst fracture. Note the large bony fragment
retropulsed into the vertebral canal *(arrow)*. **B,** a CT scan
shows this fragment of bone placed into the vertebral
canal. **C,** MRI examination (TR 300 ms, TE 35 ms) shows
encroachment of the subarachnoid space and spinal cord
at T12 *(arrow)*.

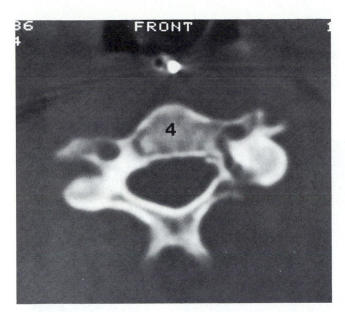

FIG 40–9.
Pillar fracture extending into intervertebral foramen on the left (same patient as in Fig 40–7; this fracture was also unsuspected).

formed from CT examinations. This is particularly useful when evaluating fractures at the cervicothoracic junction or in the high thoracic region, where lateral radiographs are often suboptimal (Figs 40–11 and 40–12). In such instances, CT examination can eliminate the necessity of obtaining conventional lateral tomograms to evaluate a fracture.[7]

Three-dimensional (3-D) reconstruction is now available as the result of CT software programs through several manufacturers. The advocates of 3-D imaging find these programs useful in determining the spatial relationships of bone fragments, particularly when the fragments must be manipulated at surgery (Fig 40–13). The initial CT programs for providing this information were time-consuming or required transfer of data to a free-standing computer system, and this detracted from their usefulness.[34] However, newer programs allow these reconstructions to be obtained in a relatively short period of time to speed the information to the clinician who finds it most useful. The true value of 3-D reconstruction, however, remains to be determined.[7]

In many institutions, particularly when MRI is not available, CT is combined with myelography using water-soluble contrast to demonstrate the encroachment on the subarachnoid space and spinal cord by fragments of bone or herniated intervertebral disks (Figs 40–14 and 40–15). CT myelography is also useful in diagnosing traumatic dural tears and nerve root avulsions (Fig 40–16),[26, 28]

spinal cord contusion with swelling (Fig 40–17), and post-traumatic cystic myelopathy (Fig 40–18). In our institution, we utilize MRI for these diagnoses unless the patient is too unstable for the study to be performed. In those rare instances, we utilize CT and myelography.

The radiographic determination of vertebral stability or instability has been based upon five criteria: vertebral displacement, widening of the interspinous space, widening of the vertebral canal in either the sagittal or coronal planes (usually assessed by a widening of the interpedicular distance), wide facet joints, and disruption of the posterior vertebral body line.[7, 12] Denis proposed a system for identifying a patient with unstable injuries by dividing the vertebral column into three compartments. The anterior compartment extends from the anterior longitudinal ligament to the midpoint of the vertebral body. The middle compartment extends from that part caudally to the posterior longitudinal ligament. The posterior compartment extends caudally from the posterior longitudinal ligament to the supraspinous ligament. Denis found in his investigation that instability resulted from disruption of any two contiguous compartments.[9, 10] Gehweiler et al., working without CT,[12] and Daffner, working with CT,[7] were able to confirm Denis' initial observations.

The five plain-film signs of displacement may easily be demonstrated by CT. Displacement can be shown when axial images of two contiguous vertebrae are superimposed one upon the other and the malalignment is clearly visible (Fig 40–19). Widening of the interspinous space implies significant injury to the posterior ligamentous structures that extend as far anteriorly and include the posterior longitudinal ligament. While this sign is quite apparent on plain films, it may also be demonstrated on axial CT by the absent laminar and spinous process shadows on two or more contiguous sections. This has been termed the "absent-spine sign" (Fig 40–20).[7, 27] Widening of the vertebral canal usually occurs in burst or crush fractures. This finding implies that there is total disruption of the body of the vertebra (usually in a sagittal plane) that is combined with a fracture through the lamina at the same level (Fig 40–21). These findings explain the widening of the interpedicular distance often seen on plain films. Widening of the facet joints implies ligamentous disruption and is often associated with widening of the interspinous space. Widened facet joints may

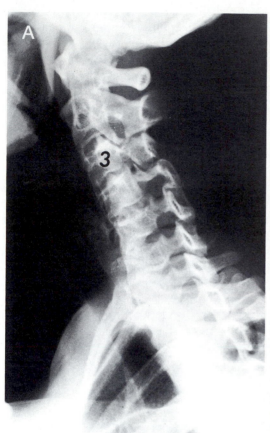

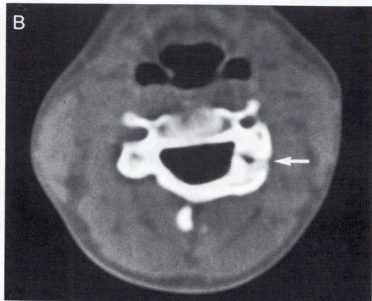

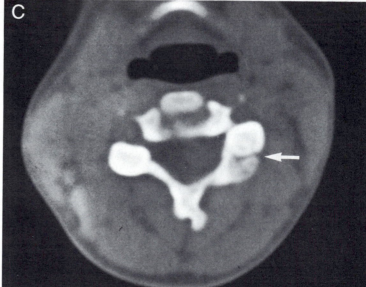

FIG 40–10.
Locked facets. **A,** an oblique radiograph shows
locking of the facets of C3 on C4. **B** and **C,** CT scans
clearly show the point of locking *(arrows).* Note the
rotation to the right. (From Daffner RH: *Imaging of
Vertebral Trauma.* Aspen Publishers, Inc, 1988. Used
by permission.)

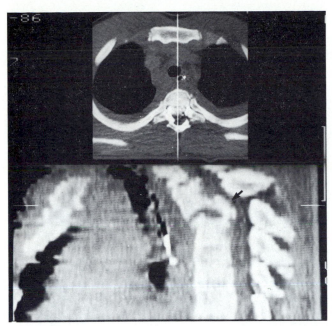

FIG 40–11.
Use of sagittal reconstruction in a fracture dislocation of C3 on C4. A reconstructed image of the CT scan shows a bone fragment *(arrow)* within the vertebral canal. (From Daffner RH: *Imaging of Vertebral Trauma.* Aspen Publishers, Inc, 1988. Used by permission.)

be clearly identified on CT (Fig 40–22). Finally, disruptions of the posterior vertebral body line, the vertical bony shadow visible on lateral radiographs, occurs primarily in bursting injuries and in grinding injuries in which there is a bursting component. Distraction of the line may also occur in flexion injuries as the result of the use of lap-type seat belts. These plain-film findings may also be confirmed by CT (Figs 40–23 and 40–24).

There are a number of pitfalls and limitations to CT that fall into two categories: patient related and technical. Patient-related pitfalls are the result of motion, patient size, and artifacts due to metallic implants. Motion on any radiographic study will

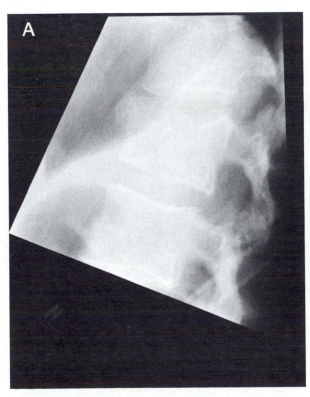

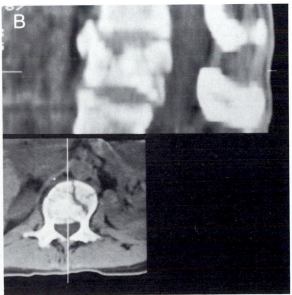

FIG 40–12.
Use of sagittal reconstruction. **A,** a lateral radiograph shows a burst fracture of L1. **B,** sagittal reconstruction shows the findings to better advantage.

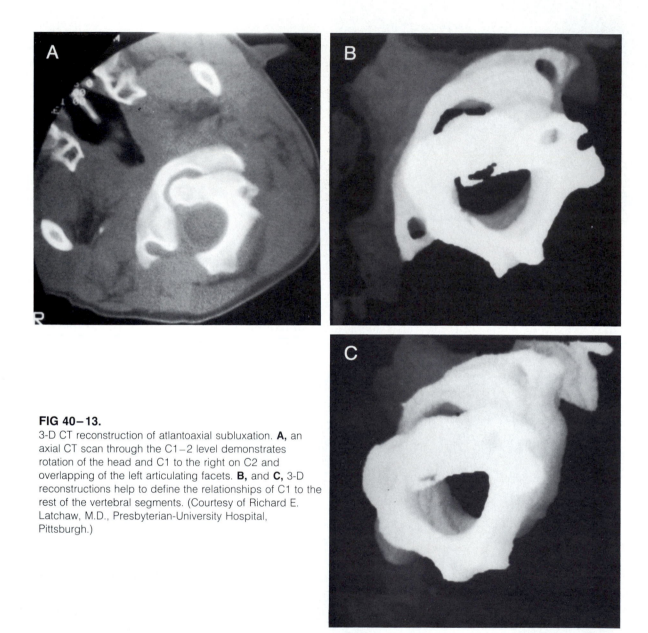

FIG 40–13.
3-D CT reconstruction of atlantoaxial subluxation. **A,** an axial CT scan through the C1–2 level demonstrates rotation of the head and C1 to the right on C2 and overlapping of the left articulating facets. **B,** and **C,** 3-D reconstructions help to define the relationships of C1 to the rest of the vertebral segments. (Courtesy of Richard E. Latchaw, M.D., Presbyterian-University Hospital, Pittsburgh.)

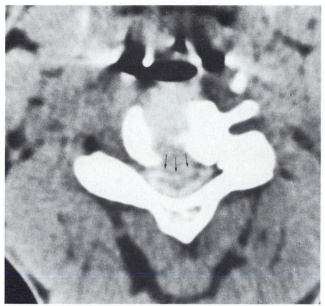

FIG 40—14.
Post-traumatic herniated intervertebral disk. A CT scan following water-soluble contrast myelography shows compression of the subarachnoid space and a herniated intervertebral disk *(arrows)*. (From Daffner RH: *Imaging of Vertebral Trauma.* Aspen Publishers, Inc, 1988. Used by permission.)

produce blurred images with the concomitant possibility of a missed diagnosis. We have not found this to be a serious problem in our practice. Patient size, however, is a more serious consideration. Most of the current CT machines available today have a weight limit of 300 lb on the table because of the way in which the table projects into the gantry. In addition, an extremely large patient who makes physical contact with the gantry ring will often produce results with many artifacts. Fortu-

nately, the manufacturers have been responsive to these problems and have constructed machines of greater weight limit with larger gantry sizes. A patient with implanted orthopedic hardware causes different problems. In most instances, these have been the result of Harrington or Luque rods that have been used for spinal stability. These metal rods cause a serious artifact that degrades the CT image. Artifacts from dental fillings may interfere with the images of the upper cervical column.

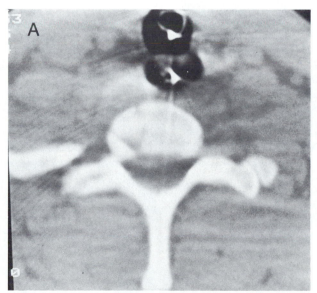

FIG 40—15.
Post-traumatic herniated intervertebral disk. **A,** a CT scan at a bone window shows a fracture of the body of T1. **B,** a soft-tissue window following CT myelography shows the herniated disk com-pressing the vertebral canal *(arrows)*. (From Daffner RH: *Imaging of Vertebral Trauma.* Aspen Publishers, Inc, 1988. Used by permission.)

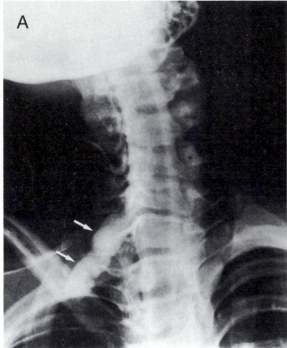

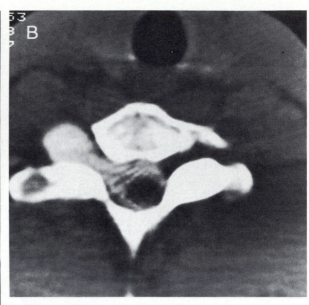

FIG 40–16.
Post-traumatic nerve root avulsion. **A,** an oblique radiograph following water-soluble contrast myelography shows extravasation of contrast along the root sheath of C7 on the right side *(arrows).* **B,** CT myelography shows the same findings. (From Daffner RH: *Imaging of Vertebral Trauma.* Aspen Publishers, Inc, 1988. Used by permission.)

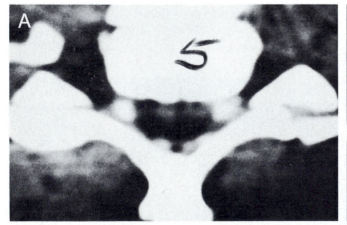

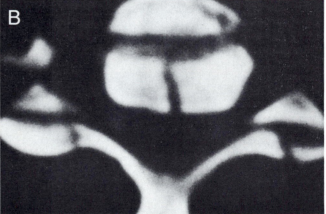

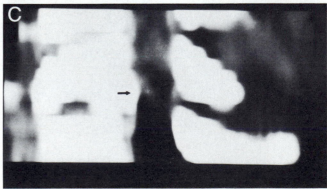

FIG 40–17.
Cord contusion with swelling. **A,** CT scanning at the C5 level following cervical myelography demonstrates narrowing of the AP diameter of the spinal canal and a widened cord shadow. **B,** Bone windowing at the same level demonstrates the fractures of the C5 vertebral body and the bilateral laminar/facetal fractures. **C,** a sagittal midline reconstruction centered at the C5 level demonstrates the swelling of the cord shadow at the level of the upper aspect of C5, with posterior displacement of a C5 fracture fragment *(arrow),* posterior displacement of the opacified subarachnoid space overlying the displaced fracture fragment, and a block to the caudad movement of contrast material. The spinal cord widening is indicative of cord swelling and/or hematoma, with the more inferior compression and block due to the bony fragment. (Courtesy of Richard E. Latchaw, M.D., Presbyterian-University Hospital, Pittsburgh.)

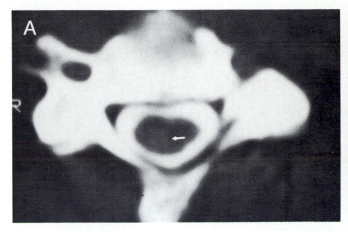

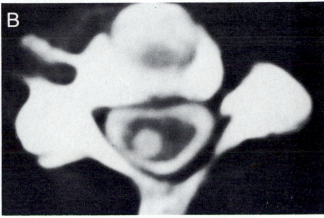

FIG 40–18.
Post-traumatic cystic myelopathy demonstrated on postmyelographic CT. **A,** CT scanning at the C4 level 1 hour following cervical myelography demonstrates very subtle contrast within the right side of a normal-sized spinal cord *(arrow)*. **B,** scanning at the same level 6 hours later demonstrates dense, homogeneous contrast in the right side of the spinal cord. The sharp margination and homogeneous high density is indicative of a post-traumatic cyst rather than myelomalacia. (Courtesy of Richard E. Latchaw, M.D., Englewood, Colo.)

Three technical pitfalls—averaging effect, poor level calibration, and fractures in the plane of the scan—may result in substandard results. Partial volume averaging effect is a well-known CT pitfall. The CT image represents an average of the radiographic densities of all of the structures included in the section of scan. Any structure that is not completely included within the scanning plane may either be distorted or totally discarded from the final image. We have encountered several patients in whom an abnormality has been identified on one view only. In each of these instances, we were dealing with particularly thin structures such as the laminae and the posterior arch of C1 (Fig 40–25). Fortunately, in most instances a fracture will be identified on more than one section. Less of a problem is a situation where there is normal overlap of structures from adjacent vertebrae.[2] In these instances, lines of interruption in the bony shadow will be identified. However, correlation with the scout views can identify where the section was obtained.

Faulty annotation on the scout film as a result of either "table creep" or malalignment of the centering system may result in erroneous information being obtained regarding the level of injury. We have not found this to be a significant problem since we rely on plain films to determine the level of fractures. Finally, fractures that are oriented in the plane of the CT examination may not always

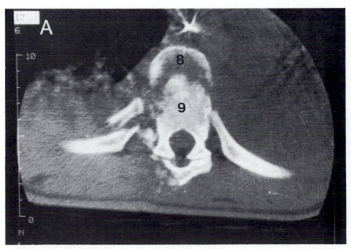

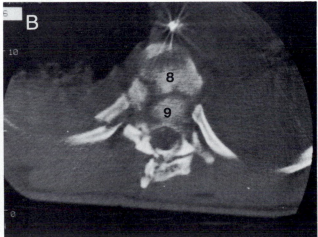

FIG 40–19.
A and **B,** T8–9 fracture dislocation. CT images clearly show portions of more than one vertebra on each section.

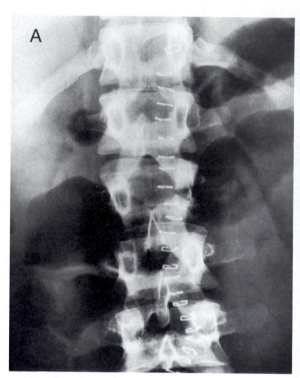

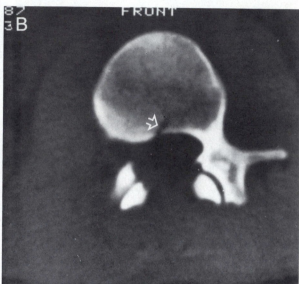

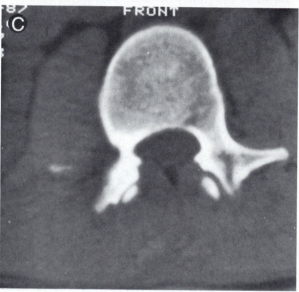

FIG 40–20.
Widening of the interspinous space in a distraction injury of
L1–2. **A,** a frontal radiograph shows widening of the
interspinous space between L1 and L2. Note the bare area
between the pedicles of L2. **B,** and **C,** contiguous CT
scans show an absence of laminar structures of L2, which
indicates the severe distraction. In **B,** note the fracture of
the upper portion of the body of L2 *(arrow).* (From Daffner
RH: *Imaging of Vertebral Trauma.* Aspen Publishers, Inc,
1988. Used by permission.)

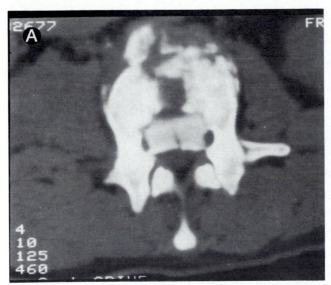
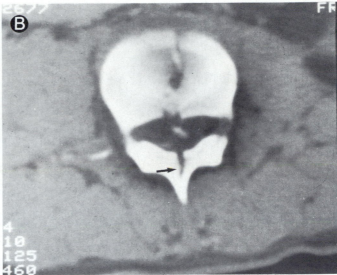

FIG 40–21.
Burst fracture with a sagittal split. **A,** a CT image through the upper portion of the involved vertebral body shows fracture fragments extending in a sagittal plane all the way to the vertebral canal. Note the large intracanalicular bone fragment. **B,** a lower section shows the fracture extending through the lamina into the spinous process *(arrow).*

be demonstrated. We have found this to occur most commonly with fractures of the dens or the body of C2 (Fig 40–26). When this pitfall is encountered, it may be necessary to tilt the gantry to bring the fracture out of the plane of the scan. Conventional tomography may be necessary if tilting the gantry is not successful.[7]

Dislocations that occur in the transverse plane may not always be apparent on the CT examination. In many instances, the plane of examination

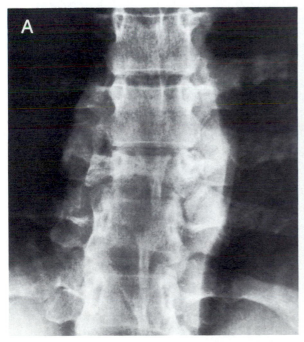
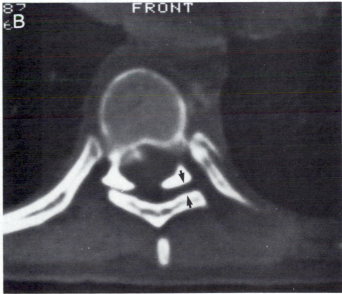

FIG 40–22.
Wide facet joint in a patient with T7–8 dislocation. **A,** a frontal radiograph shows compression of T7 with luxation of T7 on T8 to the left side. **B,** a CT scan shows widening of the facet joints, particularly on the left side *(arrows).* (From Daffner RH: *Imaging of Vertebral Trauma.* Aspen Publishers, Inc, 1988. Used by permission.)

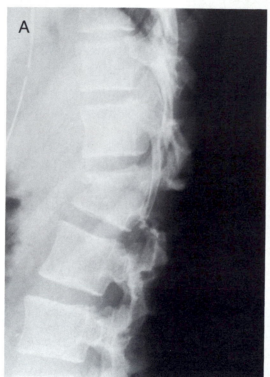

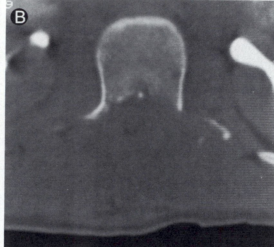

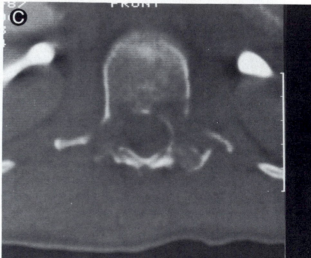

FIG 40–23.
Chance fracture of L1 as a result of lap-type seat belt use. **A,** a lateral radiograph shows a distraction injury through L1. **B,** and **C,** CT images through L1 show fractures involving the transverse processes and pedicles. Note the absence of spinous process images.

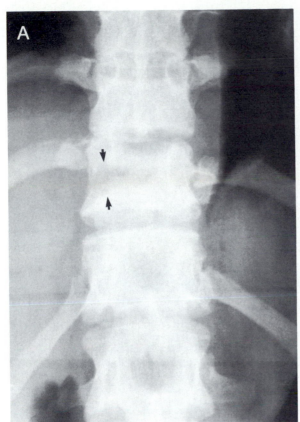

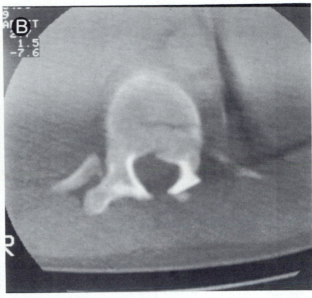

FIG 40–24.
Chance fracture at T11 from the use of lap-type seat belts. **A,** a frontal radiograph shows a fracture of the body of T11 that extends into the pedicle on the right side *(arrows)*. Note the distraction between the 11th and 12th ribs. **B,** a CT scan shows fractures through the body of T11. Note the absence of posterior structures as evidence of the distraction nature of this injury.

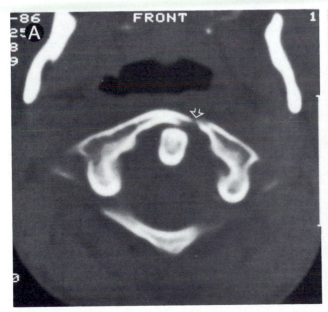

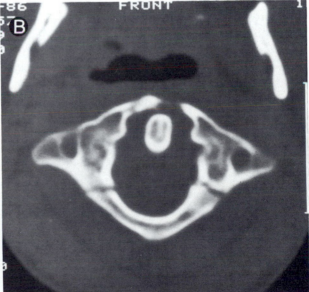

FIG 40–25.
Jefferson fracture of C1. **A,** a high section through C1 shows a fracture of the anterior arch *(arrow)*. The fracture is seen only in this view. **B,** a section slightly lower shows fractures through the posterior arch. These were seen only on this image. (From Daffner RH: *Imaging of Vertebral Trauma.* Aspen Publishers, Inc, 1988. Used by permission.)

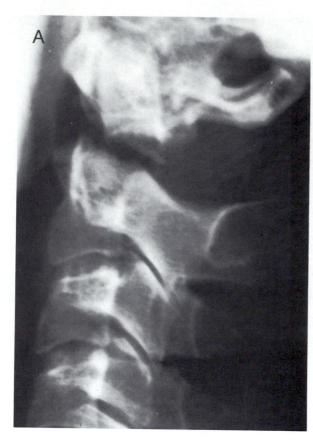

FIG 40–26.
Fractured dens. **A,** a lateral radiograph shows a fracture of the base of the dens with posterior displacement of the fragment. **B,** a CT image through the body of C2 shows the fracture line *(arrows).* The degree of distraction is not as apparent as on the plain film. In this instance, plain films offered more information than did CT. (From Daffner RH: *Imaging of Vertebral Trauma.* Aspen Publishers, Inc, 1988. Used by permission.)

does not include portions of the adjacent vertebra on any one section. In these cases, if the CT examination alone were relied upon to make a diagnosis, dislocation would not be identified. Once again, the authors stress the need to consult plain films before doing an examination.

MAGNETIC RESONANCE IMAGING

CT revolutionized the practice of diagnostic radiology. One of its many benefits was that it ushered in the age of computerized imaging. In less than 10 years, the field of nuclear magnetic resonance utilizing high magnetic fields and radiowaves was applied to medicine in the form of MRI. Abnormalities of the vertebral column were among the first areas to be evaluated by this new imaging technique. Initial interest centered upon the diagnosis of diseases of the intervertebral disk. However, it soon became apparent that MRI would also be useful in patients who had suffered vertebral trauma.[22, 31] By altering the technical factors of echo time (TE) and repetition time (TR) and by developing newer imaging menus with fancy acronymic names such as FISP (fast imaging steady-state precession), FLASH (fast low-angle shot), GRASS (gradient-refocused acquisition in a steady state), and CHESS (chemical shift selective), it became apparent that images could be obtained rapidly in these patients and provide details of bone position and disk hydration, as well as the interface between cerebrospinal fluid and the extradural spaces.

A discussion of the principles and physics of MRI is beyond the scope of this chapter. Even as this is being written, there are new developments occurring almost on a daily basis. The technical aspects for obtaining vertebral column images will be discussed briefly. The exact scanning parameters will vary from institution to institution and will depend upon the type of machine used, the strength of the magnet, the type of coil used, and the patient's condition. In our institution, all studies are performed either on a Siemens Magnetom, 0.5 Tesla, or a second Siemens Magnetom, 2.0 Tesla, operated at 1.5 Tesla. The usual vertebral column examination on the lower-field machine consists of a short spin-echo sequence utilizing a TE of 15 to 90 ms with a TR of 300 to 600 ms in the sagittal plane. In our institution, we have chosen T1-weighted parameters of 15 to 35 ms TE at a TR of 300 to 500 ms with four repetitions and 5-mm slice thickness. Special surface coils are used for the cervical, thoracic, and lumbar regions. The time of examination for five slices is approximately 9 minutes. T1-weighted technique is most useful for demonstrating normal vertebral alignment as well as bony relationships to the spinal canal (Fig 40–27).[6, 16, 18, 22–24, 33] It is also useful for demonstrating syringomyelia and bone marrow infiltration in malignant disease.[7, 8, 31]

A longer spin-echo sequence utilizing a TE of 35 to 100 ms and a TR of 2,000 to 3,000 ms at T2 and proton density weighting on the lower-field unit is obtained to evaluate the state of disk hydration as well as the interface between the cerebrospinal fluid and the extradural space. This sequence results in a higher signal intensity of the cerebrospinal fluid and thus is useful for evaluating patients with suspected extradural compression from bone fragments (Fig 40–28). This sequence is performed in the sagittal plane as well. Only one acquisition is made at these parameters and approximately nine slices at 7-mm intervals

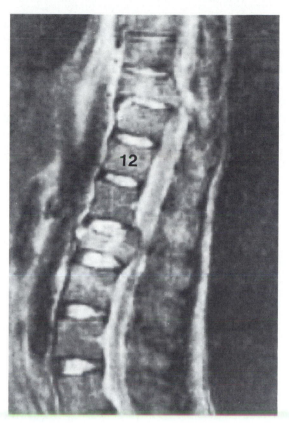

FIG 40–28.
Same patient as in Figure 40–27. Sagittal MRI (TR 2,100; TE 90) shows the abnormalities to better advantage. Note the encroachment of the subarachnoid space and thecal sac and contents at each level. On T2-weighted images, the intervertebral disks are of high signal, as is the cerebrospinal fluid.

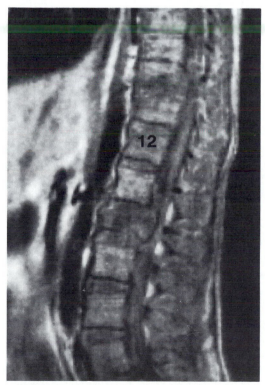

FIG 40–27.
Burst fractures of T10 and L2 as demonstrated on sagittal MRI at T1-weighted parameters (TR 500, TE 17). Although the abnormalities can be identified, intimate detail is missing. The subarachnoid space is of low signal; the spinal cord, a uniform gray. Compare with Figure 40–28.

are obtained. The sequence also takes approximately 9 minutes to perform. A third sequence performed in the axial plane is also obtained by using the same scanning parameters. This provides an additional study for correlation with CT.

When scans are performed by using the 1.5-Tesla unit, we obtain T1-weighted images in the sagittal plane at a TE of 15 ms and a TR of 500 ms for sagittal images. This sequence using two acquisitions produces nine slices in 4½ minutes. T2-weighted images utilize a TE of 22 and 90 ms with a TR of 2.1 seconds. This will produce nine slices in approximately 18 minutes. If axial images are desired, we utilize a T1-weighted sequence of 15 ms and a TR of 1 second. This produces 19 slices in 9 minutes.

"Fast scans" have been advocated for demonstrating injuries in the transverse plane. These studies must be performed on a high field-strength magnet (1.5 Tesla or greater) by utilizing extremely short sequences (TE 11 ms, TR 400 to

1,500 ms). Under these conditions, the cerebrospinal fluid has a high signal, which helps to outline the cord.

It is imperative to use surface coils to examine the vertebral column. Surface coils result in improved images with increased signal-to-noise ratios (Figs 40–29 and 40–30). Surface coils will vary from manufacturer to manufacturer.

The ideal candidate for examination by MRI is one in whom a vertebral injury is the only serious abnormality. In these patients, we utilize the short and long TR sagittal sequences. If we are able to obtain only one set of images, we prefer the longer sequence, which takes the same amount of time. The sagittal images are preferred, and these are used to determine the degree of encroachment of the subarachnoid space and the spinal cord (Figs 40–31 to 40–33). In our institution, MRI has nearly completely replaced myelography in the evaluation of vertebral trauma.

MRI has a number of distinct advantages over other forms of imaging and is able to provide addi-

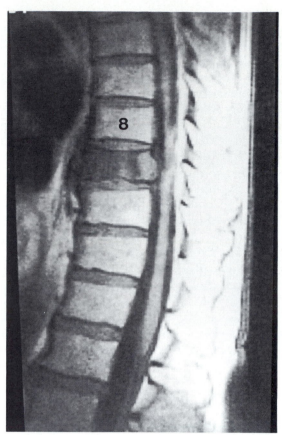

FIG 40–30.
Same patient as in Figure 40–29, but MRI with a spine surface coil (TR 500, TE 35). Note the improvement in overall image quality and detail.

tional information on the extent of injury that previously had to be implied from clinical findings. The foremost advantage is the ability of MRI to demonstrate the relationship of bone fragments that may have been displaced into the vertebral canal to the spinal cord (Figs 40–34 and 40–35). Of particular interest is the ability to assess the vertebral alignment and anatomy at the cervicothoracic junction (Figs 40–36 and 40–37).[14] This is one of the most difficult areas for diagnosing vertebral column injuries because of the overlying shoulders. Prior to the advent of MRI, sagittal images could be obtained either by polydirectional tomography or by sagittal reconstruction from a CT examination.[7] The ease with which MRI can be performed in this region has resulted in improved diagnosis and near-complete abandonment of polydirectional tomography in the region.[7, 14]

A fracture is, in reality, a soft-tissue injury in which a bone is broken. MRI is particularly useful in demonstrating the extent of soft-tissue damage associated with an injury (Figs 40–38 and 40–39).

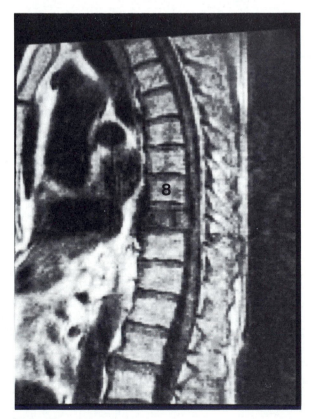

FIG 40–29.
Pathologic fracture of T9 with canal encroachment. T1-weighted MRI (TR 500, TE 35) with a body coil shows the abnormality. However, the image is considerably noisy. Compare with Figure 40–30.

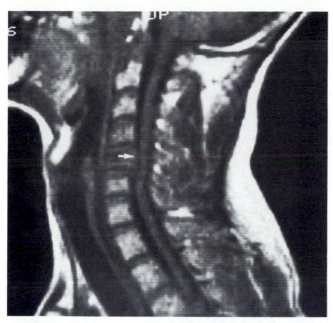

FIG 40–31.
Vertebral canal encroachment from a C5 burst fracture. A T1-weighted image (TR 500, TE 35) shows compression of the subarachnoid space *(arrow)*. (From Daffner RH: *Imaging of Vertebral Trauma*. Aspen Publishers, Inc, 1988. Used by permission.)

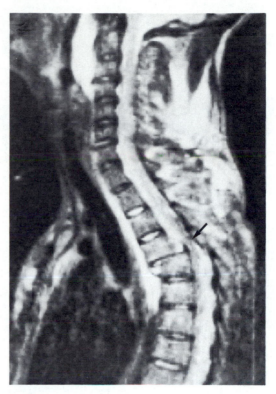

FIG 40–33.
Severe canal compromise in a patient with T4–5 dislocation. A T2-weighted image (TR 2,100; TE 90) shows the point of cord transection *(arrow)*.

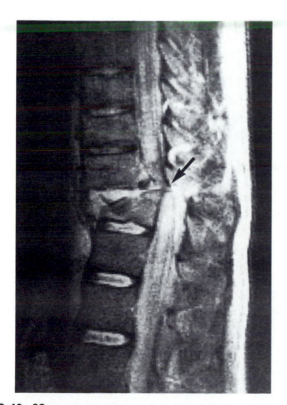

FIG 40–32.
Fracture-dislocation of T9–10 and transection of the spinal cord. A T2-weighted (TR 2,100; TE 90) image shows transection of the cord at the point of dislocation *(arrow)*.

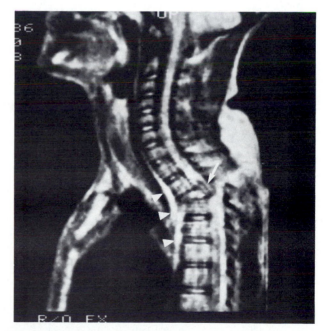

FIG 40–34.
Bone fragment *(arrow)* in the vertebral canal in the same patient as in Figure 40–11. A T2-weighted image (TR 2,100; TE 35) shows areas of hemorrhage in the prevertebral space as evidenced by high signal *(arrowheads)*. (From Daffner RH: *Imaging of Vertebral Trauma*. Aspen Publishers, Inc, 1988. Used by permission.)

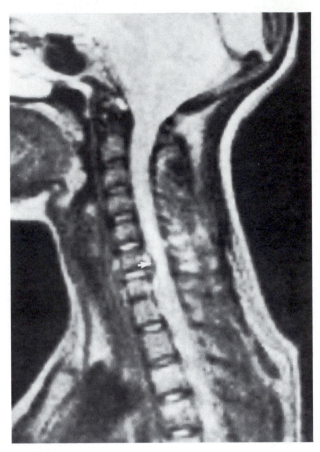

FIG 40–35.
Burst fracture with canal encroachment by a bone fragment *(arrow)*. The area adjacent to the bone fragment has higher signal due to cord hemorrhage (TR 1,500; TE 90).

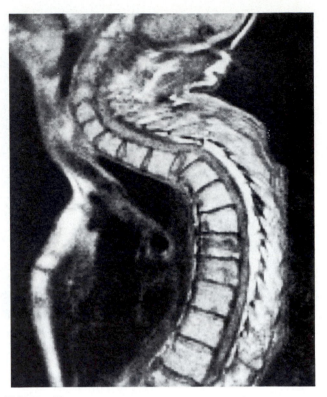

FIG 40–36.
T3 fracture-dislocation with canal encroachment. This T1-weighted image (TR 150, TE 35) easily demonstrates the cervicothoracic region. This area is normally extremely difficult to image by other means.

In particular, considerable attention has been focused on the demonstration of acute spinal cord injury.[6, 16–18, 20, 24, 33] In addition to identifying transection of the spinal cord, it is now possible to diagnose spinal cord hemorrhage and edema and to differentiate between those entities.[6, 15, 20, 24] As a rule, acutely traumatized spinal cords expand to fill the vertebral canal. The epidural fat becomes obliterated as the result of either hemorrhage or edema. Characteristically, acute spinal cord hemorrhage produces diminished signal intensity on T2-weighted images within 24 hours of injury.[6, 16, 20, 24] Paraspinal hemorrhage, on the other hand, produces high signal on T2-weighted images within and after 24 hours (Fig 40–40). On the other hand, edema and contusion of the cord result in high signal intensity on T2-weighted images (Fig 40–41).[6, 16, 20, 24] Scanning a few days later demonstrates the characteristic hyperintensity of methemoglobin-containing subacute blood similar to that seen with cerebral hemorrhage (Figs 40–42 and

40–43). The MRI appearance of the injured spinal cord has been demonstrated by Kulkarni et al. to correlate directly the recovery of neurologic function. His group found that those patients with cord edema or contusion recovered significant function, whereas those with hemorrhage did not.[20]

MRI is useful for the follow-up examination of patients with vertebral trauma. In addition to demonstrating signal changes in a damaged spinal cord as mentioned previously, MRI can help establish the diagnosis of post-traumatic spinal cord cysts or syringomyelia (Figs 40–44 and 40–45) and/or spinal cord atrophy (Figs 40–46 and 40–47). As a result, MRI has replaced myelography in our institution for these patients.[7]

No discussion of the benefits of MRI for the "spine-injured" patient would be complete without a comparison of the advantages of MRI over CT. MRI is able to manipulate inherent tissue contrast by changing the TE and TR. Furthermore, applying different scanning sequences including flip angle and proton density studies allows us to enhance certain structures while "suppressing" others. High-strength MRI units (1.5 Tesla) can dem-

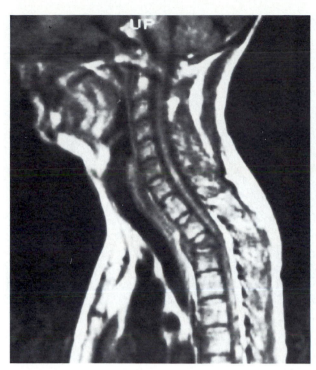

FIG 40–37.
Canal encroachment. A T1-weighted image (TR 500, TE 35) shows the
ease with which the cervicothoracic region may be demonstrated. (From
Daffner RH: *Imaging of Vertebral Trauma.* Aspen Publishers, Inc, 1988.
Used by permission.)

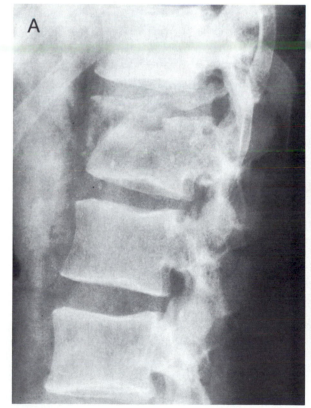

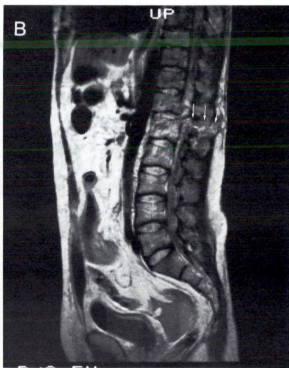

FIG 40–38.
Extent of soft-tissue injury. **A,** a lateral radiograph shows a horizon-
tal fracture through the upper portion of the body of L1. **B,** sagittal
MRI (TR 2,100; TE 35) shows the image to extend far posteriorly
(arrows). (From Daffner RH: *Imaging of Vertebral Trauma.* Aspen
Publishers, Inc, 1988. Used by permission.)

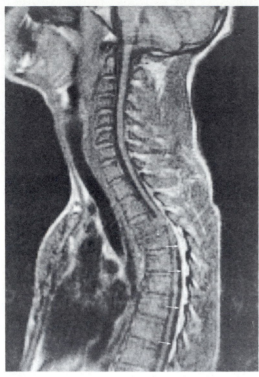

FIG 40–39.
Extent of soft-tissue damage in the same patient as in Figure 40–33. In this T1-weighted image (TR 150, TE 35) note the area with high signal, which indicates epidural hemorrhage *(arrows)*.

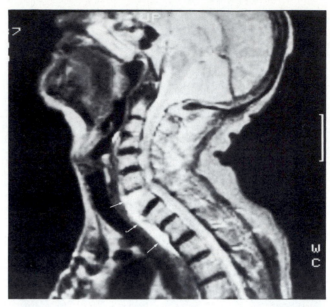

FIG 40–40.
Prevertebral hemorrhage as the result of an extension injury at C6–7 with a high-signal area in the prevertebral region *(arrows)* (TR 2,100; TE 90).

FIG 40–41.
Epidural hemorrhage *(arrows)* and cord edema in a patient with a fracture dislocation at C5–6 (TR 2,100; TE 35). Epidural hemorrhage extends from the disk space posterior to C5. The area of high signal within the spinal cord immediately behind the point of disruption indicates cord edema and contusion.

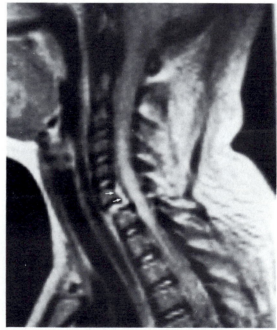

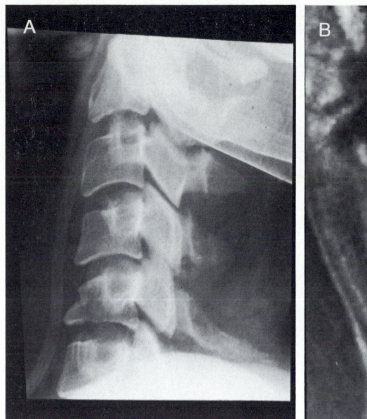

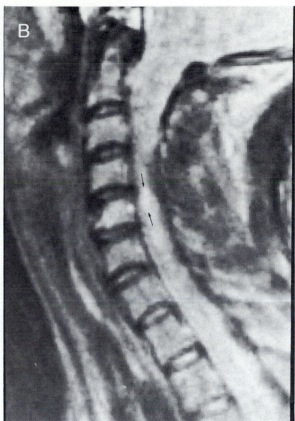

FIG 40–42.
Cord hemorrhage secondary to a burst fracture. **A,** a lateral radiograph shows buckling of the C5 vertebra. The patient is quadriplegic. **B,** a T2-weighted sagittal image (TR 1,500; TE 90) shows an area of high signal *(arrows)* within the spinal cord at C5.

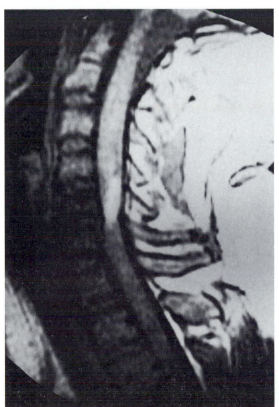

FIG 40–43.
Cord hemorrhage secondary to C5 fracture. A sagittal T1-weighted image demonstrates the fractured C5 vertebral segment and high intensity of the subacute hemorrhage within the spinal cord. This examination was performed 5 days following trauma. (Courtesy of Richard E. Latchaw, M.D., Englewood, Colo.)

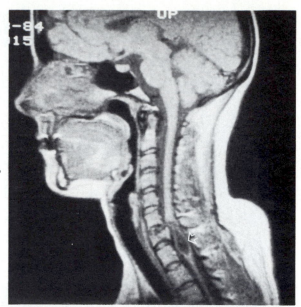

FIG 40–44.
Post-traumatic syringomyelia in a patient following a burst fracture of C7.
Note the cystic area of low signal *(arrow)* in the C7–T1 region (TR 500, TE
35). (From Daffner RH: *Imaging of Vertebral Trauma.* Aspen Publishers, Inc,
1988. Used by permission.)

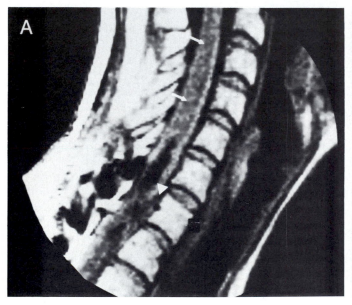

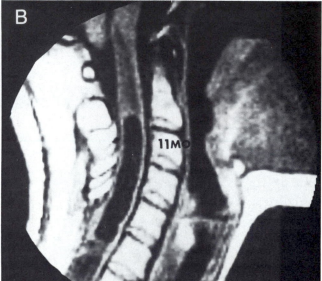

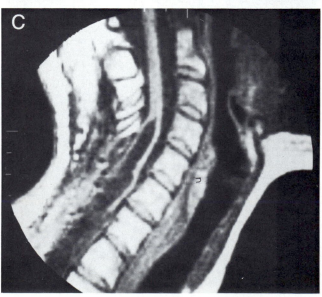

FIG 40–45.
Evolution of a post-traumatic cord cyst. **A,** a sagittal T1-weighted MR
scan 5 months after a C6–7 fracture dislocation demonstrates a
small cyst *(arrowhead)* at the level of trauma, with myelomalacia
(arrows) extending above this. The myelomalacia is more intense
than the cyst but less intense than the normal cord on the
T1-weighted sequence. **B,** 11 months following the initial MRI, the
cyst has increased in size as the myelomalacic cord continues to
cavitate. A cyst-subarachnoid shunt was inserted and markedly
decreased the size of the cyst. **C,** 11 months following
decompressive shunting, the patient's spasticity began to increase.
The T1-weighted image demonstrates recurrence of the cyst with
cord atrophy above the cyst. (Courtesy of Richard E. Latchaw, M.D.,
Englewood, Colo.)

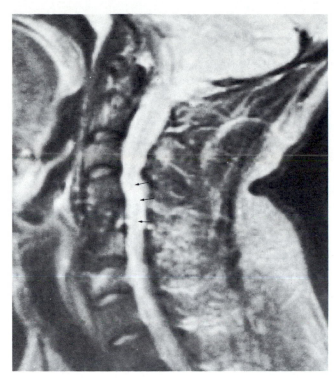

FIG 40–46.
Post-traumatic spinal cord atrophy. A T2-weighted image shows the ribbon-like atrophic cord *(arrows)* (TR 2,100; TE 90).

onstrate the loss of the gray-white matter interface as the result of injury.[6, 20, 24] One of the biggest advantages of MRI over CT is its ability to perform direct multiplanar imaging in virtually any plane. As mentioned previously, this can allow us to eval- uate anatomy and alignment, particularly in areas such as the cervicothoracic junction where such an assessment is difficult to make.[14] Finally, MRI does not produce bone artifact or signal loss in the imaging of obese patients. Indeed, in obese pa-

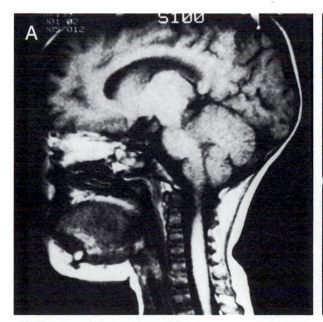
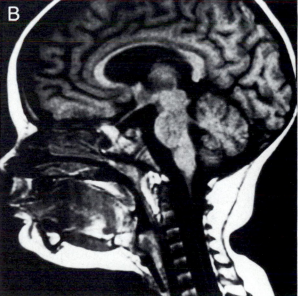

FIG 40–47.
Spinal cord hemorrhage and post-traumatic cord atrophy following suspected child abuse. **A,** a T1-weighted image of the head and cervical spine demonstrates marked hyperintensity of the cervical cord from C2 through T1, that is indicative of subacute hemor- rhage. **B,** a T1-weighted image 1 month later demonstrates pronounced atrophy of the cord. (Courtesy of Richard E. Latchaw, M.D., Presbyterian-University Hospital, Pittsburgh.)

tients, adipose tissue provides a favorable background for imaging the subarachnoid space and spinal cord.

There are disadvantages to imaging trauma patients by MRI. Primary among these is the fact that detailed skeletal anatomy cannot be obtained. However, plain films and CT should be relied upon in these instances. Patients who require life support equipment that is paramagnetic cannot be studied. This is becoming less of a problem with improved equipment that is magnet-compatible. Many trauma surgeons, on the other hand, are reluctant to have their patient within the gantry of a magnet where they may not be readily accessible for resuscitation. In some instances this may be overcome by the use of closed-circuit television monitoring of the patients in the gantry. Furthermore, it is possible for support personnel to remain in the room with the patient while the study is being performed since there is no ionizing radiation involved. Finally, patients with a cervical halo or other paramagnetic surgical implant may not be studied because of the artifacts produced. This problem is being overcome by the development of nonmagnetic halo material.[23]

In 1862, archeologist Edwin Smith discovered an Egyptian surgical papyrus dated at about 1600 B.C. at Thebes. This papyrus methodically discussed a number of surgical problems, among them vertebral injuries.[5] The method of diagnosis was purely clinical: "If thou examinist a man having a crushed vertebra in his neck . . . his falling head downward has caused that one vertebra crush into the next one . . . he is unconscious of his two arms and his two legs. . . ." In the 3600 years since that was written, we have come long way in diagnosing and treating vertebral injuries. CT and MRI are the diagnostic tools that allow us to look beyond the patient to establish the diagnosis.

REFERENCES

1. Acheson MB, Livingston RR, Richardson ML, et al: High-resolution CT scanning in the evaluation of cervical spine fractures: Comparison with plain film examinations. *AJR* 1987; 148:1179–1185.
2. Boechat MI: Spinal deformities and pseudofractures. *AJR* 1987; 148:97–98.
3. Brant-Zawadzki M, Jeffrey RB, Minagi H, et al: High resolution of thoracolumbar fractures. *AJNR* 1982; 3:69–74.
4. Brant-Zawadzki M, Miller EM, Federle MP: CT in the evaluation of spine trauma. *AJR* 1981; 136:369–375.
5. Breasted JH: *The Edwin Smith Papyrus.* Chicago, University of Chicago Press, 1930.
6. Chakeres DW, Flickinger F, Bresnahan JC, et al: MR imaging of acute spinal cord trauma. *AJNR* 1987; 8:5–10.
7. Daffner RH: *Imaging for Vertebral Trauma.* Baltimore, Aspen Publishers, Inc, 1988.
8. Daffner RH, Lupetin AR, Dash N, et al: MRI in the detection of malignant infiltration of bone marrow. *AJR* 1986; 146:353–358.
9. Denis F: Spinal instability as defined by the three-column spine concept in acute spinal trauma. *Clin Orthop* 1984; 189:65–76.
10. Denis F: The three-column spine and its significance in the classification of acute thoracolumbar spinal injuries. *Spine* 1983; 8:817–831.
11. Fielding JW, Stillwell WT, Chynn KY, et al: Use of computed tomography for the diagnosis of atlanto-axial rotatory fixation. *J Bone Joint Surg [Am]* 1978; 60:1102–1104.
12. Gehweiler JA Jr, Osborne RL Jr, Becker RF: *The Radiology of Vertebral Trauma.* Philadelphia, WB Saunders Co, 1980.
13. Gellad FE, Levine AM, Joslyn JN, et al: Pure thoracolumbar facet dislocation: Clinical features and CT appearance. *Radiology* 1986; 161:505–508.
14. Goldberg AL, Rothfus WE, Deeb ZL, et al: The impact of magnetic resonance on the diagnostic evaluation of acute cervicothoracic spinal trauma. *Skeletal Radiol,* 1988; 17:89–94.
15. Guerra J Jr, Garfin SR, Resnick D: Vertebral burst fractures: CT analysis of the retropulsed fragment. *Radiology* 1984; 153:769–772.
16. Hackney DB, Asato R, Joseph PM, et al: Hemorrhage and edema in acute spinal cord compression: Demonstration by MR imaging. *Radiology* 1986; 161:387–390.
17. Handel SF, Lee YY: Computed tomography of spinal fractures. *Radiol Clin North Am* 1981; 19:69–89.
18. Kaydoya S, Nakamura T, Kobayashi S, et al: Magnetic resonance imaging of acute spinal cord injury: Report of three cases. *Neuroradiology* 1987; 29:252–255.
19. Keene JS, Goletz TH, Lilleas F, et al: Diagnosis of vertebral fractures: A comparison of conventional radiography, conventional tomography and computed axial tomography. *J Bone Joint Surg [Am]* 1982; 64:586–594.
20. Kulkarni MV, McArdle CB, Kopanicky D, et al: Acute spinal cord injury: MR imaging at 1.5 T. *Radiology* 1987; 164:837–843.
21. Manaster BJ, Osborn AG: CT patterns of facet fracture dislocations in the thoracolumbar region. *AJNR* 1986; 7:1007–1012.
22. McArdle CB, Crofford MJ, Mirfakhraee M, et al:

Surface coil of MR of spinal trauma: Preliminary experience. *AJNR* 1986; 7:885–893.

23. McArdle CB, Wright JW, Prevost WJ, et al: MR imaging of the acutely injured patient with cervical traction. *Radiology* 1986; 159:273–274.

24. Mirvis SE, Geisler FH, Jelinek JJ, et al: Acute cervical spine trauma: Evaluation with 1.5-T MR imaging. *Radiology* 1988; 166:807–816.

25. Montana MA, Richardson ML, Kilcoyne RF, et al: CT of sacral injury. *Radiology* 1986; 161:499–503.

26. Morris RE, Hasso AN, Thompson JR, et al: Traumatic dural tears: CT diagnosis using metrizamide. *Radiology* 1984; 152:443–446.

27. O'Callaghan JP, Ullrich CG, Yuan HA, et al: CT of facet distraction in flexion injuries of the thoracolumbar spine: The "naked" facet. *AJNR* 1980; 1:97–102.

28. Petras AF, Sobel DF, Mani JR, et al: CT myelography in cervical nerve root avulsion. *J Comput Assist Tomogr* 1985; 9:275–279.

29. Post MJD, Green BA: The use of computed tomography in spinal trauma. *Radiol Clin North Am* 1983; 21:327–375.

30. Post MJD, Green BA, Quencer RM, et al: The value of computed tomography in spinal trauma. *Spine* 1982; 7:417–431.

31. Quencer RM, Sheldon JJ, Post MJD, et al: Magnetic resonance imaging of the chronically injured cervical spinal cord. *AJNR* 1986; 7:457–464.

32. Steppé R, Bellemans M, Boven F, et al: The value of computed tomography scanning in elusive fractures of the cervical spine. *Skeletal Radiol* 1981; 6:175–178.

33. Tarr RW, Drolshagen LF, Kerner TC, et al: MR imaging of recent spinal trauma. *J Comput Assist Tomogr* 1987; 11:412–417.

34. Wojcik WG, Edeiken-Monroe BS, Harris JH Jr: Three-dimensional computed tomography in acute cervical spine trauma: A preliminary report. *Skeletal Radiol* 1987; 16:261–269.

35. Yetkin Z, Osborn AG, Giles DS, et al: Uncovertebral and facet joint dislocations in cervical articular pillar fractures: CT evaluation. *AJNR* 1985; 6:633–637.

41

Post-traumatic Spinal Cord Cysts: Characterization With CT, MRI, and Sonography

Robert M. Quencer, M.D.

As a result of significant trauma to the spinal cord, specifically an episode that has left the patient with either an incomplete or complete paraplegia or quadriplegia, changes occur within the cord that may lead to the development of a spinal cord cyst. The pathologic abnormalities within the cord and adjacent subarachnoid space in concert with the dynamic alterations of cerebrospinal fluid (CSF) pulsations can lead to the formation of an expanding intramedullary cyst[1] months to years following the initial spine trauma. When these cysts form in areas of cord tissue that are nonviable or dissect into areas of cord tissue that are nonfunctional, new symptoms are unlikely; however, when a cyst expands into previously functional neural tissue, new and progressive symptoms may occur. Typically, these new symptoms include one or a combination of the following: pain, motor or sensory loss, dysesthesias, or hyperhidrosis. Such neurologic deterioration can be devastating, particularly when function of previously uninvolved spinal segment is lost or when an incomplete quadriplegic or paraplegic patient loses motor function.

Prior to the widespread use of water-soluble agents in conjunction with computed tomography (CT), the presence of an expanding intramedullary cyst in previously injured patients, although recognized as a possible sequela of cord trauma,[2] was not felt to be a very common occurrence. Little in terms of surgical intervention was offered to patients with worsening symptoms typical of a cord cyst because the means of detecting and characterizing such lesions were not available.

CT following the instillation of water-soluble contrast into the thecal sac offered the radiologist his first opportunity to visualize these intramedullary cysts in a clinically acceptable manner. It shortly became apparent that such cysts were far more common than previously presumed,[1, 3] and surgical procedures were then undertaken to decompress these cysts either by fenestration or more commonly by shunting the cysts via an indwelling catheter into the peritoneal cavity or into the distal subarachnoid space. Initially it was felt that a dense accumulation of contrast within the cord indicated the presence of a cyst, but as more cases were studied, it became apparent that false-positive examinations were possible (Fig 41–1). Specifically, contrast could accumulate within gliotic and scarred cord tissue that had been previously traumatized but that, at present, contained no shuntable cyst. There was in essence no absolutely reliable method of distinguishing myelomalacia from a cord cyst with preoperative neuroimaging. Only at surgery with intraoperative sonography[4] was this differentiation certain. Having to make such a distinction at the time of surgery and not prior to it was clearly undesirable. With the devel-

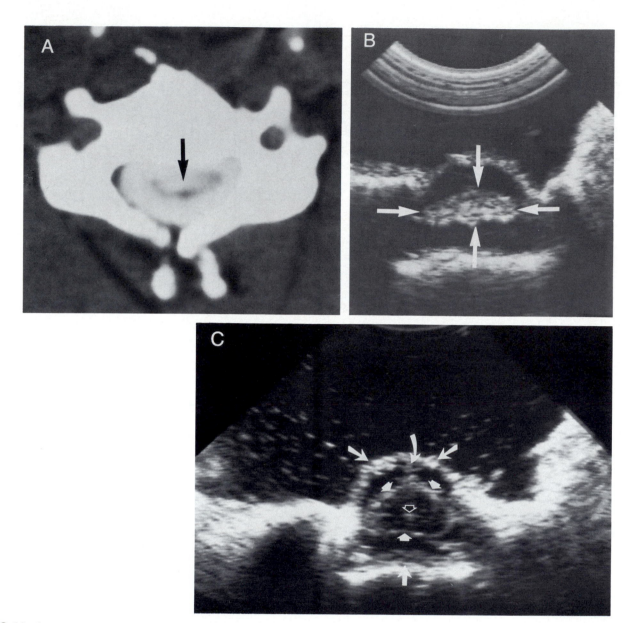

FIG 41–1.
Myelomalacia simulating an intramedullary cyst. At the C5 level, CT performed 5 hours following metrizamide myelography showed a dense collection of intramedullary contrast (*arrow* in **A**) within the spinal cord. The diagnosis of a post-traumatic spinal cord cyst in an atrophic cord was made in this quadriplegic patient who was injured 10 years prior to her present evaluation. Because of increasing spasticity, increasing upper extremity weakness, and hyperhidrosis, a C3–5 laminectomy was performed with the intent of shunting the cord cyst. At surgery, however, intraoperative sonography showed an atrophic cord (between the *arrows*) with no evidence of a cyst. Note the hyperechoic nature of the cord tissue,

absence of a central echo, and loss of the normal echogenic surface of the cord. These feelings are consistent with myelomalacia. The findings in **B** should be compared with a transverse sonogram of a normal cervical cord **(C).** Note in **C** the dorsal dura-arachnoid layer *(oblique arrows),* the dorsal arachnoid septations or septum posticum *(curved arrow),* the posterior border of the C5 vertebral body *(straight arrow),* the hyperechoic borders of the spinal cord *(solid arrowheads),* the central echo *(open arrowhead),* and the normal low-level echoes of the spinal cord. The cord can be seen surrounded by CSF. (Parts **A** and **B** from Quencer RM, Morse BM, Green BA, et al: *AJNR* 1984; 5:71–79. Used by permission.)

opment of magnetic resonance imaging (MRI), a new and more accurate method of determining the internal derangement of a traumatized cord became possible. MRI has therefore supplanted myelographic CT in the preoperative evaluation of the previously injured cord.

Before considering the changes observed with MRI in post-traumatic spinal cord cysts, it is important to understand the pathologic and physiologic abnormalities that occur in patients who have suffered cord injuries in the past because understanding these ongoing dynamic changes helps in the interpretation of MRI scans. Theories that have been espoused to explain the development of cord cysts include the sequela of hematomyelia and/or necrosis of myelomalacic spinal cord tissue. Myelomalacia as a consequence of the injury may result from ischemia or the action of enzymes released from disrupted cord tissue. Once an initial cavity within the cord is formed, progressive enlargement of the cyst in either a cephalad or caudal direction may occur as a result of intermittent, abnormally elevated increases in CSF pressure. In normal people, the rise and fall of CSF pressure results from everyday activities such as Valsalva maneuvers, straining, etc, and can be dissipated evenly throughout the entire subarachnoid space. However, in the spine-injured patient, these episodic rises of CSF pressure are focused directly at the level of the injured cord because of the surrounding scarring and adhesions within the subarachnoid space. The tethering of the cord by these adhesions to the adjacent dura also causes the neural tissue to be less pliable and therefore more suspectible to slight shearing or stretching forces. The additive effect of these repetitive CSF pulse waves can cause coalescence of what initially were small microcysts within an area of myelomalacia. Gradual expansion of the resultant cyst may ensue over months to years and cause extensive intramedullary cyst formation.[1] CSF enters these enlarging cysts from abnormally dilated Virchow-Robin spaces that connect the subarachnoid space to the cyst itself. Post-traumatic spinal cord cysts occur most commonly in expanded spinal cords, but they may also be seen in normal or atrophic-appearing cords. Why cord enlargement occurs in one case but not in another is not clear, but experience has shown that gradual expansion of these intramedullary cysts may occur in any sized cord. This dynamic information is worth bearing in mind because now with MRI techniques the motion of CSF flow or stagnation of fluid within these

cysts can be evaluated. Such imaging has an important effect on clinical management.

MRI of the previously injured cord may require a multilevel examination, particularly when an intramedullary cyst is found. These cysts may be quite large and extend well beyond the site of the original injury; therefore these patients are

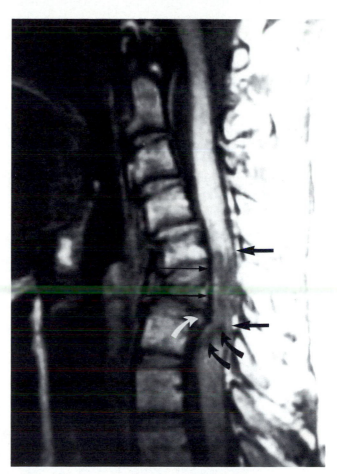

FIG 41–2.
Myelomalacia and a small adjacent cyst. Ten months prior to the present evaluation, this patient suffered a C6 burst fracture and a subluxation at the C6–7 level. MRI (600/20) shows two areas of signal hypointensity within the cord. The first is an ill-defined and heterogenous hypointensity extending from the lower C5 level ot the upper C7 level *(between the straight black arrows)*. These findings are consistent with myelomalacia. At the mid-C7 level a second area of signal hypointensity is seen *(curved black arrows)*. These features are consistent with a spinal cord cyst that would not be considered for decompression because of its small size. This cyst most likely formed in an area of microcystic myelomalacia. Note the compression of the myelomalacic cord *(long thin arrows)* from C5 through C6 by a combination of the subluxation and the retropulsed bone fragment at C6. A herniated disk at C6–7 is shown by the *curved white arrow*. In a patient with an incomplete cord injury or in a patient with partial root dysfunction with these findings, an anterior decompression with interbody fusion would be performed.

routinely examined first with a body coil (45-cm field of view) utilizing a short repetition time (TR), short echo time (TE) pulse sequence. This immediately gives an indication of whether a multilevel examination will be necessary. Surface-coil imaging for better detail is then performed at all appropriate levels. Our protocol then depends on what the initial sagittal T1-weighted images demonstrate. If there is no evidence of an intramedullary cyst, sagittal surface-coil T2-weighted images utilizing motion-compensating gradients and T1-weighted images are obtained. These are then supplemented by either T1-weighted images or gradient-echo images in the axial plane. If on the other hand the initial T1-weighted image demonstrates a well-defined, low density area within the cord, two sets of sagittal T2-weighted images are performed, first with motion-compensating gradients to suppress motion artifacts and second as a single-echo T2 study in which no effort is made to suppress CSF motion. The latter is done in order

to assess the possibility of fluid movement or turbulence within these cysts.

The evolution of MRI signal abnormalities arising from the injured cord over a period of months to years is understood best in light of the pathophysiologic and dynamic changes described above. The need to distinguish between a myelomalacic spinal cord, i.e., one that contains scarring, neuronal degeneration, and microcystic formation, from one that contains a shuntable cyst is crucial. The former is clearly not a surgical lesion, whereas the latter may be, providing it can explain the patient's present neurologic status. To begin with, virtually all patients who have had serious cord injuries with permanent sequelae will demonstrate abnormal signals on T1 and/or T2 images. In myelomalacia as with most pathologic processes, there is prolongation of the T1 and T2 relaxation times that results in a variable degree of hypointensity on T1-weighted images and a hyperintense signal on T2-weighted images. As Figures 41–2

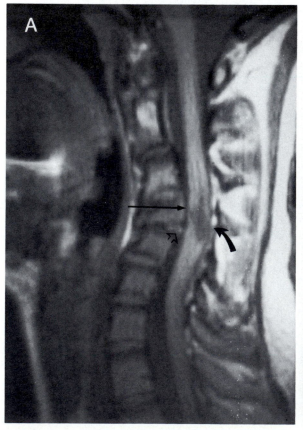 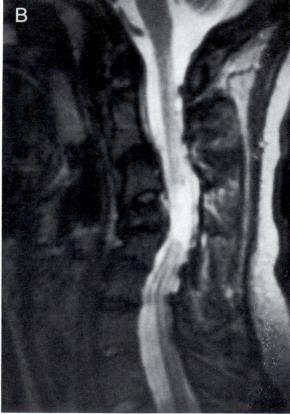

FIG 41–3.
Myelomalacia. **A,** a T1-weighted image (691/20) shows an area of ill-defined diminished intensity *(curved arrow)* consistent with myelomalacia at the level of the C4 fracture/dislocation. Cord compression by the retropulsed bone at C4 is indicated by the *long arrow*. Herniated disk material at C4–5 is also present *(open arrow)*. An artifactual linear hyperintensity is identified within the cord at the C3 level directly above the area of myelomalacia. **B,** a T2-weighted image (2,300/100) shows that the area of myelomalacia shown in **A** is now hyperintense. A nonpulsatile cyst could have a similar appearance on T2-weighted images, so the ill-defined hypointensity seen in **A** is the finding that favors the diagnosis of myelomalacia.

and 41–3 illustrate, myelomalacia involves a relatively short segment of the cord directly adjacent to the level of prior injury. In addition, although hypointensity of the area is present, it is less hypointense than CSF, and a distinct interface with surrounding normal cord is not present. Within or adjacent to areas of myelomalacia, early formation of a cord cyst can be seen (Fig 41–2). The distinction between a small (1 cm or less) nonpulsatile cyst from an area of myelomalacia is of limited clinical importance because cysts of that small a size are not shunted and patients with myelomalacia alone are not surgical candidates.

Post-traumatic spinal cord cysts can vary in size[5] from small collections that may (Fig 41–4) or may not cause cord expansion to large multilevel cysts (Figs 41–5 to 41–9). Small cysts (<2 cm) are always located at the level of prior trauma, whereas the multilevel cysts can extend inferiorly (Fig 41–5 to 41–7), superiorly (Fig 41–9), or both inferiorly and superiorly (Fig 41–8) from the level of injury. As opposed to myelomalacia, spinal cord

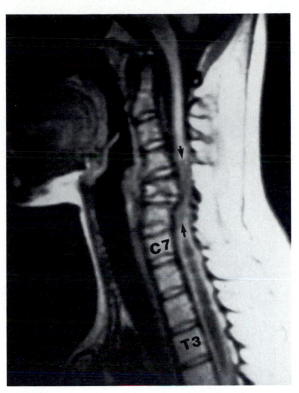

FIG 41–5.
Myelomalacia and a spinal cord cyst. On a T1-weighted image (800/26) an old fracture of C5 with cord compression and an ill-defined moderately hypointense signal from C4 to C6 *(between the arrows)* are seen. This finding is consistent with myelomalacia. From C7 to T4, however, the signal from within the cord is more hypointense, and the edges of the hypointensity are well defined. Note also the expansion of the cord in the upper thoracic area and the small intracystic septations indicative of fibroglial scarring. These findings plus the fact that the latter abnormality extends over many levels are consistent with a cord cyst. Under the proper clinical circumstances, for example, progressive loss of function is an incomplete quadriplegia, such a cyst may be shunted even though it is present below the injury level. Likewise, if nerve root symptoms are present, delayed bony decompression via an anterior approach (C5 corpectomy and a C4 to C6 interbody fusion) may help in restoring some neurologic function, despite the fact that the injury is chronic.

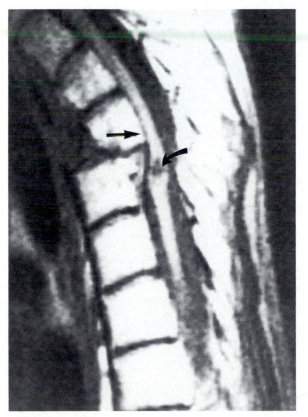

FIG 41–4.
Small intramedullary cyst. MRI of the thoracic spine (500/30) shows an old fracture/subluxation at the T3–4 level, cord compression at T3 *(straight arrow),* and a small intramedullary cyst at T4 *(curved arrow).* Cysts of this size are not shunted despite the fact that local cord expansion may be present, as in this case.

cysts on T1-weighted images offer a sharp interface with the normal surrounding cord tissue and a markedly hypointense (CSF equivalent) signal. It is important to remember, however, that a patient may have radiologic evidence of a cord cyst but may have no clinical evidence of neurologic deterioration. Close correlation between the MRI findings and the patient's clinical status is therefore necessary. In addition, when a cord cyst is found in a patient with no progressive deficit and the cyst is of relatively small size, surgery may not be indicated, but clinical follow-up and re-evaluation with MRI is warranted.

We now increasingly rely on MRI evidence of

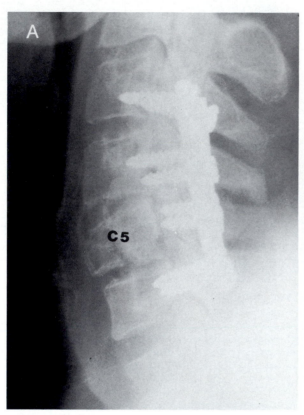

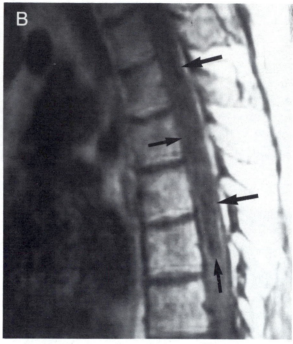

FIG 41–6.
Post-traumatic spinal cord cyst. Even with the availability of MRI, myelographic CT may occasionally be helpful. In this incomplete quadriplegic patient who had suffered a C5 fracture/subluxation, large bilateral metallic fusion plates and screws **(A)** rendered MRI in this area valueless. In the upper to midthoracic spine, however, a T1-weighted image (700/20) showed a well-defined intramedullary cyst (*between the arrows* in **B**). **C–H** *(facing page),* a T2-weighted image (2,200/80) at T4 **(C)** performed with motion-compensating gradients shows the hyperintense cyst (*curved arrow* in **C**) within the cord. A thin remnant of cord tissue is identified between the cyst and the surrounding CSF. Because the upper end of the cyst could not be identified with MRI, myelographic CT was performed at C7 **(D)** and showed a dense concentration of water-soluble contrast within the cord (*arrows* in **D**). Between these two collections of contrast is a probable intracystic scar. It was decided to perform a laminectomy at the lower end of the cyst and

shunt the cyst. At T4, longitudinal **(E)** and transverse **(F)** views show a large spinal cord cyst (*arrows* in **E** and **F**). Following a dorsal myelotomy at T4, a multihole flexible-shunt catheter was advanced into the cyst, and successful collapse of the thoracic portion of the cyst resulted **(G).** In **G,** the shunt catheter can be seen within the dorsal subarachnoid space (*between the white arrows*), and the point at which the catheter enters the cord is shown *between the arrowheads.* Cephalad to that the catheter is seen (*curved arrows*) within the collapsed cord. The catheter seen in **G** was advanced within the cord to the C6 level, and intraoperative sonography at that level **(H)** showed the tip of the catheter (*curved arrow* in **H**) within a multiloculated cyst. Note also the ventral subarachnoid cyst *(open arrows)* cephalad to the intramedullary cyst. Further maneuvers of the catheter resulted in successful decompression of the spinal cord cyst; however, it was decided not to surgically approach the subarachnoid cyst.

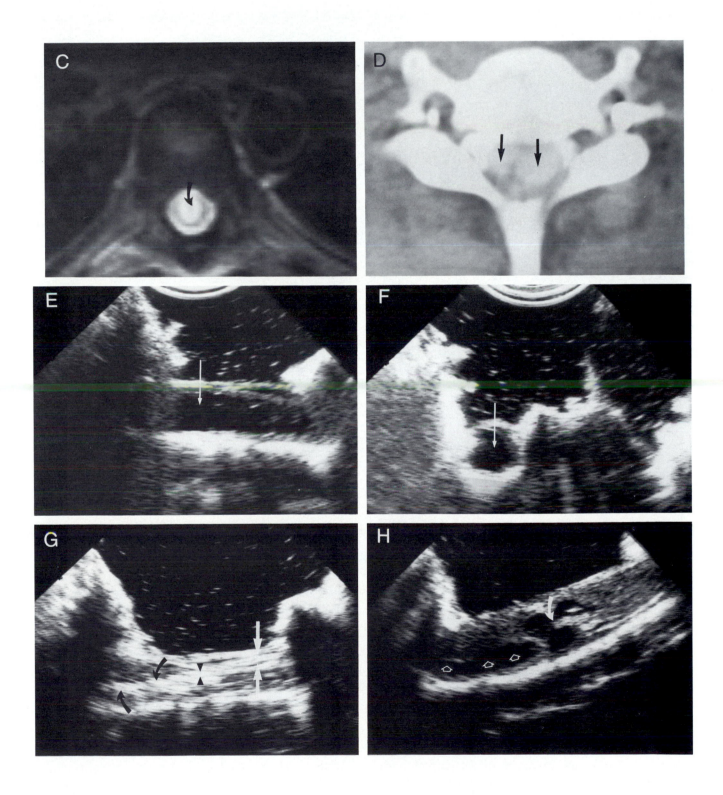

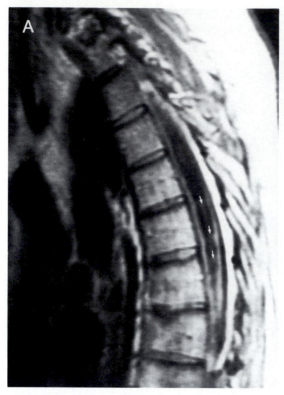

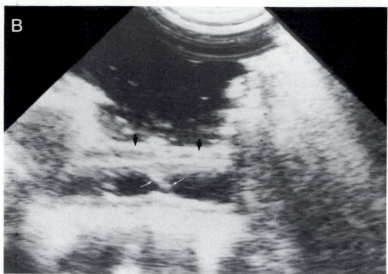

FIG 41–7.
Septated intramedullary cyst. A post-traumatic spinal cord cyst extending inferiorly from an old cervical injury is clearly seen on a T1-weighted image **(A).** Within the cyst are faintly visualized linear structures that cross the cyst at multiple levels (*arrows* in **A**). Following a thoracic laminectomy at the level of the lower end of the cyst, intraoperative sonography **(B)** shows a prominant fibroglial scar traversing the cord cyst from anterior to posterior (*white arrows* in **B**). Identification of such transcystic scarring is important because these scars may have to be broken in order to achieve total cyst decompression. Following this study the dura was opened (note the intact dura—*black arrows* in **B**), a myelotomy was performed and a shunt catheter advanced into the cyst. Successful cyst decompression was achieved.

CSF flow or turbulence within the cord to diagnose an expanding spinal cord cyst. Preliminary results indicate that when significant hypointensity within the cord cyst is seen on routine T2-weighted images without motion suppression, then a stronger case for shunting such cysts can be made (Fig 41–9) because active expansion of the cyst may be occurring. Both cardiac-gated T2 images of the spine and T2 images of the spine obtained with the use of motion-compensating gradients suppress fluid motion in these cysts[6] (Fig 41–9,B), which makes the evaluation of possible cyst enlargement difficult. It is important, therefore, to supplement such examinations with routine T2 images (Fig 41–9,C) in which just a *single* echo is used since the second echo of a symmetrical dual-echo sequence rephases the effects of constant velocity.[7] Recently we have been using cardiac-gated cine-MRI on a high–field strength system (1.5-Tesla Picker Vista) in which eight repetitive sections, each 6 mm thick, are obtained through the midsagittal plane of the spinal cord. Typically, a TR of approximately 850 ms is used, the TE is 18 ms, and the flip angle is 9 degrees. The images are viewed on the monitor in a rapid-sequence mode, and abnormal fluid flow, including CSF turbulence, can be seen. This real-time mode of cord and cyst evaluation appears better than the static gradient-echo images, which have been reported to be useful in the evaluation of nonneoplastic spinal cord cysts.[8] In concert with the clinical manifestations, these findings assist in determining whether a cyst to subarachnoid space shunt is indicated.

The presence of metallic clips in a patient's spine who has been operated on in the distant past for a spinal injury should not dissuade one from using MRI. The information obtained from such a study surpasses that obtained from CT, and frequently the artifacts caused by metal obscure only a small area of the spinal cord, which allows one to assess the cord above and below the injury and prior surgical site. In these cases, a cyst may be identified (Fig 41–10), and a decision on surgery can then be made.

Once the decision is made to operate on a post-traumatic cord cyst, intraoperative sonography should always be used. This technique allows exact location of the cyst (Figs 41–6 and 41–7), and such localization prior to opening of the dura is im-

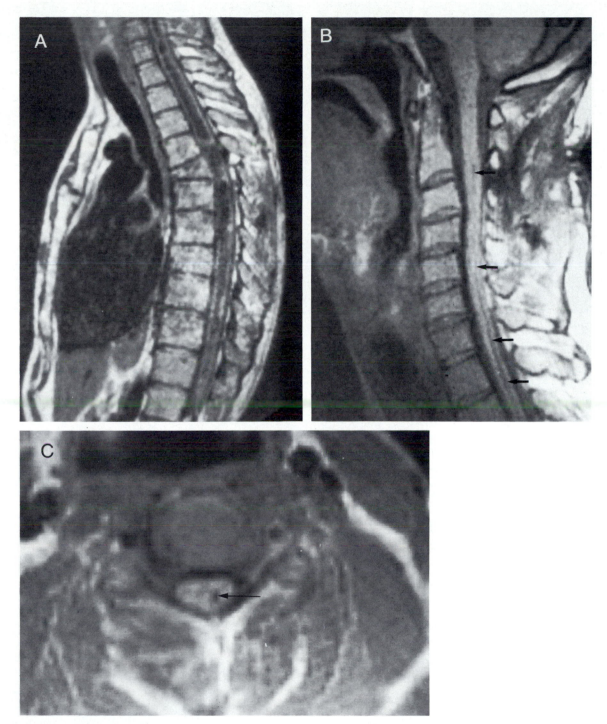

FIG 41–8.

Preshunting and postshunting of a cord cyst. **A,** T1-weighted MRI shows a cord cyst extending above and below the fracture at the T4 level. A low thoracic laminectomy was performed, and a shunt catheter was put into the cyst and advanced the entire length of the cord to the upper end of the cyst (to C2). Two months later the status of the cyst was checked by repeat MRI **(B and C),** and the study revealed no evidence of a significant residual cord cyst. The linear hypointensity within the cord on the sagittal T1 image **(B)** represents a combination of the shunt catheter and a small amount of fluid around the catheter (*arrows* in **B**). The catheter is better seen on the axial T1-weighted image **(C)** as a well-defined, markedly hypointense structure within the cord (*arrow* in **C**).

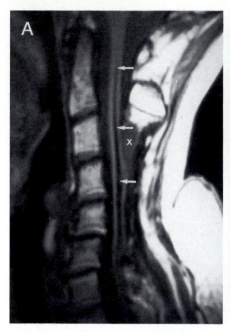
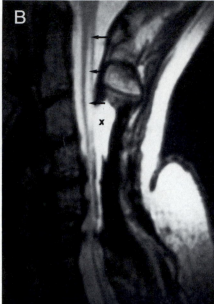
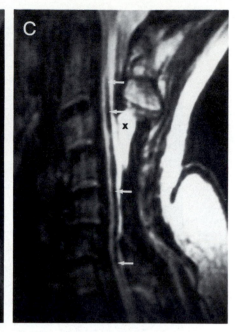

FIG 41–9.

Dephasing of cyst fluid within a post-traumatic cyst. This patient underwent a prior C3 through C6 laminectomy for a C5–6 subluxation. Because of progressive neurologic symptoms, MRI was performed and on a T1-weighted image (700/20) showed a well-defined cyst (*arrows* in **A**) within a relatively atrophic cord. T2-weighted images (2,000/100) were performed first with motion-compensating gradients **(B)** and then without these gradients **(C).**

B, note the hyperintense signal *(arrows)* in the cord extending to the C1 level. **C,** despite the use of the same TR and TE as in **B,** the cyst is hypointense, which indicates the presence of fluid flow and turbulence within the cyst. This finding indicates the probability of active cyst enlargement. The lower end of the cyst is at C7, and the upper end of the cyst is at C1. A postoperative fluid-filled "pseudomeningocoele" is indicated by an *X* in **A, B,** and **C.**

FIG 41–10.

Intramedullary cyst partially obscured by metallic artifacts. Valuable information may be obtained on MRI despite the presence of metallic artifacts as shown in this patient. Here an old fracture of T12 is present, and artifacts from prior surgical intervention posterior to the fractured vertebral body are seen. Nonetheless, an intramedullary cyst extending above and below T12 *(arrows)* that is associated with cord expansion can be identified.

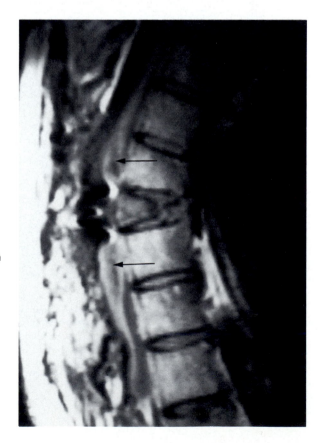

portant because a myelotomy in exactly the right position on the dorsal cord surface can then be performed. Identification of other unsuspected abnormalities (Fig 41–6,H) and confirmation of proper cyst decompression prior to surgical closure (Fig 41–6,G) are also important contributions of this technique. Fibroglial scars, which we have found in the majority of our cases, are seen by both MRI and intraoperative sonography (Fig 41–7). These transcystic fibroglial remnants divide the cyst into loculated compartments, and they can be the cause of inadequately decompressed cysts following the insertion of a shunt catheter. We have found that maneuvering the catheter may be necessary to break up these scars and convert a multiloculated cyst (Fig 41–6,H) into a single shuntable cyst. Without the use of intraoperative sonography, this type of information cannot be assessed by the surgeon at the time of the surgery. Only with ultrasound can alterations in the internal structure of the cord such as these be appreciated. Knowledge of the normal sonographic anatomy of the spinal canal and cord is necessary before this technique can be used effectively.[9] The presence of a central echo, a hyperechoic cord surface, low-level echoes from the cord, and pulsations of the CSF and cord are all features of a normal spinal cord. Myelomalacia and small spinal cord cysts, which can frequently have similar appearances on myelographic CT and occasionally on MRI, can easily be distinguished from each other via sonography. The former is associated with a hyperechoic atrophic cord (Fig 41–1,B), while cord cysts are easily identified as intramedullary anechoic areas (Figs 41–6 and 41–7).

Evaluation of patients who have had their cysts shunted should include postoperative MRI. This will ensure that the catheter is functioning properly and that the fluid is not reaccumulating in the cord cyst (Figs 41–8,B C). Typically, a slitlike remnant of the cyst is seen, which confirms proper catheter functioning, and this type of result usually correlates with an improvement in the patient's neurologic function. When a cord cyst completely collapses, the catheter can be seen as a small area of nearly complete signal void (Fig 41–8,C). The catheter is best seen in cross section (axial plane) so that partial volume averaging does not obscure the catheter.

In conclusion, the use of MRI is now indicated in all patients who have in the past suffered severe spinal cord injury and now present with increasing neurologic signs and symptoms. Flow-sensitive MRI studies give an insight into the flow dynamics of these cysts and help explain their expansion over time. Intraoperative ultrasound is an indispensible tool for characterizing these cysts and for ensuring proper cyst decompression following shunt catheter insertion. As a result of MRI evaluation preoperatively and sonography intraoperatively, these unfortunate patients may see their neurologic deterioration arrested and their rehabilitation quickened.

REFERENCES

1. Quencer RM, Green BA, Eismont FJ: Posttraumatic spinal cord cysts: Clinical features and characterization with metrizamide computed tomography *Radiology* 1983; 146:415–423.
2. Barnett HJM, Jousse AT: Syringomyelia as a late sequel to traumatic paraplegia and quadriplegia—clinical features, in Barnett HJM, Foster JB, Hudgson P (eds): *Major Problems in Neurology, Syringomyelia*, vol 1. London, WB Saunders Co, 1973, pp 129–153.
3. Seibert CE, Dreisbach JN, Swanson WB, et al: Progressive post-traumatic cystic myelopathy. *AJNR* 1981; 2:115–119.
4. Quencer RM, Morse BM, Green BA, et al: Intraoperative spinal sonography: Adjunct to metrizamide CT in the assessment and surgical decompression of post-traumatic spinal cord cysts. *AJNR* 1984; 5:71–79.
5. Quencer RM, Sheldon JJ, Post MJD, et al: Magnetic resonance imaging of the chronically injured cervical spinal cord. *AJNR* 1986; 7:457–464.
6. Hinks RS, Quencer RM: Motion artifacts in brain and spine MR. *Radiol Clin North Am* 1988; 26:737–743.
7. Quencer RM, Hinks RS, Pattany PH, et al: Improved MR imaging of the brain by using compensating gradients to suppress motion induced artifacts. *AJNR* 1988; 9:431–438.
8. Enzmann DR, O'Donohue J, Rubin JB, et al: CSF pulsations within non-neoplastic spinal cord cysts. *AJNR* 1987; 8:517–525.
9. Quencer RM, Morse BM: Normal intraoperative spinal sonography. *AJNR* 1984; 5:501–505; *AJR* 1984; 6:1301–1305.

42

Congenital Anomalies of the Spine and Spinal Cord

Charles R. Fitz, M.D.

IMAGING TECHNIQUES

Magnetic resonance imaging (MRI), the newest entry for neurodiagnosis, has replaced computed tomography (CT) and CT myelography (CTM) as the definitive procedure for spinal region anomalies.[1, 2] The sagittal view, in particular, is most valuable in that it shows a myelogram-like portrait that includes both cerebrospinal fluid (CSF) and tissues without the need for intrathecal contrast. CT continues to be better (in most cases) for bone detail. Adhesions and tethering are more accurately seen or excluded when contrast surrounds the cord, and here the combination of myelography and axial CT may give the best results even though MRI is likely to be performed in place of CT.

Bony anomalies that run in the axis of the CT image plane such as disk space narrowing or nonfusion of the odontoid are difficult to see in the axial CT image. For such abnormalities, plain films or even conventional sagittal or coronal tomography may be preferable.

Plain films are still extremely useful in the evaluation of anomalies. Spina bifida, canal widening, and abnormal vertebrae are all quickly seen on plain films. In infants and small children, it is often hard to identify which is the lowest lumbar vertebral level on sagittal MRI without plain films.

For MRI, CT, or myelography in children up to the ages of 7 or 8 years, anesthesia or sedation is likely to be needed. One does not want to prolong anesthesia, and sedation wears off, so the ethical radiologist must, in the best interest of the child, sometimes try for the best reasonable study rather than the ideal study. Even the older child, with whom one is less concerned about time, may rebel when you have exceeded his tolerance for cooperation.

Technical Aspects of CT

Very often, high-detail CT is another name for high radiation dose. In most cases, this is not needed when dealing with the high-contrast anatomy of the bony spine and water-soluble filled subarachnoid space (Fig 42–1). While there are no proved harmful effects to doses of diagnostic radiation, it is common sense to keep the dose as low as possible in a child.

When using water-soluble contrast or examining the bone, the target reconstruction technique (such as the General Electric Review) further enhances the sharpness of interfaces and clearly delineates small structures. Such techniques should be used routinely.

Direct coronal or sagittal imaging can be done in infants, but in general MRI is much better than any CT image in these planes.

NORMAL ANATOMY

Computed Tomography

Axial CT is ideally suited to reveal the size and ossification of the *child's* bony spinal canal.[3] In the

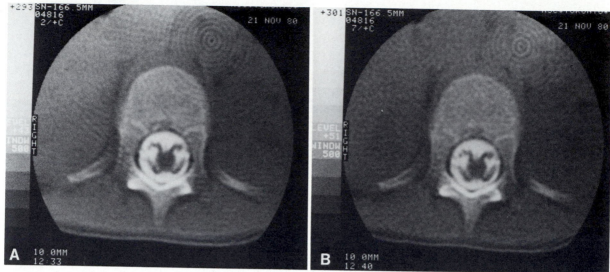

FIG 42–1.
Radiation dose. **A,** 55-mR slice CT through a normal conus after myelography. **B,** repeat slice using 200 mR. Both images have had target reconstruction that has caused a slight ring artifact. Al-though the lower radiation dose image is minimally more grainy, there is no information lost in this high-contrast image.

infant, the small size of the patient means less anatomic detail than in the older child in most scanners, but it is nonetheless sufficient for clearly revealing the contour and ossification centers of the various portions of the spine.

In spite of the lesser thickness of the bone relative to the older child and adult, visualization of the cord is quite unreliable without intrathecal contrast, with the exception of the C1 level. In the infant, the bony canal is straighter than in the older child, which makes the cord more central within the canal throughout its length. The cord takes a relatively straight course within the canal so that as the child grows the cord moves closer to the inside of each curve, which leaves it posterior in the midcervical, anterior in the upper and midthoracic, and again posterior in the lumbar area.

In early infancy, the posterior elements of the bony canal are open but curve so that if a line were drawn to continue the arc of the bone, it would complete a circle. The vertebral bodies at each level are small relative to the size of the canal and in comparison to the size of the adult. The vertebral bodies grow proportionately more in childhood than does the spinal canal diameter. In infancy, the spinal canal is relatively round, although variations are visible in each area.

In the newborn, both the anterior arch of C1 and the odontoid may have one or two ossification centers that are unfused, as are the posterior arches, which also have open neurocentral junctions (Fig 42–2). The arches are usually closed by

2 to 3 years of age but may remain open as a normal variant, especially at C1.

The neurocentral synchondroses begin to fuse at 2 years of age in the cervical region, with the line of fusion being visible into later childhood. Fusion of the odontoid to its base and the height of

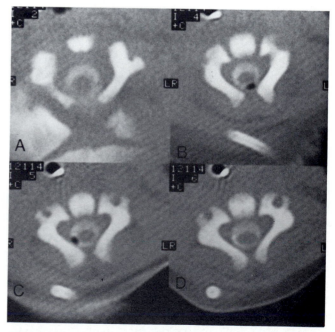

FIG 42–2.
Normal newborn cervical spine. **A,** C1. **B–D,** C2. The slices are 5 mm thick. Both the anterior ossification center of C1 and the odontoid are unfused to the laminae, which are in turn open posteriorly. A small bubble of air is present in the subarachnoid space. A shunt tube courses through the posterior subcutaneous tissue.

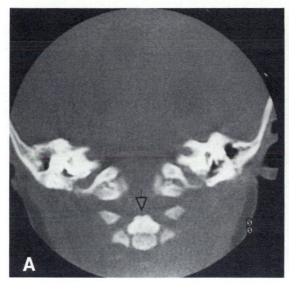

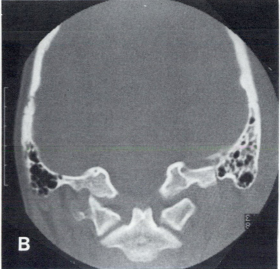

FIG 42–3.
Odontoid process, CT coronal view. **A,** in a 3-month-old child, the odontoid *(arrow)* is unfused to its base or the laminae. The separa-tion of the base and odontoid was not visible in axial slices. **B,** complete fusion of the odontoid to its base in an 8-year-old child.

the process itself are difficult to ascertain in infancy on axial CT, but they are clearly visible on coronal head sections in which the upper cervical spine is also extended into the coronal plane (Fig 42–3). The spinous processes of the cervical spine are not visible until about 2 years of age. Until the fusion of the posterior elements, the cervical canal is often somewhat triangular in shape, slowly progressing to the ovoid shape of later childhood and adulthood.

The cervical cord cross section is also slightly rounder in infancy than in the older child and shows less change with growth than do the vertebral bodies and the bony canal. With intrathecal contrast, the cord is seen to be round at C1. The remainder of the cervical cord is nearly round during the first year but becomes more ovoid, greater in the transverse diameter, by the end of the first year (Fig 42–4). Dorsal and ventral rootlets are visible, especially with 5-mm-thick slices. In the first few

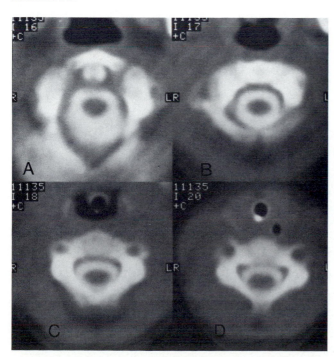

FIG 42–4.
Normal cervical cord and spine in a 1½-year-old boy. **A–D,** sequential slices from C1 through C4. The cord shape is slightly more ovoid than in Figure 42–2, the cord and subarachnoid space take a larger volume of the canal, and the canal is less triangular in shape than in Figure 42–2.

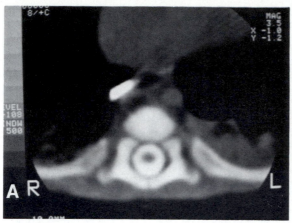
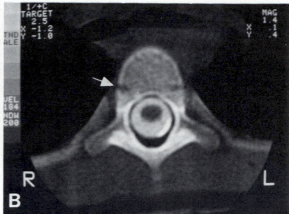

FIG 42–5.
Normal midthoracic spine and cord on CTM. **A,** 3-month-old child. **B,** 2½-year-old child. The cords are approximately equal in shape, with the younger patient having a slightly smaller and more centrally placed cord. In **A,** the neurocentral synchondroses are un-

fused. Although in close approximation, the laminae are also posteriorly unfused. In **B,** a spinous process is visible. A visible notch remains at the fusing neurocentral synchondroses *(arrow).* The bony canal is proportionately larger in the sagittal direction in **B.**

months of life, the cord is less than 50% of the spine diameter. Later, it is slightly greater than 50% of the entire transverse diameter of the bony canal in the midcervical region. As the cord approaches the thoracic level, it again becomes round.

The thoracic cord is nearly uniform in size and shape throughout its length from infancy onward. In both absolute size and size relative to the surrounding subarachnoid space and bony canal, it is smaller than the cervical cord. It occupies approximately one third of the transverse diameter of the

subarachnoid space and approximately one quarter of the transverse diameter of the canal (Fig 42–5) and enlarges slightly with growth.

The thoracic bony canal is round to slightly ovoid in outline, being largest anteroposteriorly (AP). Even in early infancy, the posterior arches approximate themselves closely at the site of the future spinous processes. With growth, both the pedicles and the laminae expand in equal proportions.

The lumbar canal is rounder in infancy than in the older child, but even in infancy becomes more

FIG 42–6.
Normal lumbosacral canal on CTM in a 1-month-old child. **A–C,** lower lumbar levels below the tip of the conus. **D,** upper sacral canal. The canal gradually becomes more triangular in cross section as it approaches the sacrum. As visible in **D,** the normal infant sacral canal is open posteriorly.

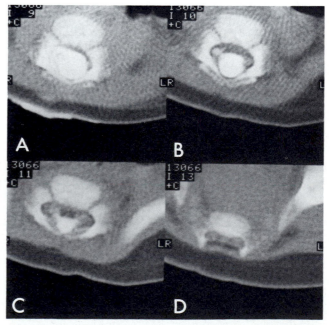

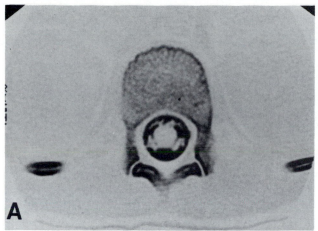
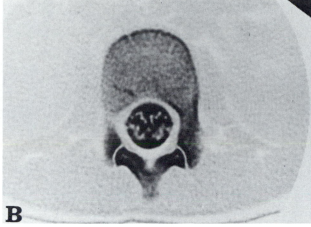

FIG 42–7.
Normal conus and cauda equina on CTM, reversed gray scale. **A,** at L1 the conus is widest. Dorsal and ventral nerve roots are visible as the exit from the conus. **B,** at the next lower vertebral body level, the small central filum is surrounded by nerve roots in a symmetrical pattern.

triangular further caudally, being wider across its base and shorter sagittally (Fig 42–6). The cord is round and widest at the T12–L1 conus expansion and tapers to the central filum, which is the size of the nerve roots that surround it in a symmetrical pattern in the upper canal (Fig 42–7).

The ring apophyses that are visible on plain-film radiographs in later childhood are not easily seen on the routine 5- or 10-mm CT slices. Because the apophyses are so close to the vertebral bodies, the space between them is averaged into the image.

NORMAL ANATOMY

Magnetic Resonance Imaging

The axial cord anatomy of CT is duplicated by MRI. Motion and pulsation artifacts, especially on T2 images, may mean that images are less crisp

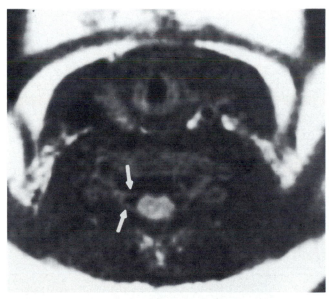

FIG 42–8.
Cervical cord in a 1-month-old infant. An axial T1 MR section shows the dorsal and ventral nerve roots unusually well *(arrows).* The outer white matter has higher signal. The apparent signal differences within the central gray matter are artifactual. The cord appears to be relatively larger within the canal than that shown by the equivalent CT of Figure 42–2 of another infant.

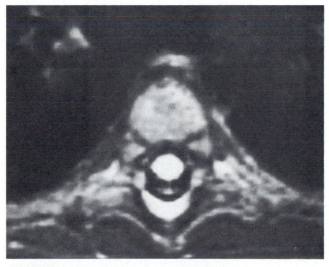

FIG 42–9.
Thoracic cord in a 14-month old. A proton-density MR image TR 2,000, TE 45 shows much of the CSF surrounding the cord still black due to pulsation artifacts. The cord is rounder than in the cervical region.

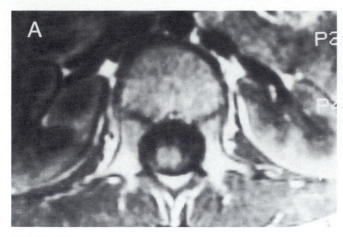

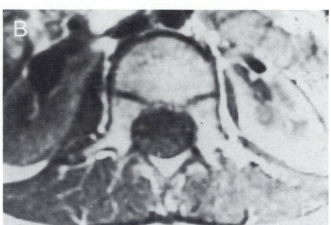

FIG 42–10.
Lumbar cord and nerve roots on MRI in a 7-year-old. **A,** an axial T1 slice through the conus shows the radiating dorsal and ventral nerve roots very well. **B,** 2 cm lower, the nerve roots can be seen within the canal, but the well-defined symmetrical pattern of CT (Fig 42–7,B) is not as clear, and the nerve root diameters look less uniform.

than on CT (Figs 42–8 and 42–9). Both dura and cortical bone have an identical lack of signal. While the conus is well seen, the nerve roots below the conus are less distinct (Fig 42–10).

Sagittal and coronal anatomy is superior to true or reconstructed CT (Fig 42–11). Because there is often a slight curve or obliquity to the spine simply from positioning, a single sagittal slice often does not identify the true midplane of the cord for any great length. Apparent changes in cord diameter must be confirmed by axial slices or obliquely angled sagittal images planned from coronal views.

The conus tip is sometimes best seen on sagittal views, sometimes with coronal ones. Axial slices are usually not necessary to confirm the level. The cauda equina is often poorly defined on sagittal images, just as the nerves are more poorly seen on lateral than AP myelography.

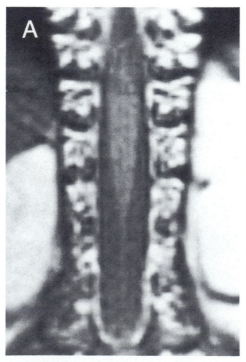

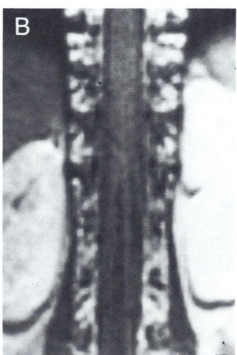

FIG 42–11.
Conus in a coronal MRI projection in a 13-month-old. **A,** the conus tip is especially well seen, with the filum being separately visible. **B,** 3 mm anteriorly, the ventral nerve roots are well seen. The conus artifactually appears to end higher.

BONY ANOMALIES

The craniovertebral junction is a common site for bony anomalies. As noted, fusions of C1 to the occiput or dens anomalies without displacement are not ideally seen on CT in the axial plane. Examination in the coronal plane or sagittal reformations may be extremely helpful in such cases (Fig 42–12).

Many isolated abnormalities such as hypoplasia of the arch or pedicle of C1 or other cervical level are of minor consequence. They are often discovered incidentally to other symptoms,[4] although a "syndrome" of pain with weakness or numbness is described.[5] Because such absence of-

ten brings up the question of erosion from tumor, CT is performed and is definitive in its findings. The lack of pedicle or arch is well demonstrated along with hypertrophy of the adjacent or contralateral structures that bear the added stress (Fig 42–13).[6, 7]

The Klippel-Feil anomaly with multiple cervical fusions probably does not warrant investigation by CT if asymptomatic. While CT may reveal unsuspected aspects of the condition (Fig 42–14), it is often less revealing than plain-film examination.

Bony anomalies without dysraphism are often discovered incidentally or may be a cause of scoliosis. While the anomalies themselves may not be significant, they should be a flag to do a complete

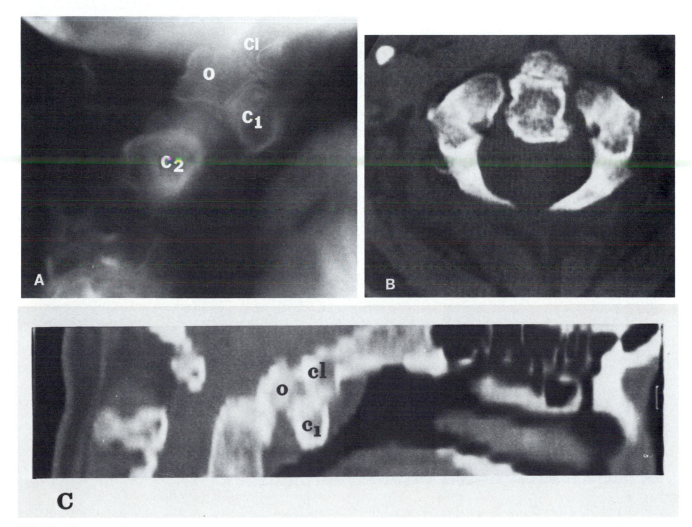

FIG 42–12.
Os odontoideum. **A,** lateral tomography demonstrates the anatomy. The os *(O)* is the odontoid ossification center that fails to fuse to the body of C2 *(C2)*. There is a bony mound, or "hillock deformity," along the superior margin of C2. The os is fused to both the anterior arch of C1, *(C1)* and the clivus *(Cl)*. **B,** an axial CT slice through C1 does not give a true appreciation of the degree of ca-

nal narrowing at this level. **C,** sagittal CT reformation is comparable to plain tomography **(A)** in anatomic clarity and shows the canal narrowing and soft-tissue compromise to good advantage (*o* = os; *c1* = C1; *cl* = clivus). (Courtesy of Richard E. Latchaw, M.D, University of Pittsburgh.)

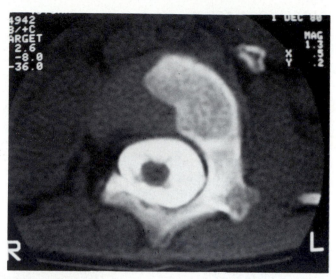

FIG 42–13.
Absent pedicle in a 3-year-old boy. CTM shows an absent right pedicle, hemivertebrae, and thickening of the left pedicle in compensation. The cord is asymmetrically positioned to the right because of mild scoliosis.

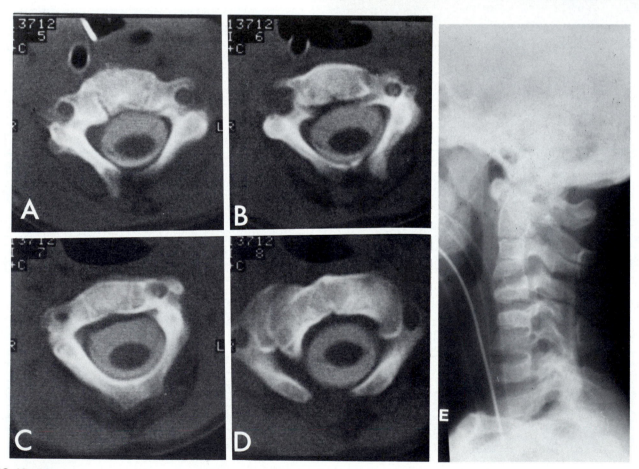

FIG 42–14.
Klippel-Feil anomaly. Axial CTM slices at C4 **(A)**, C3 **(B** and **C),** and **C1–2 (D)** show posterior spina bifida, irregularity of the verte- bral bodies, and "rotation" of C2 on C1. **E,** a lateral plain film shows fusion of C2 through C4 that is not visible on CT.

neurologic examination, which may discover minimal deficits that then are reasons to pursue further studies.

Basilar invagination is an uncommon anomaly of the craniocervical junction. Although multiple methods have been devised for measuring basilar invagination, McRae,[8] the originator of one of these, states they must be used with care. A measured mild invagination without clinical symptoms probably means nothing.

In childhood, the causes of basilar invagination are few. Although the entity is said to occur in 25% of patients with Chiari malformation,[9] it is not a significant cause of childhood symptoms in the author's experience. It is also said to be common among the Dutch.[10] Rare symptomatic diseases such as osteogenesis imperfecta, cleidocranial dysostosis, and acro-osteolysis may cause a significant amount of basilar impression. Such systemic diseases are accompanied by other signs. The degree of a marked basilar impression is not easily seen on plain films because it is hidden by the skull base itself. Either plain-film tomography or CT will demonstrate the amount of disease well, although slices no less than 3 mm apart are needed for any reconstruction of the CT image in a sagittal or coronal plane (Fig 42–15). MRI is preferable for such examinations since it gives adequate bony contrast and excellent detail of the neural structures.

DYSRAPHIC STATES

Tethered Conus

Hawass et al. found the conus tip to be at L3 or above by 25 weeks' gestational age in myelograms of 340 aborted fetuses.[11] According to postmortem studies of infants by Barson,[12] the conus tip is at the L1–2 space 2 months after birth. Reimann and Anson[13] in much earlier studies indicated that the conus tip might normally be as low as mid-L2 and

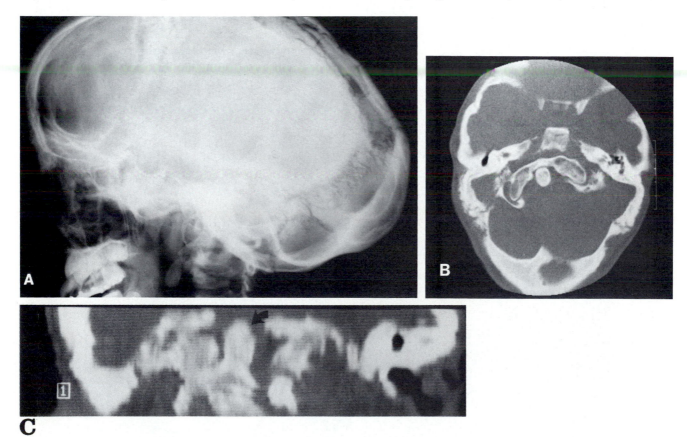

FIG 42–15.
Basilar invagination in an 11-year-old child with unclassified dysostosis and cranial nerve weakness. **A,** a lateral skull x-ray film shows the marked upward displacement of C1 into the skull. **B,** axial CT shows the upward invagination of C1 into the foramen magnum. **C,** coronal reconstruction accurately reveals the amount of displacement of the cervical spine into the skull vault. The odontoid is identified by an *arrow*.

that this was more likely in females. Work by Fitz and Harwood-Nash[14] used a practical compromise of L2–3 at the age of 2 years and the middle of the L2 level by 12 years of age as the lower limits of normal. A conus ending below those levels is considered abnormal by the author.

The embryology of the abnormality has not been examined but is presumed to be secondary to a halt in or slowing of the normal upward regression of the cord that progresses from sacrum to lumbar canal in utero. Because nearly all other forms of dysraphism have a tethering as part of their pathology and even the mildest isolated tethering has at least an occult spina bifida, the interruption of the normal regression appears to be part of a process that may be very complicated.

The clinical presentation is variable and has been dealt with by several authors.[15–17] There may be leg weakness or shortening, enuresis, back pain, or sensory changes, to name a few symptoms. Skin abnormalities such as a hairy patch or hemangioma are common. In addition to the spina bifida

that is always present, there may be a widened interpediculate distance and other dysraphic abnormalities on the plain films.

In most centers, MRI replaces myelography and CT for the evaluation of tethered conus (see Chapter 43, Fig 43–27). The mildest form has a conus only displaced by ½ to 2 vertebral body levels and a filum that is thickened (greater than 1.5-mm diameter). MRI may not easily identify such mild filum changes.

In the second type, the filum is thicker through part or all of its length, and CT or MRI of the filum indicates whether it contains fatty tissue (Fig 42–16). The third type is more complex. The conus may not be evident, with the cord gradually narrowing into a tube of variable diameter, but often 5 to 8 mm in size (Fig 42–17). This tube may be a true filum surrounded by fat but most frequently is cord neural tissue, and there is no true filum. Large lipomas are common in this type of tethering. Axial slices indicate the relationship of the lipomas to the cord and the circumference of the spinal canal, and sagittal reconstruction reveals

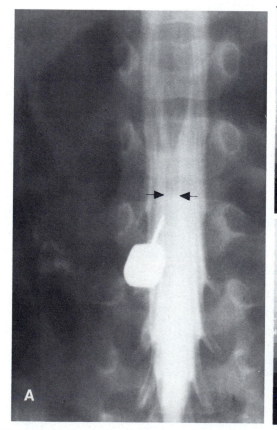

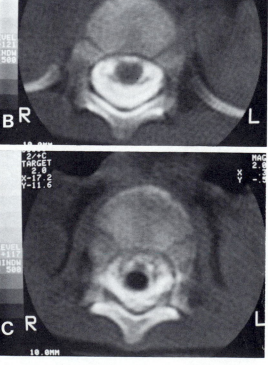

FIG 42–16.
Tethered conus, type II. **A,** a plain-film myelogram reveals thickening of the conus *(arrows).* **B,** CTM through the conus shows normal anatomy. **C,** CTM at the junction of the conus and filum shows enlargement with fatty infiltration.

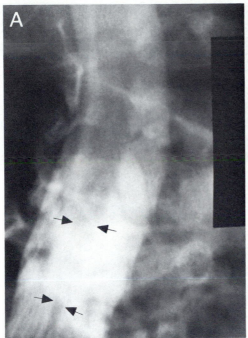
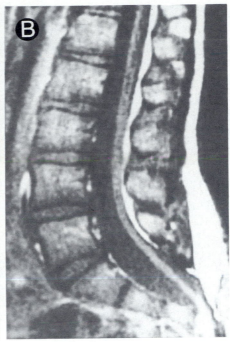

FIG 42–17.

A, tethered conus, type III-A, in a 1-year-old girl. A plain myelo-gram shows a cord with no conus enlargement that gradually nar-rows to its tip at the end of the lumbar canal *(arrows)*. Nerve roots are coming off the cord at a wider angle than is normal. CT showed no fat within the cord. **B,** sagittal T1 MRI of a 10-year-old with type III-A tethering. The cord is thinned throughout the lum-bosacral region and terminates at the end of the dural sac without an identifiable filum. The sacral subarachnoid space is enlarged.

the longitudinal extent of the abnormalities for sur-gical repair.

The lipoma is primarily on the posterior aspect of the cord. While it may simply lie dorsal to the cord, it does occasionally invade the cord itself, as seen on CT, and become intramedullary in posi-tion. With this latter type of involvement, it can be quite difficult to tell a tethered cord from a lipomy-elomeningocele (LMMC). Two CT findings are helpful. First is that the dysraphism of a tethered conus is less severe than that of a meningocele, and the laminae, although dysraphic, still tend to be arcuate in shape. Second, the lipoma is likely to remain within the bony spinal canal in the teth-ered conus (Fig 42–18). Identical findings can be seen on MRI.

Meningocele, Myelomeningocele

The spectrum of these lesions seems to be less of a continuum than does the tethered conus. This is especially so in comparing the myelomeningo-cele (MMC) with a simply meningocele or LMMC. The MMC is almost always associated with a Chiari II malformation of the brain and upper cer-vical cord and has more severe neurologic deficits.

Similar-appearing abnormalities of the cord occur with LMMC, which is usually far less symptom-atic. The main structural difference of the two le-sions is the presence of extensive fat in the LMMC. Plain meningocele, protrusion of the meninges without neural elements within, is about one tenth as common as the other varieties.

Causes of these dysraphic states are unknown, with the main theories for MMC formation being that of abnormal distension and rupture of the neu-ral tube[18] and abnormal closure of the neural tube at an even earlier time.[19] Discovery of myelo-schises of the unclosed tube in aborted fetuses by Osaka and colleagues[20] gives strength to the latter theory, even though variations of the severity of the distended neural tube give a more unified the-ory to explain associated abnormalities such as di-astematomyelia. Simple meningocele, with only a herniation of the dura through a dysraphic bony ca-nal, presumably occurs later or by a somewhat dif-ferent mechanism.

In all of these protrusions, CT clearly shows a marked posterior abnormality of the laminae, which tend to be nearly parallel and sagittally ori-ented. In MMC especially, the dysraphism usually extends over a long segment, sometimes involving

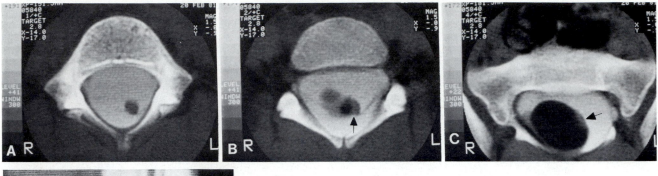

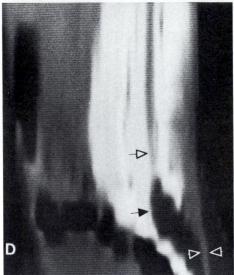

FIG 42–18.
Tethered conus, type III-B, in a 5-year-old girl. **A,** CTM through the lower lumbar level. The narrow cord is eccentric within the widened canal. Nerve roots are not visible because of their horizontal exiting from the cord. **B,** 10 mm lower, fat is visible and infiltrating the cord *(arrow)*, from which dorsal nerve roots are seen exiting. Because of averaging with surrounding metrizamide, much of the fat appears denser than the cord. Note the mild spina bifida. **C,** sacral level. The lipoma is large and distorts the cord tip *(arrow)* that surrounds the lipoma. The lipoma clearly remains in the spinal canal. **D,** sagittal reconstruction showing the cord *(open black arrow)* entering a large lipoma *(solid black arrow)* and separation between the lipoma and the more posterior subcutaneous fat by muscle and connective tissue *(open white arrowheads)*.

the entire lumbar canal or even more. Vertebral body abnormalities may also be present.

Because MMC is routinely repaired immediately after birth, neuroradiologic studies are often not done. The main goal in these operations is to cover the neural placode with dura and skin and prevent or stop any CSF leakage. The patients may return several years later with deterioration and undergo more thorough investigation at that time.[21]

Adequate investigation may be with MRI or CT with intrathecal contrast. CT has some advantage over MRI. It is usually evident on CTM whether or not contrast separates dura and neural elements, whereas adjacent position may be mistaken for posterior retethering on MRI. Lumbar puncture can usually be done either above or below the surgical repair. The canal may be wide and shallow, so an off-midline puncture with the needle angled at about 45 degrees cranially is easily accomplished if the spinous processes are deficient. Because of scarring and adhesions, the subarachnoid space may be loculated and prevent successful puncture, in which case a lateral C1–2 puncture should be carefully done while keeping

in mind that nearly all MMC patients will have a Chiari malformation.

In an MMC, the cord structure changes gradually over two or more vertebral levels until it reaches the placode area, which can be short, very disorganized, and difficult to evaluate. Contiguous 10-mm CT sections through the region of gradual change and 5-mm sections through the placode are the most efficient ways to examine the patient, with preliminary plain myelographic film and the CT digital radiograph being used as guides. Target reconstruction or its equivalent is necessary to adequately see the structural detail. Sagittal reconstruction can be useful either as comparison with or replacement for sagittal MRI (Fig 42–19).

The anatomy of such cases is complicated, and it is only since CT that such investigations have been worthwhile. The patients are often symptomatic because the placode has become retethered to the dura, but the association of congenital abnormalities should also be verified. The cord is often split, either above or uncommonly at the placode. The flattened placode, if tethered to the dura, blends with it and is barely visible (see Fig

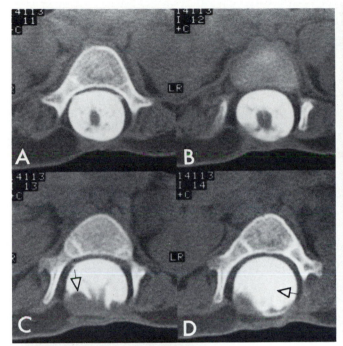
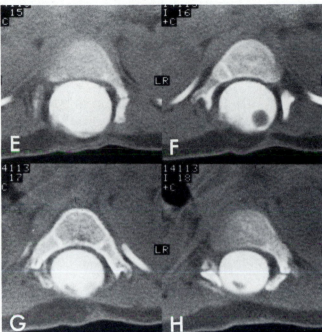

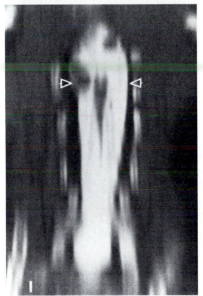

FIG 42–19.
Repaired MMC in a 5-year-old girl. Serial 5-mm CTM sections through the placode start inferiorly. **A,** midlumbar section showing a thickened reconstituted cord. **B,** end of the cleft of the cord. **C,** unusual diastematomyelic splitting of the cord in the placode, which extends across the posterior canal. A rare inclusion dermoid is visible *(arrow).* **D,** a ventral nerve root *(arrow)* visible arising from the center of the placode. **E,** the placode remaining adherent to the posterior aspect of the subarachnoid space. **F,** a second dermoid visible. **G** and **H,** the placode reforming into a dysplastic cord superiorly. **I,** coronal reconstruction revealing the two epidermoids and a portion of the splitting. Because the coronal slice cannot follow the curvature of the spine, the entire lumbar cord is not visible on a single slice. The *arrows* indicate the level of the axial slice **(C).**

42–19). Because the placode is a cord that has been sagittally split and opened from the back, the posterior surface of the placode is in fact the inside of the open cord plastered to the skin (or dura if already repaired). The anterior side of the placode is the entire outer surface of the cord. This means that the nerve roots visible off the ventral surface of a normal cord are now coming off the central portion of the placode (see Fig 42–19,D). The dorsal nerve roots exit at the lateral edges of the placode.

There can be distortions of the shape of the placode on axial projection. If the placode is at the upper lumbar level or above, the cord may also reconstitute inferiorly into a conus (see Fig 42–19,A).

Lipomyelomeningocele

LMMCs are radiologically more complicated and surgically more of a challenge. Having less neurologic symptomatology, the abnormality is in part cosmetic, but because there is much better preservation of neurologic function even with deterioration, the patient is usually fully evaluated before any surgery. There is a need to give as radical but careful a treatment as can be done to improve both function and appearance. Diagnosis can be accomplished with a high-quality water-soluble contrast myelogram with CT (CTM) or MRI.

The lipoma of the lower portion of the back that is the signal lesion is not different from surrounding subcutaneous fat. In fact, if the patient lies on his back, the external mass may be flattened and unrecognizable by CT or MRI. The mass generally blends laterally with the surrounding normal fat. It enters the wide spinal canal and affixes to the neural placode in one or two general ways. The placode itself is like that in MMC. The lipoma may attach centrally to the placode within the widened dysraphic canal, usually across the full width

of the placode. In such a case, there is usually no herniation of the subarachnoid space dorsal to the placode (Fig 42–20). If the lipoma is more laterally placed on the placode, it may rotate the placode, and there is often a subarachnoid herniation sac on the side of the canal where there is no lipoma (Fig 42–21). The lipoma is said to fix to the placode by a layer of fibrous tissue. This cannot be separated from neural tissue on CT. Although the physical distortion of the cord is precisely defined by CT, the densities of neural and fibrous tissue are alike and cannot be separated. The same is true of MRI.

As in MMC, sagittal reconstruction is useful in picturing the full longitudinal extent of the lipoma and also the water-soluble contrast–filled sac. Unless the back is unusually straight, coronal reconstruction is of limited value. Careful analysis of the

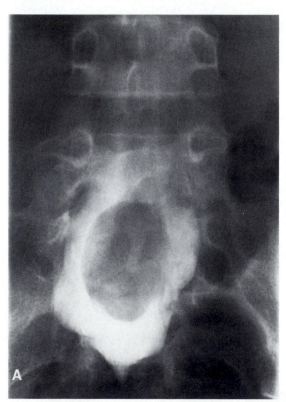

FIG 42–20.
LMMC in an 11-year-old boy. **A,** plain-film myelogram. There is a large lipoma in the sacral canal at the end of the spinal cord. **B,** CTM through the upper portion of the lipoma shows its infiltration *(arrow)* into the neural tissue. **C,** a slice through the middle of the lipoma shows infiltration similar to Figure 42–18 except that the laminae are much more widely dysraphic. **D,** further inferiorly, the lipomatous tissue *(arrow)* exits from the canal to enter the subcutaneous fat.

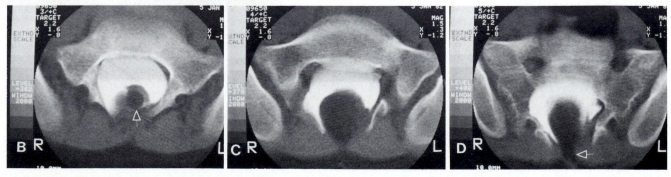

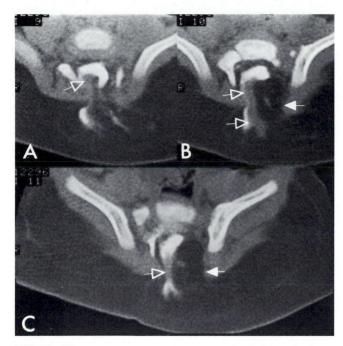

FIG 42–21.
LMMC in a 2-month old girl. **A–C,** sequential CTM slices progressing inferiorly. The laterally placed lipoma *(solid arrows)* blends with the subcutaneous fat. The cord *(open arrows)* is lateral to the portion of the lipoma that enters the spinal canal and also herniates posteriorly to form a placode.

axial sections is the most important factor in diagnosis. Except for the absence of the Chiari malformation and its associated syringomyelia, the lesions of the cord and associated anomalies are similar to those of MMC. The placode is always tethered into the lipomatous tissue.

Meningocele

Simple meningoceles, posterior protrusions of the meninges without neural elements, are uncommon compared with MMC and LMMC and are easily recognizable on plain-film myelography or CTM. No special analysis or techniques are needed to see that the sac contains no neural elements.

Anterior sacral meningoceles, although rare, constitute a more serious problem, but one ideally suited to examination by CTM. Patients usually have constipation from the mass itself, sphincter weakness, and mild neurologic dysfunction from sacral nerve pressure. Headaches from subarachnoid fluid shifts with positional changes may also occur.

Plain-film x-rays usually show the typical dys-

plastic "scimitar" or hook-shaped sacrum on the AP view. Posterior spina bifida may be present.

Intrathecal water-soluble contrast material is necessary to distinguish the meningocele from other cystic pelvic masses. There may be a neck with the meningocele protruding flasklike into the pelvis, or the base may be wide (Fig 42–22). While the sac is reportedly empty of neural tissue in most cases, nerves may pass into it[22] and should be carefully looked for on CT and distinguished from septations that are often in the sac.

Diastematomyelia

Diastematomyelia is a longitudinal splitting of the cord and a relatively common anomaly that is almost always in combination with other dysraphic conditions, especially tethering of the conus, MMC, and LMMC. Two types occur, one being a split within a single dural sac and the other associated with a double dural sac and having a spur that is usually bony.

The development of the condition has been explained by Gardner[18] as an anterior and posterior splitting of an abnormally dilated fetal cord. Another theory by Herren and Edwards[23] suggests an abnormal closure of the neural canal with the two dorsal halves of the neural plate falling ventrally without touching, thereby making two tubes. Bremer[24] suggested the possible abnormal persistence of the temporary neurenteric canal that nor-

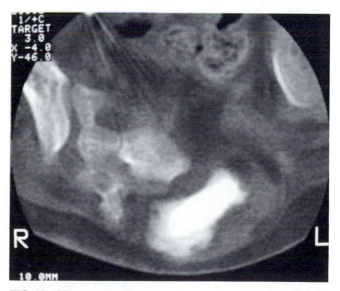

FIG 42–22.
Anterior sacral meningocele in a 2-year-old girl. CTM reveals an absence of the left side of the sacrum and a small meningocele protruding through the defect into the pelvis.

mally exists between the yolk sac and the amniotic sac through Hensen's node.

A single-sac variety was ignored and probably not recognized by most authors before the availability of water-soluble contrast and CT, although Emery and Lendon[25] found a 31% incidence in a careful autopsy series on infants with MMC and probably LMMC. The fact that it occurs more commonly than the spur variety was noted by Scotti and coworkers.[26] In my experience, it is about twice as common as the other type. While often visible on plain-film myelography, it may be obscured by contrast dilution or close proximity of the two cord parts. Therefore, CT or axial MRI are most important to secure the diagnosis. Sagittal MRI may miss the lesion.

The split usually is present over several vertebral segments of the lower thoracic or lumbar cord but may extend an even shorter distance. The majority of cases occur in association with a tethered conus, especially the milder type I or II tethers. The two cord parts are usually approximately equal in size but vary somewhat. Likewise, the two parts tend to be round on axial section but may be flattened medially, especially if in close approximation (Fig 42–23). There is occasionally a bridge between the two halves, presumably of neural tissue (Fig 42–24). The nerve roots are visible laterally and sometimes more medially, most likely as a result of cord rotation. The two halves usually rejoin before forming the filum but occasionally re-

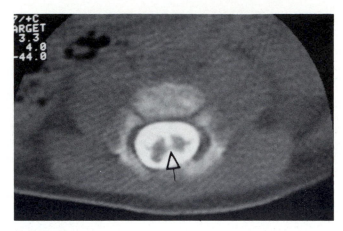

FIG 42–24.
Diastematomyelia in a 1-month-old girl. A thin bar of tissue *(arrow)* joins the two unequal halves in this single-sac variety.

main separate, and it is the presence of a second filum that may be the most important radiologic finding because the split itself seems to be non-symptomatic.

If there is no associated complicated anomaly, 10-mm axial CT sections are adequate to define this type of diastematomyelia. The exact location of its beginning and end are much less important than whether or not it ends and whether or not other pathology is also present.

When in association with LMMC or MMC, it is the author's experience that the split is above the placode in most cases. Emery and Lendon[25] found 22% to be in the placode, but no other series has found this high an incidence. They also noted a 9% incidence of one half of the cord forming a placode and the other half in a normal position within the neural canal. I believe this to be a much less common finding, although it certainly does occur.

Diastematomyelia with associated dural splitting has been well described in the radiologic literature since Neuhauser and colleagues[27] first noted the plain-film findings. An excellent review of these findings and plain-film myelography was also undertaken by Hilal and coworkers.[28] The most significant findings are spina bifida, a widened spinal canal, vertebral body and laminar anomalies, and a narrowing or absence of the disk space at the level of the spur plus visualization of the spur itself. Clinical symptoms are similar to those of the tethered conus. External skin markers such as dimples or hemangiomas are very common, and Winter and associates[29] reported hairy patches to be present in 75% of patients.

The use of CTM has been extremely helpful in

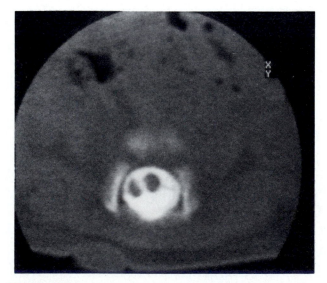

FIG 42–23.
Diastematomyelia in a 10-year-old boy. CTM in the lumbar region shows two cord halves in a single dural sac with some medial flattening of each half. The halves are slightly unequal.

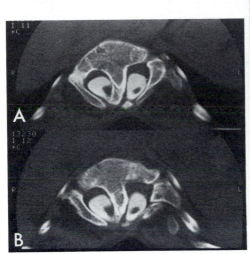

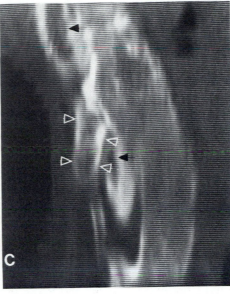

FIG 42–25.
Diastematomyelia in a 10-year-old girl. **A** and **B,** axial CTM showing a bony spur, dysraphism, and segmentation of the vertebral. **C,** sagittal reconstruction of 5-mm slices. The spur *(white arrowheads)* attaches to the back of the vertebral body rostral to its posterior tip. The intact cord above and a portion of the split cord at the spur are visible *(black arrows).*

dissecting the various parts of the sometimes complex disease, and sagittal or coronal reconstructions may be very helpful (Fig 42–25). The clear contrast between bone and other structures gives some advantage to CT. When the bony spur is oblique, it is sometimes difficult or impossible to see on plain film, as is the split cord itself on myelog-raphy. The use of CTM defines the spur, the bony anomaly, and the cord parts, which are often unequal (Fig 42–26). If scoliosis is present, as it commonly is, CT is even more valuable because the scoliosis may be locally severe and distort the diastematomyelia. Sections of 5 mm or less may be needed to analyze such cases, and it may be neces-

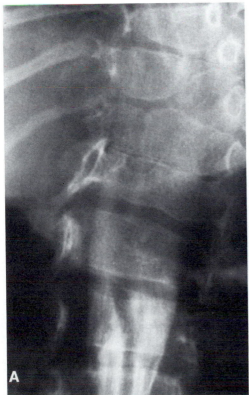

FIG 42–26.
Diastematomyelia with an oblique bony spur in a 5-year-old girl. **A,** plain-film myelogram with marked widening of the spinal canal, dysraphism, and a loss of disk spaces in the area of the bony spike, which is not seen. **B,** CTM, reversed gray scale. A large obliquely oriented spike is easily seen as it runs through the spinal canal and divides the subarachnoid space into two separate compartments in a somewhat AP manner. The cord parts are of uneven size.

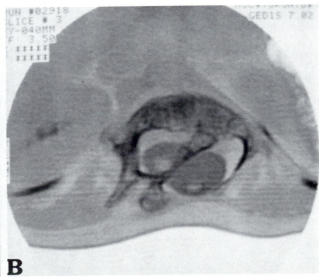

sary to do extra slices with the angle adjusted perpendicular to the curve after collecting continuous
parallel slices that are needed for reconstruction.
Cartilaginous spurs have not been encountered by
the author, with the possible exception of one case.
Partial spurs with an incomplete cleft indenting
the dura are occasionally picked up by CT and are
virtually impossible to find by any other method.

Diplomyelia, or true duplication of the cord
with full sets of nerve roots from both sides of both
hemicords, is described in a report by Herren and
Edwards,[23] but there is some doubt as to the au-
thenticity of any of the cases in that report. No
well-documented case has since been reported,
and it seems likely that the entity only exists, if it
does at all, in the rare occasion where there is a
complete duplication of a portion of the bony
spine.

Chiari Malformation

In children, the Chiari II malformation with
MMC, hindbrain malformation, and displacement of
the cervical canal is much more common than are
the Chiari I (tonsillar displacement only) or Chiari
III (hindbrain malformation with occipital encephalocele) malformations. Postulated causes for the
malformation are overgrowth of the developing
brain[30] and herniation of the hindbrain from delayed opening of the fourth ventricular foramina.[5]

The anatomic changes are complex. While axial CT easily identifies the abnormality, even with
multiplanar reconstructions the exact components
may be unclear. MRI of the craniocervical junction
more simply demonstrates the anomaly (see Chapters 43 and 24).

The cervical cord is inferiorly displaced. This
is sometimes demonstrable by visualizing the
nerve roots and lower cranial nerves traversing upward in the cervical canal. There is herniation of
the brain stem, usually only the medulla, downward and dorsally over the cervical cord. Although
the fourth ventricle is carried down with the medulla, it more often than not does not fill with water-soluble contrast material. The kink or fold that
the medulla makes atop the cord may be identifiable, especially on MRI. On top of the medulla is
the cerebellum, which is pulled down to a peglike
tip. This may be tonsil or vermis. The medulla may
be more inferior, or the cerebellum may be more
inferior.[31] At times, all three components—cord,
medulla, and cerebellum—may be identifiable
(Fig 42–27). The cord and the medulla are often
rectangular in cross section because of compression. The cervical level varies, but it is uncommon
to visualize these defects below the midcervical
region on CT.

Given the associated MMC, it is unlikely that a
Chiari II malformation will be mistaken for anything else. A Chiari I with only tonsillar displacement is much more easily demonstrated with MRI

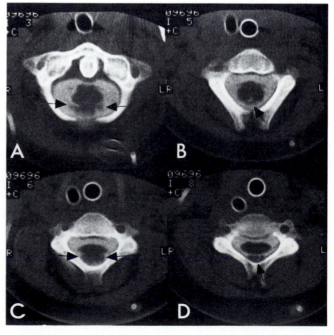

FIG 42–27.
Chiari II malformation in the same patient as in Figure 42–26. **A–D,**
axial CTM progressing inferiorly shows the cerebellum in **(A)** and **(B)**
(arrows) and, below that, a herniated medulla in **(C)** and **(D)** *(arrows)*
with a flattened cervical cord anterior to the displaced medulla.

than CT and is more commonly diagnosed now with the increasing use of MRI.[32]

Hydrosyringomyelia

Hydromyelia, enlargement of the central canal of the cord, is commonly associated with MMC. Its exact incidence is unknown because asymptomatic patients are usually not examined. Emery and Lendon[25] found a 20% incidence in their autopsy series, which again might be greater than the true incidence. Syringomyelia is a dissection of fluid out of the central canal or completely separate from the canal as a result of cord damage. Because hydromyelia itself might promote damage, it is not possible to distinguish one from the other unless the dissection or separation can be seen in the axial sections. The general term *syringomyelia* is usually used to cover both entities. While it is inaccurate in the pediatric setting, I will use the term, even though hydromyelia is almost always the primary entity.

Although Bonafe and coworkers[33] reported the diagnosis of cervical syringomyelia without the use of contrast by using a specially modified CT scanner, I believe the most reliable method of diagnosis is with water-soluble contrast plus CT (CTM) or MRI. The CT diagnosis is best made with axial sections, and reconstruction in other planes generally adds little to the diagnosis. Syringomyelia presents with a small cord, a normal-sized cord, or an enlarged cord. When the cord is small, it is flattened anteroposteriorly (Fig 42–28). Immediate

entry of contrast media into the central canal suggests communication with the fourth ventricle.

The enlarged cord, which is round in cross section, may be seen with or without contrast in the central canal. Delayed CT examination 6 to 24 hours later may show delayed filling of the central canal with water-soluble contrast material (Fig 42–29). The central canal may be relatively small, or it may be large with only a thin shell of cord tissue. Aubin and coworkers[34] reported that the vast majority of syrinxes have delayed filling. In children, about half do not fill. Aubin and coworkers[34] noted that cases with active hydrocephalus did not fill, and because most patients with MMC have hydrocephalus, this is the probable explanation for a much lower rate of central canal filling in children.

Whether delayed filling occurs via the fourth ventricle or through the cord is not clear. Even delayed filling is not conclusive evidence of syringomyelia because Kan and associates[35] have shown that this also occurs in tumor cysts. However, the knowledge of an existing Chiari malformation is strong supportive evidence of a syrinx, whereas its absence combined with a widened canal without dysraphism is equally strong support for the diagnosis of a tumor. Bonafe and colleagues[36] suggest that a small cord is evidence of a syrinx, but I believe this is more likely part of the MMC dysgenesis.

MRI is a simpler technique for the diagnosis than is CT. One must take care not to rely only on sagittal sections alone because collapsed hydromyelia may be mistaken for an atrophic cord. Like

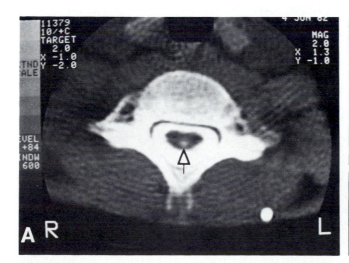

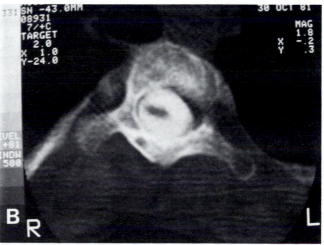

FIG 42–28.
Syringomyelia with a flattened cord. **A,** 10-year-old girl. CTM through the cervical cord reveals partial flattening and metrizamide in the enlarged central canal *(arrow).* **B,** 11-year-old boy. CTM through thoracic region shows a collapsed cord without visualization of the central canal.

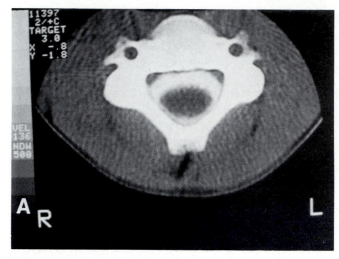
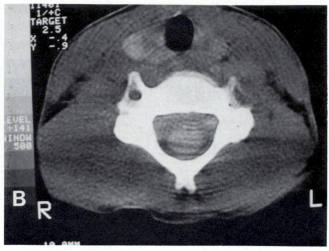

FIG 42–29.
Syringomyelia and an enlarged cord in a 12-year-old boy. **A,** initial CTM shows a dilated cervical cord surrounded by metrizamide. **B,** delayed study at 18 hours. Metrizamide has left the subarachnoid space, but some has entered the large central canal, which is now denser than the surrounding cord and subarachnoid space.

CT, axial sections are needed in many cases. MRI has found syringomyelia cavities in a high percentage of patients with Chiari I malformation, although these have been adults.[37]

CONGENITAL TUMORS

Dermoid and Epidermoid

Dermoid and epidermoid cysts are considered together in this section because there is little CT difference between them. This may not be true for MRI. Both are presumed to arise from cell rests, possibly secondary to incomplete separation of the cutaneous and neural ectoderm at the time of neural tube closure.[38] Epidermoids contain only superficial skin elements, while dermoids have glandular follicular elements. This may have some practical significance in that the dermoid may contain enough fatty material to give a low-density CT reading. Rarely, these lesions may be secondary to implantation from lumbar puncture or MMC repair. While epidermoids are evenly distributed throughout the spine, the majority of dermoids are lumbosacral.[38] The tumors may be extramedullary or intramedullary. Not all cysts are connected to a sinus tract, and likewise not all sinus tracts connect to a cyst. It is estimated that about 30% of the cysts are connected to sinuses[39, 40] and about half the sinuses end in tumors.[41] The incidence is reported to vary from 7% of pediatric spinal tumors[42] to 2.2% of all spinal tumors.[39] Epidermoids and dermoids may present with symptoms because of their mass effect or meningitis. The meningitis may be chemical from release of the contents of the cyst or infectious if there is a sinus connected to the skin.

Plain films usually will show hypoplasia of the spinous process or spina bifida, especially if there is a sinus. A sinus tract will be visible on axial CT slices, but sagittal reconstructions or sagittal MRI better reveals the usually rostral course the sinus tract takes in going from skin to dura and shows to better advantage the mass effect of the tumor (Fig 42–30). Because the tumors vary from a few millimeters to one to two vertebral body segments in size and usually have accompanying radiologic and clinical signs, they are not often confused preoperatively with other diagnoses.

In my limited experience with two infected tumors in which a total block to contrast had occurred, CTM was much less precise. While the visible sinus tract and abnormal spine denoted the site, limits of the tumor could not be determined, and intravenous contrast did not add further information.

Teratoma

Teratomas, having tissue from all three germ layers, are less common and make up 7% or less of pediatric intraspinal masses.[42] Their origin is less clear than dermoids, but they possibly arise from rests of abnormal germ cells[43] or more likely primitive somatic cells.[44] Because they are occasionally associated with diastematomyelia, the abnormal retention of the temporary neurenteric canal[24] has

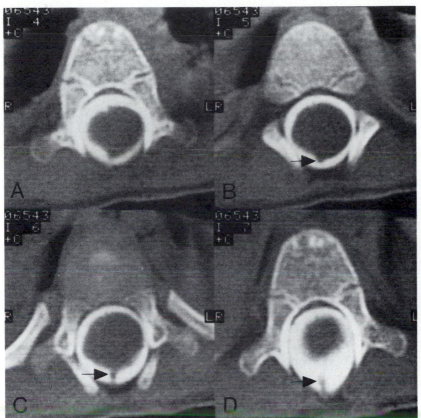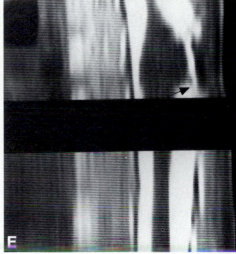

FIG 42–30.
Thoracic dermoid in a 4-year-old girl. **A–D,** inferiorly progressing sequential 5-mm CTM sections. Posterior spina bifida and cord enlargement are clearly visible. The dermoid tract *(arrows)* enters the cord from behind. **E,** sagittal reconstruction. The complete area of cord enlargement and upward passage of the tract *(arrow)* is well seen. The *black bar* in the middle of the reconstruction is due to software error that would not allow reconstruction of some of the slices.

been proposed as a cause. More often, there are no vertebral anomalies. Enlargement of the spinal canal is common.

The mass is most often small and involves one or two vertebral segments. Rarely, they have been reported to occupy the entire cord.[45] They may be intramedullary, extramedullary, or combined.

Their character is variable. They may be solid or cystic and may have fatty components or even calcification. If the nonsolid elements are identifiable, the diagnosis can be made with relative certainty. If the tumor is solid, it may be impossible to distinguish it from an acquired tumor such as astrocytoma, which will also expand the spinal canal. Because astrocytomas are frequently cystic, a cystic tumor containing no fat that expands the spinal canal may be either of these lesions. In general, astrocytomas are larger, both in cord expansion and the length of cord involved, but as noted by Pickens and coworkers,[45] the whole cord may be involved with teratoma. The limits of the tumor are

visible by CTM if there is not a complete obstruction to the flow of contrast.

Lipoma

The subject of intraspinal lipomas is difficult because they occur both as isolated lesions and in conjunction with a variety of dysraphic states, especially the tethered conus and LMMC. An isolated lipoma is uncommon and occurs in fewer than 1% of all spinal tumors.[46] The mass is most often cervical or thoracic in location,[47] and there is no dysraphism. The mass is dorsally placed within the spinal canal and may invade the cord. The author has experience with only one such lesion, which extended into the posterior fossa. Scans by CT, especially the sagittal reconstruction, gave a remarkable picture that, because of the low density of the fat, was pathognomonic (Fig 42–31). Because the cord expansion or compression occurs only at the site of the lipoma itself, it is not likely

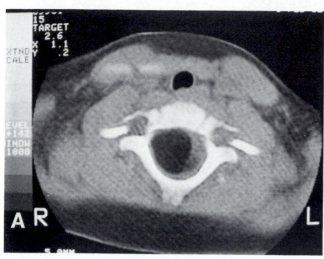

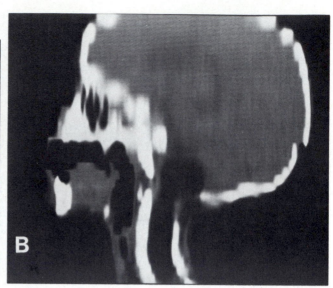

FIG 42–31.
Lipoma in a 1-year-old girl. **A,** axial CT slice through the cervical region. A large low-density lipoma has infiltrated the cord and enlarged the spinal canal. **B,** sagittal reconstruction. The lipoma occupies nearly the entire cervical canal and extrudes into the posterior fossa.

to be confused with a fat-containing tumor that is of larger dimensions.

Lipomas associated with tethering and LMMC are discussed in those sections. It is worth noting that Emery and Lenson[48] found 49 intrathecal lipomas of the filum, 26 dural lipomas, and 8 leptomyelolipomas mixed with neural tissue in 100 autopsied MMCs. The leptomyelolipomas are most likely cases of LLMC, as are perhaps some of the other lesions. CT scans of many true cases of MMC by the author have not substantiated the numbers found by Emery and Lendon, which suggests that such lipomas, if present, must be quite small.

SPLIT-NOTOCHORD SYNDROME

There are several rare gastrointestinal duplications combined with vertebral and cord anomalies that fall under the general term of *split-notochord syndrome.* The syndrome usually includes some gut duplication or cyst with an attachment to or connection through an anomalous vertebral body. The cyst can extend through the canal to the posterior wall or rarely be entirely posterior in location.[49] The origins are obscure, but theories include adhesion between the endoderm and ectoderm, which are normally separated by the advancing notochord tissue,[50] splitting of the notochord,[49] or persistence of the neurenteric canal.[24]

The majority of these lesions are neurenteric

cysts that present as intrathoracic masses with associated vertebral anomalies, usually a canal through a vertebral body. The chest mass contains gut elements at pathology. CT has the advantage of visualizing the extraspinal mass if it has not been resected, the tract through the vertebral body, and the intraspinal component. This spinal component is variable and not easily seen even with the best CTM or MRI. After it has passed through the vertebral body, the cyst may end at the dura, pass through the dura and end in an extramedullary location, or extend into the cord itself. While the extradural type is identifiable because of the normal subarachnoid space, the cyst that ends in a intradural extramedullary location attaches to the cord surface, which makes it difficult to determine intramedullary invasion. In either the intradural-extramedullary or intramedullary types, the cord and cyst make up a single "mass" that looks like an expanded and distorted cord on axial slices (Figs 42–32 and 39–30). The adherence of the tissue to the cord allows no contrast material to pass between them.

SACRAL AGENESIS

Sacral agenesis is a very rare lesion. The plain-film findings of partial or total sacral agenesis are obvious. Motor and sensory deficits and gait disturbances from abnormal hip anatomy are common

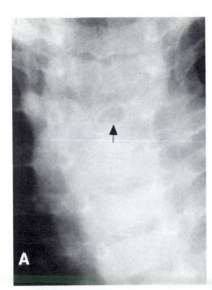

FIG 42–32.
Neurenteric cyst in a 14-year-old boy. **A,** a plain film of the thoracic spine at 3 years of age shows the typical cleft *(arrow)* through a vertebral body, which is not visible by 14 years of age because of progressive kyphosis. **B,** axial CTM at 14 years of age. The vertebrae are deformed. The cord *(solid arrow)* is deformed by the adjacent cyst *(open arrow)* that has entered the subarachnoid space. **C,** adjacent higher slice. The cord and cyst have merged into a single large mass almost completely blocking the flow of metrizamide. The cyst was thought to be intramedullary at surgery.

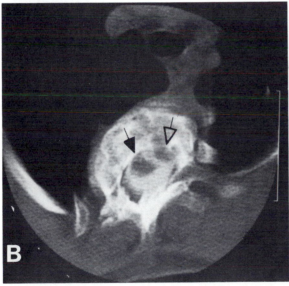

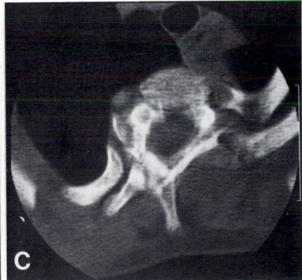

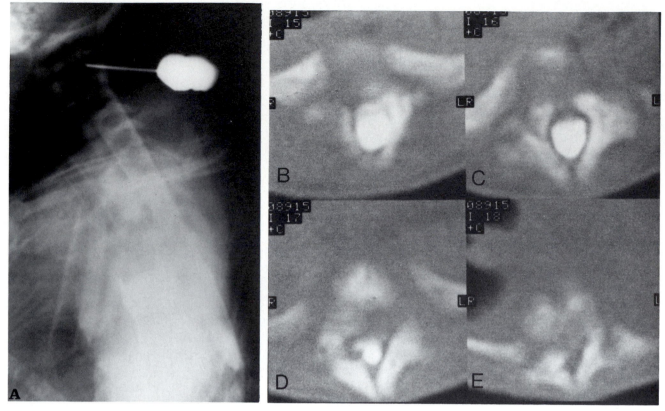

FIG 42–33.

Sacral agenesis in a 20-day-old boy. **A,** a lateral plain-film myelogram done by cervical puncture shows the short subarachnoid space ending in the lower thoracic spine. The vertebral bodies are dysplastic. **B–E,** sequential CTM slices through the lower thoracic spine. The inferior subarachnoid space contains no nerve roots. The spinal canal progressively narrows as the metrizamide-filled subarachnoid space ends.

symptoms that may be progressive. Maternal diabetes appears to be a strong factor in the occurrence of the disease, and perhaps paternal diabetes may also be causative.[51]

Two types of agenesis occur, and they can be investigated and distinguished by CTM.[52] The stenotic type has a narrow lumbar subarachnoid space that ends above the sacrum with compression of the cauda equina (Fig 42–33). This type may benefit from duraplasty. The second variety is identical to a tethered conus and may benefit from release of the conus. Both types can be distinguished by plain-film myelography. The conditions have been reported in association with MMC and other abnormalities, so each case must be individually assessed.

NONDYSRAPHIC ABNORMALITIES

Neurofibromatosis

This is one of the most complicated and diverse diseases in its manifestations. The spine is involved in both the central and mixed forms of the disease but, unlike the brain, has relatively few types of abnormalities, although they occur in a high frequency of patients. Scoliosis is the most common finding and occurs in about one half of the patients.[53] Scoliosis is clinically obvious and sometimes severe over a relatively short length of vertebrae. It often has a rotatory component. The challenge to the neuroradiologist is to decide whether the scoliosis is from bony or intraspinal abnormalities. While the bony abnormalities can be fairly well documented by plain-film tomography, the sharp angles of the scoliosis may require multiply angled series in any CTM or MRI study to provide views properly parallel or perpendicular to the cord. If a curve is severe, one may obtain a sagittal projection from an axial slice through part of the curve. The seeming distortion caused by the slicing of different parts of adjacent vertebral bodies may be confusing and require reconstructions in obliquely oriented planes. The cord, if stretched tightly along the curve, will be somewhat flattened, even though normal (Fig 42–34).

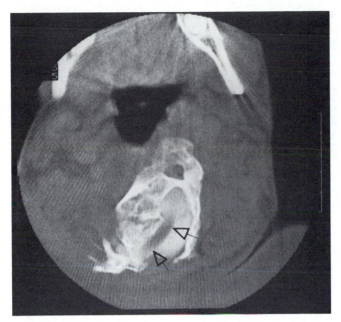

FIG 42–34.
Neurofibromatosis with scoliosis in an 18-year-old male. Axial CTM is oblique through dysplastic cervical vertebrae in a patient with severe cervicothoracic scoliosis. The cord *(arrows)* is flattened against the vertebral body through the apex of the curve.

Minor abnormalities such as scalloping of the posterior aspects of the vertebral bodies, dural ectasia, and bulging of the subarachnoid space through the foramina are easily recognized (Fig 42–35). Although these patients develop schwannomas of nerve roots in about 20% of cases,[54] this is rare in childhood.

Achondroplasia

Achondroplastic dwarfs have the misfortune of a normal-sized spinal cord in a narrowed spinal canal. The cross-sectional area of the canal throughout the spine is decreased by a combination of early fusion of the neurocentral synchondroses and abnormally thick pedicles from a hypertrophic periosteum.[55] These abnormalities narrow the lumbar canal especially, which does not have the usual physiologic widening (Fig 42–36). Further aggravating the compromised canal is the prominence of the intervertebral disks and a small "keyhole" foramen magnum (Fig 42–37). Apnea and paralysis may occur secondary to the small foramen magnum.[56, 57] About 30% of these patients also have kyphosis with vertebral body wedging.[58] All of these features are easily seen on CTM, although plain-film myelography will in fact identify the spinal canal changes fairly well. Cord compression by kyphosis is best visualized by CTM.

Mucopolysaccharidoses

The inherited group of diseases called mucopolysaccharidoses (MPS), although having similar enzymatic defects interfering with mucopolysaccharide metabolism, have marked variations in clinical severity and radiographic abnormalities. These abnormalities are primarily due to the deposition of mucopolysaccharides in bones, cartilage, ligaments, and dura. Four of the diseases have been reported to have myelographic abnormalities:

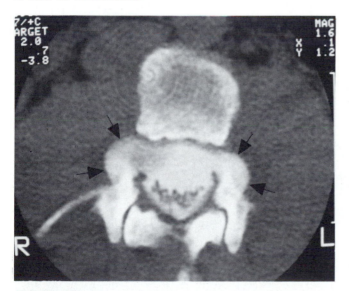

FIG 42–35.
Neurofibromatosis in a 15-year-old boy: CTM through the lumbar spine. Bulging of the subarachnoid space through the vertebral foramina *(Arrows)*, presumed to be part of the "dural ectasia," is common in this disease. The vertebra is somewhat dysplastic.

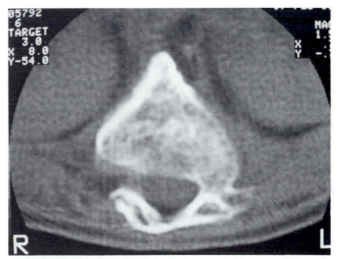

FIG 42–36.
Achondroplasia in an 11-year-old girl: CT through a lumbar vertebra. The vertebral body is anteriorly pointed. The right pedicle is thickened, and the canal is small, especially in the sagittal plane. The slice is partially through the foramen on the right.

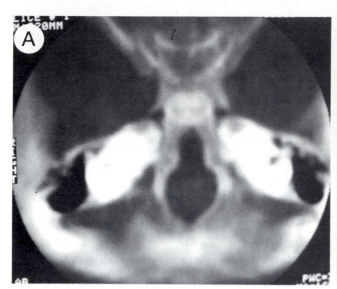 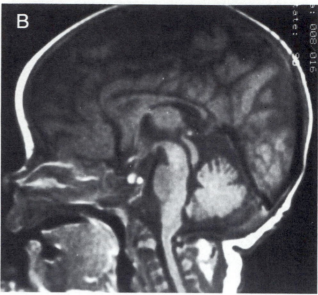

FIG 42–37.

A, Achondroplasia in a 9-month-old boy. CT through the skull base reveals the small keyhole-shaped foramen magnum. **B,** sagittal T1 MRI in a 2-month-old achondroplastic girl. There is abrupt narrow- ing at the cervicomedullary junction by the small foramen magnum, which measures 8 mm front to back.

these are Hurler's syndrome (MPS-I), Hurler-Scheie syndrome (MPS-I H/S), Morquio's syndrome (MPS-IV), and the Maroteaux-Lamy syndrome (MPS-VI).

The best-known anomalies are the flattened thoracolumbar "bullet" vertebral bodies of MPS-I and MPS-IV. Potentially more dangerous are the abnormalities that affect the cervical spine. Kennedy and colleagues[59] described a case of MPS-I H/S with compression of the cervical canal that was caused by dural deposits and ligamentous thickening, and Sostrin and coworkers[60] added an-

other case plus one with MPS-VI. Thoracolumbar compression has also been reported in MPS-VI.[61]

Cervical abnormalities in MPS-IV[62] are especially severe. These neurologically threatening abnormalities require CTM or MRI for full evaluation. The full extent of the disease in MPS-IV was described by Edwards and coworkers.[63] There is a small cervical canal with thick laminae and odontoid hypoplasia. The small C1 arch may be trapped on the posterior lip of the foramen magnum. Hypoplasia of the odontoid combined with ligament laxity causes subluxation of C1 on C2, which is fur-

FIG 42–38.

MPS-I in a 2½-year-old boy. **A,** CTM at the foramen magnum shows laminae of C1 *(1)* caught against the foramen magnum *(F)*. The slice also includes the base of C2 *(2)*. The subarachnoid space is thought to be displaced posteriorly by dural deposits. **B,** a C4 slice better shows the small cervical canal and markedly thick laminae.

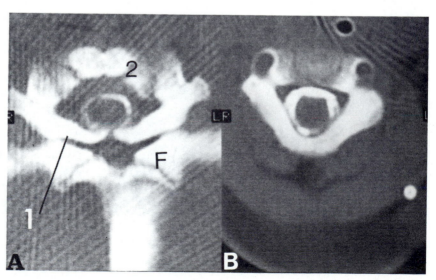

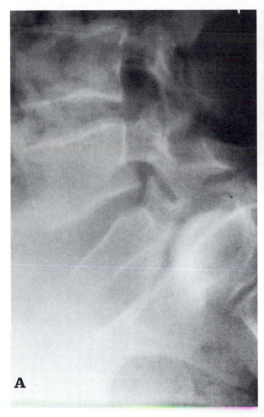

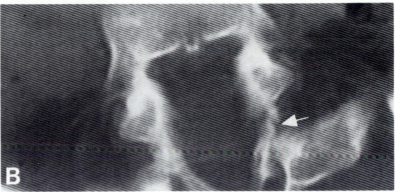

FIG 42-39.
Spondylolisthesis in a 13-year-old boy. **A,** a lateral spine film shows grade
IV displacement of L5 on S1. **B,** CT through the plane of the laminae of L5
shows elongated hypoplastic laminae with a probable congenital fracture
(arrow) on the right.

ther complicated because of the narrow cervical canal and dural deposits of the MPS. The same findings are also seen in MPS-I (Fig 42–38).

Spondylolisthesis

Spondylolisthesis, the forward slippage of one vertebral body on another, usually L5 on S1 or L4 on L5, is a fairly common pediatric entity. Its true cause is unknown. The review of McKee and colleagues[64] of 63 pediatric cases suggested that most are caused by nonunion of stress fractures, a congenital weakness of the pars, or a combination of factors. The first theory is supported by the very uncommon occurrence before children walk, and the second by a strong familial correlation.

Very few cases are truly congenital, and these are usually due to facet anomalies. The use of CT does not improve the understanding of the causations of spondylolisthesis but is well suited to the differentiation of the idiopathic and congenital types when plain films do not adequately do so. This may be combined with myelography when compression of the cauda equina causes neurologic symptoms.

The common idiopathic type of spondylolisthesis has a similar appearance on both CT and plain films. The rare congenital types are extremely difficult to analyze by plain film, and axial or near-axial CT is a much more informative imaging technique for such anomalies (Fig 42–39).

REFERENCES

1. Altman NR, Altman DH: MR imaging of spinal dysraphism. *AJNR* 1987; 8:533–538.
2. Barnes PD, Lester PD, Yamanashi WS, et al: Magnetic resonance imaging in infants and children with spinal dysraphism. *AJNR* 1986; 7:465–472.
3. Calvy TM, Segall HD, Giles FH, et al: CT anatomy of the craniovertebral junction in infants and children. *AJNR* 1987; 8:489–494.
4. Brugman E, Palmers Y, Staelens B: Congenital absence of a pedicle in the cervical spine: A new approach with CT scan. *Neuroradiology* 1979; 17:121–125.
5. Oestreich AE, Young LW: The absent cervical pedicle syndrome: A case in childhood. *AJR* 1969; 107:505–510.
6. Maldague BE, Malghem JJ: Unilateral arch hypertrophy with spinous process TIH: A sign of arch-deficiency. *Radiology* 1976; 121:567–574.
7. Lauten GJ, Wehunt WD: Computed tomography in absent cervical pedicle. *AJNR* 1980; 1:201–203.

8. McRae DL: The significance of abnormalities of the cervical spine. *AJR* 1960; 84:3–25.

9. McRae DL: Roentgenologic findings in syringomyelia and hydromyelia. *AJR* 1966; 89:695–703.

10. Caetano de Barros M, Farias W, Ataide L, et al: Basilar impression and Arnold-Chiari malformation. *J Neurol Neurosurg Psychiatry* 1968; 31:596–605.

11. Hawass ND, El-Badawi MG, Fatani JA, et al: Myelographic study of the spinal cord ascent during fetal development. *AJNR* 1987; 8:691–695.

12. Barson AJ: The vertebral level of termination of the spinal cord during normal and abnormal development. *J Anat* 1970; 106:489–497.

13. Reimann AF, Anson BJ: Vertebral level of termination of the spinal cord with report of a case of sacral cord. *Anat Rec* 1944; 88:127–138.

14. Fitz CR, Harwood-Nash DC: The tethered conus. *AJR* 1975; 125:515–523.

15. Hendrick EB, Hoffman HJ, Humphreys RP: Tethered cord syndrome, in McLaurin R (ed): *Myelomeningocele.* New York, Grune & Stratton, 1977.

16. Hoffman HJ, Hendrick EB, Humphreys RP: The tethered spinal cord: Its protean manifestations, diagnosis and surgical correction. *Childs Brain* 1976; 2:145–155.

17. Garceau GJ: The filum terminale syndrome. *J Bone Joint Surg [Am]* 35:711–716, 1953.

18. Gardner WJ: Etiology and pathogenesis of the development of myelomeningocele, in McLaurin R (ed): *Myelomeningocele.* New York, Grune & Stratton, 1977.

19. Lichtenstein BW: Spinal dysraphism. *Arch Neurol Psychiatry* 1940; 44:742–810.

20. Osaka K, Matsumoto S, Tanimura T: Myeloschisis in early human embryo. *Childs Brain* 1978; 4:347–359.

21. Heinz ER, Rosenbaum AE, Scarff TB, et al: Tethered spinal cord following meningomyelocele repair. *Radiology* 1979; 131:153–160.

22. Dyck R, Wilson CB: Anterior sacral meningocele. *J Neurosurg* 1980; 53:548–552.

23. Herren RY, Edwards JE: Diplomyelia (duplication of the spinal cord). *Arch Pathol* 1940; 30:1203–1214.

24. Bremer JL: Dorsal intestinal fistula; accessory neurenteric canal; diastematomyelia. *AMA Arch Pathol* 1952; 54:132–138.

25. Emery JL, Lendon RG: The local cord lesion in neurospinal dysraphism (meningomyelocele). *J Pathol* 1973; 110:83–96.

26. Scotti G, Musgrave MA, Harwood-Nash DC, et al: Diastematomyelia in children: Metrizamide and CT metrizamide myelography. *AJNR* 1980; 1:403–410.

27. Neuhauser EBD, Wittenborg MH, Dehlinger K: Diastematomyelia: Transfixation of the cord or cauda equina with congenital anomalies of the spine. *Radiology* 1950; 54:659–664.

28. Hilal SK, Marton D, Pollack E: Diastematomyelia in children. *Neuroradiology* 1974; 112:609–621.

29. Winter RB, Haven JJ, Moe JH, et al: Diastematomyelia and congenital spine deformities. *J Bone Joint Surg [Am]* 1974; 56:27–39.

30. Barry A, Patten BM, Stewart BH: Possible factors in the development of the Arnold-Chiari malformation. *J Neurosurg* 1957; 14:285–301.

31. Peach B: The Arnold-Chiari malformation. *Arch Neurol* 1965; 12:527–535.

32. Aboulezz AO, Sartor K, Geyer CA, et al: Position of cerebellar tonsils in the normal population and in patients with Chiari malformation: A quantitative approach with MR imaging. *J Comput Assist Tomogr* 1985; 9:1033–1036.

33. Bonafe A, Ethier D, Melancon D, et al: High resolution computed tomography in cervical syringomyelia. *J Comput Assist Tomogr* 1980; 4:42–47.

34. Aubin ML, Vignaud J, Jardin C, et al: Computed tomography in 75 clinical cases of syringomyelia. *AJNR* 1981; 2:199–204.

35. Kan S, Fox AJ, Vinuela F, et al: Delayed CT metrizamide enhancement of syringomyelia secondary to tumor. *AJNR* 1983; 4:73–78.

36. Bonafe A, Manelfe C, Espagno J, et al: Evaluation of syringomyelia with metrizamide computed tomographic myelography. *J Comput Assist Tomogr* 1980; 4:797–802.

37. Sherman JL, Barkovich AJ, Citrin CM: The MR appearance of syringomyelia: New observations. *AJNR* 1986; 7:985–995.

38. List CF: Intraspinal epidermoids, dermoids and dermal sinuses. *Surg Gynecol Obstet* 1941; 73:525–538.

39. Guidetti B, Gagliardi FM: Epidermoid and dermoid cysts. *J Neurosurg* 1977; 47:12–18.

40. Bailey IC: Dermoid tumours of the spinal cord. *J Neurosurg* 1970; 33:676–681.

41. Cardell BS, Laurence B: Congenital dermal sinus associated with meningitis: A report of a fatal case. *Br Med J* 1951; 2:1558–1561.

42. Harwood-Nash DC, Fitz CR: *Neuroradiology in Infants and Children.* St Louis, CV Mosby Co, 1976.

43. Newcastle NB, Francouer J: Teratomatous cysts in the spinal canal. *Arch Neurol* 1964; 11:91–99.

44. Kaplan CG, Askin FB, Benirschke K: Cytogenetics of extragonadal tumours. *Teratology* 1979; 19:261–266.

45. Pickens JM, Wilson J, Myers CG, et al: Teratoma of the spinal cord. *Arch Pathol* 1975; 99:446–448.

46. Rubinstein LJ: Tumours of the Central Nervous System, in *Atlas of Tumour Pathology.* Armed Forces Institute of Pathology, 1972, series 2, fasc 6.

47. Giuffre R: Intradural spinal lipomas. *Acta Neurosurg* 1966; 14:69–95.

48. Emery JL, Lendon RG: Lipomas of the cauda equina and other fatty tumours related to neurospi-

nal dysraphism. *Dev Med Child Neurol Suppl* 1969; 20:62–70.

49. Bentley JFR, Smith JR: Developmental posterior enteric remnants and spinal malformations. *Arch Dis Child* 1960; 35:76–86.

50. Beardmore HE, Wiglesworth FW: Vertebral anomalies and alimentary duplications. *Pediatr Clin North Am* 1958; 5:457–473.

51. Pang D, Hoffman HJ: Sacral agenesis with progressive neurological deficit. *Neurosurgery* 1980; 7:118–126.

52. Brooks BS, El Gammal T, Hartlage P, et al: Myelography of sacral agenesis. *AJNR* 1981; 2:319–323.

53. Casselman ES, Mandell GA: Vertebral scalloping in neurofibromatosis. *Radiology* 1979; 131:89–94.

54. Casselman ES, Miller WT, Lin SR, et al: Von Recklinghausen's disease: Incidence of roentgenographic findings with a clinical review of the literature. *CRC Crit Rev Diagn Imaging* 1977; 9:387–419.

55. Duvoisin RC, Yahr MD: Compressive spinal cord and root syndromes in achondroplastic dwarfs. *Neurology* 1962; 12:202–207.

56. Fremion AS, Garg BP, Kalsbeck J: Apnea as the sole manifestation of cord compression in achondroplasia. *J Pediatr* 1984; 104:398–401.

57. Yamada H, Nakamura S, Tajima M, et al: Neurological manifestations of pediatric achondroplasia. *J Neurosurg* 1981; 54:49–57.

58. Galanski M, Herrmann R, Knoche U: Neurological complications and myelographic features of achondroplasia. *Neuroradiology* 1978; 17:59–63.

59. Kennedy P, Swash M, Dean MF: Cervical cord compression in mucopolysaccharidosis. *Dev Med Child Neurol* 1973; 15:194–199.

60. Sostrin RD, Hasso AN, Peterson DI, et al: Myelographic features of mucopolysaccharidosis: A new sign. *Radiology* 1977; 125:421–424.

61. Wald SL, Schmidek HH: Compression myelopathy associated with type VI mucopolysaccharidosis (Maroteaux-Lamy syndrome). *Neurosurgery* 1984; 14:83–88.

62. Lipson SJ: Dysplasia of the odontoid process in Morquio's syndrome causing quadriparesis. *J Bone Joint Surg [Am]* 1977; 59:340–344.

63. Edwards MK, Harwood-Nash DC, Fitz CR, et al: CT metrizamide myelography of the cervical spine in Morquio syndrome. *AJNR* 1982; 3:66–69.

64. McKee BW, Alexander WJ, Dunbar JS: Spondylolysis and spondylolisthesis in children: A review. *J Assoc Can Radiol* 1971; 22:100–109.

43

Spinal Dysraphism: Magnetic Resonance Imaging

James A. Brunberg, M.D.

The term *spina bifida* was first utilized by the anatomist Nicolas Tulp in 1685 in his description and illustration of the lumbosacral lesion of a child with meningomyelocele.[1] Such dysraphic lesions of the spine are now understood to represent imperfect developmental fusion or closure of dorsal midline mesenchymal, neural, or osseous structures. Dysraphic spinal lesions are classified as spina bifida cystica (spina bifida aperta) if any portion of the spinal contents visibly protrudes through an anterior or posterior defect in midline fusion of bony elements. Examples include meningocele, meningomyelocele, and occasionally lipomeningomyelocele. Dysraphic spinal lesions are classified as occult if an associated anterior or posterior bifid defect in the bony spine (spina bifida occulta) is covered by skin, if there is no exposed neural tissue, and if there is no visible cystic mass or protrusion other than an occasional superficial subcutaneous lipoma. Occult dysraphic processes include diastematomyelia, hydromyelia, syringomyelia, spinal lipoma, tight filum terminale or other tethered cord syndromes, split-notochord syndrome, dorsal dermal sinus, neurenteric cyst, dermoid, and lipomeningomyelocele if there is no superficial mass. Spina bifida cystica and occult spinal dysraphic lesions may each be associated with static or progressive neurologic deficits requiring diagnostic evaluation and surgical intervention to minimize the severity of persisting neurologic deficits and to prevent further neurologic deterioration.

Radiographic procedures for the evaluation of spinal dysraphism have included myelography for lateral and anterioposterior (AP) imaging and computed tomography (CT) with or without intrathecal contrast for definition of axial or cross-sectional relationships and for tissue characterization based on x-ray attenuation.[2-4] Ultrasound has been found to be useful prior to ossification of the posterior spinal elements[5-7] and is effective in the antenatal detection of dysraphic spinal lesions.[8] Precise imaging is essential both for the establishment of a definitive initial diagnosis and for the evaluation of symptoms of persistent cord or nerve root dysfunction occurring spontaneously or following surgical repair of meningomyelocele or other dysraphic lesions.[9] Early surgical intervention is considered essential for the prevention of progressive neurologic or orthopedic deficits[10-12] in patients with potentially symptomatic dysraphic spinal lesions. Magnetic resonance imaging (MRI) is being increasingly utilized as the definitive diagnostic procedure in the evaluation of dysraphic spinal lesions.[13-18] MRI techniques allow the patient to avoid possible myelographic complications including neurotoxicity associated with the intrathecal administration of contrast, to avoid the occasional necessity for general anesthesia for optimal pediatric myelographic imaging, and to avoid the risk of trauma to a tethered or otherwise dysraphic spinal cord that is associated with needle placement. MRI in sagittal and axial planes demonstrates precise regional structural contours and generally allows for tissue distinction between the spinal cord, nerve roots, spinal fluid, fat, and soft tissue.

IMAGING TECHNIQUE

Imaging sequence parameters utilized in the MRI evaluation of spinal dysraphic lesions will vary depending on system field strength, pulsing sequence availability, patient size, and the size and types of surface coils that are available. Our experience has been predominately with a 1.5-Tesla General Electric Signa system with prototype and commercially available 14.6- and 7.6-cm round receive-only surface coils. Spin-echo pulsing sequences (repetition time/echo time [TR/TE]) are used for T1-weighted, short TR, single-echo images (600 to 800 ms/20 to 25 ms), which provide superior anatomic definition, and for long TR multiecho images (2,500 to 3,000 ms/25, 50, 75, and 100 ms), which assist in tissue characterization. Slice thickness is 4 to 5 mm with two excitations, and either a 128 × 256 or a 256 × 256 acquisition matrix is utilized. The field of view varies from 8 to 24 cm, depending on surface-coil size, axis of imaging, pulsing sequence, patient size, and matrix size. T1-weighted images are obtained first by using a 14.6-cm coil centered at the region of interest for patients over the age of 4 years and then using a 7.6-cm coil for patients less than 5 years of age. Sagittal images are obtained by using a skip factor of 1 mm, with subsequent axial images using a skip factor of 1 to 5 mm. Repositioning of the coil is occasionally necessary to allow visualization of the more rostral portions of the lumbar spinal canal and conus. Larger surface coils are utilized to visualize the remaining portions of the spinal axis. Patient positioning relative to the isocenter of the magnet is important in some MRI systems for selection of the field of view and is important because it relates to "fold-over" artifact, to visualization of the anterior border of the sacrum, and to visualization of bladder size on at least one image.

On axial images the phase-encoding gradient is utilized in the horizontal axis to avoid aorta or vena cava flow-induced signal deposition over the spine and to diminish "ghosting" of anterior abdominal wall subcutaneous fat over the spine secondary to respiratory movement if respiratory gating or spatial presaturation sequences are not available. On sagittal images the phase-encoding gradient can be utilized for the longitudinal axis to diminish respiration movement artifact. Respiratory and cardiac gating have not been routinely utilized in our experience.

Patients less than 5 years of age generally require sedation. In our experience a reliable regimen for patients over 6 months of age has been a combination of secobarbitol, 4 mg/kg intramuscularly (IM), and meperidine, 2 mg/kg IM. An alternative procedure in patients over 6 months of age has been the intravenous (IV) administration of pentobarbitol in a dosage of 2 to 6 mg/kg.[19] Pentobarbitol is administered IV over a period of several minutes with close monitoring of vital signs and with administration discontinued when adequate sedation has been achieved. The IV line is left in place during the study, and the initial sedation is generally effective for 45 to 60 minutes. Oral chloral hydrate, 50 to 70 mg/kg, is utilized for patients less than 6 months of age. Sedation of any type is utilized only if there has been adequate time for gastric emptying following the last feeding. The availability of resuscitation equipment and personnel trained in its utilization is necessary. A pulse oximeter (Nelcor) has been utilized for monitoring the pulse rate and tissue oxygen saturation on sedated patients while in the magnet. Respiratory and cardiac MRI gating equipment can be utilized for patient monitoring even when the studies are not gated. Most MRI studies of suspected spinal dysraphism can be completed within 45 to 60 minutes in a high–field strength imaging system.

MENINGOMYELOCELE

Meningomyelocele is a relatively common spinal dysraphic process occurring in 1 in 2,000 live births and characterized by an exposed region of neural tissue derived from the embryogenic neural plate. The exposed neural tissue, termed the *placode*, is most commonly in the lumbosacral region but may be at any location along the spinal axis. The embryogenesis of myelomeningocele relates to failure of closure of the neural tube and persistence of a regional superficial neural platelike structure or placode. This failure of neurulation occurs at about the 25-somite stage when the fetus is 26 to 30 days postconception and has a crown-rump length of 3 to 5 mm.[4, 20, 21] The placode subsequently becomes elevated above surrounding paraspinal soft tissue secondary to overexpansion of the subarachnoid space in the caudal dural sac anterior to the placode. If expansion of the subarachnoid space and elevation of the placode above surrounding skin surfaces does not occur, the malformation is termed a *myelocele*. Both myelocele and meningomyelocele are associated with secondary defects in spinal bony fusion.

With MRI the placode is readily demonstrated in either the postoperative or preoperative spine (Fig 43–1). The primitive neural groove that is often seen clinically in the central rostral portion of the placode may be seen with MRI. The neural groove may be in continuity with the central canal of the more rostral cord, or it may be in continuity with a cord syrinx. The origin of sensory nerve roots from the lateral aspect of the placode and of motor nerve roots from the medial ventral surface

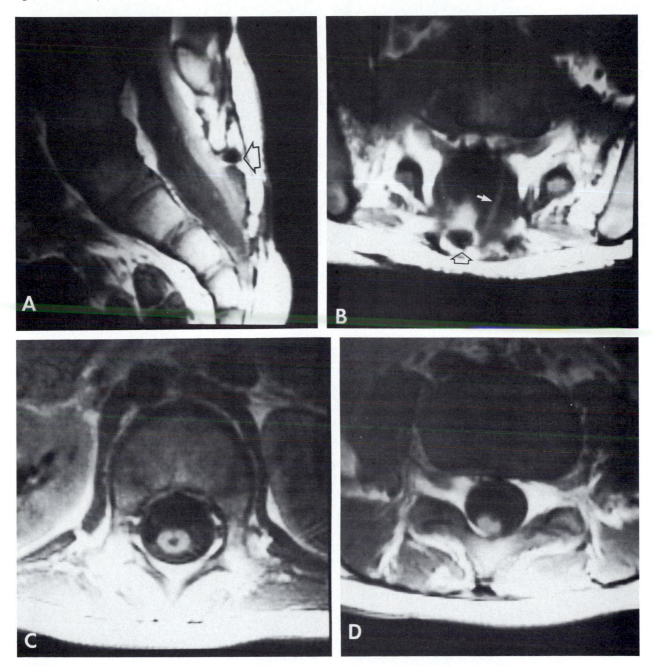

FIG 43–1.
Fifteen-month-old with a previously repaired sacral meningomyelocele and gait abnormality. **A,** a sagittal 600/20-ms image shows posterior positioning of the placode that was demonstrated at surgery to be tethered at the site of primary repair. **B–D,** axial 800/20-ms images demonstrate horizontal coursing of nerve roots originating laterally *(arrow)* and medially from the placode surgically replaced in the spinal canal. There is absence of posterior spinal elements **(B)** and an apparent arachnoid or dural cyst *(open arrow)* posterior to the placode **(B).** Enlargement of the central canal is shown **(C).** Posterior positioning of the cord in the thecal sac at the L4–5 level **(D)** was not associated with local tethering at surgery. (From Brunberg JA, Latchaw RE, Kanal E, et al; Magnetic resonance imaging of spinal dysraphism. *Radiol Clin North Am* 1988; 26:181–205. Used by permission.)

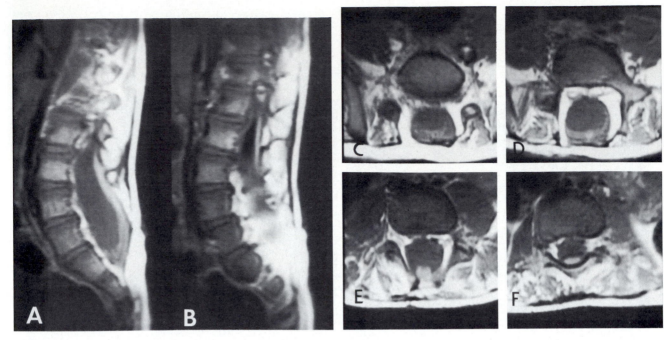

FIG 43–2.
Four-year-old with meningomyelocele repair as a neonate and gait deterioration over several months. Sagittal and axial (600 to 800/20-ms) images demonstrate posterior positioning of the placode **(A, C–E),** horizontal coursing of nerve roots **(C and D),** and ab-sence or dysgenesis of posterior spinal elements **(A–E).** There is posterior positioning of the cord at the site of the lowest intact pos-terior spinal arch **(F).** Tethering at this location cannot be ex-cluded.

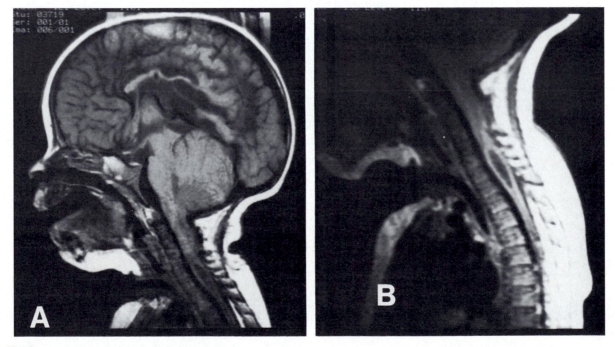

FIG 43–3.
One-month-old with a repaired meningomyelocele, shunted hydro-cephalus, Chiari II malformation, and recent onset of vocal cord paralysis. There is an abnormal gyral pattern, hypoplasia of the corpus callosum, a keel-shaped mesencephalon, aqueductal ste-nosis, a distorted and caudally displaced medulla and fourth ven-tricle, and caudal displacement of the cerebellar tonsils. A cord syrinx is demonstrated from the C5 to the T1 levels (600/20 ms).

of the placode can be demonstrated (Fig 43–1). Nerve roots course in a relatively horizontal direction through the subarachnoid space preoperatively because of tethering of the cord to surrounding cutaneous structures at the placode, and postoperatively there may be tethering of the placode to dura and subcutaneous structures at the operative site (Figs 43–1,B and 43–2). There may also be associated regional congenital structural anomalies such as a lipoma or thickened filum terminale. Preoperatively the margins of the posteriorly incomplete dura are seen to blend with subcu-

taneous fatty or fibrous tissue at the lateral margins of the placode, and there is interruption of the thoracodorsal fascial planes.

In addition to structural changes occurring at the site of the placode, MRI allows a demonstration of the almost invariably associated developmental alterations at other levels of the neuraxis. Such changes include Chiari II malformation with its associated aqueductal stenosis, hydrocephalus, gyral alteration, anomalies of the corpus callosum, keel-shaped mesencephalon, and inferior displacement of the cerebellar tonsils, medulla, and fourth

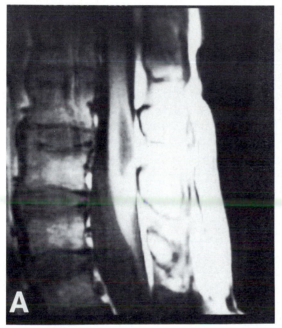

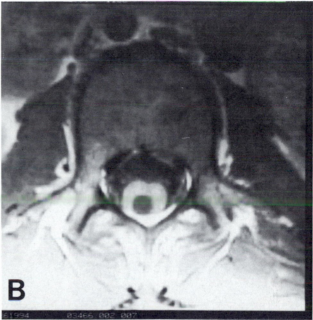

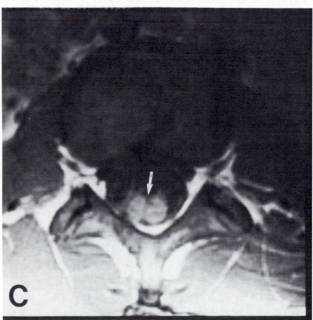

FIG 43–4.
Seven-year-old with a repaired meningomyelocele and recent gait alteration. **A,** a saggital 600/20-ms image demonstrates caudal and posterior positioning of the conus with a central syrinx and widening of the AP diameter of the terminal cord. Axial 800/20-ms images demonstrate the syrinx and horizontal coursing of nerve roots **(B).** At the L2–3 interspace level a central fissure or diastematomyelia *(arrow)* is demonstrated just above the level of the syrinx **(C)**. (From Brunberg JA, Latchaw RE, Kanal E, et al: Magnetic resonance imaging of spinal dysraphism. *Radiol Clin North Am* 1988; 26:181–205. Used by permission.)

ventricle (Fig 43–3). Diastematomyelia, with or without a bony or fibrous spur, is frequently demonstrated above (Fig 43–4,C), at, or below the level of the placode and may be present at more than one level. Irregularity of spinal cord contour in axial imaging may reflect partial cord dysgenesis or myelodysplasia, and duplication of the central canal may occur.[22] Hydromyelia or syringomyelia is commonly associated with meningomyelocele,[23] possibly secondary to obstruction of the central canal at the rostral margin of the placode following surgical repair (Figs 43–4 and 43–5) or secondary to an alteration in cerebrospinal fluid (CSF) flow at the foramen magnum due to an associated Chiari malformation (see Fig 43–3).[16, 24] Because of the occurrence of syrinx formation proximal to the site of the placode it is necessary to image the spinal cord along its entire length to exclude a significant lesion. Intraspinal lipomas occasionally are associated with meningomyelocele and occur along the course of the filum terminale or in extradural or intradural locations where they may be associated with tethering of the cord (Fig 43–6).

Cord tethering associated with spina bifida cystica may occur either as an initial or primary component of the dysraphic developmental process or may develop as a secondary process following sur-

gical repair due to adhesions at the operative site (see Figs 43–1 and 43–2).[23, 25, 26] Tethering is clinically manifested following a period of clinical stability by deterioration of bladder, bowel, motor, or sensory function, by back or leg pain, and by scoliosis or foot deformity,[23, 25, 26] or it may be more subtly manifested by failure of the child to achieve expected developmental milestones. MRI can identify several processes that may be responsible for cord tethering in preoperative or postoperative patients with spina bifida cystica. The initial cause of tethering in unoperated meningomyelocele patients is the fixation of the spinal cord or of the exposed placode to cutaneous and subcutaneous structures at the meningomyelocele site. In addition, there may be primary tethering of the cord due to an associated dysraphic structural alteration such as a thickened filum terminale, lipoma, or diastematomyelia. A third reported cause of primary tethering is membrana reuniens where a neural band courses posteriorly from the filum or cord to attach to the posterior meninges.[25] Finally, a fibrovascular or cartilaginous band may connect bifid spinal laminae at the upper or lower levels of the spina bifida.[4, 27] The spinal cord may be tethered to these transverse bands at a point where spinal cord, placode, and nerve roots herniate posteriorly through

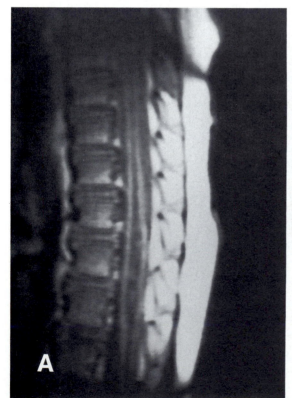

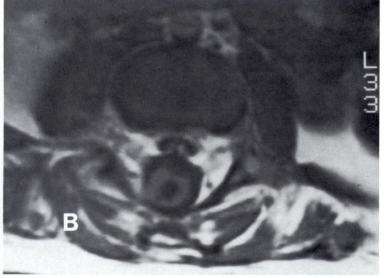

FIG 43–5.
Thirteen-month-old with a meningomyelocele repaired at birth. Sagittal and axial 600/20-ms images demonstrate a syrinx extending from the T9 through the L3 levels **(A)**. An axial image at the L3 level demonstrate central positioning of the syrinx cavity within the cord.

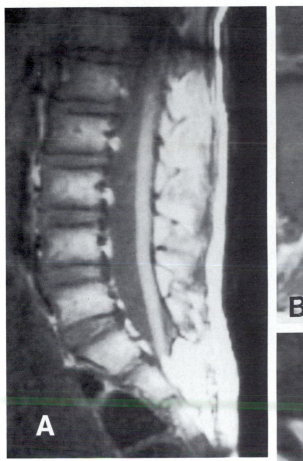

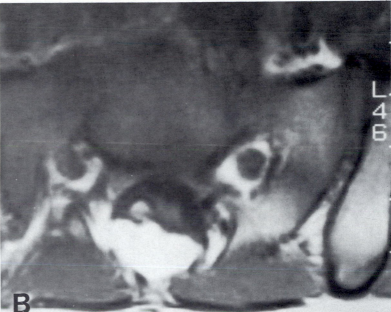

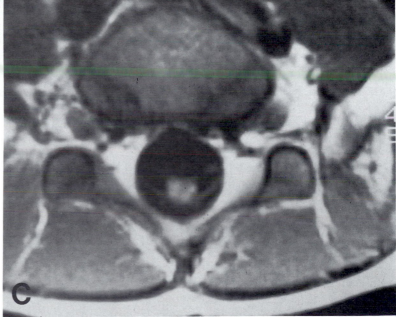

FIG 43–6.
Five-year-old with a lipoma at the site of meningomyelocele repair. The cord is tethered at the S2 level. **A–C,** 600/25-ms images demonstrate the lipoma posterior to the cord at the S2 level **(A and B)** and horizontal coursing of nerve roots adjacent to the caudally positioned cord at the L5 level **(C).**

the dysraphic dural and bony defects. The necessity for release of the tethering associated with meningomyelocoele at each of these potential locations either at the time of early surgical repair or with subsequent surgical procedures has been emphasized.[23, 25, 26] Following primary repair of a meningomyelocele, during which the placode is surgically replaced within the spinal canal, the most common cause of secondary tethering is the postoperative adherence of the placode to surrounding dura, to a dural graft, or to subcutaneous tissue at the repair site.[25]

When MRI demonstrates posterior positioning of the placode or cord at the site of previous surgical meningomyelocele repair, it is our experience that surgical exploration will demonstrate the presence of cord tethering (Figs 43–1, 43–2, 43–7, and 43–8). Posterior positioning of the cord above the site of operative repair and above the most caudal bifid posterior elements may, however, be positional and relate to a "bowstring" effect of the lordotic curvature of the spine rather than to actual tethering (see Fig 43–1,A and D). Neither short nor long TR images allow definitive characteriza-

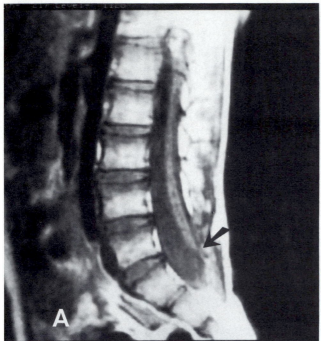
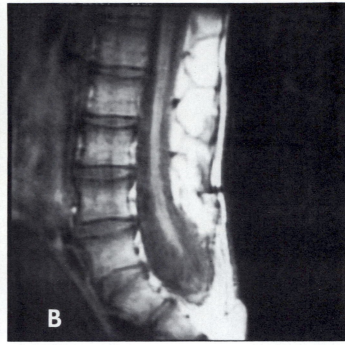

FIG 43–7.
Seven-year-old with a lumbosacral meningomyelocele repaired as an infant and with declining motor and bladder function. **A,** a pre-operative sagittal 600/20-ms image demonstrates tethering of the caudal cord and placode at the operative site *(arrow)*. The spinal cord is posteriorly situated in the widened spinal canal. **B,** a post- operative image demonstrates the cord to be more centrally positioned in the spinal canal following operative release. (From Brunberg JA, Latchaw RE, Kanal E, et al; Magnetic resonance imaging of spinal dysraphism. *Radiol Clin North Am* 1988; 26:181–205. Used by permission.)

tion of the presence or absence of CSF between the posterior surface of the cord and the dura. The demonstration of such fluid would exclude the presence of tethering of the posterior cord to the dura at a given site. The absence of CSF signal posterior to the cord may, however, be due to tethering or may be due to cord pulsation and a CSF flow phenomenon, with flow or turbulence appearing as a region of low MRI signal intensity mimicking a region of fibrous tethering. Axial CT studies with intrathecal contrast may therefore be more sensitive than MRI in defining the presence of a thin layer of CSF posterior to the cord at a site of suspected tethering. If distal cord pulsations are evident on ultrasound evaluation, tethering at the site of pulsation is unlikely. Sufficient MRI experience has not yet been gained with cardiac-gated and gradient-refocused short TR sequences to determine whether these pulsing sequences will be useful for purposes of excluding sites of tethering above the area of surgical repair.

Deterioration in neurologic function in patients with previously repaired meningomyeloceles may occur at the end of the first or in the early second decade of life secondary to tethering, but it may also occur due to growth of a dermoid tumor at the site of operative repair.[28] The presence of a dermoid may result from incomplete excision of dermal elements at the time of initial surgical repair or may represent congenital dermal rests anterior to the placode. The occurrence of a teratoma at the site of meningomyelocele repair and an ependymoma at the site of meningocele repair[29] has been reported. Such tumors may represent neoplastic transformation of regional primordial tissue elements.[29] Symptoms in all cases were those of a spinal mass lesion.

Structural alterations in bone associated with spina bifida cystica are demonstrated with MRI (Figs 43–1 to 43–8) and include widening of interpedicular distances and widening of the spinal canal. The pedicles may rotate from a normal sagittal to a coronal orientation, and transverse processes may rotate into an anterior orientation. The laminae are incomplete at the site of spina bifida and generally are directed downward and posteriorly or are rudimentary. Additional osseous structural alterations include absence of spinous processes, scoliosis, kyphosis, and anomalies of segmentation of the posterior elements and vertebral bodies.

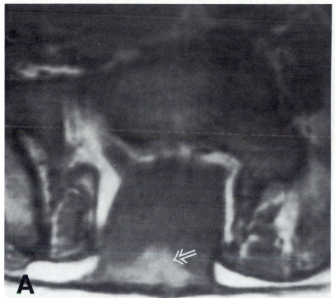

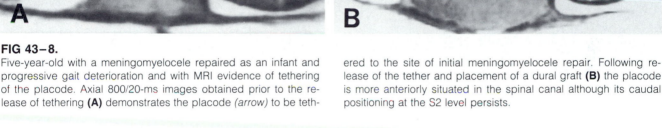

FIG 43–8.
Five-year-old with a meningomyelocele repaired as an infant and progressive gait deterioration and with MRI evidence of tethering of the placode. Axial 800/20-ms images obtained prior to the release of tethering **(A)** demonstrates the placode *(arrow)* to be tethered to the site of initial meningomyelocele repair. Following release of the tether and placement of a dural graft **(B)** the placode is more anteriorly situated in the spinal canal although its caudal positioning at the S2 level persists.

There is lateral displacement of paraspinal musculature at the level of the meningomyelocele. The fibrovascular or cartilaginous band described as connecting bifid spinal laminae at the upper or lower levels of the spina bifida[4, 27] has not been imaged with MRI techniques, possibly because of its blending with cortical bone, periosteum, or other fibrous structures.

LIPOMENINGOMYELOCELE

Lipomeningomyeloceles are characterized by lipomatous tissue that extends ventrally from the subcutaneous region through dysraphic posterior spinal bony elements and through unfused dura to abut on the dorsal aspect of the conus or terminal portion of a dysplastic spinal cord.[4, 27] There is an associated CSF-containing meningocele of varying size. Lipomeningomyeloceles may occur as an occult lesion or may be manifested as cystic spina bifida. Lipomeningomyeloceles are approximately one fourth as common as meningomyeloceles, represent 20% of skin-covered lumbosacral masses, and may represent up to 50% of occult spinal dysraphic lesions.[12] Lipomeningomyeloceles are diagnosed most commonly in infancy, but in the absence of neurologic symptoms or an obvious mass,

the diagnosis may not be made until adulthood. A fatty midline subcutaneous lumbosacral mass is the most common clinical manifestation and occasionally is the only finding. The subcutaneous lipoma may be located off midline, or rarely, there may be no superficial manifestations. Cutaneous anomalies including a skin dimple, dermoid sinus, hypertrichosis, hemangioma, or other cutaneous vascular alterations may be associated. Although there may be no neurologic or orthopedic deficits if the process is diagnosed early, the majority of patients will develop such symptomatology if appropriate early surgical repair is not completed.[12, 30] MRI is therefore suggested for all patients with lumbosacral subcutaneous lipomatous masses, even in the absence of additional anomalous physical findings, to determine whether an underlying spinal dysraphic process exists.

With MRI the lipomatous component of the lipomeningomyelocele is demonstrated as an area of high intensity on T1-weighted images and low intensity on T2-weighted images (Figs 43–9 and 43–10). The lipoma merges with subcutaneous fat and extends through a structural defect in the lumbodorsal fascia; through paraspinal musculature, ligaments, and posterior spinal bony elements; and through a defect in the posterior dura (Fig 43–9). At the level of the defect in the posterior dura the

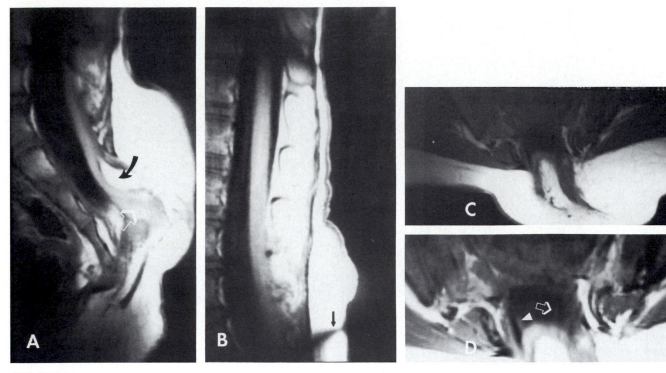

FIG 43–9.
Sixteen-month-old with a low lumbar subcutaneous soft-tissue mass and normal neurologic findings. **A,** a sagittal 600/20-ms image demonstrates the subcutaneous lipoma and caudal fixation of the spinal cord to the S3–4 level with dysplastic enlargement of the terminal cord *(open arrow)*. There is extension of fatty tissue *(curved arrow)* into the spinal canal immediately posterior to the spinal cord. **B,** the cord is posteriorly positioned in the spinal canal due to a "bowstring" effect at the L4–5 level. Note the artifact from the edge of the surface coil *(arrow)*. There is widening of the AP diameter of the spinal canal. **C–H,** axial 800/20-ms images through the sacral region. **C** is windowed to demonstrate the fibrovascular strands within the lipoma as it indents the posterior aspect of the placode. **D,** a magnified image at the same location as

C, demonstrates extension of the lipoma to the dorsal surface of the placode, with motor nerve roots *(open arrow)* arising medially and sensory roots *(arrowhead)* arising laterally from the placode. Horizontal coursing of nerve roots through the subarachnoid space is demonstrated at all levels. **E–H** *(facing page),* a central region of decreased intensity in the cord parenchyma **(F–H)** demonstrates increased intensity on long TR sequences, which is consistent with syrinx formation or duplicated central canal. Dysplasia of posterior spinal elements is noted **(D–G),** with continuity of laminae at more rostral levels **(H)**. (From Brunberg JA, Latchaw RE, Kanal E, et al: Magnetic resonance imaging of spinal dysraphism. *Radiol Clin North Am* 1988; 26:181–205. Used by permission.)

lipoma may indent, infiltrate, and widen the placode (Fig 43–9) and may extend rostrally or caudally under intact posterior vertebral elements, predominately as an extradural but occasionally as an intradural mass. The emergence of the dorsal nerve roots laterally and of ventral nerve roots medially from the anterior aspect of the placode into the subarachnoid space can be demonstrated (Fig 43–9). At the lateral margins of the placode there may be a confluence of tissues including dura, neural tissue, fibrous tissue, and lipoma. The dorsal surface of the placode may be covered with fibrous tissue, fat, and neuroglia. With appropriate image windowing, strands of this tissue can be seen to project into the immediately adjacent lipoma as linear bands of low intensity (Fig

43–9,C). The dorsal surface of the placode is thus covered with lipoma in lipomeningomyelocele, as compared with meningomyelocele where the placode is exposed to air on its dorsal surface. There may be expansion of the subarachnoid space anterior to the placode, with posterior displacement of both the placode and the lipoma and with kinking of the cord and meningocele by intact bridging posterior spinal elements or fibrous bands above or below the lipomeningocele (Fig 43–10). If the lipoma is off midline in its location, the CSF-containing meningocele will protrude posteriorly on the opposite side and rotate the placode into a more vertical position. The CSF-containing meningocele within the subcutaneous lipoma is demonstrated as an area of decreased intensity on T1- and

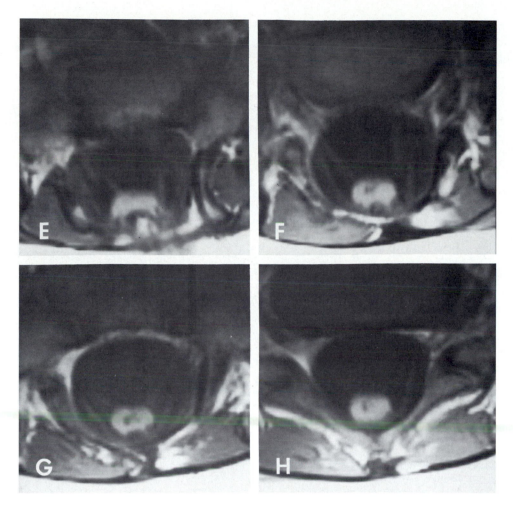

increased intensity on T2-weighted images (Fig 43–10). Communication of the meningocele with the spinal subarachnoid space may be demonstrable with MRI because it is in 60% of patients studied with myelography.[12] The spinal cord is invariably tethered in its position by the lipoma and may also be tethered by the transverse fibrovascular or fibrocartilaginous bands bridging the dysraphic posterior spinal elements above and below the lipomeningomyelocele. Distal to the placode there may be an absence of spinal cord, or there may be a reconstituted cord segment that terminates in a thickened or tethered filum. MRI often demonstrates an enlarged bladder, which correlates with the abnormal urodynamic study results[31] often seen in otherwise neurologically intact patients with lipomeningomyeloceles. The routine radiography of lipomeningomyelocele has been reviewed.[4, 12, 27]

Posterior spinal elements demonstrate structural changes varying from a failure of midline fusion and absence of spinous processes at the most rostral level to marked hypoplasia, relative AP orientation, and a complete absence of posterior elements at the site of the lipoma and meningocele. Anomalies of development and segmentation of vertebral bodies frequently coexist, and there is an association of lipomeningomyelocele with sacral agenesis. A fibrovascular or fibrocartilagenous band extending transversely between the dysplastic laminae, as with meningomyelocele, may be a point of tethering of the cord and of the meningocele.

Surgical repair is not urgent for patients with lipomeningomyelocele. Progressive neurologic dysfunction does, however, occur and appears to relate to growth of the spine in association with cord tethering to the lipoma, to dermal elements, or to a transverse fibrous band extending between bifid posterior spinal elements above and below

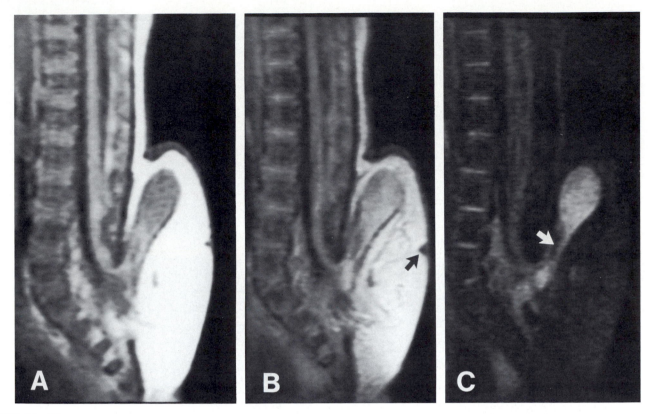

FIG 43–10.

Two-month-old with a soft-tissue mass in the lower lumbar region and normal neurologic findings. **A,** a sagittal 600/20-ms image demonstrates caudal fixation of the spinal cord with neural tissue extending into the large meningeal sac within the rostral portion of the subcutaneous lipoma. The cord makes an abrupt angle around the intact posterior spinal elements at the L4 level. Variation in intensity of spinal fluid within the sac and anterior to the cord may relate to a flow phenomenon or to altered protein content. **B,** a sagittal 2,500/25-ms image demonstrates caudal fixation of the cord and demonstrates the dura surrounding the meningocele within the lipoma. Fibrous septa within the lipoma and a central cutaneous dimple *(arrow)* are demonstrated. **C,** a sagittal 2,500/100-ms image demonstrates spinal fluid within the meningomyelocele. Dysraphic neural elements extending into the meningocele cavity are characterized as a filling defect of low intensity *(arrow).* (From Brunberg JA, Latchaw RE, Kanal E, et al: Magnetic resonance imaging of spinal dysraphism. *Radiol Clin North Am* 1988; 26:181–205. Used by permission.)

the lipomeningomyelocele. Direct trauma to the subcutaneous lipoma may also correlate with the development of symptoms.[32] The development of symptoms may also relate to increasing bulk and complexity of the lipomatous component of a lipomeningomyelocele with age, with the incorporation of additional cord parenchyma or additional nerve roots making resection more difficult.[32] Other congenital anomalies associated with lipomeningomyelocele that may have a role in the development of neurologic dysfunction include diastematomyelia, terminal hydromyelia, syringomyelia associated with Chiari I malformation, dermoid or epidermoid cyst, proliferation of neuroglial hamartomatous tissue adjacent to the cord (Fig 43–11), dermal sinus, and tethered filum. In a series of 97 patients with lipomeningomyeloeceles described by Hoffman et al., 35 of 56 patients less than

6 months of age were neurologically normal preoperatively. Only 12 of 41 patients over 6 months of age and none of the 14 patients over 4 years of age were neurologically normal if the structural defects associated with lipomeningomyelocele had not been surgically repaired.[33] Symptoms of neurologic impairment develop gradually, over months or years, and include bowel and bladder dysfunction, lumbosacral sensory alteration, motor deficits, loss of muscle bulk, lumbar pain radiating into the lower extremities, orthopedic deformities of the feet, and scoliosis. A skin dimple is often present, and in Hoffman and associates' series 5 of 97 patients were demonstrated to have a skin tag or tail-like appendage.[33] Early surgical management is advocated to prevent neurologic deterioration and include the release of tethering at the site of the lipoma, at the filum, and at the site of posterior pro-

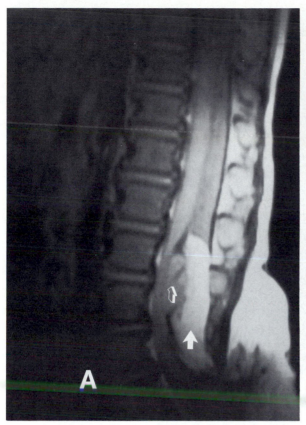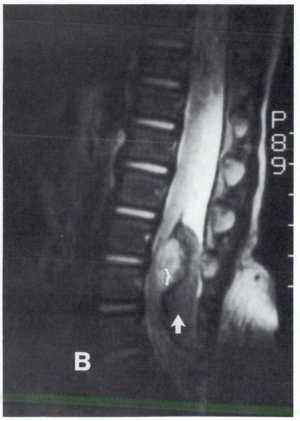

FIG 43–11.
Seven-month-old with a lipomeningomyelocele. Sagittal 3,000/30-ms **(A)** and 3,000/120-ms **(B)** images demonstrate extension of the lipoma into the spinal cord. The mass *(open arrows)* between the lipoma *(arrow)* and the spinal cord was demonstrated at surgery to represent a neural-glial hamartoma.

trusion of neural elements past a transverse cartilaginous or fibrovascular bands above and below the site of dysraphism.[12, 27, 32, 33] The lipomatous elements are excised, and the meningocele is repaired. In a series of 75 patients with lipomeningocele Edwards noted reversal of function loss in 26% and stabilization of a course of progressive function loss in 74% following operative intervention.[32]

MENINGOCELE

Meningocele is the extension of nonneural tissue including spinal fluid, dura, and arachnoid through a bony defect in the spine (Fig 43–12). The extension is most commonly through posterior bony elements into paraspinal or subcutaneous tissues but may develop anteriorly into the retroperitoneum, thorax, or skull base. Structural bone alterations are generally less prominent in meningocele than in meningomyelocele. Regional nerves may herniate into and become adherent to the wall of the sac, and there may be fusion of the dura and arachnoid at the neck of or throughout the entire sac. Fibrous or glial septa may traverse the sac and may be most prominent at the neck. Lipomas, glial and smooth muscle heterotopias, and myelodysplasia (Fig 43–13) may occur in association with meningocele and are demonstrable with MRI.

SYRINGOMYELIA

Syringomyelia is a spinal cord abnormality characterized by a longitudinal intramedullary cavitary lesion that is surrounded by gliosis. The distinction between hydromyelia as an enlargement of the ependyma-lined central canal and syringomyelia as cavitation of the cord involving other than the central canal is clinically unnecessary, and the inclusive term *syringohydromyelia* is increasingly utilized.[16, 34, 35] There are two major types of syringomyelia, communicating and non-

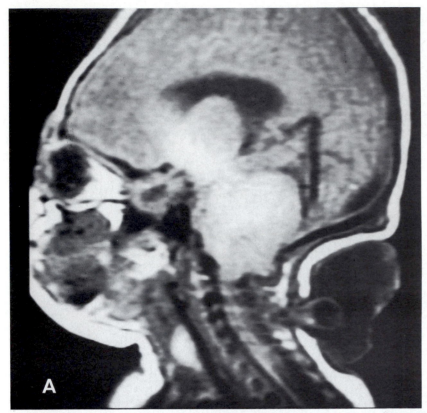

FIG 43–12.
Two-day-old with a cervical meningocele and normal neurologic findings. **A,** a sagittal 600/20-ms image demonstrates a cervical meningocele at the C3 level with central meningeal and glial tissue that cannot be distinguished from the spinal cord or nerve roots with MRI. A Chiari malformation is demonstrated at the foramen magnum on this slightly off midline view. **B** and **C,** coronal 600/20-ms images demonstrate the meningocele cavity and the central tissue within it as they extend toward the cervical cord. Nerve roots are demonstrated to extend from the cord *(open arrow)*, which has a central posterior fissure. A right subgaleal hematoma and altered contour of the calvarium is demonstrated *(arrow)*. (From Brunberg JA, Latchaw RE, Kanal E, et al: Magnetic resonance imaging of spinal dysraphism. *Radiol Clin North Am* 1988; 26:181–205. Used by permission.)

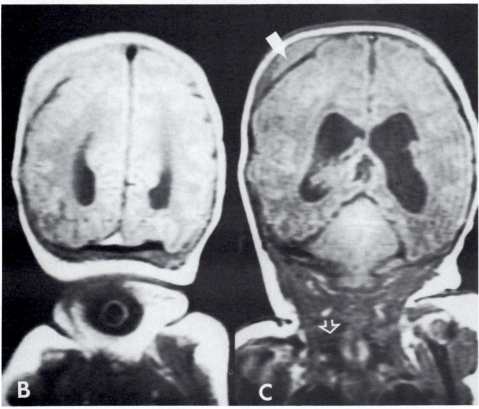

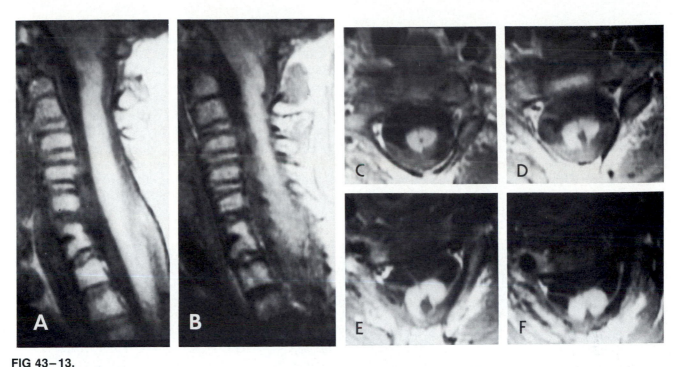

FIG 43–13.
Four-year-old with previous cervical meningocele repair. **A** and **B,** sagittal 600/20-ms images demonstrate suspected cord tethering manifested by posterior positioning of an enlarged spinal cord. There is abnormal segmentation and a narrowed AP diameter of the C6 and C7 vertebral bodies. **C–F,** axial 800/20-ms images demonstrate myelodysplasia with an enlarged central canal at the C3 level **(C)** in continuity with a posterior clefting of the cord at the C4 to C7 levels **(D–F).** There is horizontal coursing of the nerve roots. Poorly defined regions of increased intensity posterior to the cord most likely represents postoperative fibrosis or gliosis. (From Brunberg JA, Latchaw RE , Kanal E, et al: Magnetic resonance imaging of spinal dysraphism. *Radiol Clin North Am* 1988; 26:181–205. Used by permission.)

communicating. Communicating syringomyelia, implying a patent communication with the ventricular system through the central canal, is generally associated with a congenital or acquired lesion in the region of the foramen magnum. Normal CSF pulsations in the fourth ventricle are propagated through the obex and into the central canal. CSF may then be trapped in the central canal due to a ball-valve effect induced by structural change at the foramen magnum.[36] Chiari I and II malformations with mass effect on the cervical cord at the foramen magnum from caudally displaced tonsillar tissue are the most common correlates of syringomyelia in patients with spinal dysraphism (see Fig 43–3). Posterior fossa cysts, occipital encephaloceles (Fig 43–14), acquired mass lesions in the posterior fossa, and basal arachnoiditis may produce syringomyelia by the same mechanism. In a patient with an unrepaired meningomyelocele, a flow of CSF from the central canal can occasionally be observed on the rostral unruptured surface of the placode. Following surgical repair of the meningomyelocele, flow of caudally diverted CSF in the central canal becomes obstructed at the site of re-

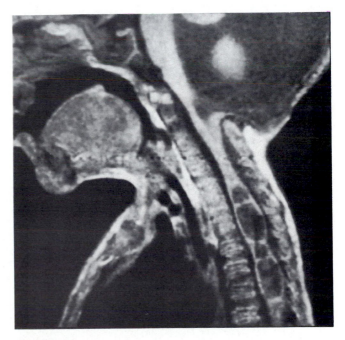

FIG 43–14.
Two-month-old with a repaired posterior fossa encephalocele. CSF is seen to extend into the central medulla, and there is an associated cervicothoraxic cord syrinx.

pair, and a communicating syrinx may result (see Figs 43–4 and 43–5).

Noncommunicating syringomyelia does not communicate with the ventricular system. CSF is thought to enter a noncommunicating syrinx through enlarged parenchymal perivascular spaces, along dorsal or ventral nerve roots, or through macroscopic direct communications with the subarachnoid space. Fluid may enter via these pathways during a transient increase in intraspinal pressure such as may occur with a Valsalva maneuver when the pressure is not transmitted to the cranial vault because of a blockage at the foramen magnum. CSF

forced into the cord parenchyma may remain there if a "ball-valve" effect exists at the site of fluid entrance. This second mechanical process for noncommunicating syrinx formation may thus also be occurring in patients with Chiari malformations described above. Trauma,[37] spinal arachnoiditis, and fluid secretion or necrosis occurring in association with a spinal cord tumor are additional causes of noncommunicating syringomyelia. The primary congenital formation of a large central canal may also be responsible for the presence of a cord syrinx. Once a syrinx has formed by any mechanism, the syrinx may be maintained by fluid secretion from its ependy-

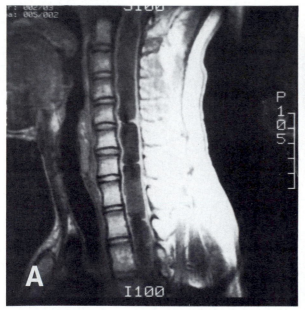

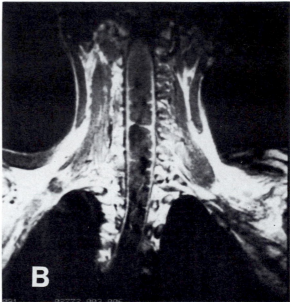

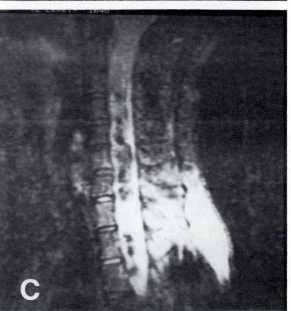

FIG 43–15.
Eighteen-year-old with progressive spasticity and a suspected spinal cord tumor. **A,** a sagittal 600/20-ms image demonstrates a syrinx extending from C1 through the upper thoracic cord with incomplete transverse septations. A Chiari I malformation was demonstrated on separate images. **B,** a coronal 800/20-ms image demonstrates the transverse extent of the syrinx cavity within the spinal cord. Regions of lowest intensity within the syrinx cavity relate to CSF flow. **C,** a sagittal 3,000/120-ms image demonstrates areas of flow or turbulence within the syrinx as regions of low intensity. (From Brunberg JA, Latchaw RE, Kanal E, et al: Magnetic resonance imaging of spinal dysraphism. *Radiol Clin North Am* 1988; 26:181–205. Used by permission.)

mal or glial surface. Symptoms of syringomyelia include pain, loss of muscle bulk, disassociated sensory alteration, paraparesis, scoliosis, trophic skin changes, and neuropathic joints.

Syrinx location and size are best characterized with MRI sequences utilizing T1-weighted images (Figs 43–15 and 43–16). The intensity of the syrinx cavity on T1-weighted images is usually low relative to that of cord parenchyma but depends on the TR and TE of the pulsing sequence, on the protein content of the cyst, on the presence of hemoglobin metabolites, and on flow or turbulence. Characteristics of the syrinx cavity including size, eccentricity of position, and the intensity of surrounding cord parenchyma on T1- and T2-weighted images do not allow a distinction between the potential causes of syrinx formation. Increased parenchymal intensity surrounding a syrinx on T2-weighted images may be from gliosis or edema in communicating syringomyelia or may represent tumor or residuals of trauma. Initial reports indicate that gadolinium–diethylenetriamine pentaacetic acid (Gd-DTPA) may be useful in defining the presence of a cord parenchymal tumor associated with syrinx formation.[38] CSF flow or turbulence is seen as areas of decreased intensity within the syrinx cavity on routine T1- and T2-weighted images in patients with communicating syringomyelia (see Fig 43–11). Such flow or turbulence has also, however, been demonstrated in patients with a noncommunicating syrinx.

Surgical management of syringomyelia is based on the apparent etiology and may include syrinx shunting to the subarachnoid space or peritoneal cavity, cyst fenestration, foramen magnum decompression with lysis of adhesions or membranes, placement of a ventriculoperitoneal shunt, and placement of a tissue plug in the obex. MRI is useful following foramen magnum decompression (Fig 43–17) or after shunting of a syrinx to demonstrate changes in syrinx size, to demonstrate the position of shunt tubing, and to demonstrate the possible presence of septations in the syrinx that may prevent adequate drainage. Subsequent studies are also useful in confirming the absence of an associated cord tumor.

SPINAL LIPOMA

Spinal lipomas are fat and fibrous tissue deposits within the spinal canal that may invade or ad-

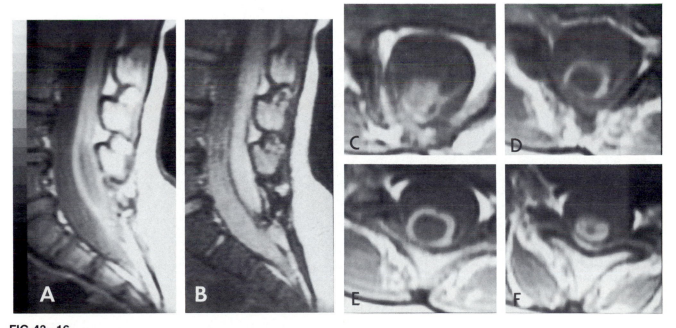

FIG 43–16.
Sixteen-month-old with a lumbosacral fatty soft-tissue mass, no previous surgical procedures, and normal neurologic findings. **A,** a sagittal 800/20-ms image demonstrates a central syrinx in a tethered cord with a subcutaneous lipoma that does not extend into the spinal canal. **B,** a sagittal 3,000/100-ms image demonstrates the syrinx fluid to be of high intensity. **C–F,** axial 800/20-ms images confirm the central location of the syrinx and the caudal location of the conus. (From Brunberg JA, Latchaw RE, Kanal E, et al: Magnetic resonance imaging of spinal dysraphism. *Radiol Clin North Am* 1988; 26:181–205. Used by permission.)

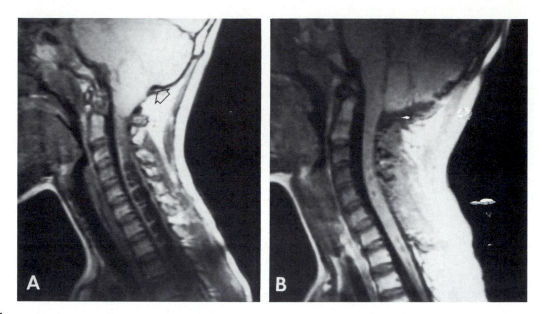

FIG 43–17.
Eleven-year-old with Chiari I malformation and progressive weakness of the left upper and left lower extremities. **A,** a sagittal 600/20-ms image demonstrates inferior displacement of the cerebellar tonsils past the posterior rim of the foramen magnum *(arrow).* A syrinx of the cervical cord extends from the C2–3 level beyond the field of imaging into the upper thoracic cord. **B,** following occipital and cervical decompression the syrinx cavity has almost completely collapsed. Note the absence of posterior spinal elements through the C6 level and the occipital craniectomy site. (From Brunberg JA, Latchaw RE, Kanal E, et al: Magnetic resonance imaging of spinal dysraphism. *Radiol Clin North Am* 1988; 26:181–205. Used by permission.)

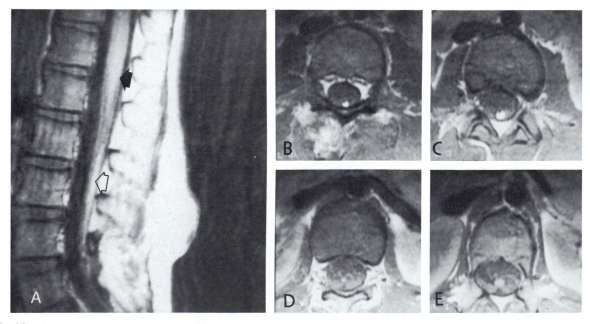

FIG 43–18.
Three-year-old with a lumbar subcutaneous soft-tissue mass, a cutaneous dimple, and otherwise normal examination findings. **A,** a sagittal 600/25-ms image demonstrates the conus to be in a normal position *(closed arrow)* and demonstrates a linear region of increased intensity that is consistent with lipomatous tissue involving the filum terminale *(open arrow).* **B–F,** axial 800/25-ms images demonstrates a small region of increased intensity in the posterior thecal sac caudal to the conus that appears to be indented by glial tissue of the filum and is consistent with lipoma of the filum terminale **(B and C).** The conus is at the L1–2 level **(D)**. (From Brunberg JA, Latchaw RE, Kanal E, et al: Magnetic resonance imaging of spinal dysraphism. *Radiol Clin North Am* 1988; 26:181–205. Used by permission.)

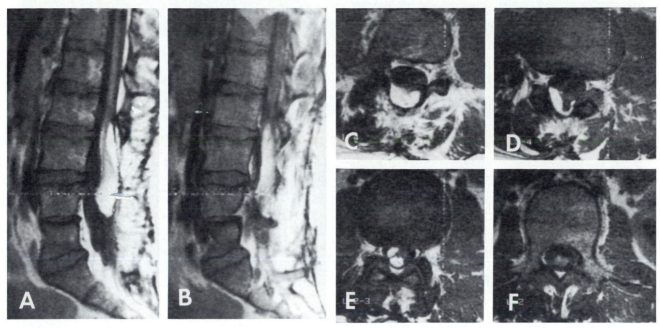

FIG 43–19.
Seventeen-year-old with low back pain and normal neurologic findings. **A** and **B,** adjacent sagittal 800/20-mms images demonstrate an intradural lipoma surrounding the cauda equina and conus. Nerve roots are seen as linear bands of relatively low intensity extending through the lipoma. **C–F,** axial images demonstrate clustering of nerve roots within the posteriorly positioned lipoma. (From Brunberg JA, Latchaw RE, Kanal E, et al: Magnetic resonance imaging of spinal dysraphism. *Radiol Clin North Am* 1988; 26:181–205. Used by permission.)

here to spinal cord, cauda equina, or meninges. With MRI spinal lipomatous tissue is characterized by relatively high signal on T1- and spin-density weighted images and by relatively diminished signal intensity on T2-weighted images. Fibrous tissue, vessels, calcification, meningeal elements, and neural elements, when associated with the lipoma, are seen as regions of decreased MRI signal intensity crossing through or encapsulating the lipoma (Figs 43–18 to 43–23). A fibrous capsule may be imaged as surrounding the lipoma but must be differentiated from chemical shift artifact (Fig 43–23).

Spinal lipomas are postulated to arise during embryologic development from cutaneous ectodermal cell rests that become isolated from the surrounding ectoderm at the time of neural tube closure. Spinal lipomas may also arise from perivascular mesenchyma accompanying the initial vascularization of the embryonic spinal cord. Persisting mesenchyma on the dorsal surface of the unclosed neural tube may also prevent closure of the neural tube or prevent fusion of both the dura and posterior spinal elements with lipomeningomyelocele formation.[4]

Spinal lipomas may be found in any compartment within the spinal canal. They may be intradural or extradural or may be both intradural and extradural in location, with MRI demonstrating the site of passage of the lipoma through the dura. Intradural lipomas may be confined to the filum terminale (see Fig 43–18), may be intermixed with the nerve roots of the cauda equina (Fig 43–19), may be well circumscribed and situated in a juxtamedullary position generally posterior or posterolateral to the spinal cord (Figs 43–20 and 43–21), or may represent a portion of a bone or fibrous spur occurring in association with diastematomyelia. Lipomas may also be entirely intramedullary in location. Intradural lipomas may invade the spinal cord but are more commonly adherent via a fibrous capsule to the posterior aspect of the spinal cord and/or to the meninges where they may represent a potential cause of tethering. Cord tethering can occur in association with an intraspinal lipoma, with the conus caudally fixed at the tip of the sacral canal by the lipoma (Fig 43–22). Although lipomas may be adherent to the surface of the cord, chemical shift artifact may erroneously suggest the presence of a thick fibrous tissue plane between the cord and the lipoma that may not exist (Fig 43–23). Lipomas may extend extradurally to intra-

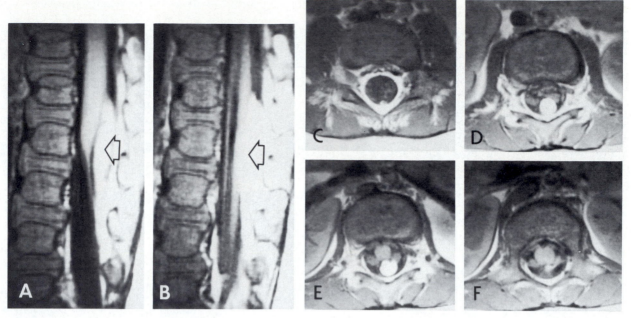

FIG 43-20.
Six-month-old with a sacral subcutaneous lipoma and normal neurologic findings. **A** and **B,** adjacent sagittal 600/25-ms images demonstrate the presence of a lipoma *(arrow)* posterior to the terminal spinal cord. The off-midline sagittal image **(B)** demonstrates clumping of dorsal and ventral nerve roots, which, in the absence of axial or a true midline sagittal image, could be mistaken for a tethered cord. **C-F,** axial 800/20-ms images extending superiorly to be positioned posterior to the terminal spinal cord **(F).** (From Brunberg JA, Latchaw RE, Kanal E, et al: Magnetic resonance imaging of spinal dysraphism. *Radiol Clin North Am* 1988; 26:181–205. Used by permission.)

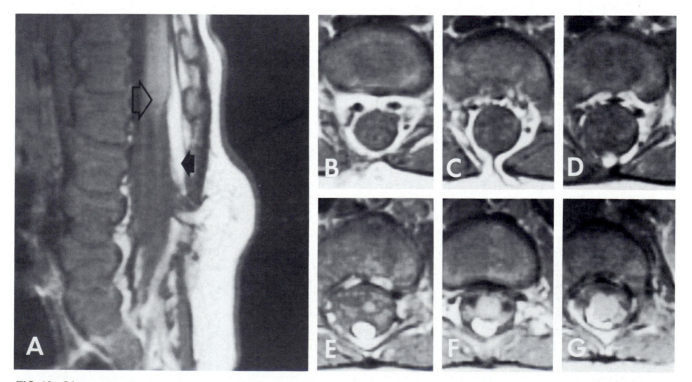

FIG 43-21.
Ten-month-old with a subcutaneous lumbar lipoma and normal neurologic findings. **A,** a sagittal 600/20-ms image demonstrates a well-demarcated intradural lipoma *(closed arrow)* situated posteriorly in the thecal sac and extending rostrally behind the conus *(open arrow).* **B-G,** axial 800/20-ms images at L1–4 demonstrate a fibrous strand continuous with the lumbodorsal fascia and with the dura at L4, and nerve roots are seen in cross section in the thecal sac **(C).** The lipoma pierces the dura at L3 **(D)** and extends superiorly within the dura **(E-G)** posterior to the conus at the L1–2 level **(E** and **F).** Clusters of nerve roots surround the conus **(E** and **F).**

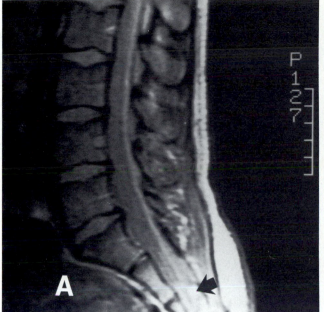

FIG 43–22.
Fifteen-year-old with sensory alteration involving both lower extremities. There is no history of previous surgical procedures. Sagittal 3,000/25-ms **(A)** and 3,000/100-ms **(B)** images demonstrate a small lipoma *(arrow)* at the tip of an enlarged sacral canal. There is associated cord tethering.

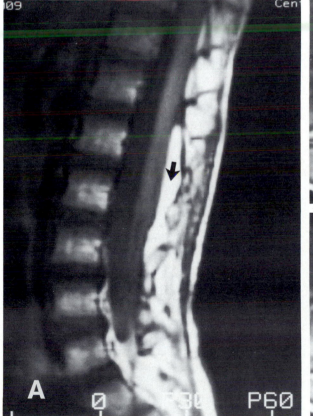

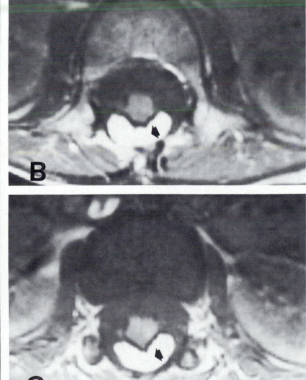

FIG 43–23.
Five-year-old male with an intradural lipoma. **A–C,** 600 to 800/20-ms images demonstrate the intradural lipoma *(arrows)* extending from L1 to L3. There is an undulating posterior border of the lipoma adjacent to dysplastic posterior spinal elements. The region of low intensity between the cord and the lipoma **(B** and **C)** was thought to result from a chemical shift effect and to not represent fibrous tissue in these axial images obtained with a horizontally oriented, phase-encoding gradient. At surgery the lipoma was easily removed from the dorsal surface of the spinal cord.

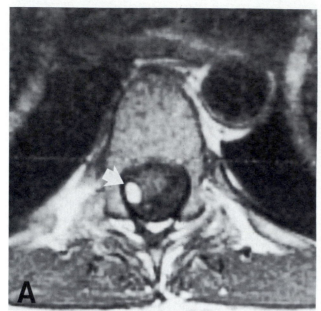
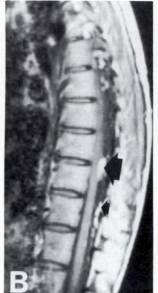
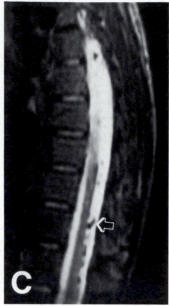

FIG 43–24.
Thirty-nine-year-old with a suspected thoracic spine lesion. **A,** an axial 800/20-ms image demonstrates a well-demarcated region of increased intensity *(arrow)* posterolateral to the cord. **B,** a sagittal 600/20-ms image demonstrates a high-intensity region *(large arrow)* and similar intradural regions inferiorly *(small arrow).* **C,** a sagittal 3,500/100-ms image, slightly more medial in position than

B, demonstrates the areas to be of low intensity *(arrow).* Correlative roentgenograms demonstrated the region to be iophendylate (Pantopaque) from a previous myelogram. (From Brunberg JA, Latchaw RE, Kanal E, et al: Magnetic resonance imaging of spinal dysraphism. *Radiol Clin North Am* 1988; 26:181–205. Used by permission.)

durally through a dorsal defect in the dura (Fig 43–21) and may be associated with an extradural mass effect. Associated dysraphic alterations in vertebral elements are well demonstrated with MRI since cortical bone has essentially no signal and fat in medullary bone has high signal intensity on T1-weighted images. Bone changes occurring secondary to the mass effect of the lipoma include widening of the spinal canal, erosion of pedicles, and thinning of the posterior elements.

Although intradural lipomas are reported to occur most commonly at dorsal and cervical levels, in our experience intradural lipomas unassociated with lipomeningomyeloceles have occurred most commonly in the lumbosacral region. Although most patients with spinal lipomas are asymptomatic at birth or have only a lumbosacral subcutaneous lipoma, symptoms generally develop with age. Combining their experience with 73 cases and a review of five major published series, Pierre-Kahn et al. reported progressive neurologic deficits in 56% of cases of intraspinal lipomas.[39] Early surgical intervention is generally favored to avoid sequelae that relate to the effect of tethering of the cord or nerve roots by the lipoma,[39] to a mass effect from the lipoma, or to the effect of associated spinal congenital anomalies.

Iophendylate (Pantopaque) persisting in the spinal canal may be difficult to distinguish from the presence of a lipoma, and a localized region of bright signal on short TR or spin-density weighted images requires correlation with routine radiographic images (Fig 43–24).[40]

TETHERED CORD

Tethering or fixation of the spinal cord can occur either as an isolated phenomenon or in association with the other dysraphic spinal lesions described in this chapter. Tethering most commonly involves the lumbar cord or conus, but may occur at any location and has been described at cervical[41] and thoracic[42] levels. Caudal tethering of the cord unassociated with other dysraphic processes most commonly relates to the presence of a short or thickened filum terminale. Caudal tethering or inferior positioning of the conus from any cause is defined as positioning of the conus below the L3 vertebral body level in patients less than 6 years of age and below the L2–3 interspace level in patients over 12 years of age.[4, 43, 44] A rapid relative ascent of the spinal cord occurs at 9 to 18 weeks of gestation, and by 48 weeks of gestational age the conus is usually at the L3 level. Caudal fixation of the conus in the absence of other dysraphic processes may occur secondary to early intrauterine focal caudal perispinal hemorrhagic or inflammatory processes involving all three germ layers.[45]

Symptoms of tethering may be manifested in childhood or may not present until adult life.[11, 43, 44] Symptoms include sensory or motor alteration involving the lower extremities, bladder or bowel dysfunction, scoliosis, or orthopedic deformities of the feet. Cord symptoms most likely relate to stretching of spinal pathways and to ischemia from arterial and venous stretching.[46]

Radiographic findings of caudal tethering demonstrated with MRI include a caudally positioned conus, posterior positioning of the caudal spinal cord within the spinal canal, and occasionally a long tapering of the conus or thick filum terminale (Fig 43–25). MRI allows definitive localization of the normal conus on axial images, although there may be some ambiguity in defining the conus in patients with a thick filum terminale. With a tethered cord, horizontal coursing of nerve roots is well demonstrated. On sagittal MRI it is occasionally difficult to distinguish the conus from nerve roots of the cauda equina, which cluster in four groups around the conus and terminal cord (see Fig 43–20). Axial MRI is imperative in establishing the level of the conus.

While operative intervention usually relieves symptoms of pain associated with the tethered cord syndrome, bladder and bowel dysfunction is often unimproved postoperatively.[25] There may be an incomplete recovery of motor function, although there is generally an arrest in progression of symptomatology. Early diagnosis and surgical intervention appear to favorably influence long-term function.[11]

DIASTEMATOMYELIA

Diastematomyelia is characterized by a longitudinal division of the spinal cord, most commonly occurring between the T9 and S1 cord levels. The embryogenesis of diastematomyelia is not fully understood but may relate to a split of the notochord with associated ventral invagination of endoderm and dorsal invagination of neural ectoderm, to failure of dorsal midline fusion of the neural plate with

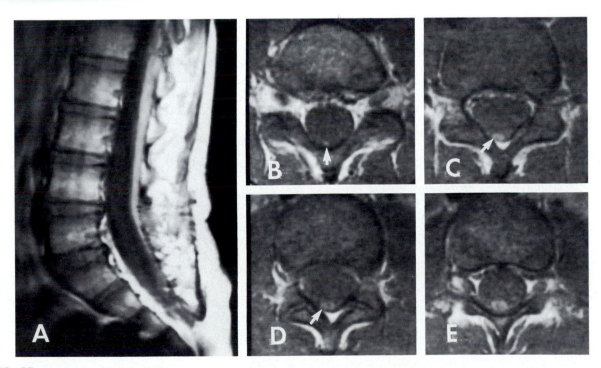

FIG 43–25.
Three-year-old with sacral lipomeningocele repair as an infant and a 4-month history of bilateral anterior thigh pain. **A,** a sagittal 600/20-ms image demonstrates the caudal positioning of the cord and fatty tissue in the lumbar subcutaneous region. **B–E,** axial 800/20-ms images demonstrate a thickened filum *(arrow)* at L5–S1 **(B)** and a tapered posteriorly situated conus *(arrow)* at L5 **(C)** and L4 **(D)** and L3–4 vertebral levels. (From Brunberg JA, Latchaw RE, Kanal E, et al: Magnetic resonance imaging of spinal dysraphism. *Radiol Clin North Am* 1988; 26:181–205. Used by permission.)

continued incurving of the plate margins resulting in two separate neural tubes, or to a primary mesodermal abnormality that splits the neural plate.[4, 10] In approximately half of diastematomyelia cases there is a single, undivided dural tube (Figs 43–26 and 43–27). In the remainder there is a splitting or longitudinal division of the dural sac[47] with a fibrous, cartilaginous, or bony septum between the cord divisions (Fig 43–28). The septum is most commonly located at the L1 to L4 level and appears as a linear band of decreased intensity on T1-, spin-density, and T2-weighted images. The spur and the division of the cord may be asymetrically or obliquely positioned. The cord segments may be rotated up to 90 degrees, and the spur may be continuous with the anterior and/or the posterior aspects of either the dura or the periosteum of the spinal canal. In those patients in whom the dural sheath is not divided, a spur is generally not radiographically demonstrated between the cord segments (Figs 43–26 and 43–27).[47] Apart from the spur at the site of clefting, there may be fibrous bands, as described by James and Lassman, that extend from the cord to the dura and cause a tethering effect on the cord or nerve roots.[48] These bands have not been demonstrated with MRI. A tethered conus or thick filum terminale is frequently found in association with diastematomyelia, as are meningomyelocele (see Fig 43–4), dermal sinus, lipoma, myelodysplasia, and syringomyelia. In most cases of diastematomyelia there is a narrowed AP diameter of the spinal canal and narrowing of the intervertebral disk space at the level of the diastematomyelia (Fig 43–28). There are frequently associated anterior or posterior bony fusion defects, butterfly vertebrae, hemivertebrae, or vertebral body fusions (Figs 43–26 and 43–28).

Diastematomyelia is three times more frequent in females than males. Symptoms are nonspecific, do not allow clinical distinction of diastematomyelia from other dysraphic processes, and do not accurately predict the level of involvement or the degree of laterality of the cord division.[47] Clinical features include skin changes with a hairy patch, local hyperpigmentation, subcutaneous lipoma, and occasionally the presence of an associated meningomyelocele or dermal sinus. There is frequent muscle wasting with hyporeflexia of one lower extremity and occasional hyperreflexia in the

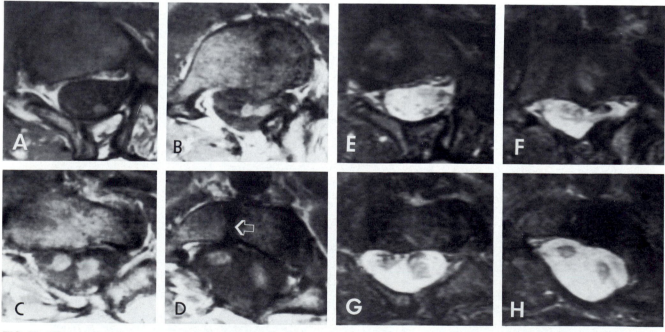

FIG 43–26.
Diastematomyelia in a 15-year-old with a repaired thoracolumbar meningomyelocele. **A–D,** axial 800/20-ms images, and **E–H,** 3,500/100-ms images at correlating locations. **A** and **E** at the L3–4 interspace demonstrate the caudal rejoining of the cord segments. **B** and **F** are at the L3 level and **C** and **G** at the L2 level. **D** and **H,** at the L1 level, demonstrate a wide CSF-containing space between the segments without a fibrous or bony septum. A cleft through which a meningocele does not extend is seen in the vertebral body at L1 **(D)** *(arrow)*. (From Brunberg JA, Latchaw RE, Kanal E, et al: Magnetic resonance imaging of spinal dysraphism. *Radiol Clin North Am* 1988; 26:181–205. Used by permission.)

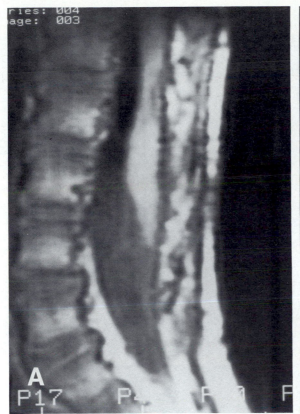

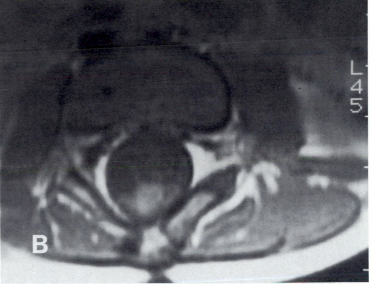

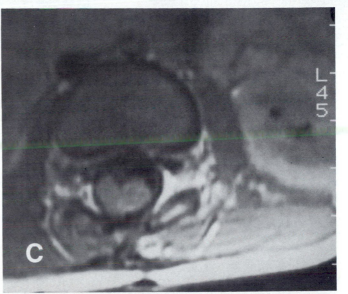

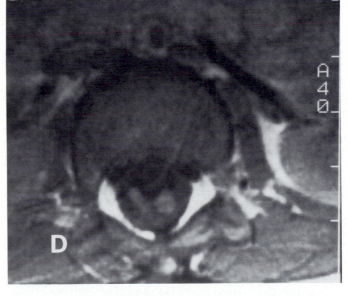

FIG 43–27.
One-year-old with a tethered cord and diastematomyelia.
A–D, 600 to 800/20-ms. The conus is caudally positioned
at the L3–4 interspace level (**A** and **B**) where there is
narrowing of the AP diameter of the verebral bodies and
widening of the spinal canal. At the L3 level (**C**) there is
an anterior fissure in a somewhat enlarged cord. The
diastematomyelia in a single dural sleeve unassociated
with a central septum is demonstrated at the L2 level
(**A** and **D**) where there is narrowing of the AP diameter of
the cord over the one segment length of the
diastematomyelia.

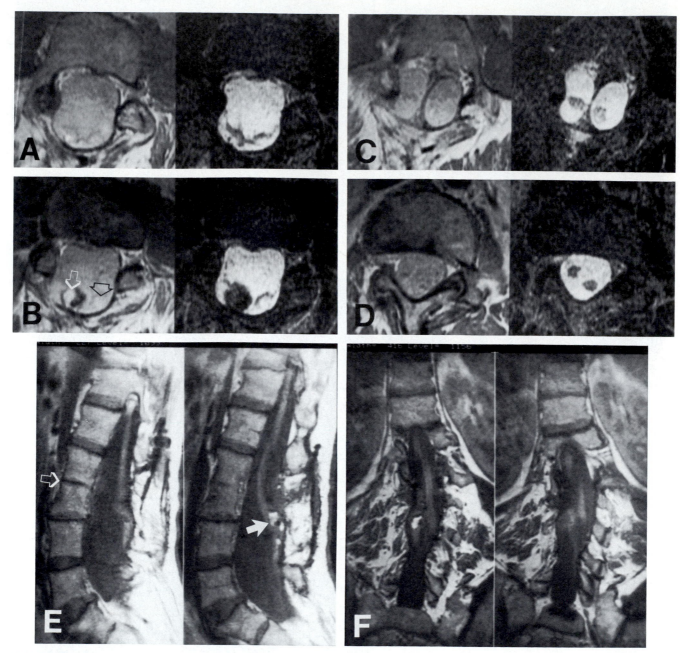

FIG 43–28.

Thirty-two-year-old with diastematomyelia. **A–D,** axial images at 2,500/25-ms on the *left*, 2,500/100-ms on the *right*. At the L4 level **(A)** the diastematomyelia rejoins at the conus, which is caudally positioned. A lipoma in the enlarged right segment of the diastematomyelia *(open white arrow)* is of high intensity on the 25-ms echo and of low intensity on the 100-ms echo **(B).** In the left segment a syrinx *(open black arrow)* is isointense with CSF on both echoes **(B).** A fibrous or bony spur is present at the L3–4

level **(C). E,** adjacent sagittal 600/20-ms images demonstrate decreased height of the L2–3 interspace *(open arrow)* and decreased AP diameter of the L2 and L3 vertebral bodies. The lipoma in the *right* cord segment is demonstrated *(arrow).* **F,** coronal images demonstrate the diastematomyelia and the lipoma in the *right* cord segment. (From Brunberg JA, Latchaw RE, Kanal E, et al: Magnetic resonance imaging of spinal dysraphism. *Radiol Clin North Am* 1988; 26:181–205. Used by permission.)

opposite extremity. Symptoms of bladder dysfunction are common. There is often scoliosis, diminished range of motion of the lumbar spine, and cavovarus deformity of a foot.[10, 47, 49]

Although the patient may be neurologically in-

tact at the time of diagnosis, there is such a high risk of developing cord symptoms of spinal cord dysfunction by adolescence that anticipatory surgical intervention is generally advocated.[10] Progressive deterioration in the unoperated patient may relate to traction on the lower end of the spinal cord cleft by the spur, to compression of the surrounding cord and distortion of spinal fiber tracts by the spur, or to the occurrence of ischemia or metabolic alteration by regional compression.[10] The fibrous bands described by James and Lassman that cause a tethering effect on the cord or nerve roots[48] may also be responsible for progressive symptomatology. Progressive neurologic deficits may also relate to the associated dysraphic spinal lesions described above. Although patients with established motor dysfunction may demonstrate postoperative improvement, sensory deficits and bladder dysfunction will generally persist after surgical repair.[10] MRI allows a specific diagnosis of diastematomyelia, defines the presence of a bony or cartilaginous spur, and demonstrates the presence or absence of surgically approachable associated dysraphic processes. Fibrous bands between the cord surface and dura, potentially responsible for cord tethering, and thin fibrous or glial strands extending between the diastematomyelia segments may be missed with MRI.

SACRAL AGENESIS

Sacral agenesis (sacral dysgenesis) is a form of caudal regression or caudal dysplasia characterized by a congenital absence of caudal vertebral elements. It varies in severity and may involve the coccyx, sacrum, and lumbar spine or may extend into the lower thoracic region. Sacral agenesis occurs in an estimated 1% of children of diabetic mothers, and 16% of infants with caudal dysplasia have diabetic mothers. The roles of insulin, sulfur-containing substances, and altered carbohydrate metabolism in its pathogenesis have been reviewed.[50] The necessity for the combination of a teratogenic insult and genetic susceptibility in the production of sacral dysgenesis has been postulated.[50]

Classification of sacral agenesis can be based upon the extent of structural involvement of the caudal spine or upon the configuration of the dura surrounding terminal spinal neural elements. Smith differentiates three types of sacral dysgenesis, including total sacrococcygeal agenesis characterized by articulation of the ilia with each other below the last lumbar vertebrae, subtotal sacrococcygeal agenesis characterized by the absence of only the most caudal segments, and hemisacrum where there may be total or subtotal unilateral absence of sacral vertebral bodies and lateral

masses.[51] Myelography and MRI allow a further classification of patients with sacral agenesis into those with high termination of the subarachnoid space at an area of dural sac stenosis and into those patients with a widened or normal dural sac extending to the expected site of termination of the sacrum.[52] The latter group frequently has associated tethered cord, anterior or posterior meningocele, or subcutaneous lipoma (Fig 43–29).

Structural changes demonstrated with MRI relate embryologically to failed induction of vertebral body formation by the notochord and to an altered reciprocal inductive relationship between the primitive neural ectoderm and adjacent mesoderm with resultant dysplastic changes in the spinal cord, nerve roots, and posterior spinal elements.[50] Initial symptoms most commonly relate to orthopedic and genitourinary dysfunction. Neurologic deficits are most common in the L5 through S2 nerve root distributions, and sensory deficits are less prominent than motor findings of flaccid paresis and loss of muscle bulk. Sacral nerve roots may fail to develop caudal to the level of agenesis with complete absence of sensory and motor function below the level of bone hypoplasia. A neurogenic bladder is almost invariable, and MRI demonstrates enlargement of the bladder. The extent of the neurologic deficit cannot be definitively predicted from the radiographic findings.

Progressive orthopedic, motor, sphincteric, and sensory dysfunction may occur in patients with sacral agenesis secondary to spinal canal stenosis rostral to hypoplastic vertebral body levels (Fig 43–30) or secondary to compression of nerve roots by dysplastic bone elements projecting into the cauda equina or terminal cord at the level of dysgenetic vertebral segments. Progressive deficits may also relate to dural sac stenosis, a process that is distinct from spinal canal stenosis, or may relate to the presence of a tethered cord. Dural sac stenosis may benefit from duroplasty. Sacral agenesis may occur in combination with diastematomyelia, lipomeningomyelocele, intradural lipoma, dermoid cyst, dermal sinus, or a syrinx (Fig 43–31), any of which may cause progressive neurologic impairment or failure to achieve anticipated milestones. Neurologic deficits resulting from associated spinal cord dysplasia or dysplasia of lumbosacral roots is generally nonprogressive and is not surgically approachable. MRI in association with routine radiographic imaging can provide a definitive diagnosis of sacral agenesis, with characterization of tissue types and associated developmental structural anomalies to aid in early surgical intervention.

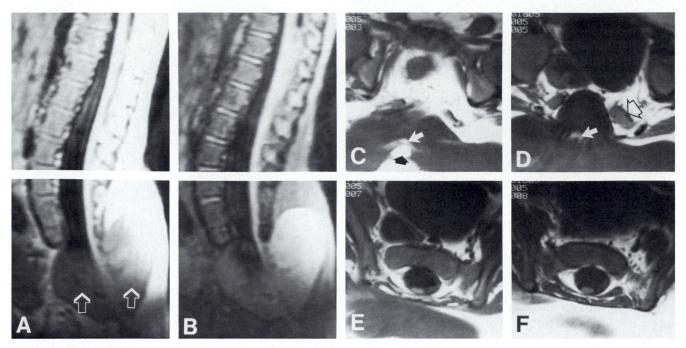

FIG 43–29.
Eleven-month-old with sacral agenesis and an imperforate anus. **A** and **B,** sagittal 600/20-ms **(A)** and 2,500/100ms **(B)** images demonstrate an absence of the sacrum with anterior and posterior meningoceles *(arrows)*. **C–E,** axial 600/20-ms images demonstrate the terminal cord *(white arrow)* adjacent to a lipoma *(black arrow)* **(C)** and an absence of the sacrum. **D,** the spinal cord *(white arrow)* courses through the enlarged thecal sac, and rudimentary sacral vertebral bodies are demonstrated *(open arrow)*. The S1 vertebral body is widened **(E** and **F),** and horizontal nerve roots emerge from the spinal cord. (Courtesy of Hagop Tookoian, M.D., Fresno Imaging, and John Slater, M.D, Fresno, Calif.)

Pang and Hoffman have stressed the necessity for early surgical intervention to prevent or arrest potentially progressive neurologic dysfunction.[50]

Total sacrococcygeal agenesis is most commonly associated with complex gastrointestinal, genitourinary, and respiratory anomalies. A complex of anomalies may include a bifid or absent scrotum, anorectal malformation, and a presacral meningocele or teratoma. There is a strong correlation between this combination of anomalies and maternal diabetes, and there is a strong association with mental retardation.

SPLIT-NOTOCHORD SYNDROME

A group of developmental anomalies termed the *split-notochord syndrome* is thought to result from the sagittal splitting of embryogenic notochord and of surrounding mesoderm, endoderm, and neural ectoderm, with the formation of a communicating tract between the gut and the skin over the dorsal spine. Such anomalies may result when the primitive notochord fails to cause separation of endoder-

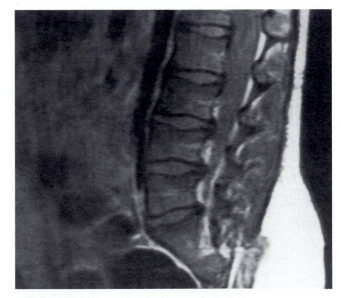

FIG 43–30.
Nine-year-old male with sacral agenesis. Sagittal 600/20-ms images demonstrate marked stenosis of the lower lumber and sacral spinal canal in this image through the widest portion of the canal. There is nonvisualization of the thecal sac below the L5–S1 level that is consistent with stenosis of the dural sac.

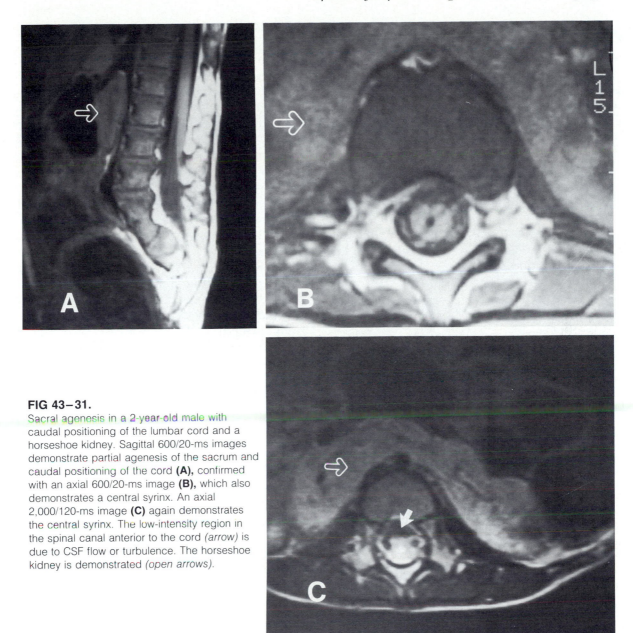

FIG 43–31.
Sacral agenesis in a 2-year-old male with caudal positioning of the lumbar cord and a horseshoe kidney. Sagittal 600/20-ms images demonstrate partial agenesis of the sacrum and caudal positioning of the cord **(A),** confirmed with an axial 600/20-ms image **(B),** which also demonstrates a central syrinx. An axial 2,000/120-ms image **(C)** again demonstrates the central syrinx. The low-intensity region in the spinal canal anterior to the cord *(arrow)* is due to CSF flow or turbulence. The horseshoe kidney is demonstrated *(open arrows).*

mal and ectodermal surfaces, with a connection thus persisting between these two surfaces. Mesoderm normally proliferates around the notochord but does not do so at the site of persistent mesodermal-ectodermal adhesion. A communication or tissue tract thus forms between ectodermal and endodermal surfaces. Theories of embryodysgenesis of the split-notochord syndrome have been reviewed.[4, 53]

Among the disorders included under the heading of split-notochord syndrome is dorsal enteric fistula. This disorder is characterized by a continuity between endodermal and ectodermal surfaces as a fistulous passage through the vertebral body, spinal canal, and/or spinal cord. The fistulous tract connects the gastrointestinal tract and the dorsal cutaneous surface. A small circle of bowel mucosa is demonstrated on the skin surface, and there is passage of gastrointestinal contents onto the skin of the dorsal paraspinal region. Bone changes consisting of anterior and posterior spina bifida may be present at the level of the dorsal enteric fistula. Associated spinal cord anomalies may include diastematomyelia and spina bifida cystica. Remnants or lesser forms of a dorsal enteric fistula may occur in locations anterior or posterior to the spine or within the spinal canal. Such remnants have been termed enteric cysts (neurenteric cyst), enteric sinuses, enteric fistulas, or enteric diverticula. MRI demonstrates the cystic nature of the intraspinal and/or paraspinal mass lesion and demonstrates the associated structural alterations involving the vertebrae and spinal cord (Fig 43–32). There may be MRI evidence of recent or remote hemorrhage into the cysts. The cysts may extend into the cord parenchyma and are frequently adherent to the ventral surface of the cord. Enteric cysts are most commonly found as a mediastinal mass on a chest film, but may be found in mesentery, spinal canal, or posterior perivertebral locations. Teratoma within the spinal canal may be associated with the split-notochord syndrome.

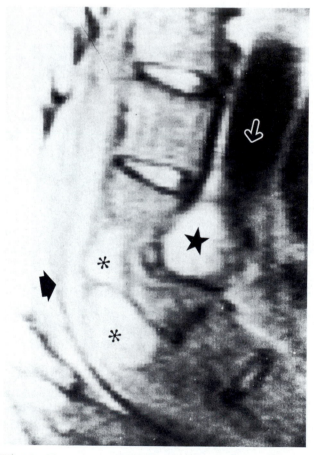

FIG 43–32.
Intradural neurenteric cyst. A sagittal T2-weighted image of the thoracic spine demonstrates a focal kyphosis at the T6–7 level where there is anomalous vertebral segmentation as a block vertebrae. The spinal cord is flattened and displaced posteriorly *(arrow)* by two intraspinal cysts *(asterisks)*. A third intrathoracic cyst *(star)* is anterior to the block vertebrae and posterolateral to the aorta *(open arrow)*. (Courtesy of Marsha J. Crofford, M.D., Division of Neuroradiology, University of Texas Medical Branch, Galveston.)

DERMAL SINUS

Dermal sinuses are congenital dorsal midline squamous epithelial-lined tracts that extend centrally from the skin. The tract may terminate in subcutaneous tissue or in the colorectal region as with the relatively common sacrococcygeal pilonidal sinus. Lumbar dermal sinus tracts and the rare thoracic and cervical dermal sinus lesions may, however, extend further centrally, enter the spinal canal, perforate the dura, and terminate within a nerve root, the spinal cord, or the filum. The more centrally extending tracts may serve as conduits for recurring episodes of meningitis or for abscess formation, which may involve soft tissue, osseous structures, the epidural space, or the spinal cord. Anywhere along its course or at its termination, the tract may be associated with a dermoid or epidermoid with associated mass effect. Centrally extending dermal sinuses most commonly occur in the lumbar and occipital regions, locations that are similar to the sites of occurrence of myeloceles and meningomyeloceles. They extend in a rostral direction and tend to follow a segmental or dermatomal distribution. Their embryogenesis is thought to relate to incomplete separation of cutaneous ectoderm from neural ectoderm at the site of the anterior and posterior neuropores.

MRI has been of limited utility, in our experience, for evaluation of the subcutaneous and central extent of the tract itself but has been useful for determining the presence of an associated central dermoid or epidermoid. The tract appears on T1-weighted sequences as a region of low signal intensity that may be only 2 to 4 mm in diameter. MRI may fail to demonstrate the tract in sagittal or axial planes because of its tortuous course or because of a partial volume effect if thick slices are utilized or overlapping slices are not obtained.

SPINAL DERMOIDS, EPIDERMOIDS, AND TERATOMAS

Epidermoids are mass lesions that are generally cystic and are lined by squamous epithelium. Dermoids may be solid, cystic, or multicystic and are composed of dermal elements including squamous epithelium, sweat glands, sebaceous glands, hair follicles, and the products of these cutaneous structures. Teratomas are rare complex intraspinal masses that contain derivatives of more than one germ cell layer. Teratomas are derived from totipotential germ cells that are sequestered in the dorsal midline mesenchyma during their migration from the yolk sac to the gonadal ridge. Dermoids and epidermoids arise within the spinal canal either from isolated congenital cell rests or as the result of local overgrowth of cutaneous elements anywhere along the course of a dermal sinus as described above. Intraspinal dermoids or epidermoids may also arise from tissue implanted in the spinal canal at the time of lumbar puncture or from cutaneous structures adhering to the margins of the placode at the time of meningomyelocele repair.[54] Spinal dermoids and epidermoids most commonly present as intraspinal mass lesions but may present with a chemical meningitis if there has been leakage of cystic fluid into the subarachnoid space.

Epidermoids on T1-weighted images may be hyperintense or isointense relative to CSF, while T2-weighted images demonstrate intensity patterns similar to CSF (Fig 43–33). Dermoid tumors are variable in their MRI appearance, with imaging characteristics depending upon foci of fatty tissue or cystic components within the mass. Intraspinal dermoids and epidermoids are slow growing and are generally conspicuously large relative to

the contents of the spinal canal at the time of their clinical presentation. Teratomas may be intradural extramedullary or may be intramedullary in location. MRI of a teratoma demonstrates the heterogeneity of the tissues composing the lesion, with intensity patterns consistent with regions of cyst formation, fat, fibrous tissue, or bone[55] (Fig 43–34).

CONCLUSION

High–field strength MRI with surface coils has dramatically altered the diagnostic evaluation of the patient with suspected spinal dysraphism. MRI obtained in sagittal and axial planes demonstrates precise regional structural contours and allows a distinction between the spinal cord, nerve, spinal fluid, fat, and soft tissue. It allows a distinction between these normal tissues and abnormal parenchyma such as a tumor and syrinx. Such distinction is based on anatomic information best demonstrated in short TR sequences and is based on tissue intensity differences in T1-, proton spin-density, and T2-weighted series. Optimal pulsing

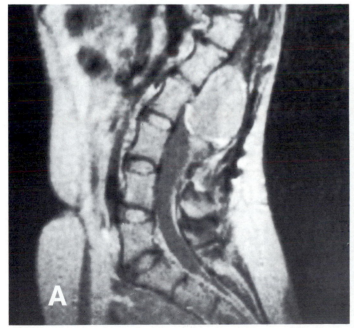 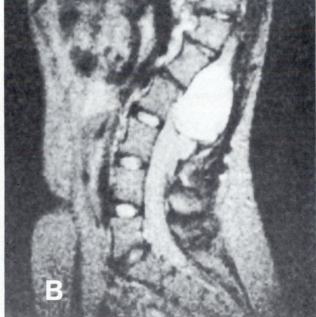

FIG 43–33.
Epidermoid cyst in a 31-year-old female with a previous partial resection of a lumbar intraspinal lipoma. Symptoms included increasing weakness and sensory alteration of the left lower extremity with progressive bladder dysfunction. Sagittal 2,000/30-ms **(A)** and 2,000/90-ms **(B)** images demonstrate a cystic intraspinal mass with an apparent central fluid-fluid level in this supine patient. The long TR/long TE image demonstrates the cyst to be of higher intensity than surrounding CSF. Lipomatous tissue is seen at the inferior aspect of the epidermoid cyst.

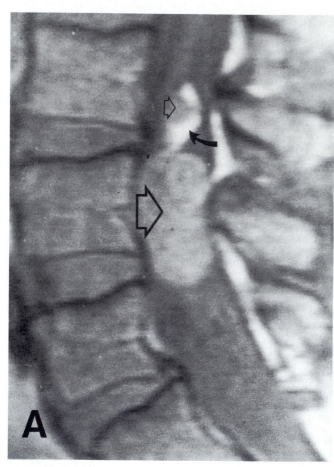
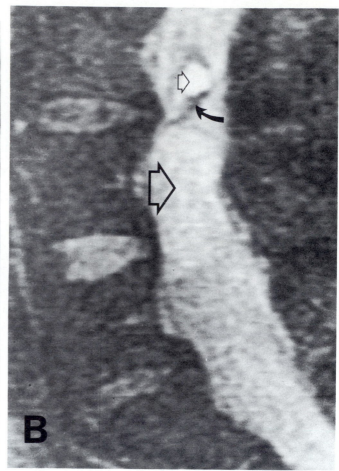

FIG 43–34.
Fifty-two-year-old with back pain radiating into the right lower extremity. **A,** (1,000/25 ms) and **B** (2,000/80 ms) demonstrate a cystic *(small open arrow)* and lipomatous component *(curved arrow)* of the upper segment of the tumor. The larger and lower keratin-

containing segment of the tumor *(large open arrow)* is only slightly hyperintense relative to CSF on the long TR, late TE image. (Courtesy of Ahmad Monajati, M.D., Section of Neuroradiology, Rochester General Hospital, NY.)

sequences vary depending upon the field strength of the imaging system utilized, upon the size and type of surface coils utilized, and upon the size and area of the body to be imaged. Developmental defects in fusion of osseous and neural structures are routinely imaged, as are associated mesenchymal midline alterations involving muscular, fibrous, and fatty elements. With MRI alone, it is generally possible to either localize and characterize the anatomic alterations associated with dysraphism or to exclude the presence of surgically remedial spinal dysraphism as a cause of the patient's symptomatology. High–field strength MRI utilizing surface coils is now the primary imaging modality in patients with suspected spinal dysraphism.

REFERENCES

1. Furukawa T: First description of spina bifida by Nicolas Tulp. *Neurology* 1987; 37:1816.
2. Harwood-Nash DC: Computed tomography of the pediatric spine: A protocol for the 1980's. *Radiol Clin North Am* 1981; 19:479–494.
3. Naidich TP, Harwood-Nash DC, McLone DG: Radiology of spinal dysraphism. *Clin Neurosurg* 1983; 30:341–365.
4. Naidich TP, McLone DG, Mutluer S: A new understanding of dorsal dysraphism with lipoma (lipomyeloschisis): Radiologic evaluation and surgical correction. *AJR* 1983; 140:1065–1078.
5. Sarwar M, Virapongse C, Bhimani S: Primary tethered cord syndrome: A new hypothesis of its origin. *AJNR* 1984; 5:234–242.
6. Scott RM, Wolpert SM, Bartoshesky LE, et al: Dermoid tumors occurring at the site of previous men-

ingomyelocele repair. *J Neurosurg* 1986; 65:779–783.

7. Naidich TP, Rodkowski MA, Britton J: Real time sonographic display of caudal spinal anomalies. *Neuroradiology* 1986; 28:512–527.

8. Lindfors KK, McGahan JP, Tennant FP, et al: Midtrimester screening for open neural tube defects: Correlation of sonography with amniocentesis results. *AJR* 1987; 149:141–145.

9. Tadmor R, Ravid M, Findler G, et al: Importance of early radiologic diagnosis of congenital anomalies of the spine. *Surg Neurol* 1985; 23:493–501.

10. Humphreys RP, Hendrick EB, Hoffman HJ: Diastematomyelia. *Clin Neurosurg* 1983; 30:436–456.

11. Pang D, Wilberger JE: Tethered cord syndrome in adults. *J Neurosurg* 1982; 57:32–47.

12. Schut L, Bruce DA, Sutton LN: The management of the child with a lipomeningocele. *Clin Neurosurg* 1982; 30:464–476.

13. Brunberg JA, Latchaw RE, Kanal E, et al: Magnetic resonance imaging of spinal dysraphism. *Radiol Clin North Am* 1988; 26:181–205.

14. Bale JF, Bell WE, Dunn V, et al: Magnetic resonance imaging of the spine in children. *Arch Neurol* 1986; 43:1253–1256.

15. Barnes PD, Lester PD, Yamanashi WS, et al: MRI in infants and children with spinal dysraphism. *AJR* 1986; 147:339–346.

16. Sherman JL, Barkovich AJ, Citrin CM: The MR appearance of syringomyelia: New observations. *AJNR* 1986; 7:985–995.

17. Walker HS, Dietrich RB, Flannigan DB, et al: Magnetic resonance imaging of the pediatric spine. *Radiographics* 1987; 7:1129.

18. Altman NR, Altman DH: MR imaging of spinal dysraphism. *AJNR* 1987; 8:533.

19. Kanal E, Burk DL, Brunberg JA, et al: Pediatric musculoskeletal MRI. *Radiol Clin North Am*, in press.

20. French BN: The embryology of spinal dysraphism. *Clin Neurosurg* 1983; 30:295–340.

21. Lemire RJ: Neural tube defects: Clinical correlation. *Clin Neurosurg* 1983; 30:165–177.

22. Emery JL, Lendon RG: The local cord lesion in neurospinal dysraphism (meningomyelocele). *J Pathol* 1973; 110:83–96.

23. Park TS, Cail WS, Maggio WM, et al: Progressive spasticity and scoliosis in children with meningomyelocele. Radiological evaluation and surgical treatment. *J Neurosurg* 1985; 62:367–375.

24. Williams B: Current concepts in syringomyelia. *Br J Hosp Med* 1970; 4:331–342.

25. Heinz ER, Rosenbaum AE, Scarff TB, et al: Tethered spinal cord following meningomyelocele repair. *Radiology* 1979; 131:153–160.

26. Venes JL, Stevens JA: Surgical pathology in tethered cord secondary to meningomyelocele repair. *Concepts Pediatr Neurosurg* 1983; 4:165–185.

27. Naidich TP, McLone DG, Mutluer S: A new understanding of dorsal dysraphism with lipoma (lipomyeloschisis). Radiologic evaluation and surgical correction. *AJR* 1983; 140:1065–1078.

28. Pierre-Kahn A, Lacombe J, Pichon J, et al: Intraspinal lipomas with spina bifida. *J Neurosurg* 1986; 65:756–761.

29. Gregorios JB, Green B, Page L, et al: Spinal cord tumors presenting with neural tube defects. *Neurosurgery* 1986; 19:962–966.

30. Hoffman HL, Taecholarn C, Hendrick EB, et al: Lipomeningomyeloceles and their management. *Concepts Pediatr Neurosurg* 1985; 5:107–117.

31. Hellstrom WJ, Edwards MSB, Kogen BA: Urologic aspects of the tethered cord syndrome. *J Urol* 1986; 135:317–320.

32. Edwards MSB: Management of lipomeningomyelocele in childhood. *Int Pediatr* 1987; 2:120–123.

33. Hoffman HJ, Taecholarn C, Hendrick EB, et al: Management of lipomeningomyelocele. *J Neurosurg* 1985; 62:1–8.

34. Harwood-Nash DC, Fitz CR: Myelography and syringomyelia in infancy and childhood. *Radiology* 1974; 113:661–669.

35. Peerless SJ, Durward QJ: Management of syringomyelia: A pathophysiological approach. *Clin Neurosurg* 1983; 30:531–576.

36. Gardber WJ, McMurry FG: "Non-communicating syringomyelia": A non-existent entity. *Surg Neurol* 1976; 6:251–256.

37. Post MJD, Quencer RM, Green BA, et al: Radiologic evaluation of spinal cord fissures. *AJNR* 1986; 7:329–355.

38. Slasky SB, Bydder GM, Nicrdorf IIP, et al: MR imaging with gadolinium DTPA in differentiating tumor, syrinx and cyst of the spinal cord. *J Comput Assist Tomogr* 1987; 11:845–850.

39. Pierre-Kahn A, Lacombe J, Pichon J, et al: Intraspinal lipomas with spina bifida. *J Neurosurg* 1986; 65:756–761.

40. Braun IF, Malko JA, Davis PC, et al: The behavior of Pantopaque on MR: In vivo and in vitro analysis. *AJNR* 1986; 7:997–1001.

41. Eller TW, Bernstein LP, Rosenberg RS, et al: Tethered cervical spinal cord. *J Neurosurg* 1987; 67:600–602.

42. Bruce DA: Typical and atypical forms of the tethered spine syndrome, in Holtzmann RNN, Stein BM (eds): *The Tethered Spinal Cord*. New York, Thieme-Stratton, Inc, 1985.

43. Fitz CR, Harwood-Nash DC: The tethered conus. *AJR* 1975; 125:515–523.

44. Hendrick EB, Hoffman HJ, Hunphreys RP: The tethered spinal cord. *Clin Neurosurg* 1983; 30:457–463.

45. Sarwar M, Virapongse C, Bhimani S: Primary tethered cord syndrome: A new hypothesis for its origin. *AJNR* 1984; 5:234–242.

46. Sarwar M, Crelin ES, Virapongse C: Experimental cord stretchability and the tethered cord syndrome. *AJNR* 1983; 4:641–643.

47. Scotti G, Musgrave MA, Harwood-Nash DC, et al: Diastematomyelia in children: Metrizamide and CT metrizamide myelography. *AJNR* 1980; 1:403–410.

48. James CCM, Lassman LP: *Spinal Dysraphism; Spina Bifida Occulta*. New York, Appleton-Century Crofts, 1972.

49. Chehrazi B, Haldeman S: Adult onset of tethered cord syndrome due to fibrous diastematomyelia: Case report. *Neurosurgery* 1985; 16:681–685.

50. Pang D, Hoffman HJ: Sacral agenesis with progressive neurologic deficit. *Neurosurgery* 1980; 7:118–126.

51. Smith ED: *Congenital Malformations of the Rectum Anus and Genito-Urinary Tracts*. London, E & S Livingston, 1963.

52. Brooks BS, Gammal TE, Hartlage P, et al: Myelography of sacral agenesis. *AJNR* 1981; 2:319–323.

53. Batson RA, Scott RM: Neurenteric cysts, in Hoffman HJ, Epstein F, (eds): *Disorders of the Developing Nervous System*. Boston, Blackwell Scientific Publications, 1986.

54. Scott RM, Wolpert SM, Bartoshesky LE, et al: Dermoid tumors occurring at the site of previous meningomyelocele repair. *J Neurosurg* 1986; 65:779–783.

55. Monajati A, Spitzer RM, Wiley L, et al: MR imaging of a spinal teratoma. *J Comput Assist Tomogr* 1986; 10:307–310.

PART XIII

Therapeutic Techniques Using MR and CT

44

The Use of Image-Guided Stereotaxy in Morphologic and Functional Surgery of the Brain

L. Dade Lunsford, M.D.

The revolution in medical imaging over the past 10 years demanded a resurgence in the field of stereotaxy, or guided brain surgery. The earlier ability to diagnose multiple lesions of the brain led to the construction and utilization of tools capable of reaching the depths of the brain with precision and reliability. The advances in imaging have been paralleled by similar advances in therapy administered with stereotactic instruments made of imaging-compatible materials. At present, stereotactic technique may be used in as much as 30% of all intracranial surgery. The resulting safety and efficacy has had a profound effect on the practice of modern neurosurgery.

HISTORICAL PERSPECTIVE

Guided brain surgery first was introduced into the English language scientific literature in 1908 by Horsley and Clark, who created a stereotactic device to study the structure and function of the monkey cerebellum.[1] Although Kirschner successfully used guiding devices for electrode coagulation of the trigeminal ganglion in 1933,[2] intracranial surgery remained dormant until Spiegel and associates developed human stereotaxy in 1947.[3] The technique was refined and expanded by many surgeons in Europe and the United States, including Leksell,[4] Riechert,[5] Talairach et al.,[6, 7] Cooper,[8] and Van Buren and MacCubbin.[9]

For many years, the major use involved functional surgery of the brain, especially for Parkinson's disease and other dyskinesias. Radiologic definition of the brain was dependent upon contrast encephalography or cerebral angiography and the use of anatomic landmarks as reference points for determination of intracranial targets. To many surgeons, the technique remained too abstruse, sophisticated, and impractical to use in routine neurosurgical practice. Nonetheless, through the 1950s and 1960s, instruction in stereotactic technique was widespread in major teaching programs in the United States. After the introduction of dopaminergic agents to treat Parkinson's disease, the number of patients referred for stereotactic surgery declined rapidly, and interest waned in the technique as a whole. The current enthusiasm for stereotaxy awaited the development of sophisticated new imaging techniques, with their promise of early recognition of intracranial pathology and the direct visualization of intracranial targets.

Seeing promise even in the early computed tomographic (CT) diagnostic units, several intrepid investigators demonstrated that CT could be used to visualize appropriate targets for neurosurgical intervention and to guide catheters or biopsy instruments to these lesions. Bergström and Greitz devised an interchangeable base ring adapted to an EMI scanner and Leksell stereotactic frame that permitted actual stereotactic procedures in 1976.[10]

The first major problem encountered by early workers in the field of CT-guided intracranial surgery was how to relate the target shown on a horizontal CT image to external skull landmarks or skull radiographs. Accordingly, various investigators developed a series of localizing grids[11-13] that could be used to orient the target in space. Evolution of the scanners led to evolution of surgical technique. The problems first encountered have been eliminated by an enlarged scanner aperture, reduced imaging and reconstruction times, improved resolution, and accurate electronic radiographic localization using the scanner x-ray tube.[14] Increasingly earlier recognition of lesions and more detailed assessment of their relationship to the normal brain convincingly demonstrated the need for accurate guiding devices fully compatible with CT and, subsequently, magnetic resonance imaging (MRI).

Accumulated evidence has shown that image-guided stereotaxis is safer, more accurate, and more reliable than image-guided techniques that do not rely on stereotactic instrumentation.[15] Both CT and MRI have become important imaging devices to the stereotactic surgeon and have replaced other radiographic imaging techniques in most cases. Only cerebral angiography, often in digital format, has withstood the transition; however, it usually is used in conjunction with other computer-assisted imaging tools.

IMAGE-GUIDED STEREOTACTIC DEVICES

Technical Achievements

The conceptual problem in image-guided stereotaxis was the need to convert two-dimensional horizontal or coronal images into three-dimensional stereotactic targets. Coordinates identified on the image required conversion to stereotactic frame coordinates. The need to transpose stereotactic coordinates visualized with CT onto lateral skull radiographs was eliminated by the development of entirely new devices for stereotaxis or the modification of existing devices for newer imaging tools. The Leksell (Fig 44–1),[16] Riechert,[17] and Todd-Wells[18] frames are among the devices that have been modified for image-guided stereotaxis. Entirely new devices integrated with sophisticated computer programs for coordinate determination include those developed by Brown,[19] Perry et al.,[20] Gouda et al.,[21] Patil,[22] and Koslow et al.[23] Each apparatus has its own relative merits, but the choice of instruments ultimately depends on the surgeon's needs and training and the goals of the procedures for which it will be used. Several perti-

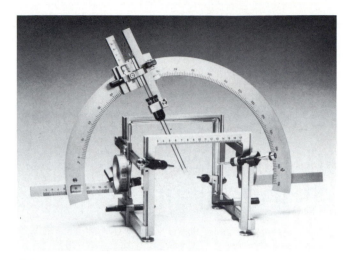

FIG 44–1.
The Leksell model D CT- and MRI-compatible stereotactic frame.

nent questions should be considered before a device is chosen:

1. Is it *complete* system (i.e., are the necessary instruments for imaging, biopsy, or lesioning fully integrated within the system)?
2. Is it *simple* (i.e., does the user understand the concept of coordinate determination and the manipulations that are necessary to obtain the surgical coordinates)?
3. Is it *versatile* (i.e., are multiple approach trajectories available, including temporal, posterior fossa, and trans-sphenoidal routes)?
4. Is it *accurate*?
5. Is it *compatible only with CT* (i.e., can the same instrument be used with other radiographic techniques, including contrast encephalography, angiography, and MRI)?
6. Is it *computer dependent* (i.e., can coordinates be determined only with the use of sophisticated computer programs)?
7. Is it *adaptable for the future* (i.e., will the device be useful in the burgeoning study of human brain function determined by positron emission tomography (PET), ultrasound, or microwave scanning)?

Requirements of Stereotactic Devices

Table 44–1 demonstrates the requirements of modern stereotactic systems. The completion of any CT stereotactic procedure requires integration of a sophisticated and precise stereotactic surgical instrument with an equally sophisticated x-ray imaging device. Stereotactic instruments must be

TABLE 44–1.

Image-Guided Stereotactic Surgery: System Requirements

Stereotactic instrument
  Rigid skull fixation (glass for MRI, carbon fiber for CT)
  Low atomic number construction (CT image compatibility)
  Magnetically isolated
  Mechanical accuracy: ±0.6 mm
  Rapid detachability
  Smooth mechanisms
  Completely sterilizable
Computer hardware
  High spatial resolution (0.75 mm)
  Variable collimation (slice thickness, 1.5–1.0 mm)
  Low image noise
  Low radiation dosage per slice (2–5 cGy)
  Accurate remote-controlled bed assembly (0.1 mm)
  Megabyte disk storage
  High-speed computer
  Laser localization
  Sagittal electronic radiographic localization
  High matrix display (360 × 360)
Computer software
  Multiplanar reconstruction
  Target coordinate calculation
  Probe trajectory preview

TABLE 44–2.

Comparison of MRI and CT for Stereotactic Imaging

Stereotactic MRI	Stereotactic CT
1. Superior contrast resolution	1. Superior spatial resolution (0.8 mm)
2. Direct multiplanar imaging and target determination	2. Direct axial imaging; multiplanar reformatted imaging
3. Artifact free (modified coordinate frame has no magnetic resonance signal)	3. Artifact created by skull fixation pins and any metal in the image
4. Lesion depiction by varying T1 and T2 relaxation times in spin-echo sequence	4. Lesion enhancement by IV contrast
5. Longer imaging times (approximately 1 hr)	5. Shorter imaging time (less than 20 min)
6. Impractical for intraoperative imaging at present (1.5 tesla) magnetic field strength	6. Excellent tool for intraoperative imaging
7. No ionizing radiation	7. Ionizing radiation

8. Magnetic susceptibility concerns
  Spatial displacement
  Image distortion
  Local field effects
	8. Accuracy related to slice thickness

constructed of rigid, low–atomic number material to maintain CT image quality.[24] MRI-compatible devices must be magnetically isolated to reduce image distortion from magnetic susceptibility artifacts.[25] The role of these artifacts in MRI stereotactic surgery is being evaluated.[25] Although we have not found significant variation between CT- and MRI-determined target localization in the same patient, concerns about accuracy with MRI are still real. Table 44–2 compares CT and MRI stereotactic target definition techniques.

Firm skull fixation must be provided by imaging-compatible pins, immobile and strong, placed into the outer table of the skull. The pins should be made of material that will reduce image degradation (e.g., carbon fiber for CT or fiberglass for MRI) or should be adjustable so that they can be placed outside the region of interest containing the intracranial target.

The instrument should provide full access to the head to enable the surgeon to manipulate the frame satisfactorily under sterile conditions and still allow the supporting nursing and anesthesia staffs easy approach to the patient. The frame should be rapidly detachable. The device should be easily cleaned, smooth in mechanism, and readily sterilized by conventional steam or gas autoclaving techniques.

Advanced-generation CT scanners have the necessary requirements for CT stereotaxis. The increased quality and number of detectors has pushed spatial resolution to the virtual theoretical limit. Compatible frames do not degrade image resolution significantly. Slice thickness can be reduced to 1.5 mm if necessary for accurate coordinate determination and detailed reconstructed images. Megabyte disk storage and a high-speed computer allow the image manipulation necessary to fully define the lesion or target in near real time. Laser localization and sagittal electronic radiographic techniques have fully oriented surgeons to their standard domain, the extracranial topography and lateral skull radiographs with which they are most familiar.

Computer software techniques are of paramount importance during all procedures. Multiplanar reconstructions and reformatted images provide minute detail of the lesion, permit subsequent verification of the target coordinate calculations, and allow previews of trajectories prior to the actual passage of the instruments.[26–28]

The team approach must be emphasized, with the surgeon and radiologist working hand in hand to maximize clinical safety and quality. Whether surgery is performed within the scanner[29–31] or in the operating room or is divided between these two units[32] becomes the option of the surgeon and the radiologist, given the facilities available and the time required.

Cost

The expense of commercially available imaging-compatible stereotactic devices remains relatively high. Three competitive units available in the United States can be purchased for between $30,000 and $50,000. Most devices are freely adaptable to commercially available CT scanners. Comparable neurosurgical devices currently in widespread use, including lasers, ultrasonic aspirators, and counterbalanced operating microscopes, are all considerably more expensive than CT stereotactic devices. In addition, the safety and efficacy associated with stereotactic technique significantly reduces the morbidity and mortality associated with freehand-guided biopsies.[33-40]

Use of the Leksell Stereotactic System

Because of its utility and versatility in both morphologic and functional neurosurgery, the use of the Leksell stereotactic device (Elekta Instruments, Decatur, Ga) will be described in detail. The low–atomic number, lightweight aluminum frame can be used without modification for CT, MRI, and standard stereotactic procedures requiring ventriculography or angiography.[25] The following modifications have been made for image compatibility.

1. Skull fixation pins (two frontal, two suboccipital) are adjustable in location to minimize the image artifacts (see Fig 44–1). Four steel drill bits with accompanying drill sleeves are used to penetrate the scalp and anchor the frame to the external table of the skull. The steel sleeves and bits are replaced later by four fiberglass or carbon fiber pins, which fit snugly into the small drill holes placed in the skull. Low–atomic number carbon fiber is ideal for use with CT, whereas fiberglass is necessary for MRI.

2. The chucks used to house the pins are made of low-artifact plastic.

3. Plastic earplugs are used for precise application of the frame but are removed during the localization and surgical aspects of the procedure.

Operation of the Leksell system is simple: the chosen target is placed at the center of a semicircu-

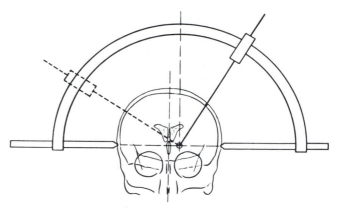

FIG 44–2.
In the Leksell stereotactic system the stereotactic target represents the center of a spherical arc attached to the coordinate frame. The target can be approached through any functionally safe trajectory.

lar arc, which is attached to the coordinate frame at the chosen x, y, and z target coordinates (Fig 44–2). The target selected is defined by three-dimensional rectilinear coordinates, where x is defined as the patient's left-right coordinate, y as the patient's anterior-posterior coordinate, and z as the patient's inferior-superior coordinate (Fig 44–3). This coordinate system was based on the standard

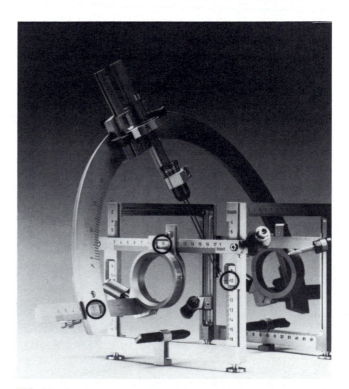

FIG 44–3.
The center of the stereotactic coordinate frame is defined as 10 for the x (left-right), y (anterior-posterior), and z (superior-inferior) coordinates of the frame.

axial plane of the brain. With the Leksell system, the target can be approached by any anatomically and functionally safe trajectory described by the semicircular arc and the probe holder. The frame center is defined as x, y, and z = 100; left-right or negative and positive values are eliminated (Fig 44–4).

The Leksell coordinate frame is applied after the patient is given local anesthesia and the entire head is prepared with antiseptic solution. General anesthesia is required for children or very anxious adults. Generally, it is easiest to apply the frame with the patient sitting comfortably in a chair. Prior images are reviewed to assess the general region of interest. This allows the surgeon to place the skull fixation pins above or below the general region of interest to further reduce CT image artifacts. MRI artifacts are less important because neither the frame nor the pins have a magnetic resonance signal. The frame is centered on the head with plastic ear bars, which are positioned in the (unanesthetized) external auditory canals. The ear bars are adjusted so that the x = 100 coordinate of the frame roughly corresponds to the midline of the patient. The earplugs are rotated to lock them firmly in position, and the stereotactic frame then

can be angled up or down to select the needed and desired relationship to the orbitomeatal plane.

After local anesthesia is administered, the four steel sleeves and pins are advanced through the scalp until they rest against the outer table of the skull. A battery-powered drill is used to insert the pins into the outer table of the skull. After all four steel pins are placed suitably, they are removed sequentially and replaced with fiber pins. When proper tension has been ensured and the frame has been checked for secure application to the head, the earplugs are removed. The frame is extremely lightweight and is supported easily by the patient, who is free to sit or move about with the frame attached.

Next, the patient is taken to the CT table, and the steel footplates of the coordinate frame are attached to the CT adapter, which substitutes for the standard headrest on the bed of the CT scanner (Fig 44–5). The frame remains attached to the adapter by magnetic footplates, which allow rapid detachment if necessary. During MRI the steel footplates are replaced by aluminum feet that snap into a plastic adapter designed especially for the commercial MRI unit being used.

For CT studies, intravenous contrast medium can be administered during the application of the frame. The gantry is not tilted because the horizontal CT images should be taken parallel to the z =

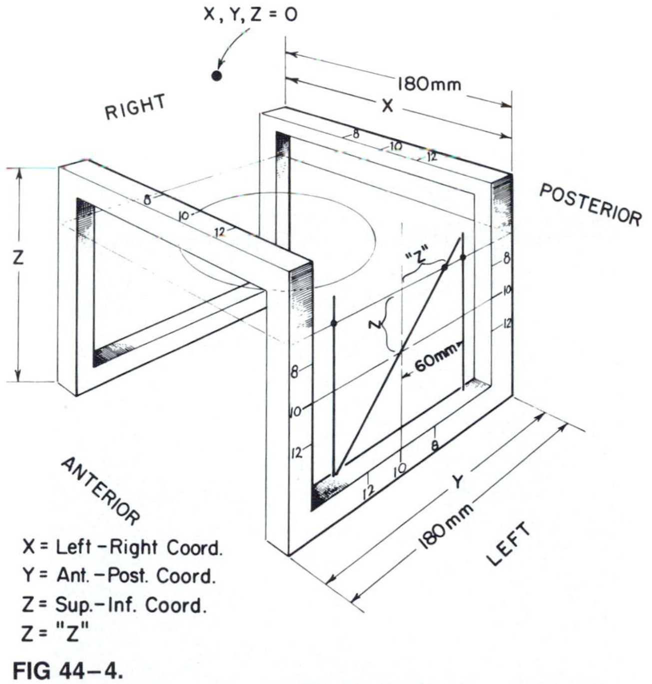

X, Y, Z = 0

RIGHT

180mm
X

POSTERIOR

Z

"Z"

60mm

180 mm

ANTERIOR

LEFT

X = Left –Right Coord.
Y = Ant. –Post. Coord.
Z = Sup.–Inf. Coord.
Z = "Z"

FIG 44–4.
Schematic diagram of the Leksell coordinate frame defining the x-, y-, and z-coordinates. The position of the slice (z-coordinate) is determined by fiducial markers that are placed on side plates located on both sides of the stereotactic frame. (From Lunsford LD (ed): *Modern Stereotactic Neurosurgery.* Boston, Martinus Nijhoff, 1988. Used by permission.)

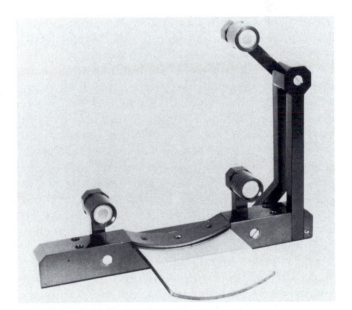

FIG 44–5.
The GE 9800 CT coordinate adapter that is used to interface the coordinate frame and the CT scanner table. (From Lunsford LD (ed): *Modern Stereotactic Neurosurgery.* Boston, Martinus Nijhoff, 1988. Used by permission.)

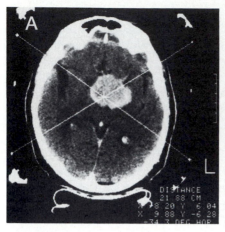
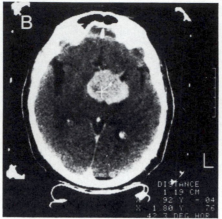
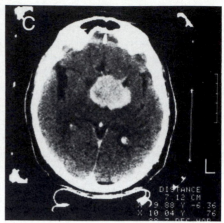

FIG 44–6.
A, the center of the stereotactic coordinate frame is defined on an axial CT scan image by drawing diagonal lines between the fiducial markers. **B,** the axial CT scan image, the stereotactic target *(small cross)* is defined in reference to the center of the frame *(large cross)*. The x- and y-coordinates are determined directly from the CT scan image. **C,** the z-coordinate is determined by measuring the position of the diagonal fiducial marker. By adding 4 to the actual distance measured (7.12), the actual z-coordinate on the stereotactic frame is obtained (11.1).

100 plane. Collimator size is selected so that each slice thickness provides sufficient anatomic detail. The reconstructed CT image should be sufficiently large to include the patient's head and the stereotactic frame (with the 9800 CT scanner [General Electric Medical System, Milwaukee], medium body, a 25-cm field of view should be selected).

During CT imaging, two plastic sideplates are attached to the CT coordinate frame. Side plates are used for coordinate determination, whether using the CT scanner computer software or a specially scaled grid for determining the target coordinates.[16] Each plastic coordinate indicator plate has two vertical 2-mm-wide aluminum strips connected by a diagonal horizontal bar, which is attached to the frame so that the diagonal bar always descends from the posterior to the anterior parts of the frame (Fig 44–4). The distance between the two vertical bars is 120 mm. The middle of the diagonal bar, 60 mm from each vertical bar, represents the center of the stereotactic frame (z = 100 plane). All axial CT images will demonstrate three small radiopaque indicators on each side, which are used to determine the x-, y-, and z-coordinates.

Software options on currently available CT scanners differ among manufacturers. However, simple distance-measuring functions using a cursor generally are included. No additional computer software must be added to the system to determine the coordinates of the target located on the horizontal CT image. It is important to remember that CT body scanners have images reversed so that the patient's left is right on the CT image. General

principles of computer coordinate determination using the Leksell CT system have been established[15, 25] (Fig 44–6). For MRI stereotactic surgery, the fiducial side plates are replaced with those containing hollow tubes filled with a dilute copper sulfate solution (or other suitable material that can be seen on T1- and T2-weighted images) (Fig 44–7).

The Leksell stereotactic frame is equipped with a plastic target coordinate grid scaled for the

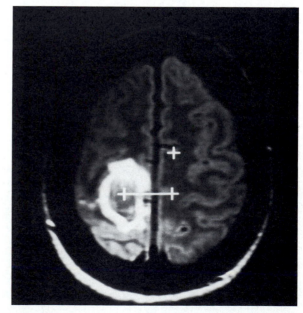

FIG 44–7.
Stereotactic MRI of a patient with a glioblastoma in the right parietal region. The determination of the x-coordinate is shown.

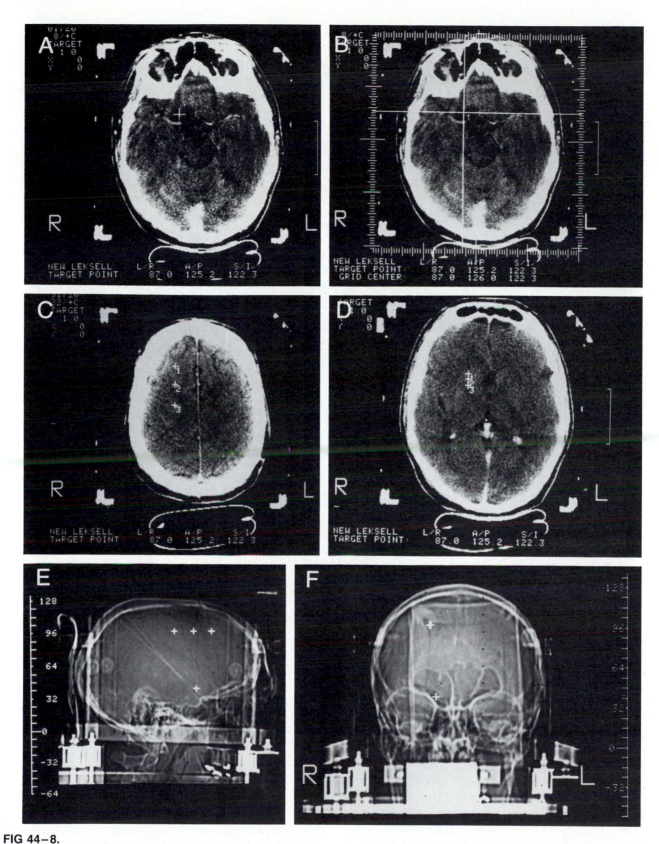

FIG 44–8.
By using special computer software programs for the GE 8800 CT scanner, the actual Leksell stereotactic coordinates can be calculated and displayed on the target image **(A)**. A stereotactic coordinate scale can be displayed over the image to define the target in a similar way **(B)**. Possible entry points can be displayed in the superior image **(C)** and the pathways to the target displayed in intervening images **(D)**. The possible entry points and target points can be displayed on the lateral **(E)** and frontal scout **(F)** views.

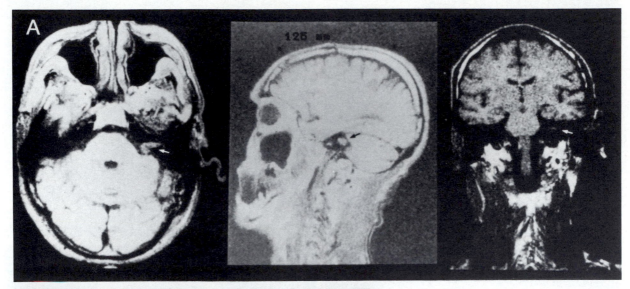

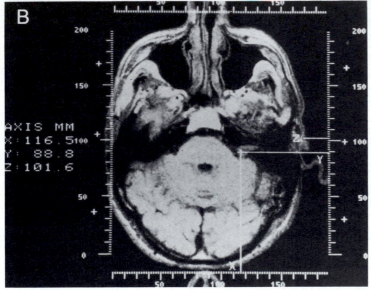

FIG 44–9.
A, stereotactic MRI used to define a target for radiosurgical ablation using the gamma knife in axial, sagittal, and coronal planes. **B,** stereotactic localization using a specially designed computer software program for the Siemens MRI unit. (From Lunsford LD (ed): *Modern Stereotactic Neurosurgery.* Boston, Martinus Nijhoff, 1988. Used by permission.)

user's own CT or MRI scanner and resultant image size. This grid can be used to read the coordinates directly, so targets can be determined from a single image that contains the target, without the use of the computer software. Both computer and grid techniques can be used to verify the accuracy of target determination. Special stereotactic computer programs have been created for the Siemens CT and MRI units as well as the GE 8800 CT scanner (Fig 44–8).[28] However, standard software available on all commercially sold units (containing deposit-cursor and measure-distance functions) will allow accurate target determination without the need to rely on specially designed programs (Fig 44–9).

After imaging has been completed and the coordinates determined and confirmed, the surgical procedure can begin. The procedure can be performed in the CT scanner (Fig 44–10), or the patient can be moved to the operating room. Surgery in high–field strength MRI units is not practical but may be possible in resistive devices that can be "turned off." The plastic side plates are removed and kept in the scanner suite. The magnetic adapter for the stereotactic frame can be used on the operating room table itself. The stereotactic frame and the patient's head are cleansed again with antiseptic solution, with care taken to sanitize the entire frame (including the pins). In the operating room, the surgeon sits or stands at the head of the operating room table, whereas in the scanner, the surgeon sits at the back of the CT aperture (Fig 44–11).

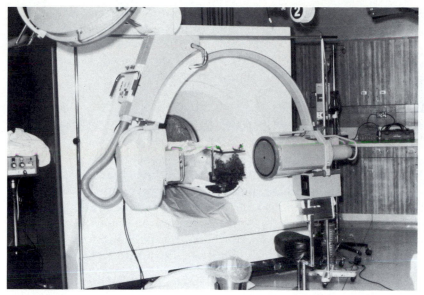

FIG 44–10.
Dedicated CT stereotactic operating room at Presbyterian-University Hospital, Pittsburgh. A ceiling-mounted sea arm fluoroscopic device with angiographic capabilities is interfaced with the CT scanner for intraoperative imaging.

After suitable preparation and draping, the semicircular arc is attached to the side bars, which have been set at the determined y- and z-coordinates. The x-coordinate is set on the spherical arc. The site of the burr hole or twist drill hole is selected. Because the target is the center of the spherical arc, any functionally safe trajectory can be selected. However, in the lateral approach to lesions in the temporal lobe, it is important to place the burr hole virtually in the center of the spherical rings that attach the arc to the side bars of the frame. Because of the location of certain targets and the relationship of the pins, the coordinate frame, and the semicircular arc, it may be necessary to reverse the semicircular arc on the side bars. The appropriate values must be switched accordingly so that the correct side is selected. This allows a full range of trajectories to reach targets from supraorbital and low frontal to coronal, vertex, parietal, occipital, suboccipital, temporal, and even trans-sphenoidal approaches. The radius of the Leksell spherical arc is 190 mm. When the probe stop is set at 0, the probe tip (190-mm probe) will be at the target. The probe stop on the spherical arc can be set between 50 mm above the target and 20 mm below the target; thus, serial biopsy specimens, for example, can be taken along the line of that trajectory (Fig 44–12).

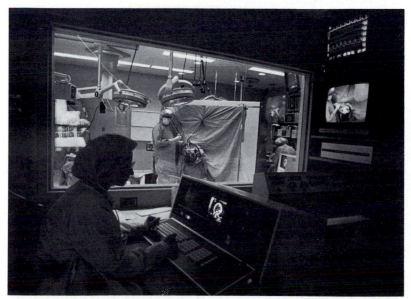

FIG 44–11.
Surgery itself is performed in the CT scanner. During the imaging portions of the procedure, the patient can be seen and monitored through the adjacent console room.

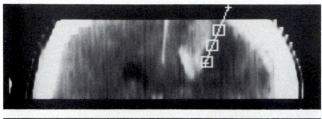

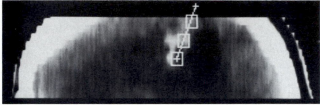

FIG 44–12.
Frontal and sagittal reformatted imaging techniques are useful to display various biopsy sites.

Intraoperative Imaging

The desire to repeat CT imaging during the stereotactic procedure[29, 30, 41, 42] stemmed from the need to (1) confirm target accuracy by visualizing the probe tip at the target site; (2) assess the results of therapeutic intervention, such as biopsy or aspiration; and (3) immediately assess the possibility of operative complications, such as postoperative hemorrhage.

Because the spherical arc of the Leksell system produces intolerable image artifacts, a probe holder was constructed that anchors the stereotactic probe in position to allow removal of this arc and the side bars (Figs 44–13 and 44–14). With this device, artifact-free intraoperative CT imaging

is possible. The elimination of artifacts has proved to be of paramount importance during the stereotactic aspiration of colloid cysts of the third ventricle (Fig 44–15)[43, 44] and mechanical aspiration of deep intracerebral hematomas.[45–49]

MORPHOLOGIC SURGERY OF THE BRAIN

Stereotactic technique can be used for both diagnostic exploration of various brain lesions and individual therapy. Such procedures can be described as explorative (biopsy procedures), decompressive (puncture or aspiration techniques), therapeutic (injection or implantation of specific therapeutic agents), or radiosurgical (Table 44–3).

Explorative Stereotactic Surgery

The need to perform accurate biopsies of brain lesions recognized with advanced imaging tools has been the primary stimulus of renewed interest in stereotactic surgery (Fig 44–16). Stereotactic tumor biopsy has been shown to be an accurate, precise, and safe method to obtain correct histologic diagnoses and to direct appropriate therapy.[33, 50] The introduction of CT guidance in stereotactic technique not only increased the number of biopsies but also reduced patient morbidity and mortality. Centers that have long relied upon stereotactic biopsy technique for tumor diagnosis have demonstrated that mortality should be less than 1% and significant morbidity less than 3%.[33, 39]

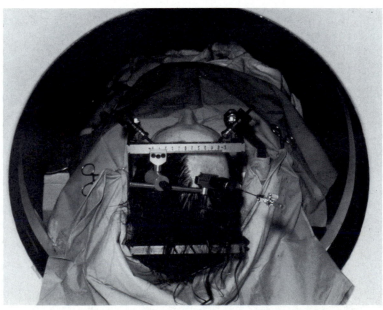

FIG 44–13.
Intraoperative CT scan imaging is accomplished by using a probe holder attached to the stereotactic frame to eliminate potential image artifacts.

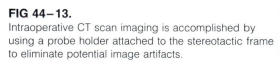

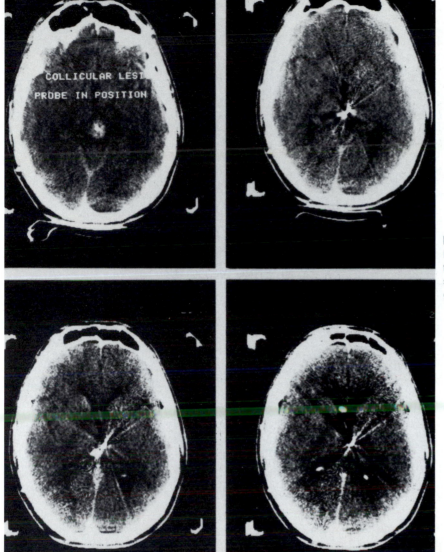

FIG 44–14.
Intraoperative CT scan imaging can be used to confirm the position of a probe at the stereotactic target (collicular plate germinoma).

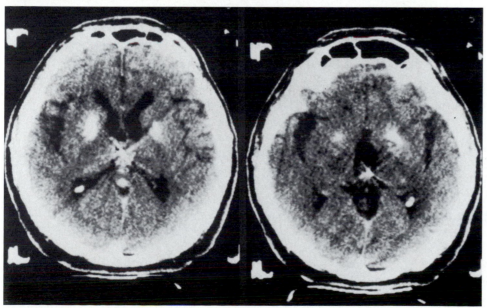

FIG 44–15.
Intraoperative stereotactic imaging is very important during the stereotactic aspiration of colloid cysts not only to confirm accurate probe placement *(left)* but also adequate evacuation of the cyst *(right)*.

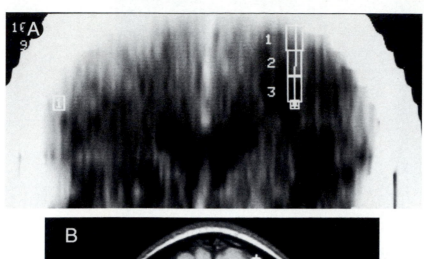

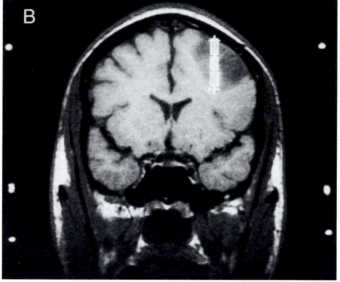

FIG 44–16.
A, biopsy sites through a low-attention mass lesion are demonstrated on a reformatted coronal CT scan. **B,** Stereotactic MRI (T1 weighted) on the same patient on the same day defines the margins of the neoplasm much more clearly. The fiducial markers used for target localization can be seen surrounding the image.

Patients are referred after imaging has disclosed the brain abnormality. The need for cerebral angiography is based on the location and the size of the tumor. At the present time, we still regard angiography as a valuable adjunct in the evaluation of deep midline, intraventricular, pineal region, or parasellar masses. We have found little correlation between the vascularity demonstrated by either contrast-enhanced CT scans or angiography and the occurrence of a hemorrhagic complication after tumor biopsy. The additional use of various T1- and T2-weighted MR sequences can provide data about the vascularity of a neoplasm in many cases and obviate the need for angiography (Fig 44–17). With gadolinium-diethylenediamine pentaacetic acid (DTPA)–enhanced MRI, tumors can be identified with at least the same degree of specificity and with better resolution than provided by intravenously iodine-enhanced contrast CT scans.

CT Scan Biopsy Technique

After the Leksell frame is applied, serial axial CT images are taken to determine the target slice and to obtain the necessary coordinates. Contrast enhancement is used in all cases. Patients with iodine allergies are treated in advance with intravenous corticosteroids and antihistamines. Images are taken at 5-mm intervals to localize the target area and preplot the probe trajectory and biopsy sites (Fig 44–18). Both sagittal and coronal reconstructions are then performed to further define the lesion and to plan the approach of a phantom

TABLE 44–3.

Image-Guided Stereotaxy: Morphologic Surgery of the Brain

Procedure Type	Conditions
Explorative (biopsy)	Primary glial neoplasm
	Metastasis
	Pituitary adenoma
	Degenerative diseases
	Leukemic infiltrate
	Sarcoidosis
	Lymphoma
	Pineal region tumors
	Acoustic neurinoma
	Herpes simplex encephalitis
	AIDS*
Decompressive (puncture, aspiration)	Brain abscess
	Arachnoid cyst
	Colloid cyst
	Intracerebral hematoma
Therapeutic (injection, implantation)	Intracystic irradiation
	Interstitial irradiation
	Tumor chemotherapy or immunotherapy
Stereotactic radiosurgery	AVM,* tumors

*AIDS = acquired immunodeficiency syndrome; AVM = atrioventricular malformation.

probe. Multiplanar reconstructions have been very helpful not only to define the lesion fully but also to select a probe trajectory that appears the safest. Serial biopsies of various regions of the tumor can be correlated histologically with the biopsy site demonstrated by CT or MRI. Reconstructed CT images also can be used with the scout image to demonstrate the location of a preselected burr hole and probe pathway.

After the patient is moved to the operating room, the scalp and frame are prepared and draped, and the side bars are attached at the chosen coordinates. Serial biopsy specimens are taken in the trajectory of the probe shown by the CT images. Many biopsy instruments have been created for stereotactic devices, including suction or aspiration devices[51–55] and microforceps.[39] We prefer to use a "corkscrew" spiral instrument developed by Backlund and associates.[54] With this technique, a corkscrew spiral (inner cannula) is advanced 1 cm beneath the tip of the probe (outer cannula, 2.1-mm outer diameter). The outer probe then is advanced over the spiral to amputate tissue within the spiral. Both the spiral and the outer cannula are removed, and a small 10×0.2-mm core of the lesion is unscrewed between the thumb and forefinger of the surgeon. These specimens are placed immediately in formalin. Frozen sections are not made, having proved frustrating to both the surgeon and the pathologist. Touch preparation specimens also can be performed, lightly affixed to slides, and stained.

On the day after surgery, the surgeon reviews the case and the x-ray films with the neuropathologist. This has resulted in a strong working relationship with the neuropathologist and has allowed a highly positive diagnostic biopsy rate (96% of our cases).

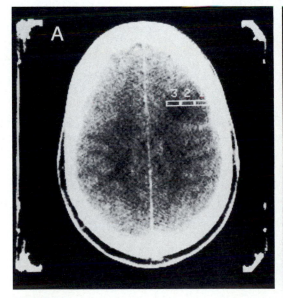
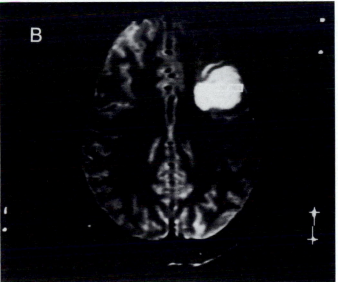

FIG 44–17.
A, stereotactic biopsy sites are depicted on the CT scan. **B,** these biopsy sites can be compared to the T2-weighted MRI images in an attempt to define tumor margins.

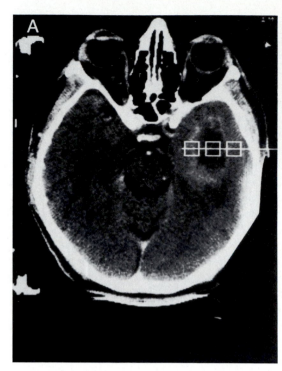

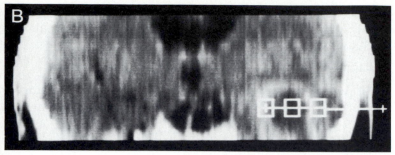

FIG 44–18.
A, axial CT scan showing the sites for biopsy of a left temporal glioblastoma.
B, reformatted CT scan displaying the same targets.

MRI Localization: Technique and Uses

The patient is attached to the appropriate adapter designed for the radiofrequency head coil of the magnet in use. We have used a 1.5-Tesla unit for our MRI studies in both patients and experimental animals. Initial T1- and T2-weighted images supplemented by coronal scans are used for target determination (Fig 44–19). The entire MRI time has been reduced to 45 minutes after frame application. We later perform stereotactic CT to compare target location determined by these independent techniques.

Stereotactic MRI has two major roles. The first is to identify appropriate targets that cannot be de-

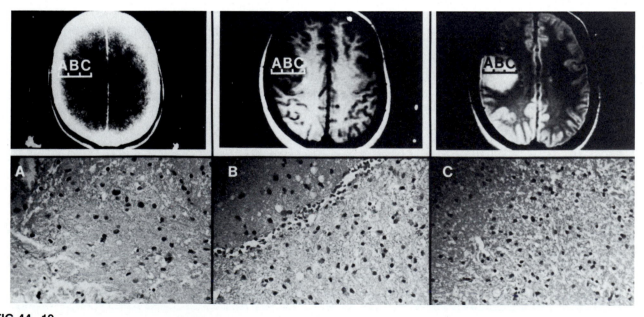

FIG 44–19.
With stereotactic CT and T1- and T2-weighted MRI biopsy site specimens can be compared with the histologically defined neo-plasm (astrocytoma). The margins of the neoplasm in this case corresponded to the margins defined by T2-weighted MRI.

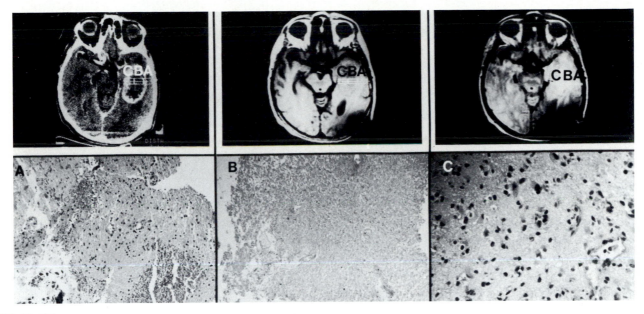

FIG 44–20.
Stereotactic comparison using CT and T1- and T2-weighted MRI to define the various components of a glioblastoma of the left tempo-ral lobe. Glioblastoma was confirmed in sites *A* and *C*, with central necrosis at site *B.*

fined (or seen at all) on high-resolution CT images; these are almost always small brain astrocytomas. Second, MRI is valuable in attempting to define the histologic margins of a neoplasm (Fig 44–20). We have compared the definition of tumors by CT, MRI, and histologic studies. Like Kelly and his co-workers,[56] we have identified tumor in and even beyond the high T2 signal that is commonly identified as perilesional "edema," especially in patients with malignant glial tumors (Table 44–4).[57] Gd-DTPA–enhanced MRI is a superior technique to define the lesion, but the blood-brain barrier disruption identified by this paramagnetic contrast agent is not specific.

Results of Stereotactic Intervention

Modern stereotactic imaging using the Leksell system was introduced at Presbyterian-University Hospital in February 1981.[20, 40] During the next 7 years, 817 patients underwent imaging-guided stereotactic procedures (see Table 44–3). The majority of the procedures were done to answer specific questions posed by the clinical and preoperative neuroimaging examinations. Diagnostic biopsy was performed in 591 patients (72.3% of the total). The histologic definition of glial neoplasms accounted for many of these cases.

Overall, a firm histologic diagnosis was made in 92% of patients; in an additional 4% of biopsy procedures, suspected tumors were ruled out. The diagnosis of these lesions had a major impact on subsequent therapy, frequently leading to changes in planned treatment strategies such as irradiation or the addition of antibiotics in cases of unrecognized brain abscess.[58] Our results in 96 patients with malignant gliomas indicated that stereotactic

TABLE 44–4.
A Comparison of the Histologic Borders of Tumors Defined by Stereotactic CT, MRI, and Biopsy

| Diagnosis | No. of Cases | Histologic Definition of Tumor (No. of Cases) | | |
		CT Margin	MRI Margin	Beyond CT and MRI Margin
Glioblastoma	4	4	4	4
Anaplastic astrocytoma	3	3	3	1
Well-differentiated astrocytoma	6	6	6	1

biopsy followed by external beam irradiation was often the most appropriate treatment strategy and resulted in median survival rate equaling or surpassing reported results from multicenter trials of tumor debulking, irradiation, and chemotherapy.[59]

Stereotactic biopsy performed in conjunction with aspiration of cystic tumors often has led to early relief of preoperative deficits. This technique also has been useful for the recognition of Alzheimer's disease, intracranial lymphoma, granulomatous diseases, and more recently, the various manifestations of AIDS. Because an increasing number of AIDS patients are referred for diagnosis of cerebral lesions, these patients are currently treated empirically for toxoplasmosis. If they fail to respond to appropriate therapy, a biopsy is done. We have defined primary central nervous system (CNS) lymphoma and cryptococcal abscesses in several such patients. The role of stereotactic surgery in AIDS patients must be assessed critically insofar as new data can be expected to lead to significant changes in therapy that are likely to enhance useful survival.

Patients with herpes simplex encephalitis have been diagnosed rapidly and efficiently with stereotactic technique.[42] We have had no difficulty in defining the virus either by histologic technique or by culture from stereotactic biopsy specimens. Other, rarer lesions of the brain stem and pons can be diagnosed, which often leads to major changes in therapy.[58, 60-62] Either a parietal or frontal approach is used for pineal region tumors.[55] If a germinoma is diagnosed, no further surgery is indicated, and irradiation can be started.

Complications

The high morbidity associated with freehand nonstereotactic biopsy techniques can be traced to several features:

1. Poor localization of the lesion before CT scanning.
2. Numerous attempts to reach the target (multiple probe passages using different trajectories).
3. Attempts to secure large pieces of tumor tissue to bolster the positive biopsy rate, usually fostered by the frustrating experience of frozen sections and the mistaken belief that large specimens of tissue are required to reach a diagnosis.

These complications can be avoided by using stereotactic technique, which provides precise tar-

get identification, allows multiple biopsies in a single trajectory, and has rigid probe and skull fixation. In 591 consecutive stereotactic biopsies at our institution between February 2, 1981, and February 1, 1988, no patient died as a result of the surgery. Fewer than 3% of patients had transient worsening of neurologic signs such as hemiparesis or aphasia in the absence of a postoperative intracerebral hemorrhage. Such signs resolved over several days after the patients were given temporarily higher doses of corticosteroids.

Nine patients (1.5%) had postoperative intracerebral hemorrhages leading to increased neurologic deficits; four patients required craniotomy and evacuation of the clot because of a mass effect and developing neurologic deficits. Two intracerebral hematomas occurred in a delayed fashion (more than 6 hours after surgery); in both patients, brain abscesses had been aspirated vigorously (a practice to be avoided). All other intracerebral hematomas were recognized on the immediate postbiopsy CT scan (Fig 44–21).

Two patients died between 30 and 45 days after surgery, partially as a consequence of postoperative hematomas and partially from their underlying diseases (lymphoma and periarteritis nodosa). One patient died suddenly en route to the hospital after sustaining a generalized seizure. Five days previously, the patient had undergone stereotactic biopsy of a parietal anaplastic astrocytoma and had been discharged from the hospital to begin outpatient radiation therapy.

The risk of intracerebral hemorrhage during stereotactic biopsy has been reduced by the elimination of multiple probe passages to the target. Percutaneous techniques through high-risk areas such as the lateral temporal lobe and sylvian fissure also may increase morbidity. In the present series, percutaneous techniques not requiring an open burr hole and exposure of the cortex were reserved for patients with lesions that could be approached via frontal or occipital trajectories, which presented little likelihood of encountering major arterial feeders. In most other cases, an appropriately located burr hole should be placed so that the cortex is visible and the pial vessels can be coagulated prior to passage of the biopsy probe.

After the last biopsy specimen is obtained, the probe with the stylet removed is left at the deepest site to allow observation for any bleeding. The probe must remain in position until all bleeding ceases, which indicates that any hemorrhage has

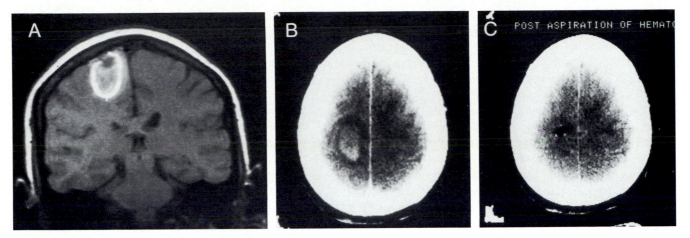

FIG 44—21.
Stereotactic MRI can define a right parietal hemorrhage **(A).** An axial-plane CT scan of the MRI site defines the lesion, **(B)** which can be removed by stereotactic aspiration **(C).**

coagulated at the tip of the probe. Applying coagulating current to the biopsy probe itself is not advocated because uncontrolled current spread is dangerous and can provoke unwanted rupture of nearby small tumor vessels. Immediate postoperative CT has enabled rapid identification of hematoma formation leading to early therapy. Postoperative CT scans rarely show small clinically insignificant hematomas at the biopsy site. In addition, a tiny air defect introduced by the probe can be used to confirm accurate location of the biopsy target site (Fig 44—22).

Decompressive Stereotactic Surgery

Brain Stem Stereotactic Surgery

Lesions of the brain stem, including the pons and midbrain, can be approached by stereotactic technique.[58, 60] In a previous study, we found that as many as 30% of brain stem lesions first diagnosed by clinical and imaging criteria alone ultimately had diagnoses not even considered before surgery. Mass lesions above the level of the middle cerebellar peduncle are approached by a transfrontal percutaneous technique proceeding along

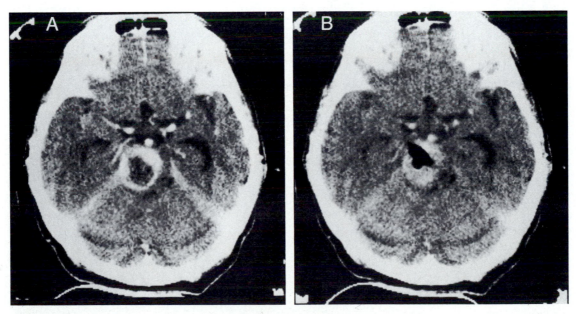

FIG 44—22.
A, stereotactic CT demonstration of a pontine glioblastoma with 3 cc of intratumoral cystic fluid. **B,** postaspiration stereotactic images reveal collapse of the lesion and a typical "air" marker.

the long axis of the brain stem (Fig 44–22). Masses at the level of the middle cerebellar peduncle or below usually are reached via a percutaneous transcerebellar approach. Cystic masses such as neuroepithelial cysts, brain abscesses, and hematomas can be aspirated with minimal morbidity. When such lesions also obstruct the sylvian aqueduct, aspiration and, if necessary, simultaneous placement of a ventricular drain can alleviate hydrocephalus. We do not advocate transtentorial biopsy of pontine lesions because the dura is vascular and, in general, lesions are best approached by the shortest trajectory to the target that will minimize dural or pial punctures.

At present, empirical therapy even of brain stem lesions is not warranted because misdiagnosis results in either delayed or inappropriate therapy. Histologic grading of brain stem glial neoplasms can provide valuable insights into both prognosis and treatment options. Although diagnostic images can confirm the presence of an intrinsic mass lesion, no significant features of either CT or MRI emerged during our series that enabled us to make a firm histologic diagnosis. For example, in some cases, iodine contrast enhancement was associated with a more aggressive neoplasm, but in other cases, we could not confirm the presence of tumor anaplasia despite contrast opacification.[57]

Benign Brain Cysts

To exclude a diagnosis of neoplastic lesion, brain cysts require diagnosis with stereotactic biopsy when possible. We recently studied an interhemispheric arachnoid cyst that had retained metrizamide for up to 6 months after stereotactic injection designed to assess the anatomic location. The cyst resolved after a delayed hemorrhage and infection occurred within the cyst; these were associated with removal of an infected cystoperitoneal shunt.

Colloid Cysts of the Third Ventricle

Between 1979 and 1988, we performed stereotactic surgery on 19 patients with colloid cysts of the third ventricle. These lesions can be defined well by preoperative imaging (Fig 44–23). The ability to recognize these benign but often diffi-

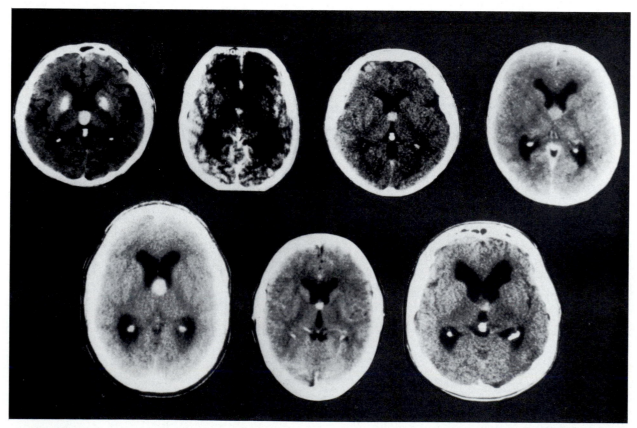

FIG 44–23.
Axial-plane CT scan images of seven patients with colloid cysts. Stereotactic aspiration was performed in all cases.

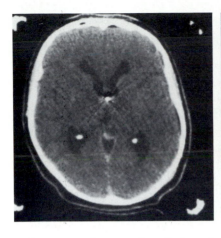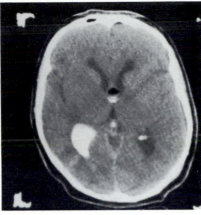

FIG 44–24.
Intraoperative CT scan imaging confirms the presence of the probe in the colloid cyst and a small remnant of contrast in the cyst *(right)* after injection of contrast into the ventricular system.

cult-to-treat lesions has led to the need to find less invasive means to eliminate them. Recently, these cysts have been diagnosed after a CT or MRI scan of the brain was done for unrelated reasons. In contrast to reports from other centers,[43] we have been successful in the stereotactic removal of the intracystic colloid material in 66% of our patients.[44] The reasons for failure of stereotactic aspiration are two: the cyst is displaced from the puncture needle itself (a problem greatest in small lesions, i.e., less than 1 mL), or the intracystic colloid material is too viscous to be aspirated through available needles.

Our preliminary data suggest that when preoperative MRI discloses a colloid cyst of very high signal (bright) on T1 studies and similarly bright on T2 scans, successful aspiration is less likely (presumably due to the high protein content). Aspiration is more apt to succeed with lesions that have low signal on T1 and are bright on T2 images. CT scans have not been predictive of success, except that the larger lesions are most often successfully aspirated.

At present, we approach colloid cysts in a step-wise fashion: we plan to proceed first with stereotactic technique using intraoperative CT scans to assess the degree of success (Figs 44–24 and 44–25). If percutaneous transfrontal aspiration fails, we attempt stereotactic endoscopic removal using instruments designed especially for this procedure. If this fails, we continue with stereotactic microsurgical removal. Few other benign cysts warrant such an aggressive approach, especially in the absence of significant neurologic deficits; however, the risk of sudden death is real in patients with colloid cysts. Stereotactic surgery has proven advantages for this condition: most patients can remain awake and mildly sedated, which facilitates treatment in otherwise high-risk patients. At the conclusion of the procedure, we have performed CT contrast ventriculography in some patients to assess the patency of the ventricular system. Even with successful aspiration, hydrocephalus (almost universally present) is not always relieved, and patients may still need cerebrospinal fluid diversion later. In two patients, isosmotic contrast agent injected into the lateral ventricle after cyst aspiration was retained in the colloid cyst remnant and simu-

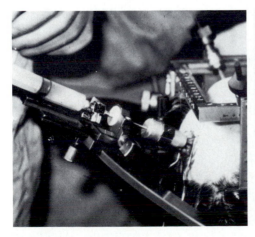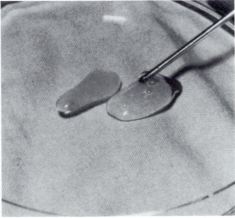

FIG 44–25.
Stereotactic aspiration of a colloid cyst can be performed if the material is of sufficiently low viscosity to come out through a needle.

lated the original cyst. In both cases, delayed aspiration of the retained intracystic contrast material was required. As a result, we no longer routinely perform postaspiration CT ventriculography.

Successful aspiration obviates the need for craniotomy. Most patients are discharged within 2 days after surgery and do not require postoperative anticonvulsants. To date, no patient has needed reaspiration for recurrent cyst formation, even though the cyst wall itself was not removed. We have encountered no postoperative morbidity from stereotactic surgery, in contrast to our previous experience with both transfrontal and transcallosal surgical removal.[44]

Intracerebral Hemorrhage

The role of stereotactic aspiration in the treatment of deep intracerebral hemorrhages is poorly defined at present.[45–48] A multicenter randomized, prospective study is currently underway in Japan. This study is designed to assess the relative advantages of surgical removal via craniotomy, stereotactic aspiration, or conservative treatment of such hematomas.

A specially designed instrument based on the principle of the Archimedes screw can be used to remove even acute, firmly coagulated blood from targets deep in the basal ganglia, pons, cerebellum, or thalamus.[45] Estimating the volume of the intracerebral hemorrhage with CT region-of-interest techniques can be quite helpful in predicting patient outcome since patients with hemorrhages larger than 100 mL rarely survive. Because few data support aggressive removal of deep hypertensive hemorrhages, we generally have followed the policy of performing stereotactic aspiration only when the patient's level of consciousness begins to deteriorate and suggests a progressive mass effect.

We use CT intraoperatively to assess the degree of volume reduction during aspiration and to monitor the development of new hemorrhage at the operative site. Complete aspiration is neither practical nor desirable; the goal of surgery is to remove enough blood to take the patient off the steep portion of the pressure-volume curve of intracranial hypertension. In some patients, we believe that neurologic improvement was hastened by our intervention, but our ability to improve on the natural history of recovery remains conjecture.

Brain Abscess

We treat brain abscess preferentially with stereotactic technique.[41, 61] Its precision and safety have enabled us to treat both deep and subcortical abscesses, many of which were unsuspected before stereotactic intervention. Seventeen patients have been treated by stereotactic biopsy, aspiration, and when needed, catheter drainage. In this way, fungal, bacterial, nocardial, and parasitic abscesses have been diagnosed, and appropriate antimicrobial therapy instituted.

When the total lesion volume is 2 mL or less, simple aspiration is sufficient; when the lesion volume is greater, we also insert a drainage tube in the abscess cavity. This tube is left in place for 2 to 3 days and gradually advanced out. Earlier experience with two patients who suffered intracerebral hemorrhages after overly vigorous aspiration led us to abandon such an approach in favor of simple aspiration (enough for cytologic and bacteriologic studies) followed by catheter drainage in larger abscesses.[63]

Culture technique is very important in brain abscess diagnosis. We request that a bacteriologic specialist come to the operating room to pick up the specimens and ensure that proper plating techniques are used. Antibiotics are adjusted on the basis of final organism identification.

All 17 of our patients were cured of their brain abscesses, which included two nocardial abscesses and one tuberculous abscess. To date, one patient with an *Aspergillus* brain abscess, diagnosed by stereotactic technique and treated with amphotericin B, has survived 14 months after diagnosis in the face of chronic myelogenous leukemia. In contrast to our present policy for AIDS patients (see above), we do not advocate stereotactic biopsy in cases of suspected slow-virus infection because the sterilizing solution necessary to cleanse the instruments (dilute hypochlorite solution) frequently destroys the instruments. In addition, patients infected with suspected slow virus rarely have a deep or subcortical lesion identified as a target suitable for biopsy.

THERAPEUTIC STEREOTACTIC TECHNIQUE

In addition to biopsy diagnosis and aspiration, image-guided stereotaxis can be used for a variety of interventional procedures, which include implantation of radioactive agents and intratumoral chemotherapy.[64]

Intracavitary Irradiation

Cystic irradiation is designed to eliminate cyst secretion and result in cyst involution. Backlund has pioneered the use of intracystic irradiation to treat craniopharyngiomas.[51–54] From 1965 to 1980, Backlund treated more than 100 cases of craniopharyngioma by a program of stereotactic irradiation. The majority of tumors were solitary cystic or, occasionally, multicystic lesions, which were treated by the stereotactic implantation of a β-ray–emitting isotope (yttrium 90 colloid) into the cyst and radiosurgery (see below).

The use of CT promoted early recognition of these tumors and enabled an accurate determination of the cyst volume before surgery.[65] When using stereotactic techniques, the craniopharyngioma cyst is punctured, and 1 mL of fluid is removed for examination and confirmation of the nature of the cyst. The isotope injection is designed to provide an optimal dose of 20,000 cGy of irradiation to the cyst wall. The cyst is aspirated later if neurologic symptoms warrant. Yttrium 90 has a half-life of 2.3 days, and essentially, the full dose of irradiation is delivered by 2 weeks. Yttrium 90 is not available in the United States, where we have used phosphorus 32 colloid instead.

Gradual involution of the cyst is shown by serial CT examinations. The greatly reduced mortality and morbidity with this procedure are in contrast with the results after frontal craniotomy and radical or subtotal tumor excision. Stereotactic technique is associated with a lower incidence of postoperative visual loss, endocrine dysfunction, and development of diabetes inspidus.[66] These results warrant the more widespread use of this technique in the treatment of craniopharyngioma and cystic glial tumors that are refractory to conventional surgery or irradiation.[67]

Interstitial Irradiation

Stereotactic technique has been used throughout the world for the biopsy of various malignant brain tumors and the subsequent implantation of radioactive isotopes for interstitial irradiation (brachytherapy).[17, 68–71] Isotopes that have been used include gold 198, iridium 192, and iodine 125. Radium is difficult to work with because it is toxic to the person performing the implantation. Iodine 125 seeds have attractive features that have allowed the development of both afterloading techniques using "high-dose" or "low-dose" seeds (less than 1 mCi).[69] The use of CT stereotaxis has proved to be a necessary adjunct for accurate isotope placement (Fig 44–26). Unfortunately, the definition of the tumor margin has been illusory, even with MRI with or without contrast agents. Therefore, the volume that must receive the implant to arrest tumor growth is rarely known.

Our experience (as of February 1988) consists of 32 patients with malignant gliomas (anaplastic astrocytoma and glioblastoma), all of whom previously had external beam therapy to a total dose of 5,000 to 6,000 cGy (Fig 44–27). Patients with lobar anaplastic astrocytoma receiving "boost" interstitial radiation therapy appear to live significantly longer (median life expectancy of more than 156 weeks).[59] Approximately 25% of patients developed delayed radiation necrosis of the brain that required craniotomy and debulking. The histologic examination usually disclosed residual viable tumor as well.

The results obtained by Mundinger and colleagues,[71] Ostertag and coworkers,[39] and Gutin

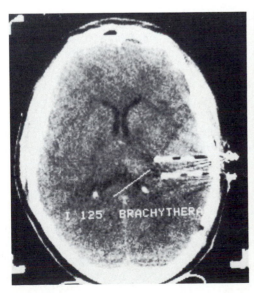 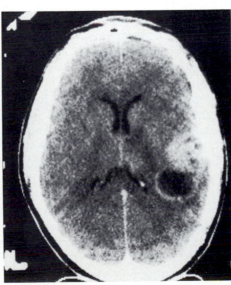

FIG 44–26.
Stereotactic placement of parallel ^{125}I-loaded catheters for brachytherapy. The preoperative tumor volume is identified on the *right,* including a cyst that was aspirated at the time of implantation.

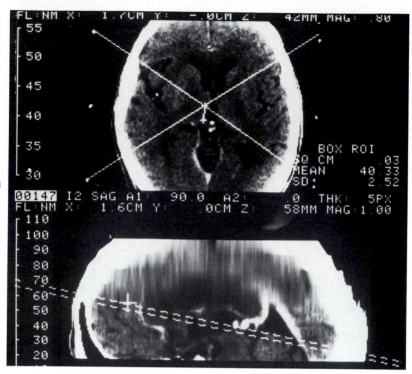

FIG 44–27.
Stereotactic definition of the foramen of Monro–pineal gland target used during creation of a reformatted plane during functional neurosurgical intervention.

and associates[70] have been promising enough to warrant continued development of interstitial irradiation as a treatment for malignant brain tumors. Volume implantation techniques using iodine 125 remain investigational at present but are an exciting frontier in the field of tumor therapy as well as stereotactic technique.

Functional Surgery of the Brain

Surgical treatment of symptoms (disordered physiology) caused by neurologic disease and treated at a site remote from the origin of the disease constitutes the field of functional neurosurgery. Marino has stated, "The aim and objective of functional neurosurgery are to treat, correct, or balance the functions of the brain that are altered toward either hyperfunctional or hypofunctional states."[72] Intracranial functional neurosurgery has long relied upon presumedly stable anatomic landmarks such as the posterior-anterior commissural (intercommissural) line or the foramen of Monro–pineal line to define the sites or targets for surgical intervention (Fig 44–27). These targets have been defined carefully in various neurosurgical atlases of the brain and were derived from the study of pooled anatomic specimens.[6, 9, 73] The target sites themselves, which cannot be visualized with conventional radiographic techniques, have been defined in relationship to the intercommis-

sural line. During surgery, electrophysiologic recording or stimulation has been used to precisely confirm or to adjust the target site; radiographic anatomic detail has been insufficient to delineate the target successfully.

The integration of CT and functional neurosurgery has become one of the remaining frontiers for radiologic-neurosurgical interaction.[40] High-resolution images on advanced-generation CT and MRI scanners provide graphic anatomic detail of the brain that enables the recognition of normal ventricular landmarks as well as the important white matter tracts (e.g., the internal capsule) (Fig 44–28). However, physiologic monitoring remains necessary for understanding and treatment of disordered physiology managed by functional neurosurgery.

The ability to obtain artifact-free CT images while a stereotactic frame is attached to the patient coupled with advanced CT software has improved resolution sufficiently to define the known anatomic landmarks of the brain.[26] Serial high-resolution scans can be used for sagittal reconstruction of the midline third ventricle. Oblique reformatted images (Arrange, General Electric Corp, Milwaukee) can be used to define the intercommissural plane from a midline sagittal formation of the third ventricle and to identify the anterior and posterior commissures. From the formatted image, the target coordinates can be derived of, for example, a ven-

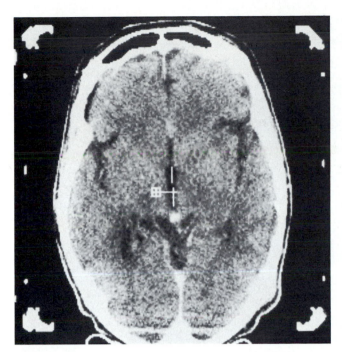

FIG 44–28.
Determination of a thalamic target referable to the intercommissural line.

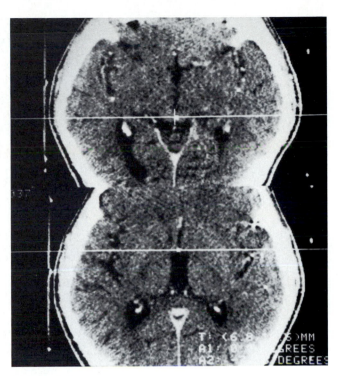

FIG 44–29.
Posterior and anterior commissures are identified to define the intercommissural plane.

tral lateral nucleus thalamotomy for dyskinesia. Alternatively, the actual axial images containing the posterior and anterior commissures can be used to format the oblique plane containing, for example, both the anterior and posterior commissures (Fig 44–29). The image can be reconstructed at different angles to define a target plane containing both commissures (Fig 44–30). When stereotaxis is performed within the CT scanner, the probe can be placed initially into the third ventricle and metrizamide injected (1 mL, 170 mg I/mL). A sagittal computed radiograph (Scoutview, General Electric Corp, Milwaukee) can be used to define the anterior and posterior commissures, after which the appropriate axial CT images can be taken superior or inferior to the intercommissural plane.

More recently, MRI has proved advantageous because of its superior contrast resolution (Fig 44–31). Narrow slices reveal the midsagittal and intercommissural planes dramatically and allow direct visualization of the appropriate deep brain nucleus (Fig 44–32). At present, we prefer to confirm MRI-derived targets with CT studies done immediately afterward, at least until future computer programs eliminate magnetic susceptibility (Fig 44–33).

One major advantage of intracranial image-based stereotaxis lies in the ability to identify the

internal capsule. Stereotactic targets can be selected to avoid this critical pathway, which represents the lateral border of the thalamus. Conventional ventriculography techniques have relied upon the width of the third ventricle as a guide to the lateral location of the target within the brain. The use of CT has demonstrated no clear relation-

TABLE 44–5.
Imaging-Guided Stereotactic Surgery at Presbyterian-University Hospital—March 1981 to February 1988

Type of Procedure		No. of Patients	Percentage
Diagnostic biopsy/aspiration*		591	72.3
Therapeutic (total)		78	10.8
Interstitial irradiation	30		
Intracavitary irradiation	20		
Colloid cyst evacuation	17		
Catheter implantation	11		
Functional (total)		70	8.6
Thalamotomy	24		
Depth electrodes (epilepsy)	32		
Depth electrodes (pain)	10		
Other pain	4		
Gamma knife radiosurgery		68	8.3
Total		817	100

*Includes brain abscess and hematoma patients.

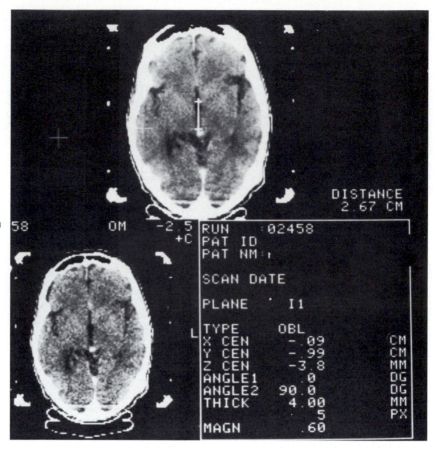

FIG 44–30.
Intercommissural distance can be measured from the reformatted oblique intercommissural plane.

ship between the width of the third ventricle and the thalamic width. Kelly and coworkers spearheaded the computerized digitization of the Schaltenbrand and Bailey stereotactic atlas integrated within the CT scanner.[74] The digitized atlas can be scaled to each patient's CT images, thereby allowing specific labeling of the various brain nuclei and tracts.

The usage of CT stereotaxic and functional surgery of the brain can be subdivided into neuroab-

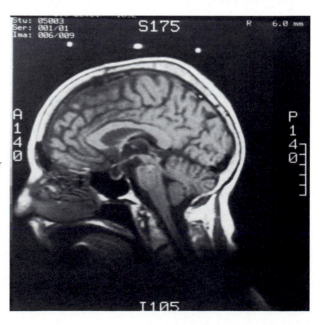

FIG 44–31.
Midsagittal stereotactic MRI used to define the anterior and posterior commissures.

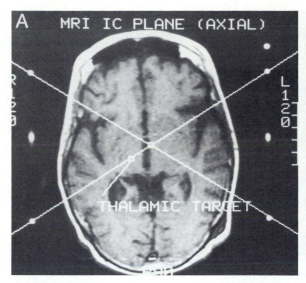
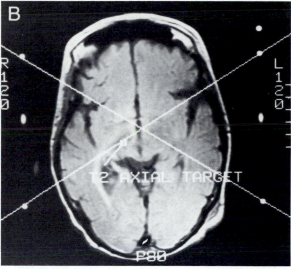

FIG 44–32.
A, determination of the probe tip targets for thalamotomy in a patient in whom the anterior and posterior commissures can be demonstrated on axial MRI. **B,** a T2-weighted image discloses the ab-

normality in the thalamic nucleus in this patient with a prior infarct of the midbrain and thalamus.

lative, neurostimulative, and neurorecording techniques (Table 44–5).

Neuroablative Techniques

The introduction of dopaminergic agents in the treatment of Parkinson's disease resulted in an immediate and profound reduction in the number of

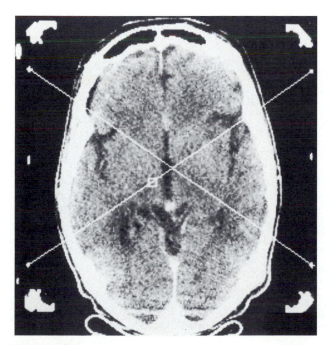

FIG 44–33.
An axial CT scan performed on the same patient with stereotactic technique is used to verify the target slice.

patients referred for stereotactic surgery. Recent evidence has rekindled interest in stereotactic treatment for dyskinesias and is based on the recognition that dopaminergic precursors often fail to significantly improve tremor or rigidity and that long-term dopa treatment can result in excessive dyskinesias.[75] Stereotactic thalamotomy again may become a first-line treatment for unilateral parkinsonian tremor and ridigity, cerebellar outflow tremor related to benign essential tremor or multiple sclerosis, and dystonia. The common target site for these disparate diseases is the ventrolateral nucleus of the thalamus. The effects of a right ventrolateral nucleus thalamotomy are shown in Figure 44–34. The use of early postoperative CT has shown that these lesions are not just simple pale areas of a coagulation but, instead, are frequently hemorrhagic.[76]

CT has afforded the recognition of precise areas for stereotactic intervention in patients with profound psychiatric neuroses unresponsive to conventional psychiatric or medical intervention. Both the anterior limb of the internal capsule and the cingulum have been ablated in the treatment of severe depression and obsessive-compulsive and anxiety neuroses.[77] Currently, psychotic behavior is not treated by behavioral surgery.

Neurostimulative Procedures

Electrode implantation for the purpose of chronic deep-brain stimulation has been used pri-

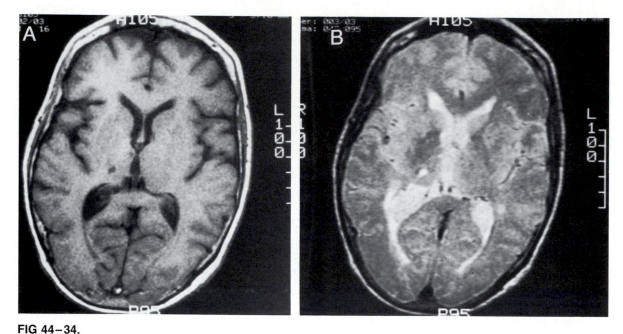

FIG 44–34.
A, 6 weeks after thalamotomy the thalamic lesion can be seen in the right ventrolateral nucleus of the thalamus. **B,** T2-weighted MRI shows the lesion to advantage.

marily to treat both nociceptive (somatic) and deafferentation pain syndromes.[78–84] Bipolar platinum electrodes have been implanted into the medial thalamus and periaqueductal gray matter to treat patients with somatic pain, especially those with cancer involving upper extremity, head and neck,

or midline structures (Fig 44–35). The target site is visualized well with CT or MRI alone because the periventricular target area has been identified as 2 mm anterior to the posterior commissure and 2 mm lateral to the wall of the third ventricle. The ability to define this target when using CT or MRI

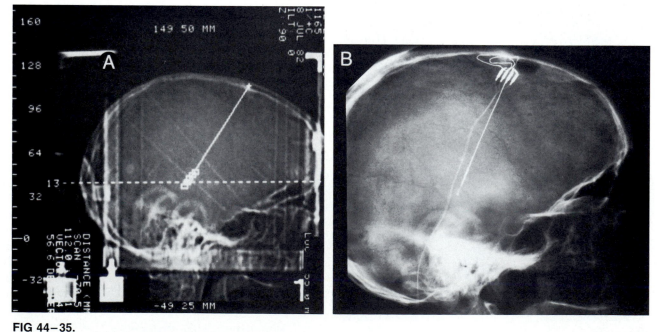

FIG 44–35.
A, sagittal scout CT scan disclosing the pathway of a deep-brain electrode into the periventricular gray matter. **B,** actual postoperative skull x-ray film disclosing the stereotactic electrode.

demonstrates that functional neurosurgery can be performed without ventriculography.[27] Follow-up CT scans can confirm that the electrode has been placed successfully at the target.

Electrodes have been implanted in the thalamic sensory nuclei and the posterior limb of the internal capsule in patients suffering such deafferentation pain syndromes as thalamic pain and anesthesia dolorosa.[79, 80] Although the site of implantation can be seen (e.g., the posterior limb of the internal capsule target is 15 mm lateral to the posterior commissure), confirmation of the appropriate target area still depends upon pertinent intraoperative stimulation findings as well as poststimulation pain relief. Surgery has been more successful in the treatment of somatic pain than in deafferentation pain, which is notoriously difficult to treat by neurosurgical technique.[84] Pain relief obtained with deep-brain stimulation has been related to increased production of endogenous morphinelike substances (endorphins) and to augmentation of descending serotonergic inhibitory pathways.[81]

Implantation of electrodes for the treatment of dyskinesia has been reported by Siegfried and Rea.[85] Target sites for implantation have been identified in the dentate nuclei and the pulvinar nucleus of the thalamus. Thus far, the long-term results of deep-brain stimulation for movement disorders have not been gratifying enough to warrant widespread adoption of this technique in the treatment of dyskinesias.

Neurorecording

Long-term depth recording has been shown to be a valuable modality in the treatment and identification of epileptogenic foci within the brain (Fig 44–36). When using stereotactic technique coupled with angiography, multiple electrodes have been inserted into various cortical and subcortical areas of the brain.[6] We have placed bilateral intracerebral electrodes to study patients with temporal lobe epilepsy and before considering surgical resection, temporal lobectomy, or stereotactic intervention for intractable seizure disorders. The sites for electrode implantation can be identified with CT and the pathway of a phantom probe plotted on the CT images prior to actual stereotactic implantation in the brain. Such depth recordings have enabled differentation between primary and "mirror" epileptogenic foci.

STEREOTACTIC RADIOSURGERY

Stereotactic radiosurgery refers to single-treatment, closed-skull destruction of an intracranial target by using ionizing beams of irradiation (Fig 44–37).[4, 86] The location of the target is defined in stereotactic space by advanced imaging techniques. Leksell defined the term *stereotactic radiosurgery* in 1951; he first used a cyclotron-generated proton beam and later a linear accelerator.[86] These techniques were abandoned because of their complexity, cost, and inefficiency. Instead, Leksell arranged for construction of the first gamma knife, a device containing 179 sources of cobalt 60 focused at a point. This instrument was used to create fine lesions within deep-brain tracts or nuclei to treat movement disorders or psychiatric conditions. A second-generation gamma knife was installed at the Karolinska Hospital, Stockholm, in 1975; it had been redesigned to treat cerebral neoplasms and arteriovenous malformations (AVMs). More than 2,000 patients were treated with this technique between 1968 and 1988. The technique was long delayed in entry into the United States for several reasons: insufficient familiarity of physicians with the uses and results, cost, and major regulatory agency hurdles.

The first U.S. gamma knife designed for treatment of cerebral tumors and AVMs was installed at the University of Pittsburgh in 1987. Four and one-

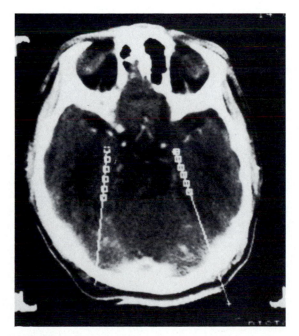

FIG 44–36.
Axial CT scan demonstrating the pathway of bitemporal electrodes inserted for epilepsy recordings.

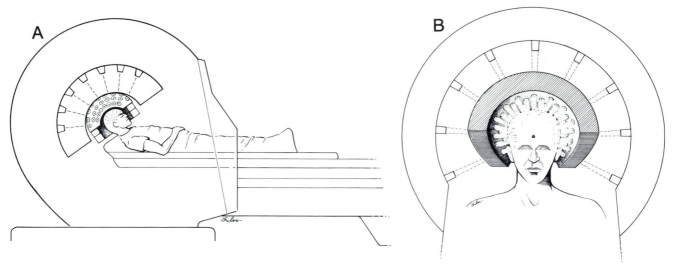

FIG 44–37.

A, the Leksell stereotactic radiosurgical gamma knife. Two hundred one Cobalt sources are focused on a point within the patient's skull by stereotactic technique (side view). **B,** anteroposterior view demonstrating the concept of radiosurgical treatment using 201 sources of cobalt 60 irradiation focused on a target point.

half years of analyzing results, health care planning, and health care agency review preceded the installation. The need to load the approximately 6,000 Ci of cobalt 60 on site, within the hospital, was a major radiologic physics challenge. The design of the Pittsburgh gamma knife suite is shown in Fig 44–38. This unit (Fig 44–39), the fifth one built in the world, had substantial changes in design to enable the treatment of larger tumors and to incorporate major advances in computer isodose planning that had become available with high-speed data processing. The gamma knife now con-

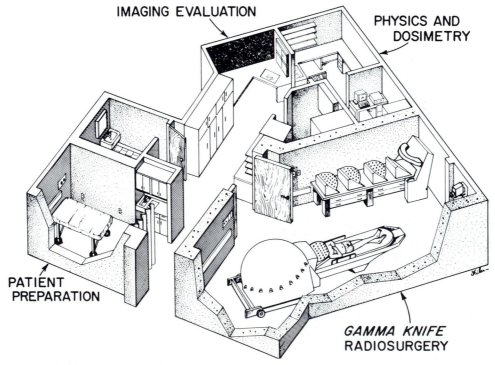

FIG 44–38.

Schematic drawing of the Presbyterian-University stereotactic radiosurgical unit. The gamma unit itself is housed in a heavily shielded room.

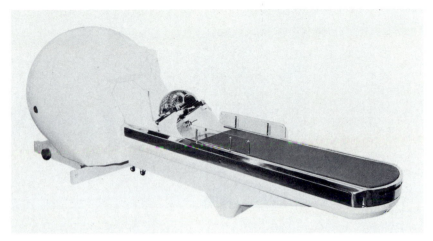

FIG 44–39.
The Leksell stereotactic gamma knife.

tains 201 cobalt sources in a hemispherical array that are directed at a target point, which is brought into the focus. The target is defined in stereotactic space with CT, MRI, or cerebral angiography. A specially constructed coordinate head frame is used to visualize the target; the frame has interchangeable fiducial markers to calculate the target location, depending on the imaging tool used.[87] Four interchangeable helmets have collimators of either 4, 8, 14, or 18 mm to vary the diameter of the

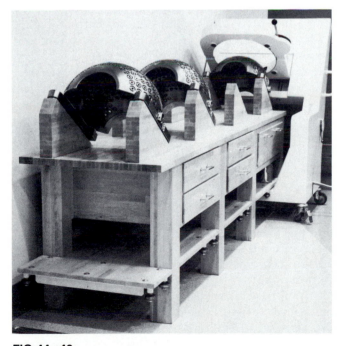

FIG 44–40.
The diameter of the focus of the gamma unit can be varied by using interchangeable collimator helmets. Each helmet weighs 500 lb and must be moved with a hydraulic unit.

radiosurgical lesion (Fig 44–40). By combining a series of irradiation "shots," lesions of larger size and more unusual configuration can be treated.

The gamma knife historically has been used to treat a variety of intra-axial AVMs[88] and extra-axial, histologically benign neoplasms, including acoustic neurinomas,[89] meningiomas, pituitary tumors, craniopharyngiomas,[51] and pineal region tumors.[55] Steiner has treated more than 900 AVMs. In a series of optimally treated AVMs (600 cases, personal communication, 1988), Steiner was able to achieve angiographically defined obliteration in 50% of cases 1 year after treatment, 87% 2 years after treatment, and 97% by 3 years after radiosurgery (Fig 44–41). No patient died as a result of treatment; 3.2% of patients had delayed onset of a new neurologic symptom, which could be related to delayed radiation injury to the brain surrounding the AVM. Norén has treated more than 200 cases of acoustic neurinomas; in a series of 120 patients followed for up to 4 years, 90% had controlled tumor growth and did not require surgical removal.[89]

Seventy-one patients were treated in the first 6 months of operation of the Pittsburgh gamma knife, beginning in August 1987. The majority of patients had AVM (Fig 44–42). We have embarked cautiously on a program to treat more aggressive malignant tumors if the tumor border can be defined by perioperative imaging and histologic studies. For example, solitary metastatic brain tumors can undergo gamma knife treatment in conjunction with external beam irradiation if the lesion is less than 25 mm in diameter. Many of our patients have already exhausted conventional neurosurgical and irradiation techniques or have intracerebral lesions

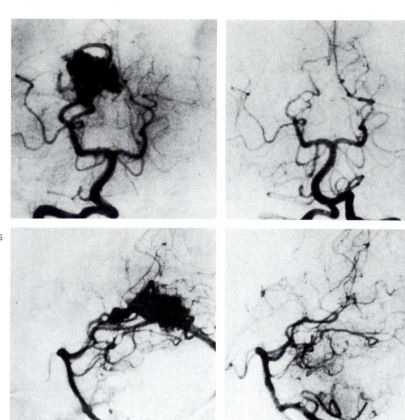

FIG 44–41.
Preoperative and postoperative angiographic views of a right posterior temporal arteriovenous malformation obliterated 2 years after stereotactic radiosurgical treatment. (Courtesy of L. Steiner, M.D., Ph.D.)

considered unresectable by standard microsurgical tools.

At present, angiography remains the imaging tool of choice to define intracranial AVMs for radiosurgery (Fig 44–43). We are using protocols in

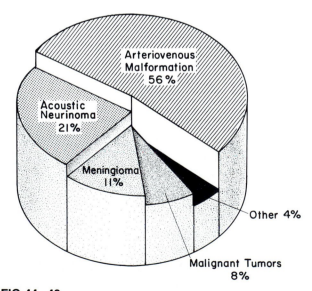

FIG 44–42.
The spectrum of patients currently being treated with the Presbyterian-University Hospital gamma knife in Pittsburgh.

which we can evaluate MRI as an adjunct to angiography to confirm obliteration. Patients with AVMs less than 25 to 30 mm in greatest diameter currently are referred for radiosurgical treatment directly. For those patients with larger AVMs, we proceed first with endovascular embolization to reduce the nidus size to less than 25 to 30 mm. One or more embolization sessions may be necessary. This combined venture provides a logical end point for AVM size reduction with embolization techniques since final obliteration with the gamma knife is now possible. The goal is to cover the malformation's nidus in one or more shots so that the margin of the lesion receives 2,000 to 2,500 cGy in a single treatment session. The gamma knife provides a much higher dose to the target center, a feature that may be critical in producing delayed obliteration.

Skull base tumors such as acoustic neurinomas can be treated with the gamma knife as an alternative to surgical removal (Fig 44–44). This option can be especially valuable in bilateral cases (e.g., neurofibromatosis). Initially, postoperative hearing is preserved at preoperative levels in every patient, but over time, more than 70% of patients have hearing deterioration leading to deafness.[89]

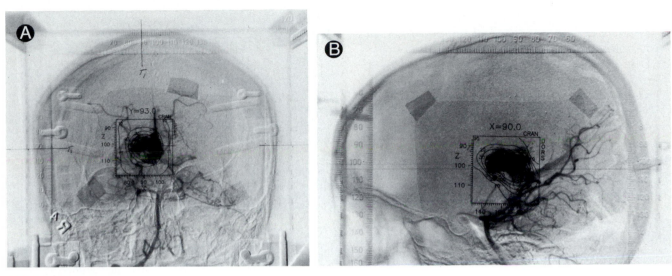

FIG 44–43.
Left anterior-posterior **(A)** and lateral **(B)** stereotactic imaging of a midbrain and thalamic AVM. The computer-generated isodose plans are displayed over the stereotactic images.

No patient has sustained a permanent facial palsy after treatment, however. We also have treated skull base meningiomas and pituitary tumors. Stereotactic radiosurgery is a valuable alternative for patients considered too infirm or elderly to undergo conventional operations.

Rapid, computer-based radiation dose planning for gamma knife treatment has facilitated expeditious treatment of patients. The isodose plans are integrated with the stereotactic images and scaled for the magnification of the study used to define the target. These isodose plots provide a three-di-

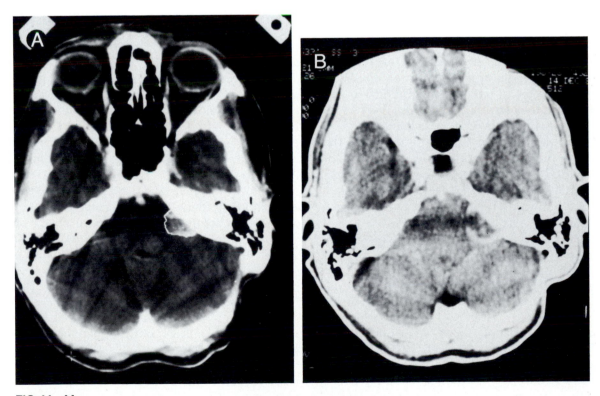

FIG 44–44.
A, Preoperative stereotactic imaging of a left cerebellopontine angle acoustic neurinoma. **B,** 3 months after radiosurgical ablation, reduced contrast opacification can be seen within the tumor.

mensional view of the target and surrounding brain. Newer techniques to target tumors are being investigated; for example, we have confirmed that gadolinium-enhanced MRI is a superior way to demonstrate a recurrent pituitary tumor prior to radiosurgery.

To date, several techniques analogous to gamma knife radiosurgery have been proposed. A combination of stereotactic guiding devices with linear accelerators has progressed to the point of patient treatment[90]; however, at present, no radiologic physics data or patient results substantiate the equivalency of such linear accelerator technique to the gamma knife. The precise and small (4 mm) collimation available with the gamma knife has made possible the destruction of even very small tumors such as intracanalicular acoustic tumors. Our experimental primate studies have begun to define the developmental rate of the radiosurgical lesion and to determine which imaging and electrophysiologic studies can predict the development of the lesion over time (Fig 44–45).

IMAGE-GUIDED STEREOTACTIC SURGERY: THE FUTURE

Radiologic vs. Surgical Sites

CT-guided stereotaxis can be performed entirely in the scanner or can begin in the scanner, with the actual surgery performed in the operating room. The time constraints imposed by busy radiologic imaging sites often make it impractical to reserve large blocks of time for stereotactic surgery. If surgery is done in the CT scanning suite, the unit must be fully equipped with all necessary anesthesia and life support facilities, and the traditional aseptic environment of the operating room must be maintained. The additional time required for intermittent electrophysiologic monitoring and testing further reduces the likelihood that extensive time can be devoted to CT stereotaxis in the diagnostic scanner.

To circumvent these problems, a CT unit dedicated to stereotactic surgery was developed at the University of Pittsburgh (Fig 44–46). In this new operating room concept, the CT scanner is reversed in location so that the rear of the scanner opens onto the larger part of the room. The patient is placed supine on the scanner bed and advanced through the scanner aperture after attachment of the stereotactic frame. In this way, the surgeon has

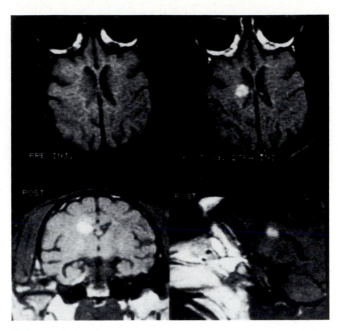

FIG 44–45.
Demonstration of an 8-mm stereotactic radiosurgical lesion (150 Gy) performed 6 weeks prior to gadolinium-enhanced MRI. The lesion can be seen in advantage in multiple planes in this 33-lb baboon.

free access to the head of the patient. At any time during the procedure, CT images can be taken by retracting the patient into the scanner aperture. An intriguing potential exists for development of other surgical procedures guided by images performed in body scanners.

Percutaneous cervical cordotomy is one spinal procedure during which CT guidance may provide superior definition of the spinal cord. Xenon-enhanced CT for determining cerebral blood flow can be performed during surgical revascularization of the brain or during particulate embolization of AVMs. It has become incumbent upon neurosurgeons to fully grasp and use the advanced radiologic imaging techniques currently available to diagnostic radiologists lest neurosurgeons remain dependent upon outmoded, inadequate radiographic techniques.

Certainly not all centers reasonably can be expected to finance the cost of surgical CT units. Kelly and associates have advocated the use of diagnostic imaging centers but equipped his operating room with independent display consoles to facilitate remote targeting.[91, 92] In our experience, intraoperative imaging has been crucial to the success of certain procedures and has allowed the early recognition of potential complications in virtually all other procedures.

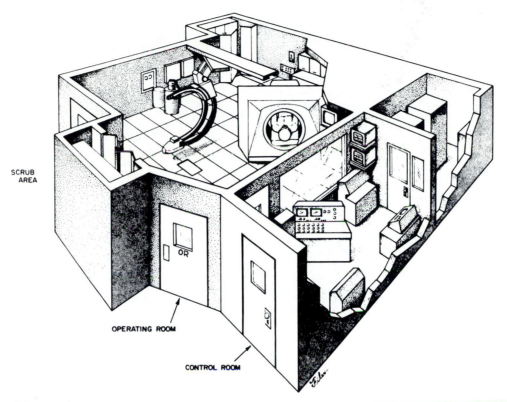

FIG 44–46.
The stereotactic operating room suite at Presbyterian-University Hospital contains a dedicated CT scanner and ceiling-mounted sea arm fluoroscope.

New Devices

Entirely new devices have been constructed for integration with new imaging tools. Techniques have been developed to resect tumors by using laser adaptations[92] and endoscopic "resectoscopes."[93–96] "Frameless" stereotactic systems integrated with the operating room microscope promise more precise removal of lesions with less trauma to the brain.[97] Recently, the introduction of robotic technique for target access has been used by Young.[98] In this technique, a robotic mechanism replaces the stereotactic frame. Modern stereotactic frames are made for image compatibility regardless of the tool selected for target definition. Entirely new frames compatible with either open or closed (radiosurgical) treatment of brain tumors have been built,[99] and intraoperative ultrasound has been advocated.[100]

New Indications

A primary outgrowth of our ability to see and diagnose brain lesions much earlier in clinical disease states is the need for a concomitant reassessment of when and how to treat these lesions. The goal of enhancing neurologic function and reducing risks has been realized by the incorporation of stereotactic technique in routine neurosurgical practice. The field continues to enlarge with the addition of new indications. For example, stereotactic surgery can be used to restore cerebrospinal fluid pathways via third ventriculostomy[91] or aqueduct of Sylvius reconstruction.[101]

Transplantation of neuroendocrine or fetal tissue[102] to restore deficient neurtransmitter function is likely to be done best by stereotactic technique, whereby damage to brain surrounding the target implantation site can be avoided.[103] Such innovative transplantation techniques represent a new frontier for neurosurgery and may emerge as one of the most important indications for imaging-guided stereotactic surgery. Morphologic definition of the brain deficiency using MRI or PET, anatomic resolution of the target area, and stereotactic delivery of the replacement tissue to restore integrity of a more normally functioning nervous system will ensure the permanent union of modern imaging tools and their surgical counterparts.

Acknowledgments

The author expresses his gratitude to Helene Hochman who edited the manuscript and to Phyllis Shoemaker and Mary Ann Vincenzini who helped prepare it. The work was supported in part by a grant from the W.I. Patterson Charitable Trust.

REFERENCES

1. Horsley V, Clark RH: The structure and functions of the cerebellum examined by a new method. *Brain* 1908; 31:45–124.
2. Kirschner M: Die Punktionstechnik und Elektrokaogulation des Ganglion gasseri: Uber "gezielte" Operationionen. *Arch Klin Chir* 1933; 176:581–620.
3. Spiegel EA, Wycis HJ, Marks M, et al: Stereotaxic apparatus for operations on the human brain. *Science* 1947; 106:346–350.
4. Leksell L: *Stereotaxis and Radiosurgery: An Operative System.* Springfield, Il, Charles C Thomas, Publishers, 1971, p 69.
5. Riechert T: *Stereotactic Brain Operations, Methods, Clinical Aspects, Indications.* Bern, Switzerland, Hans Huber, 1980, p 387.
6. Talairach J, David M, Tournoux P: *L'Exploration Chirurgicale Stereotaxique du Lobe Temporal dans l'Epilepsie Temporale.* Paris, Masson, 1958, p 136.
7. Talairach J, Szikla G: Stereotactic neuroradiological concepts applied to surgical removal of cortical epileptogenic areas, in Rasmussen T, Marino R (eds): *Functional Neurosurgery.* New York, Raven Press, 1979, pp 219–242.
8. Cooper IS: *Parkinsonism: Its Medical and Surgical Therapy.* Springfield, Il, Charles C Thomas, Publishers, 1961, p 239.
9. Van Buren JM, MacCubbin DA: An outline of the human basal ganglia with estimation of anatomical variants. *J Neurosurg* 1962; 19:811–839.
10. Bergström M, Greitz T: Stereotaxic computed tomography. *AJR* 1976; 127:167–170.
11. Levinthal R, Winter J, Bentson JR: Technique for accurate localization with the CT scanner. *Bull Los Angeles Neurol Soc* 1976; 41:6–8.
12. Piskun WS, Stevens CA, LaMorgese JR, et al: A simplified method of CT assisted localization and biopsy of intracranial lesions. *Surg Neurol* 1979; 11:413–417.
13. Maroon JC, Bank BO, Drayer BP, et al: Intracranial biopsy assisted by computerized tomography. *J Neurosurg* 1977; 46:740–744.
14. Lunsford LD, Maroon JC: CT localization and biopsy of intracranial lesions, in Schmidek HH, Sweet WH (eds): *Operative Neurosurgery.* New York, Grune & Stratton, 1982, pp 403–418.
15. Lunsford LD, Martinez AJ: Stereotactic exploration of the brain in the CT era. *Surg Neurol* 1984; 22:222–230.
16. Leksell L, Jernberg B: Stereotaxis and tomography: A technical note. *Acta Neurochir (Wien)* 1980; 52:1–7.
17. Mundinger F, Birg W: CT stereotaxy in the clinical routine. *Neurosurg Rev* 1984; 7:219–224.
18. Kelly PJ, Alker GJ: A stereotactic approach to deep-seated central nervous system neoplasms using the carbon dioxide laser. *Surg Neurol* 1981; 15:331–334.
19. Brown RA: A computerized tomography–computer graphics approach to stereotactic localization. *J Neurosurg* 1979; 50:715–720.
20. Perry JE, Rosenbaum AE, Lunsford LD, et al: CT guided stereotactic surgery: Conception and development of a new methodology. *Neurosurgery* 1980; 7:376–383.
21. Gouda KI, Friedberg SR, Larsen CR, et al: Modification of the Gouda frame to allow stereotactic biopsy of the brain using the GE 8800 CT scanner. *Neurosurgery* 1983; 13:176–181.
22. Patil AA: Computed tomography-oriented stereotactic system. *Neurosurgery* 1982; 10:370–374.
23. Koslow M, Abele MG, Griffith RC, et al: Stereotactic surgical system controlled by computerized tomography. *Neurosurgery* 1981; 8:72–82.
24. Lunsford LD, Rosenbaum AE, Perry J: Stereotactic surgery using the "therapeutic" CT scanner. *Surg Neurol* 1982; 18:116–122.
25. Lunsford LD, Martinez AJ, Latchaw RE: Stereotactic surgery with a magnetic resonance and computerized tomography system. *J Neurosurg* 1986; 64:872–878.
26. Latchaw RE, Lunsford LD, Kennedy WH: Reformatted imaging to define the intercommissural line for CT-guided stereotactic functional neurosurgery. *AJNR* 1985; 6:429–433.
27. Lunsford LD, Latchaw RE, Vries J: Stereotaxic implantation of deep brain electrodes using computed tomography. *Neurosurgery* 1983; 13:280–286.
28. Lunsford LD, Listerud JA, Rowberg AH, et al: Stereotactic software for the GE 8800 CT scanner. *Neurol Res* 1987; 9:118–122.
29. Lunsford LD: Advanced intraoperative imaging for stereotaxis. The surgical CT scanner. *Acta Neurochir Suppl (Wien)* 1984; 33:573–575.
30. Lunsford LD: A dedicated CT system for the stereotactic operating room. *Appl Neurophysiol* 1982; 45:374–378.
31. Lunsford LD, Nelson PB: Stereotactic aspiration of a brain abscess using the "therapeutic" CT scanner. *Acta Neurochir (Wien)* 1982; 62:25–29.

32. Gildenberg PL, Kaufman HH, Murthy KSK: Calculation of stereotactic coordinates from the computed tomographic scan. *Neurosurgery* 1982; 10:580–586.

33. Edner G: Stereotactic biopsy of intracranial space occupying lesions. *Acta Neurochir (Wien)* 1981; 57:213–234.

34. Bosch DA: Indications for stereotactic biopsy in brain tumors. *Acta Neurochir (Wien)* 1980; 54:167–179.

35. Boëthius J, Bergström M, Greitz J: Stereotactic computerized tomography with a GE 8800 scanner. *J Neurosurg* 1980; 52:794–800.

36. Boëthius J, Collins VP, Edner G, et al: Stereotactic biopsies and computerized tomography in gliomas. *Acta Neurochir (Wien)* 1978; 40:223–232.

37. Apuzzo MCJ, Chandrasoma P, Cohen D, et al: Computed imaging stereotaxy. Experience and perspectives related to 500 procedures applied to brain masses. *Neurosurgery* 1987; 20:930–937.

38. Moran CJ, Naidich TP, Gado MH, et al: Central nervous system lesions biopsied or treated by CT-guided needle placement. *Radiology* 1979; 131:681–686.

39. Ostertag CB, Mennel HD, Kiessling M: Stereotactic biopsy of brain tumors. *Surg Neurol* 1980; 14:275–283.

40. Rosenbaum AE, Lunsford LD, Perry JH: Computerized tomography guided stereotaxis: A new approach. *Appl Neurophysiol* 1980; 43:171–173.

41. Lunsford LD: Stereotactic drainage of brain abscesses. *Neurol Res* 1987; 9:270–274.

42. Lunsford LD, Martinez AJ, Latchaw RE, et al: Rapid and accurate diagnosis of herpes simplex encephalitis by stereotaxic computed tomography. *Surg Neurol* 1984; 21:249–257.

43. Bosch DA, Rahn T, Backlund EO: Treatment of colloid cysts of the third ventricle by stereotactic aspiration. *Surg Neurol* 1978; 9:15–18.

44. Hall WA, Lunsford LD: Changing concepts in the treatment of colloid cysts in the computed tomography era. *J Neurosurg* 1987; 65:186–191.

45. Backlund EO, Van Holst H: Controlled subtotal evacuation of intracerebral hematomas by stereotactic technique. *Surg Neurol* 1987; 9:99–101.

46. Broseta M, Gonzalez-Dareler J, Barcia-Salorio JL: Stereotactic evacuation of intracerebral hematomas. *Appl Neurophysiol* 1982; 45:443–448.

47. Higgins AC, Nashold BS, Cosman E: Stereotaxic evacuation of primary intracerebral hematomas: New instrumentation. *Appl Neurophysiol* 1982; 45:438–442.

48. Kandel EI, Peresedov VV: Stereotaxic evacuation of spontaneous intracerebral hematomas. *J Neurosurg* 1985; 62:204–213.

49. Matsamoto K, Hondo H: CT guided stereotaxic evacuation of hypertensive intracerebral hematomas. *J Neurosurg* 1984; 61:440–448.

50. Levander R, Bergström M, Boëthius J, et al: Stereotactic computed tomography for biopsy of gliomas. *Acta Radiol* 1978; 19:867–888.

51. Backlund EO: Stereotactic radiosurgery in intracranial tumors and vascular malformations, in Krayenbuhl H (ed): *Advances and Technical Standards in Neurosurgery*, vol 6. New York, Springer-Verlag NY, Inc, 1979, pp 1–37.

52. Backlund EO: Stereotaxic treatment of craniopharyngiomas. *Acta Neurochir (Wien)* 1974; 21:177–183.

53. Backlund EO: Studies on craniopharyngiomas: IV. Stereotactic treatment with radiosurgery. *Acta Chir Scand* 1972; 139:344–351.

54. Backlund EO, Johansson L, Sarby B: Studies on craniopharyngiomas: II. Treatment by stereotaxis and radiosurgery. *Acta Chir Scand* 1972; 749–759.

55. Backlund EO, Rähn J, Sarby B: Treatment of pinealomas by stereotaxic radiation surgery. *Acta Radiol* 1974; 13:368–376.

56. Kelly PJ, Daumas-Duport C, Kispert DB, et al: Imaging-based stereotaxic serial biopsies in untreated intracranial glial neoplasms. *J Neurosurg* 1987; 66:865–874.

57. Lunsford LD, Martinez AJ, Latchaw RE: Magnetic resonance imaging does not define tumor boundaries. *Acta Radiol Suppl* 1986; 369:154–156.

58. Coffey RJ, Lunsford LD: Stereotactic surgery for mass lesions of the midbrain and pons. *Neurosurgery* 1985; 17:12–18.

59. Coffey, RJ, Lunsford LD: Survival after stereotactic biopsy of malignant gliomas. *Neurosurgery* 1988; 22:465–473.

60. Hood TW, Gebarski SS, McKeever PE, et al: Stereotaxic biopsy of intrinsic lesions of the brain stem. *J Neurosurg* 1986; 65:172–176.

61. Hall WA, Martinez AJ, Dummer JS: Nocardial brain abscess: Diagnostic and therapeutic use of stereotactic aspiration. *Surg Neurol* 1987; 28:114–118.

62. Wise BL, Gleason CA: CT-directed stereotactic surgery in the management of brain abscess. *Ann Neurol* 1979; 6:467.

63. Lunsford LD: Stereotactic drainage of brain abscesses. *Neurol Res* 1987; 9:270–274.

64. Bosch DA, Hindmarsh T, Larsson S, et al: Intraneoplastic administration of bleomycin in intracerebral gliomas: A pilot study. *Acta Neurochir Suppl (Wien)* 1980; 30:441–444.

65. Lunsford LD, Levine G, Gumerman LW: A comparison of computed tomographic and radionuclide methods to determine intracranial cystic tumor volumes. *J Neurosurg* 1985; 63:740–744.

66. Pollack IF, Lunsford LD, Slamovits TE, et al: Ste-

reotactic intracavitary irradiation for cystic craniopharyngiomas. *J Neurosurg* 1988; 68:227–233.

67. Kobayashi T, Kageyama N, Ohara K: Internal irradiation for cystic craniopharyngioma. *J Neurosurg* 1981; 55:896–903.

68. Coffey RJ, Friedman WA: Interstitial brachytherapy of malignant brain tumors using CT-guided stereotaxis and available imaging software: Technical note. *Neurosurgery* 1987; 20:4–7.

69. Gutin PH, Dormandy R: A coaxial catheter system for afterloading radioactive sources for interstitial irradiation of brain tumors. *J Neurosurg* 1982; 56:734–735.

70. Gutin PH, Leibel SA, Wara WM, et al: Recurrent malignant gliomas: Survival following interstitial brachytherapy with high activity iodine-125 sources. *J Neurosurg* 1987; 67:864–873.

71. Mundinger F, Birg W, Ostertag CB: Treatment of small cerebral gliomas with CT aided stereotaxic curietherapy. *Neuroradiology* 1978; 16:564–567.

72. Marino R: Introduction: Functional neurosurgery as a specialty, in Rasmussen T, Marino R (eds): *Functional Neurosurgery*, New York, Raven Press, 1979, pp 1–5.

73. Schaltenbrand G, Wahren W: *Atlas for Stereotaxy of the Human Brain*. Chicago, Year Book Medical Publishers, Inc, 1977.

74. Goerss S, Kelly PJ, Kall B, et al: A computed tomography stereotactic adaptation system. *Neurosurgery* 1982; 10:375–379.

75. Kelly PJ, Gillingham FJ: The long-term results of stereotaxic surgery and L-dopa therapy in patients with Parkinson's disease. A ten year study. *J Neurosurg* 1980; 53:332–337.

76. Passerini A, Broggi G, Giorgi G: CT studies in patients operated with stereotaxic thalamotomies. *Neuroradiology* 1978; 15:561–563.

77. Meyerson BA, Bergström M, Greitz T: Target localization in stereotactic capsulotomy with the aid of computed tomography, in Hitchcock ER, Ballantine HJ Jr, Meyerson BA (eds): *Modern Concepts in Psychiatry Surgery*. Amsterdam, Elsevier Science Publishers, 1979, pp 217–221.

78. Hosobuchi Y: The current status of analgesic brain stimulation. *Acta Neurochir Suppl (Wien)* 1980; 30:219–227.

79. Hosobuchi Y, Adams JE, Rutkin B: Chronic thalamic stimulation for the control of facial anesthesia dolorosa. *Arch Neurol* 1973; 29:158–161.

80. Hosobuchi Y, Adams JE, Fields HL: Chronic thalamic and internal capsular stimulation for the control of facial anesthesia dolorosa and dysesthesia of thalamic syndrome. *Adv Neurol* 1974; 4:783–787.

81. Meyerson BA: Biochemistry of pain relief with intracerebral stimulation: Few facts and many hypotheses. *Acta Neurochir Suppl (Wien)* 1980; 30:229–237.

82. Richardson DE, Akil H: Pain reduction by electrical brain stimulation in man: I. *J Neurosurg* 1977; 47:128–183.

83. Richardson DE, Akil H: Pain reduction by electrical stimulation in man: II. *J Neurosurg* 1977; 47:184–194.

84. Young RF, Kroenig R, Fulton W, et al: Electrical stimulation of the brain in treatment of chronic pain. *J Neurosurg* 1985; 62:389–396.

85. Siegfried J, Rea GL: Deep brain stimulation for treatment of motor disorders, in Lunsford LD (ed): *Modern Stereotactic Neurosurgery*. Boston, Martinus Nijhoff, 1988, pp 409–412.

86. Leksell L: Stereotactic radiosurgery. *J Neurol Neurosurg Psychiatry* 1983; 46:797–803.

87. Leksell L, Lindquist L, Adler JR, et al: A new fixation device for the Leksell stereotaxic system. *J Neurosurg* 1987; 66:626–629.

88. Steiner L: Treatment of arteriovenous malformations by radiosurgery, in Wilson CB, Stein BM (eds): *Intracranial Arteriovenous Malformations*. Baltimore, Williams & Wilkins, 1984, pp 295–313.

89. Norén G, Arndt J, Hindmarsh T, et al: Stereotactic radiosurgical treatment of acoustic neurinomas, in Lunsford LD (ed): *Modern Stereotactic Neurosurgery*. Boston, Martinus Nijhoff, 1988, pp 481–490.

90. Lutz W, Winston KR, Maleki N: A system for stereotactic radiosurgery with a linear accelerator. *Int J Radiat Oncol Biol Phys* 1988; 14:373–381.

91. Kelly PJ, Goerss S, Kall BA, et al: CT-based stereotactic third ventriculostomy: Technical note. *Neurosurgery* 1986; 18:791–794.

92. Kelly PJ, Kall BA, Goerss S, et al: Computer assisted stereotactic laser resection of intraaxial brain neoplasms. *J Neurosurg* 1986; 64:427–439.

93. Jacques S, Shelden CH, Lutes HR: Computerized microstereotactic neurosurgical endoscopy under direct three-dimensional vision, in Lunsford LD (ed): *Modern Stereotactic Neurosurgery*. Boston, Martinus Nijhoff, 1988, pp 185–194.

94. Jacques S, Shelden CH, McCann GD: Computerized three-dimensional stereotaxic removal of small central nervous system lesions in patients. *J Neurosurg* 1980; 53:816–820.

95. Shelden CH, McCann G, Jacques S, et al: Development of a computerized microstereotaxic method for localization and removal of minute CNS lesions under 3-D vision. *J Neurosurg* 1980; 52:21–27.

96. Shelden CH, Jacques S, McCann GD: The Shelden CT-based microneurosurgical stereotactic system: Its application to CNS pathology. *Appl Neurophysiol* 1982; 45:341–346.

97. Roberts DW, Strohbehn JW, Hatch JF, et al: A frameless stereotaxic integration of computed tomography imaging and the operating microscope. *J Neurosurg* 1986; 65:545–549.

98. Young RF: A robotic system for stereotactic neurosurgery, in Lunsford LD (ed): *Modern Stereotactic Neurosurgery.* Boston, Martinus Nijhoff, 1988, pp 259–268.

99. Peters TM, Clark JA, Olivier A, et al: Integrated stereotaxic surgery with CT, MR imaging and digital subtraction angiography. *Radiology* 1986; 161:821–826.

100. Berger MS: Ultrasound-guided stereotactic biopsy using a new approach. *J Neurosurg* 1986; 65:550–554.

101. Backlund EO, Grepe A, Lunsford LD: Stereotactic reconstruction of the aqueduct of Sylvius. *J Neurosurg* 1981; 55:800–810.

102. Perlow MJ, Freed WJ, Hoffer BJ, et al: Brain grafts reduce motor abnormalities produced by destruction of nigrostriatal dopamine system: Behavioral and histochemical evidence. *Science* 1979; 204:643–647.

103. Backlund EO, Granberg PO, Harberger B, et al: Transplantation of adrenal medullary tissue to striatum in parkinsonism: First clinical trials. *J Neurosurg* 1985; 62:109–173.

Index

middle ear and,
911–912
retinal, 887
Focal cavitation, 789, 791
Focal cerebral ischemia,
145
Focal edema, cerebral,
244
Focal hypoplasia of
cerebral
hemisphere, 784
Focal parenchymal
injury, 227–233
Foix-Chavany-Marie
syndrome, 55
Follicle-stimulating
hormone–
secreting pituitary
adenoma, 696
Follicular thyroid
adenoma, 1065
Food and Drug
Administration,
Magnevist trial
and, 103–104
Footplate of temporal
bone, 905
Foramen
cervical spine and,
1078–179
enlargement of, 948
lumbar spine and,
1082–1083
MRI imaging and,
1103–1104
stenosis and, 1135,
1136
neural, tumors
involving, 1194,
1196
orbital, 821
lucencies of orbital
wall and, 890
stenosis of, 1162
tumor spread and, 963,
965
Foramen magnum
Chiari I malformation
and, 757
CT anatomy of, 1072
meningioma of, 512
Foramina of Magendie
and Lushka, 480
Foraminotomy, 1160
Foreign bodies,
intraorbital, 831
Forking deformity with
aqueductal
stenosis, 755
Fossa
pterygopalatine, 965,
967

Fossa, cranial
middle
epidural hematoma
and, 208
nerve sheath tumor
of, 536
posterior; *see* Posterior
fossa
Fourth ventricle
Chiari II
malformation and,
757, 760
Chiari I malformation
and, 757
Dandy-Walker
complex and, 767,
768
ependymoma of, 495
isolated, 771, 772
tumors of, 478,
478–495
astrocytoma and
glioblastoma and,
483
ependymoma and,
488, 490, 495
hydrocephalus and,
480–483
medulloblastoma
and, 483–484,
487–488
Fracture
Chance, 1242, 1243
epidural hematoma
and, 206–207
facial, 985–989
nasal, 206
orbital, 833–838
skull, 204, 247–248
basal, 205
child abuse and,
257, 259
spinal
burst, 1226, 1228,
1229, 1232
CT versus MRI in,
1248, 1253
soft tissue and, 1246,
1248
temporal bone,
924–925
Fracture dislocation of
spine, 1235, 1239,
1247
Fragment
extruded intraspinal
disk, 1127
of nuclear material,
1151
spinal bone, 1247
Frame, Leksell
stereotactic, 1339,
1340, 1342

Frontal branches of
anterior cerebral
artery, 47
Frontal hematoma
aneurysm and, 272
epidural, 212
Frontal horn
agenesis of corpus
callosum and, 781
septo-optic dysplasia
and, 780
Frontal lobe
arachnoid cyst and, 527
metastasis and, 607
pulped, 218
Frontal sinus
carcinoma of, 650
tumor spread and, 961,
963
Frontoethmoid
mucocele, 980
Frontotemporal
arachnoid cyst,
528
Fungal infection
AIDS and, 326
intracranial, 317
opportunistic
candidal, 330–331
nocardiosis and, 326,
329–330
sinusitis and, 976, 978,
979
spinal, 1220
Fusion
of neurocentral
synchondrosis,
1270–1271
spinal, 1160–1161
complications of,
1177–1179

G

Gadolinium ion, toxicity
of, 97
Gadolinium–
diethylenetriamine
pentaacetic acid
scan, 95–108
acoustic neuroma and,
930
astrocytoma and, 459
basic principles of,
96–99
of cerebellar
astrocytoma, 486
cerebral infarction and,
157
cervical tumor and,
1063
of cystic cerebellar
astrocytoma, 486

detector–contrast
agent interaction
and, 99–103
in differential
diagnosis of tumor,
631
future of, 106–107
of medulloblastoma,
490, 492
of meningioma, 516
multiple sclerosis,
358–359
orbital, 829–830
uses of, 105–106
Gamma knife,
1361–1366
Ganglioglioma, 476
Ganglion
dorsal root, 1079
geniculate, 934
infarction of, 54
Ganglioneuroma, 1196
Gas CT cisternography,
928–929
Gd-DTPA; *see*
Gadolinium–
diethylenetriamine
pentaacetic acid
scan
Genetic disease
globoid cell
leukodystrophy
and, 378
mucopolysaccharidosis
and, 1293–1295
Geniculate body,, 58
Geniculate ganglion,
934
German measles, 369
Germinal matrix
intracranial
hemorrhage, 294
Germinoma
pineal, 572–574
suprasellar, 577, 578
Germinoma, suprasellar,
733, 734, 735
Gerstmann's syndrome,
56
Giant-cell astrocytoma
tuberous sclerosis and,
589
Giant-cell tumor
paranasal sinus and,
968
spinal, 1188
Giant cholesterol cyst,
918
Giant osteoid osteoma,
spinal, 1186–1187
Gigantism, 806
Gillain-Barré syndrome,
368